McGraw-Hill's

Manual of Laboratory & Diagnostic Tests

McGraw-Hill's

Manual of Laboratory & Diagnostic Tests

DENISE D. WILSON, PHD, APN, FNP, ANP

Associate Professor
Mennonite College of Nursing
Illinois State University
Normal, Illinois
Family Nurse Practitioner/Adult Nurse Practitioner
Medical Hills Internists & Pediatrics
Bloomington, Illinois

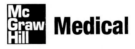 Medical

New York Chicago San Francisco Lisbon London Madrid Mexico City
New Delhi San Juan Seoul Singapore Sydney Toronto

McGraw-Hill's Manual of Laboratory & Diagnostic Tests

Copyright © 2008 by The McGraw-Hill Companies, Inc. All rights reserved. Printed in the United States of America. Except as permitted under the United States Copyright Act of 1976, no part of this publication may be reproduced or distributed in any form or by any means, or stored in a data base or retrieval system, without the prior written permission of the publisher.

1 2 3 4 5 6 7 8 9 0   CTP/CTP   0 9 8 7

ISBN: 978-0-07-148152-6
MHID: 0-07-148152-4

This book was set in Times by International Typesetting and Composition.
The editors were Quincy McDonald and Christie Naglieri.
The production supervisor was Catherine Saggese.
Project management was provided by International Typesetting and Composition.
The text designer was Cathleen Elliott.
China Translation and Printing Services was printer and binder.

This book is printed on acid-free paper.

Library of Congress Cataloging-in-Publication Data

Wilson, Denise D.
    McGraw-Hill's manual of laboratory & diagnostic tests / Denise D.
Wilson.—1st ed.
        p. ; cm.
    Includes bibliographical references and index.
    ISBN: 978-0-07-148152-6 (pbk. : alk. paper)
    MHID: 0-07-148152-4 (pbk. : alk. paper)
    1. Diagnosis, Laboratory—Handbooks, manuals, etc.   I. Title.
II. Title: Manual of laboratory & diagnostic tests.   III. Title:
McGraw-Hill's manual of laboratory and diagnostic tests.
    [DNLM: 1. Laboratory Techniques and Procedures—Handbooks.
2. Diagnostic Techniques and Procedures—Handbooks. QY 39 W747m   2008]
RB38.2.W538   2008
616.07′5—dc22
                                                                2007013305

I dedicate this book to...

...those who care for others...may you always remember that it is an honor and a privilege to be allowed to share in others' lives

...those for whom we care...may you always be treated with respect and kindness

CONTENTS

PREFACE

McGraw-Hill's Manual of Laboratory & Diagnostic Tests was developed to provide up-to-date information on the most commonly used laboratory and diagnostic tests. To provide this information quickly, the tests are provided in alphabetical order using an easy-to-follow format. New tests such as BRCA, FISH, NT-proBNP, and video capsule endoscopy are included. A unique feature of the text is the provision, when available, of selected aspects of evidence-based practice guidelines related to the particular test. Familiarity with these guidelines is essential in caring for the individual with such conditions as diabetes, hypertension, and hyperlipidemia, as well as in determining appropriate screening tests.

Following the alphabetical listing of the laboratory and diagnostic tests, five appendices have been included.

- Appendix A includes a list of common tests for particular conditions or those typically grouped for processing.
- Appendix B has been included to explain how the endocrine system works and how this foundational knowledge can be applied to understand various laboratory tests related to endocrine disorders.
- Appendix C provides information on patient safety issues. The 2007 JCAHO National Patient Safety Goals related to laboratory and diagnostic testing are discussed. Additional discussion focuses on communication of test results in light of HIPAA regulations.
- Appendix D discusses safety of the health-care provider related to universal precautions/ bloodborne pathogens.
- Appendix E discusses what evidence-based practice (EBP) is, its historical foundations, and steps of the EBP process. It also provides internet resources for clinical practice guidelines and evidence to be used in clinical decision-making.

The appendices are followed by a bibliography of sources used for this text, including the evidence-based practice guidelines, and a comprehensive index listing of all test names and abbreviations used in the text.

It is my hope that you, the reader, find this a helpful resource as you strive to provide quality patient care.

Denise D. Wilson

ACKNOWLEDGMENTS

I would like to acknowledge and thank those individuals who have, in some way, played a part in the completion of this text. Thank you to:

Quincy McDonald, Senior Acquisitions Editor for McGraw-Hill, for enthusiastically supporting this project and keeping me on track (most of the time!).

Christie Naglieri, Project Development Editor, for her diligence in developing each aspect of the text.

Sandi Burke, PhD, RN, for her thoughtful review of the appendix on evidence-based practice.

My colleagues at Mennonite College of Nursing at Illinois State University and Medical Hills Internists & Pediatrics, for their encouragement, sharing of knowledge, and friendship throughout the years.

My graduate family nurse practitioner students, for making me glad that I am a teacher of nursing and appreciating my need and desire to practice.

My patients, for making me proud that I am a nurse practitioner and being so appreciative of the care I provide.

My family and friends, for always being there to offer support.

My mother, Ida Williams, for being a loving Mom and such a supporter of my work and dreams throughout my life.

My husband, Gary Wilson, for believing in me, for doing all the things around home that I did not have time for while working on this project, and for showing his love in so many ways.

INTRODUCTION

The laboratory and diagnostic tests of *McGraw-Hill's Manual of Laboratory & Diagnostic Tests* are presented in a consistent format designed to focus on what is important for the health-care provider of today. The following format is used for each test.

NAME OF THE TEST

The primary test name is given, followed by other commonly used names and abbreviations.

TEST DESCRIPTION

The description provides a foundation for understanding the test: its purpose, how it assists in the diagnosis of various conditions, relevant physiology, and the meaning of results in conjunction with other tests which might be performed.

THE EVIDENCE FOR PRACTICE

When available, relevant evidence-based practice guidelines have been included to assist the primary care provider in clinical decision-making. Discussion about evidence-based practice can be found in Appendix E. Reference sources for these guidelines are noted here and/or in the Bibliography.

NORMAL VALUES

The normal values listed are intended to serve as general guidelines, or reference values. They are not meant to replace test norms provided by each laboratory. When available, values are given in both conventional and SI units. Conventional units, such as milligram and liter, as those which have been used historically in health-care in the United States. In an attempt to standardize the measurements world-wide, a system of international (SI) units was developed. SI units have not yet become the standard in all parts of the world, thus both conventional units and SI units are included for all tests, when available. Conversion factors for various laboratory components can be found at the website for the *Journal of the American Medical Association* (JAMA) at *http://jama.ama-assn.org/content/vol295/issue1/images/data/103/DC6/JAMA_auinst_si.dtl*

POSSIBLE MEANINGS OF ABNORMAL VALUES

This section provides a compilation of conditions which *may* account for an abnormal test result. The lists are presented alphabetically to assist the reader in quickly locating the desired information.

CONTRIBUTING FACTORS TO ABNORMAL VALUES

This section provides information regarding patient conditions, equipment or procedural peculiarities, foods, and drugs which may affect test results. Drugs are listed either as individual generic names, or, when an entire group of drugs is applicable, as a broad classification.

INTERVENTIONS/IMPLICATIONS

This section includes the patient education and preparation required during the pretest period, the steps of the test/procedure, and the posttest care of the patient. Most procedures involve potential contact with the patient's body fluids. The institution's infection control policy regarding collection and handling of specimens should be reviewed and carefully followed. This includes compliance with the universal precautions developed by the Centers for Disease Control and Prevention (CDC) discussed in Appendix D.

CLINICAL ALERTS

This section lists in bold print the possible complications of a procedure. It also includes suggested patient education, follow-up testing needed, and applicable clinical tips from practice.

CONTRAINDICATIONS

This section lists the primary types of patients upon whom a particular test should *not* be performed. In addition, the health-care provider must always assess the individual patient to determine the presence of other factors which may cause the test to be contraindicated for that particular patient.

Laboratory and Diagnostic Tests

Abdominal Aorta Sonogram
(Ultrasound of the Abdominal Aorta)

Test Description

Ultrasonography is a noninvasive method of diagnostic testing in which ultrasound waves are sent into the body with a small transducer pressed against the skin. The transducer then receives any returning sound waves, which are deflected back as they bounce off various structures. The transducer converts the returning sound waves into electric signals that are then transformed by a computer into a visual display on a monitor.

In this particular type of ultrasonography, the transducer is passed over the area from the xiphoid process to the umbilicus. The purpose is to detect and measure a suspected abdominal aortic aneurysm (AAA). It can also be used to monitor a known AAA for increase in size. The lumen of the abdominal aorta is normally less than 4 cm in diameter. It is considered to be aneurysmal if it is greater than 4 cm and at high risk of rupture if it is greater than 7 cm. This test can also be used as a follow-up evaluation after surgery for repair of an aneurysm.

THE EVIDENCE FOR PRACTICE

The U.S. Preventive Services Task Force recommends one-time screening for AAA by ultrasonography in men aged 65 to 75 who have ever smoked. The Task Force makes no recommendation for or against screening for AAA in men aged 65 to 75 who have never smoked, and recommends against routine screening for AAA in women. (See: www.ahrq.gov/clinic/uspstf/uspsaneu.htm)

Normal Values

Negative for presence of aneurysm
Abdominal aorta lumen diameter <4 cm

Possible Meanings of Abnormal Values

Abdominal aortic aneurysm

Contributing Factors to Abnormal Values

- The transducer must be in good contact with the skin as it is being moved.
- Clear imaging can be hampered by the presence of retained gas or barium in the intestine, obesity, and patient movement.

Interventions/Implications

Pretest
- Explain to the patient the purpose of the test. Provide any written teaching materials available on the subject. Note that there is no discomfort involved with this test.
- Fasting for 8 hours is required prior to the exam.

Procedure
- The patient is assisted to a supine position on the ultrasonography table.
- A coupling agent, such as a water-based gel, is applied to the area to be evaluated.

- A transducer is placed on the skin and moved as needed to provide good visualization of the structures.
- The sound waves are transformed into a visual display on the monitor. Printed copies of this display are made.

Posttest
- Cleanse the patient's skin of remaining coupling agent.
- Report abnormal findings to the primary care provider.

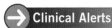

Clinical Alerts

- This test should be scheduled for completion prior to any studies requiring barium. If such studies have already occurred, 24 hours must pass prior to performing the ultrasound to allow passage of the barium beyond the area to be viewed.

Abdominal Sonogram (Abdominal Ultrasound)

Test Description
Ultrasonography is a noninvasive method of diagnostic testing in which ultrasound waves are sent into the body with a small transducer pressed against the skin. The transducer then receives any returning sound waves, which are deflected back as they bounce off various structures. The transducer converts the returning sound waves into electric signals that are then transformed by a computer into a visual display on a monitor.

In this particular type of ultrasonography, the areas evaluated include those studied in the liver and pancreatobiliary system sonogram (gallbladder, biliary system, liver, and pancreas) along with the spleen, kidneys, and aorta.

Normal Values
Normal appearance of gallbladder, biliary system, liver, pancreas, spleen, kidneys, and aorta

Possible Meanings of Abnormal Values
- Aortic aneurysm
- Ascites
- Cholecystitis
- Cholelithiasis
- Cirrhosis of the liver
- Dilation of the bile ducts
- Gallbladder carcinoma
- Gallbladder polyps

- Hematoma
- Hepatic abscess
- Hepatic tumor
- Hepatocellular disease
- Hydronephrosis
- Liver cyst
- Liver metastases
- Pancreatic carcinoma
- Pancreatitis
- Pheochromocytoma
- Pseudocyst of the pancreas
- Renal calculi
- Renal carcinoma
- Renal cysts
- Ruptured spleen
- Splenomegaly

Contributing Factors to Abnormal Values

- The transducer must be in good contact with the skin as it is being moved. A water-based gel is used to ensure good contact with the skin.
- Test results are hindered by the presence of bowel gas, retained barium, or obesity.

Interventions/Implications

Pretest
- Explain to the patient the purpose of the test. Provide any written teaching materials available on the subject. Note that there is no discomfort involved with this test.
- The patient is to eat a fat-free meal in the evening and then fast for 8 to 12 hours before the test. This promotes accumulation of bile in the gallbladder, resulting in better visualization during ultrasonography.

Procedure
- The patient is assisted to a supine position on the ultrasonography table.
- A coupling agent, such as a water-based gel, is applied to the area to be evaluated.
- A transducer is placed on the skin and moved as needed to provide good visualization of the structures.
- The sound waves are transformed into a visual display on the monitor. Printed copies of this display are made.

Posttest
- Cleanse the patient's skin of any lubricant.
- Report abnormal findings to the primary care provider.

→ Clinical Alerts

- For patients with clinical suggestion of gallbladder disease who have a negative abdominal ultrasound, a hepatobiliary iminodiacetic acid (HIDA) scan of the gallbladder may be needed.

A

Abdominal X-ray (Kidney, Ureter, and Bladder Radiography, KUB, Flat Plate X-ray of the Abdomen, Scout Film)

Test Description

The abdominal x-ray, often referred to as a flat plate of the abdomen or KUB, provides an overall view of the lower abdomen that shows the position of the kidneys, ureters, and bladder. The ureters are not normally visible on the KUB unless abnormal, as when calculi are present. The test is a simple x-ray film with the patient in a supine position. It requires no physical preparation of the patient. Renal enlargement, renal displacement, congenital anomalies, and renal or ureteral calculi are just a few of the abnormalities that may be seen as a result of this test. In addition to abnormalities of the urinary tract, the KUB may be used to assess for the presence of ascites and for gas within the intestines, which may occur with intestinal obstruction.

THE EVIDENCE FOR PRACTICE

The plain film of the abdomen may be sufficient to diagnose ureterolithiasis in patients with known stone disease and previous KUBs. The sensitivity of the KUB for ureterolithiasis in other patients is poor; such patients might benefit more from having a noncontrast CT.

Normal Values

Normal size, shape, and location of kidneys. Ureters not seen. Bladder shown as shadow. Normal intestinal gas pattern.

Possible Meanings of Abnormal Values

- Accumulation of gas in intestine
- Ascites
- Calculi
- Congenital abnormalities
- Cysts
- Hydronephrosis
- Intestinal obstruction
- Paralytic ileus
- Renal trauma
- Tumor
- Vascular calcifications

Contributing Factors to Abnormal Values

- Any movement by the patient may alter quality of films taken.
- Retained barium, gas, or stool in the intestines may alter the test results.

Interventions/Implications

Pretest

- Explain to the patient the purpose of the test. Provide any written teaching materials available on the subject. Note that the test involves no discomfort.
- No fasting is required before the test.

- The test should be completed before the patient has any diagnostic tests involving barium.

Procedure
- The patient is assisted to a supine position on the radiography table.
- The patient's arms are extended overhead.
- Films are taken of the patient's abdomen.

Posttest
- Report abnormal findings to the primary care provider.
- Schedule any additional testing for differential diagnosis as ordered.

→ Clinical Alerts

- The test should be scheduled prior to or at least 24 hours after any barium studies are conducted.

Acetylcholine Receptor Antibodies
(AChR, Anti-ACh Antibodies)

Test Description

Acetylcholine (ACh) and the catecholamines (epinephrine and norepinephrine) are the main neurotransmitters of the autonomic nervous system. In normal contraction of the muscles, ACh is released from the terminal end of the nerve into the neuromuscular junction. ACh then binds with receptor sites on the muscle membrane, resulting in the opening of sodium channels. This allows sodium ions to enter and depolarize the cell. This begins an action potential that passes along the entire muscle fiber, resulting in muscle contraction.

Myasthenia gravis (MG) is an autoimmune disease that affects neuromuscular transmission. In this disease, antibodies form that interfere with the binding of ACh to the receptor sites on the muscle membrane. This prevents muscle contraction from occurring. These antibodies are present in more than 85% of the patients with MG. Thus, this test is used for diagnosis of MG and for monitoring the patient's response to immunosuppressive therapy for the disease.

Normal Values

Negative or ≤0.03 nmol/L

Possible Meanings of Abnormal Values

Increased

Myasthenia gravis

Contributing Factors to Abnormal Values

- False-positive results may occur in patients with amyotrophic lateral sclerosis (ALS).
- Drugs that may decrease ACh receptor antibody titers: immunosuppressive drugs.

A

Interventions/Implications

Pretest
- Explain to the patient the purpose of the test and the need for a blood sample to be drawn.
- No fasting is required before the test.

Procedure
- A 7-mL blood sample is drawn in a red-top tube.
- Gloves are worn throughout the procedure.

Posttest
- Apply pressure at venipuncture site. Apply dressing, periodically assessing for continued bleeding.
- Label the specimen and transport it to the laboratory.
- Report abnormal findings to the primary care provider.

→ Clinical Alerts

- Three types of acetylcholine receptor antibodies are available for testing. The most common is the ACh receptor *binding* antibody. If this test is negative, testing for the *blocking* antibody and the *modulating* antibody should be done.
- The ACh receptor blocking antibody is especially useful in monitoring response to therapy.

Acid-Fast Bacilli (AFB)

Test Description

The acid-fast method is a special staining technique that is particularly useful when identifying mycobacteria in sputum specimens, which often contain a variety of organisms. Examples of mycobacteria are those causing leprosy, tuberculosis, and respiratory infection in patients with acquired immunodeficiency syndrome (AIDS). Mycobacteria retain stain coloring even after treatment with a decolorizing acid-alcohol solution. Once bacilli are determined to be acid-fast, a culture is done to differentiate the type of mycobacteria, along with sensitivity testing to determine appropriate pharmacologic treatment.

THE EVIDENCE FOR PRACTICE

Any patient with a cough lasting ≥2 to 3 weeks, with at least one additional symptom including fever, night sweats, weight loss, or hemoptysis, should have a chest radiograph. If suggestive of tuberculosis, three consecutive morning sputum specimens for AFB should be collected.

Normal Values

Negative for bacilli

Possible Meanings of Abnormal Values

Positive

AIDS
Leprosy
Tuberculosis

Contributing Factors to Abnormal Values

- Collection of saliva, rather than sputum, will provide inaccurate test results.

Interventions/Implications

Pretest

- The sputum should be collected before antimicrobial therapy is begun.
- Explain to the patient the purpose of the test and the need for a sputum specimen.
- Explain the procedure to the patient:
    - An early morning specimen is best, because sputum is most concentrated at that time.
    - The patient should brush the teeth and rinse the mouth with water before collecting the sputum to reduce contamination of the sample.
    - The sputum must be from the bronchial tree. The patient must understand this is different from saliva in the mouth.
    - The sample is collected in a sterile sputum container.
- If tuberculosis is suspected, three consecutive morning specimens may be ordered. This increases the chance of isolating the microbes.
- If the sputum is very thick, it can be thinned by inhaling nebulized saline or water or by increasing fluid intake the evening before sample collection. Postural drainage and chest physiotherapy may also prove helpful.

Procedure

- The patient should take several deep breaths and then cough deeply to obtain the sputum. At least one teaspoon of sputum is needed.
- If specimen collection via coughing is ineffective, endotracheal suctioning and fiber-optic bronchoscopy are other options.
- After collection of the sputum, the sample is sent to the laboratory for a Gram stain. This is used to differentiate between true sputum and saliva, which contains many epithelial cells. Decolorizing solution is used to determine acid-fastness of the bacilli.
- The sputum is then placed on the appropriate culture medium and allowed to incubate. Final reports for tuberculosis (AFB culture) may take 1 to 6 weeks.

Posttest

- Label the specimen container and transport it to the laboratory as soon as possible. Note any current antimicrobial therapy on the label.
- Gloves should be worn when handling the specimen.
- Report positive results to the primary care provider.

➔ Clinical Alerts

- A positive AFB smears indicates a likely mycobacterial infection. The AFB culture is then used to identify the specific mycobacteria.

- If the AFB smear/culture is positive after several weeks of drug treatment, this indicates ineffective treatment and that the patient is still infectious. A change of treatment regimen would be warranted.

 ## Acid Phosphatase (Prostatic Acid Phosphatase [PAP])

Test Description
Acid phosphatase, also known as prostatic acid phosphatase (PAP), is an enzyme found primarily in the prostate gland, with high concentrations found in the seminal fluid. It is found in smaller concentrations in the kidneys, liver, spleen, bone marrow, erythrocytes, and platelets. Acid phosphatase is used to diagnose advanced metastatic cancer of the prostate and to monitor the patient's response to therapy for prostate cancer.

In the past, this test has been considered a tumor marker for prostatic cancer. However, with the advent of the prostate-specific antigen (PSA) test, monitoring of the acid phosphatase is decreasing in popularity. An additional use of acid phosphatase testing is testing for its presence in vaginal secretions during the investigation of cases of alleged rape.

THE EVIDENCE FOR PRACTICE
According to guidelines of the American Academy of Pediatrics for evaluation of sexual abuse in children (http://pediatrics.aappublications.org/cgi/content/full/116/2/506), a high acid phosphatase level in a child is suggested as one criterion for reporting suspected sexual abuse.

Normal Values
2.2–10.5 U/L (37–175 nkat/L SI units)

Possible Meanings of Abnormal Values

Increased
Acute renal impairment
Bone metastases
Breast cancer
Cirrhosis
Eclampsia
Gaucher's disease
Hemolytic anemia
Hepatitis
Hyperparathyroidism
Liver tumor
Multiple myeloma
Obstructive jaundice
Paget's disease

A

Prostate cancer
Sexual abuse

Contributing Factors to Abnormal Values

- Hemolysis of the blood sample may alter test results.
- Any manipulation of the prostate gland, including rectal examination or cystoscopy, should be avoided for 2 days before the test.
- Acid phosphatase levels vary during the day. Multiple tests of acid phosphatase should be drawn at the same time each day.
- Drugs that may *increase* acid phosphatase: anabolic steroids, androgens, clofibrate.
- Drugs that may *decrease* acid phosphatase: alcohol, fluorides, oxalates, phosphates.

Interventions/Implications

Pretest

- Explain to the patient the purpose of the test and the need for a blood sample to be drawn.
- No fasting is required before the test.

Procedure

- A 7-mL blood sample is drawn in a collection tube containing a silicone gel. The tube should be kept on ice.
- Gloves are worn throughout the procedure.

Posttest

- Apply pressure at the venipuncture site. Apply dressing, periodically assessing for continued bleeding.
- Label the specimen and transport it to the laboratory immediately.
- Report abnormal findings to the primary care provider.

 Adrenocorticotropic Hormone (ACTH, Corticotropin)

Test Description

In response to a stimulus such as stress, the hypothalamus secretes corticotropin-releasing hormone. This hormone stimulates the secretion of adrenocorticotropic hormone (ACTH) by the anterior pituitary gland. ACTH, in turn, causes the adrenal cortex to release the glucocorticoid hormone cortisol. As levels of cortisol in the blood rise, the pituitary gland is stimulated to decrease ACTH production via a negative feedback mechanism. (See Appendix B for description of hormonal feedback process).

Diurnal variations in ACTH levels occur, with peak levels occurring between 6 and 8 AM and trough levels occurring between 6 and 11 PM. Trough levels are approximately one-half to two-thirds the peak levels.

Assessment of ACTH levels is used in conjunction with knowledge of cortisol levels to evaluate adrenal cortical dysfunction. For example, consider the patient with Addison's disease in which the adrenal cortex is hypoactive, thus producing

A

abnormally low levels of cortisol in the blood. The anterior pituitary gland senses the low serum cortisol levels and, as a result, increases its release of ACTH. This is an attempt to stimulate the adrenal gland to increase its production of cortisol. Thus, the combination of high ACTH and low cortisol levels indicates adrenocortical hypoactivity. Conversely, if the adrenal gland is overproducing cortisol, as in the presence of an adrenal tumor, the ACTH level will be low as the anterior pituitary gland responds to the elevated cortisol level. Should there be a high level of ACTH due to a pituitary tumor or a nonendocrine ACTH-producing tumor, there will also be an elevated cortisol level, as the adrenal gland responds to stimulation by the ACTH.

Normal Values

6.0–76.0 pg/mL (1.3–16.7 pmol/L SI units)

Possible Meanings of Abnormal Values

Increased	Decreased
Addison's disease	Cushing's syndrome
Ectopic ACTH syndrome	Hypopituitarism
Pituitary adenoma	Primary adrenocortical hyperfunction (tumor)
Pituitary Cushing's disease	Secondary hypoadrenalism
Primary adrenal insufficiency	
Stress	

Contributing Factors to Abnormal Values

- Levels of ACTH may vary with exercise, sleep, and stress.
- Testing for ACTH should be scheduled no sooner than 1 week after any diagnostic tests using radioactive materials.
- Drugs that may *decrease* ACTH levels: amphetamines, calcium gluconate, corticosteroids, estrogens, ethanol, lithium carbonate, spironolactone.

Interventions/Implications

Pretest
- Explain to the patient the purpose of the test and the need for a blood sample to be drawn. Usually one morning sample is drawn, but when ACTH hypersecretion is suggested, a second sample is drawn in the evening.
- The patient should consume a low-carbohydrate diet for 48 hours before the test.
- Fasting and limited physical activity for 10 to 12 hours before the test is required.

Procedure
- A 7-mL blood sample is drawn in either a plastic tube (because ACTH may adhere to glass), a collection tube containing heparin, or a collection tube containing EDTA.
- Gloves are worn throughout the procedure.

Posttest
- Apply pressure at venipuncture site. Apply dressing, periodically assessing for continued bleeding.

A

- The sample is to be placed on ice, labeled, and taken to the laboratory immediately.
- Report abnormal findings to the primary care provider.

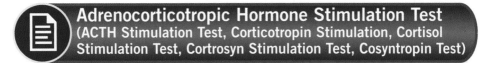

Adrenocorticotropic Hormone Stimulation Test
(ACTH Stimulation Test, Corticotropin Stimulation, Cortisol Stimulation Test, Cortrosyn Stimulation Test, Cosyntropin Test)

Test Description

The hypothalamus secretes corticotropin-releasing hormone. This hormone stimulates the secretion of adrenocorticotropic hormone (ACTH) by the anterior pituitary gland. ACTH, in turn, causes the adrenal cortex to release the glucocorticoid hormone cortisol. Problems occurring in the adrenal cortex are considered "primary" disorders, whereas those occurring in the anterior pituitary gland are known as "secondary" disorders. It is important to determine whether a patient's problem is of a primary or a secondary nature.

Various tests may be used to evaluate adrenal hypofunction through stimulation of the adrenal glands. The most common is the rapid ACTH test, for which cosyntropin (Cortrosyn) is administered. ACTH stimulation testing is especially valuable in the diagnosis of Addison's disease. If plasma cortisol levels increase after administration of ACTH, the adrenal gland has the ability to function when stimulated and the cause of the adrenal insufficiency would be due to a problem in the pituitary gland. If, however, the plasma cortisol levels do not rise or increase only minimally, the problem lies with the adrenal gland. The test can also be used to check for recovery of the hypothalamus-pituitary-adrenal (HPA) axis during tapering of steroids after long-term use.

Normal Values

Rise of at least 7 mcg/dL above baseline level with peak of >20 mcg/dL

Possible Meanings of Abnormal Values

Minimal or No Increase

Addison's disease
Adrenal insufficiency
Adrenocortical tumor

Contributing Factors to Abnormal Values:

- Levels of ACTH may vary with exercise, sleep, and stress.
- Drugs that may also affect test results: amphetamines, calcium gluconate, corticosteroids, estrogens, ethanol, lithium carbonate, spironolactone.

Interventions/Implications

Pretest

- Explain to the patient the purpose of the test and the need for multiple blood samples to be drawn.

- Fasting and limited activity for 10 to 12 hours before the test is required.

Procedure
- A 5-mL blood sample is drawn in a collection tube containing heparin for a baseline plasma cortisol level, labeled, and sent to the laboratory.
- Within 30 minutes of drawing the baseline cortisol level, cosyntropin (Cortrosyn) is administered either intravenously (preferable) or intramuscularly.
- Plasma cortisol levels are drawn at 30 and 60 minutes after cosyntropin administration.
- Gloves are worn throughout the procedure.

Posttest
- Apply pressure at venipuncture site. Apply dressing, periodically assessing for continued bleeding.
- Each blood sample must be carefully labeled as to the time it was drawn, including whether it was baseline, 30 minutes after the cosyntropin administration, or 60 minutes after the cosyntropin administration.
- Transport the specimens to the laboratory.
- Report abnormal findings to the primary care provider.

Clinical Alerts

- When testing for HPA axis recovery during tapering of steroids, if the increase in cortisol is <7 mcg/dL and/or the peak cortisol value is <20 mcg/dL, a slower steroid taper is recommended and the challenge test should be retried at a later date.

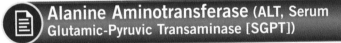

Alanine Aminotransferase (ALT, Serum Glutamic-Pyruvic Transaminase [SGPT])

Test Description
Alanine aminotransferase (ALT) is an enzyme found in the kidneys, heart, and skeletal muscle tissue but primarily in liver tissue. It functions as a catalyst in the reaction needed for amino acid production. The test is used mainly in the diagnosis of liver disease and to monitor the effects of hepatotoxic drugs.

ALT is assessed along with asparate aminotransferase (AST) in monitoring liver damage. These two values normally exist in an approximately 1:1 ratio. The AST is greater than the ALT in alcohol-induced hepatitis, cirrhosis, and metastatic cancer of the liver. ALT is greater than AST in the case of viral or drug-induced hepatitis and hepatic obstruction due to causes other than malignancy.

The degree of increase in these enzyme levels provides information as to the possible source of the problem. A twofold increase is suggestive of an obstructive problem, often requiring surgical intervention. A 10-fold increase of ALT and AST indicates a probable medical problem such as hepatitis.

THE EVIDENCE FOR PRACTICE

In managing abnormal lipids, statin medications are commonly used. One major side effect of statin use is liver toxicity, although the likelihood of liver transaminase elevations >3 times the upper limit of normal is small. Liver transaminases (ALT and AST) are obtained 6 to 12 weeks after statin therapy is initiated. (Full text of guidelines available at: http://circ.ahajournals.org/cgi/content/full/112/20/3184.)

Normal Values

Female: 7–30 U/L (0.12–0.50 µkat/L SI units)
Male: 10–55 U/L (0.17–0.91 µkat/L SI units)

Possible Meanings of Abnormal Values

Increased
Biliary obstruction
Bone metastases
Cholestasis
Cirrhosis
Congestive heart failure
Eclampsia
Hepatic ischemia
Hepatic necrosis
Hepatitis
Infectious mononucleosis
Liver cancer
Muscle inflammation
Obesity
Pancreatitis
Pulmonary infarction
Reye's syndrome
Shock
Trauma

Contributing Factors to Abnormal Values

• Hemolysis of the blood sample may alter test results.
• Drugs that may *increase* ALT levels are numerous and include: ACE-inhibitors, acetaminophen, anticonvulsants, antibiotics, antipsychotics, benzodiazepines, estrogens, ferrous sulfate, heparin, interferons, lipid-lowering agents, NSAIDs, salicylates, thiazides.

Interventions/Implications

Pretest
• Explain to the patient the purpose of the test and the need for a blood sample to be drawn.
• No fasting is required before the test.

Procedure
• A 7-mL blood sample is drawn in a collection tube containing a silicone gel.
• Gloves are worn throughout the procedure.

Posttest
- Apply pressure for 3 to 5 minutes at venipuncture site. Apply dressing, periodically assessing for continued bleeding.
- Teach the patient to monitor the site. If the site begins to bleed, the patient should apply direct pressure and, if unable to control the bleeding, return to the laboratory or notify the primary care provider.
- Label the specimen and transport it to the laboratory.
- Report abnormal findings to the primary care provider.

 Clinical Alerts

- With liver dysfunction, the patient may have prolonged clotting time.
- Liver enzymes, including ALT and AST, are routinely monitored in patients who take HMG-CoEnzyme A reductase inhibitors ("statin" medications).

 Aldolase

Test Description
Aldolase is a glycolytic enzyme that is present in all body cells. The highest concentrations of aldolase are found in the cells of skeletal muscles, the heart, and liver tissue, although the test is considered most specific for muscle tissue destruction. When damage to muscle tissue occurs, cells are destroyed, resulting in the release of aldolase into the blood. Thus, testing for aldolase is useful in monitoring the progress of muscle damage in such disorders as muscular dystrophy.

Normal Values
Adult:	0–7 U/L (0–117 nkat/L SI units)
Child:	Two times adult norms
Newborn:	Four times adult norms

Possible Meanings of Abnormal Values

Increased	Decreased
Burns	Late muscular dystrophy
Dermatomyositis	
Gangrene	
Hepatitis	
Liver cancer	
Muscle inflammation	
Muscle necrosis	
Muscle trauma	
Myocardial infarction	
Myositis	
Polymyositis	

Progressive muscular dystrophy
Pulmonary infarction

A

Contributing Factors to Abnormal Values

- Hemolysis of the blood sample falsely increases the test results.
- Recent minor trauma, including intramuscular injections, may increase the aldolase level.
- Drugs that may *increase* aldolase levels: corticotropin, cortisone acetate, hepatotoxic drugs.
- Drugs that may *decrease* aldolase levels: phenothiazines.

Interventions/Implications

Pretest
- Explain to the patient the purpose of the test and the need for a blood sample to be drawn.
- Although fasting is not required before the test, some institutions require a short fasting period to improve the accuracy of the test results.

Procedure
- A 5-mL blood sample is drawn in a collection tube containing a silicone gel.
- Gloves are worn throughout the procedure.

Posttest
- Apply pressure at venipuncture site. Apply dressing, periodically assessing for continued bleeding.
- Label the specimen and transport it to the laboratory.
- Report abnormal findings to the primary care provider.

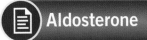

Aldosterone

Test Description

Aldosterone is a mineralocorticoid secreted by the adrenal cortex. The release of aldosterone is controlled primarily by the renin-angiotensin-aldosterone system. A decrease in extracellular fluid results in decreased blood flow through the kidneys, which in turn stimulates production and secretion of renin by the kidneys. Renin acts on angiotensinogen to form Angiotensin I which, in the presence of angiotensin-converting enzyme (ACE), is converted to Angiotensin II. Angiotensin II stimulates the adrenal cortex to increase aldosterone production. The effects of aldosterone occur in the renal distal tubule, where it causes increased reabsorption of sodium and chloride and increased excretion of potassium and hydrogen ions. The result of these actions is retention of increased water and an increase in extracellular fluid. The ultimate effect of changes in aldosterone level is regulation of blood pressure.

Measurement of aldosterone level is performed on both the plasma and the urine. This information assists in the diagnosis of *primary aldosteronism*, caused by an abnormality of the adrenal cortex, and of *secondary aldosteronism*, which may result from overstimulation of the adrenal cortex by a substance such as angiotensin or ACTH.

A

THE EVIDENCE FOR PRACTICE

Primary hyperaldosteronism may account for up to 15% of patients with hypertension, particularly in middle age. The use of the random serum aldosterone/plasma renin activity ratio (ARR) with a sufficiently high cutoff value has facilitated diagnosis at an acceptable cost and low risk.

Normal Values

Plasma, standing:	4–31 ng/dL (111–860 pmol/L SI units)
Plasma, recumbent:	<16 ng/dL (<444 pmol/L SI units)
Urinary excretion:	6–25 mcg/day (17–69 nmol/day SI units)

Possible Meanings of Abnormal Values

Increased	Decreased
Adrenal cortical hyperplasia	Addison's disease
Aldosterone-producing adenoma	High-sodium diet
Cirrhosis of liver with ascites	Hypernatremia
Congestive heart failure	Hypokalemia
Hemorrhage	Salt-losing syndrome
Hyperkalemia	Septicemia
Hyponatremia	Toxemia of pregnancy
Hypovolemia	
Low-sodium diet	
Malignant hypertension	
Nephrosis	
Nephrotic syndrome	
Potassium loading	
Pregnancy	
Primary hyperaldosteronism (Conn's syndrome)	
Stress	

Contributing Factors to Abnormal Values

- Test results may be altered by diet, exercise, licorice ingestion, and posture.
- Drugs that may *increase* aldosterone levels: corticotropin, diazoxide, diuretics, hydralazine hydrochloride, nitroprusside sodium, oral contraceptives, potassium.
- Drugs that may *decrease* aldosterone levels: fludrocortisone acetate, methyldopa, nonsteroidal anti-inflammatory drugs, propranolol, steroids.

Interventions/Implications

Pretest

- Explain to the patient the purpose of the test and the need for a blood sample to be drawn. Explain the effect of the upright position on the test results.
- No fasting is required before the test.
- Unless otherwise ordered, instruct the patient to follow a 3-g sodium diet for at least 2 weeks before the test. Explain to the patient that this is considered "normal" sodium intake.
- Explain 24-hour urine collection procedure to the patient.
- Stress the importance of saving *all* urine in the 24-hour period. Instruct the patient to avoid contaminating the urine with toilet paper or feces.

- Inform the patient of the presence of a preservative in the collection bottle.
- If possible, drugs that may affect test results should be withheld for at least 2 weeks before the test.

Procedure

Blood sampling
- A 7-mL blood sample is drawn in a plain red-top collection tube containing no gel. In hospitalized patients, one blood sample is drawn while the patient is supine and another is drawn 4 hours later after the patient has been upright and ambulating. For outpatients, the blood sample is drawn after the patient has been upright for 2 hours.
- Gloves are worn throughout the procedure.

Urine collection
- Obtain the proper container containing 1 g of boric acid as preservative from the laboratory.
- Begin the testing period in the morning after the patient's first voiding, which is discarded.
- Timing of the 24-hour period begins at the time the first voiding is discarded.
- *All* urine for the next 24 hours is collected in the container, which is to be kept refrigerated or on ice.
- If any urine is accidentally discarded during the 24-hour period, the test must be discontinued and a new test begun.
- The ending time of the 24-hour collection period should be posted in the patient's room.
- Gloves are worn whenever dealing with the specimen collection.

Posttest
- Apply pressure at venipuncture site. Apply dressing, periodically assessing for continued bleeding.
- Label the specimen and transport it to the laboratory.
- At the end of the 24-hour collection period, label and send the urine container on ice to the laboratory as soon as possible.
- Resume medications as taken before the testing period.
- Report abnormal findings to the primary care provider.

 Alkaline Phosphatase (ALP)

Test Description
Alkaline phosphatase (ALP) is an enzyme found in the liver, bone, placenta, intestine, and kidneys but primarily in the cells lining the biliary tract and in the osteoblasts involved in the formation of new bone. ALP is normally excreted from the liver in the bile. Increased ALP levels are found most commonly during periods of bone growth (as in children), in various types of liver disease, and in biliary obstruction. ALP is also considered a tumor marker that increases in the case of osteogenic sarcoma and in breast or prostate cancer that has metastasized to the bone.

A

Normal Values

Female:	30–100 U/L (0.5–1.67 μkat/L SI units)
Male:	45–115 U/L (0.75–1.92 μkat/L SI units)
Elderly:	Slightly higher norms
Children:	One to three times adult norms
Puberty:	Five to six times adult norms

Possible Meanings of Abnormal Values

Increased	Decreased
Biliary obstruction	Celiac disease
Bone metastases	Chronic nephritis
Calcium deficiency	Cystic fibrosis
Cancer of head of pancreas	Excessive vitamin D intake
Cirrhosis	Genetic defect
Eclampsia	Hypophosphatemia
Healing fracture	Hypothyroidism
Hepatitis	Lack of normal bone formation
High-fat intake	Malnutrition
Hyperparathyroidism	Milk-alkali syndrome
Infectious mononucleosis	Pernicious anemia
Leukemia	Placental insufficiency
Liver cancer	Scurvy
Osteogenic sarcoma	
Osteomalacia	
Paget's disease	
Pancreatitis	
Pregnancy	
Rheumatoid arthritis	
Rickets	
Vitamin D deficiency	

Contributing Factors to Abnormal Values

- Hemolysis of the blood sample may alter test results.
- Drugs that may *increase* ALP levels are numerous and include: ACE-inhibitors, acetaminophen, anticonvulsants, antibiotics, antipsychotics, benzodiazepines, estrogens, ferrous sulfate, heparin, interferons, lipid-lowering agents, NSAIDs, salicylates, thiazides, trimethobenzamide, variconazole.
- Drugs that may *decrease* ALP levels: arsenicals, cyanides, fluorides, nitrofurantoin, oxalates, phosphates, propranolol, zinc salts.

Interventions/Implications

Pretest
- Explain to the patient the purpose of the test and the need for a blood sample to be drawn.
- Fasting for 10 to 12 hours is usually required before the test.

Procedure
- A 7-mL blood sample is drawn in a red-top collection tube.
- Gloves are worn throughout the procedure.

Posttest
- Apply pressure 3 to 5 minutes at venipuncture site. Apply dressing, periodically assessing for continued bleeding.
- Teach the patient to monitor the site. If the site begins to bleed, the patient should apply direct pressure and, if unable to control the bleeding, return to the laboratory or notify the primary care provider.
- Label the specimen and transport it to the laboratory.
- Report abnormal findings to the primary care provider.

→ **Clinical Alerts**

- With liver dysfunction, patient may have prolonged clotting time.

 Allergen-Specific IgE Antibody
(RAST Test, Radioallergosorbent Test, Allergy Screen)

Test Description
The protein of the blood is composed of albumin and globulins. One type of globulin is the group of gamma globulins, also called immunoglobulins or antibodies. Gamma globulins are produced by certain white blood cells known as B lymphocytes in response to stimulation by antigens. There are five types of immunoglobulins: IgA, IgD, IgE, IgG, and IgM. IgE is the antibody of allergies.

Testing for allergies to various substances can be done via skin testing, however, this can be uncomfortable for the patient and carries the risk of causing an allergic reaction, since allergens are actually introduced into the body. Another way to test for such allergies is the allergen-specific IgE antibody test. This test is also called the radioallergosorbent test, or RAST test, because it involves the use of fluorescent immunoassay to identify the specific allergens that are affecting the person. The specific antigens, or allergens, are bound to a carrier substance. If the person is allergic to a particular allergen, a specific IgE antibody in the person's blood sample will react with the allergen.

Normal Values
> 0 (No IgE detected)
> 1 (Equivocal/borderline)

Possible Meanings of Abnormal Values

> **Increased**
> Positive allergy to tested substance (Values vary from 2 through 6, with higher classifications indicating higher levels of IgE).

Contributing Factors to Abnormal Values
- Test results are affected by the type of allergen, length of exposure time to the allergen, and any previous hyposensitization therapy.

Interventions/Implications

Pretest
- Explain to the patient the purpose of the test and the need for a blood sample to be drawn.
- No fasting is required before the test.

Procedure
- A 7-mL blood sample is drawn in a red-top collection tube.
- Gloves are worn throughout the procedure.

Posttest
- Apply pressure at venipuncture site. Apply dressing, periodically assessing for continued bleeding.
- Label the specimen and transport it to the laboratory.
- Report abnormal findings to the primary care provider.

→ **Clinical Alerts**

- Specific allergies found through this test should be noted in the patient's medical record.

Alpha₁-Antitrypsin Test (AAT)

Test Description
Alpha$_1$-antitrypsin (AAT) is a protein produced by the liver. It has a protective function, in that it prevents the release of proteolytic enzymes that can damage tissues such as that of the lung. AAT deficiency can be inherited or acquired. When an inherited problem, AAT deficiency is most often noted in individuals of European descent and is first noted relatively early in life. Acquired AAT deficiency is seen in patients who have protein-deficiency syndromes such as liver disease, nephrotic syndrome, and malnutrition. Regardless of the type, the deficiency of AAT allows proteolytic enzymes to damage lung tissue, resulting in severe emphysema in young adulthood.

THE EVIDENCE FOR PRACTICE
Alpha$_1$-antitrypsin (AAT) deficiency accounts for less than one percent of cases of chronic obstructive pulmonary disease (COPD). However, it may be suspected and an AAT level obtained in patients with moderate-severe COPD before the age of 50, a family history of AAT, chronic bronchitis with airflow obstruction in a person who has never smoked, bronchiectasis in the absence of clear risk factors, or cirrhosis without apparent risk factors.

Normal Values
85–213 mg/dL (20–60 µmol/L SI units)

Possible Meanings of Abnormal Values

A

Increased	Decreased
Acute inflammatory disorders	AAT deficiency
Cancer	Chronic liver disease
Chronic inflammatory disorders	Emphysema
Chronic liver disease	Malnutrition
Hepatitis	Nephrotic syndrome
Infection	Severe hepatic damage
Pregnancy	
Stress	
Systemic lupus erythematosus (SLE)	
Thyroid infection	

Contributing Factors to Abnormal Values

- Drugs that may *increase* AAT levels: estrogens, oral contraceptives, steroids.

Interventions/Implications

Pretest
- Explain to the patient the purpose of the test and the need for a blood sample to be drawn.
- No fasting is required before the test unless the patient has hyperlipidemia. If so, the patient should fast 8 to 10 hours before the test.

Procedure
- A 7-mL blood sample is drawn in a red-top collection tube.
- Gloves are worn throughout the procedure.

Posttest
- Apply pressure at venipuncture site. Apply dressing, periodically assessing for continued bleeding.
- Label the specimen and transport it to the laboratory.
- Report abnormal findings to the primary care provider.

→ **Clinical Alerts**

- Patients who are AAT deficient need to be taught to avoid smoking and employment in occupations in which air pollutants are common.
- Genetic counseling should be offered to patients with positive test results. Testing of other family members should also be conducted.

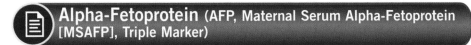

Alpha-Fetoprotein (AFP, Maternal Serum Alpha-Fetoprotein [MSAFP], Triple Marker)

Test Description
Alpha-fetoprotein (AFP) is a globulin protein formed in the yolk sac and liver of the fetus. As the fetus develops, the level of AFP found in the mother's serum increases. Only minute amounts of AFP remain in the bloodstream after birth.

A

This test is used primarily to screen for the presence of neural tube defects in the fetus, such as spina bifida and anencephaly. The test, done between 15 and 20 weeks of pregnancy, does not absolutely diagnose a birth defect. However, if the AFP is found to be abnormally high, additional testing, including ultrasonography and testing of the amniotic fluid for AFP, is needed.

In many institutions, the test for AFP is now combined with measurement of estriol and human chorionic gonadotropin. This combination testing is known by various names, including "triple marker." The measurement of these three substances provides screening for neural tube defects, trisomy 18, and trisomy 21 (Down syndrome). An accurate fetal gestational age is essential for accurate test results, because the levels of the substances all vary with gestational age. The most accurate method of assessing gestational age is ultrasonography; if unavailable, gestational age by last menstrual period is used. This testing is a screening tool; negative results do not guarantee a normal baby.

AFP is also considered a tumor marker for several types of cancer. Cancers typically are characterized by undifferentiated cells. These cells often still carry surface markers similar to those found in the fetus. The higher the AFP level, the greater amount of tumor present. Thus, AFP can also be used to assess response to cancer treatment.

THE EVIDENCE FOR PRACTICE

- Maternal serum AFP evaluation is an effective screening test for neural tube defects (NTDs) and should be offered to all pregnant women.
- Women with elevated serum AFP levels should have a specialized ultrasound examination to further assess the risk of NTDs.

Normal Values

Nonpregnant females/males: <40 ng/mL (<40 mg/L SI units)

Pregnant females: Reference laboratory provides normal values based on gestational age.

Possible Meanings of Abnormal Values

Increased	Decreased
Biliary cirrhosis	Down syndrome
Breast cancer	Fetal death
Colon cancer	
Fetal distress	
Fetal neural tube defect	
Gastric cancer	
Hepatic cancer	
Hepatitis	
Lung cancer	
Multiple fetuses	
Pancreatic cancer	
Renal cancer	
Testicular cancer	

Contributing Factors to Abnormal Values
- Hemolysis of the blood sample may alter test results.

Interventions/Implications

Pretest
- Explain to the patient the purpose of the test and the need for a blood sample to be drawn.
- No fasting is required before the test.

Procedure
- A 7-mL blood sample is drawn in a red-top collection tube. (Note: Some laboratories use a collection tube containing EDTA for the triple marker screening test.)
- Gloves are worn throughout the procedure.

Posttest
- Apply pressure at venipuncture site. Apply dressing, periodically assessing for continued bleeding.
- Label the specimen and transport it to the laboratory.
- Report abnormal findings to the primary care provider.

→ Clinical Alerts

- If the AFP is found to be abnormally high, additional testing, including ultrasonography and testing of the amniotic fluid for AFP, is needed.
- For low-risk women considering becoming pregnant, folic acid supplementation of 400 mcg per day is recommended because it has been shown to reduce the occurrence and recurrence of neural tube defects.

Ambulatory Electrocardiography (Ambulatory Monitoring, Event Monitoring, Holter Monitoring)

Test Description
Ambulatory electrocardiography involves the monitoring of the electrical activity of the heart as the patient carries out normal life activities. By continuously monitoring the patient's heart, ambulatory electrocardiography is able to detect dysrhythmias that occur only sporadically and are easily missed during periodic electrocardiographic assessments.

   Holter monitoring is performed by attaching several chest electrodes to a small recorder that is carried with the patient. The monitoring is conducted for a 24- to 48-hour period. The patient maintains a diary of activities and any symptoms experienced during the testing period.

   Event monitoring, which is conducted for a 30-day period, is used for those patients whose symptoms occur infrequently. This monitor consists of a small recorder and two electrodes that can be removed for bathing and reapplied by the patient. When symptoms such as fluttering or discomfort are experienced, the

A

patient presses the "Record" button. A recording is then made of the heart's electrical activity for the 15 seconds before the "Record" button was pushed and for 1 minute afterward. The patient maintains a diary of the symptoms experienced.

Normal Values

Normal rate, rhythm, and waveforms

Possible Meanings of Abnormal Values

Cardiac dysrhythmias

Contributing Factors to Abnormal Values

- Interferences to the recording of the electrocardiogram are shown on the recording as artifact. This may occur due to equipment failure, electrode adherence problems, or electromagnetic interference.
- The adequacy of the testing is dependent on the patient maintaining normal daily activities during the testing period and keeping a detailed diary of activities and symptoms.

Interventions/Implications

Pretest

- Explain to the patient the purpose of the test and the need for electrodes to be attached to the chest. Note that the test causes no discomfort but does require wearing a small tape recorder for 24 to 48 hours for Holter monitoring and 30 days for event monitoring.
- Instruct the patient to maintain a diary of activities and situations, such as emotional stress, that occur during the test period. Included in the diary should be any symptoms experienced and the time at which they occur. The symptoms will then be able to be correlated with the electrocardiographic pattern occurring at that time.
- No fasting is required before the test.

Procedure

- The skin is cleansed with an alcohol swab and then abraded until slightly reddened.
- The electrodes are securely applied to the skin.
- The monitor and case are positioned; then the electrode cable is attached to the monitor.
- The recorder is turned on.
- The patient is provided with the recording diary and with a telephone number of the cardiology technician who may be called with questions or problems.

Posttest

- At the end of the testing period, remove the electrodes and cleanse the skin of any residual gel or adhesive.
- Label the recording tape and send the tape and diary to the cardiologist for interpretation.
- Inform the patient that it will take several days for the electrocardiographic tape and diary to be interpreted.
- Report abnormal findings to the primary care provider.

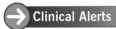

Clinical Alerts

- Caution the patient that the device must not be allowed to become wet.
- Magnets, metal detectors, electric blankets, and high-voltage areas should be avoided while wearing the monitoring device.

Aminolevulinic Acid (ALA, Delta-Aminolevulinic Acid, Delta-ALA)

Test Description

Aminolevulinic acid (ALA), a urine pigment, is the precursor to porphobilinogen (PBG) in the formation of heme of hemoglobin. Subsequent steps include: PBG leading to formation of uroporphyrinogen III/uroporphyrin III, followed by formation of coproporphyrinogen III/coproporphyrin III, then protoporphyrinogen/protoporphyrin. This process then leads to heme formation. If a problem occurs during heme formation, the ALA accumulates and is excreted in the urine. ALA is normally absent from urine.

The presence of ALA in the urine usually indicates lead poisoning. The test can be used as a screening device for detection of excessive absorption of lead before the appearance of symptoms.

Concentrations of ALA are greatly increased in many patients with acute neurological forms of porphyrias. ALA testing may be ordered in patients with symptoms suggestive of acute porphyria, such as abdominal pain, nausea, constipation, peripheral neuropathy, muscle weakness, urinary retention, confusion, and hallucinations.

Normal Values

Random specimen:	0.1–0.6 mg/dL (7.6–45.8 µmol/L SI units)
24-hour urine:	1.5–7.5 mg/dL/24 hour (11.15–57.2 µmol/24 hours SI units)

Possible Meanings of Abnormal Values

Increased
Acute porphyria
Chronic alcohol abuse
Hepatitis
Hepatic carcinoma
Lead exposure
Lead poisoning

Contributing Factors to Abnormal Values

- Failure to protect the urine from light may alter test results.
- Drugs which may *increase* ALA levels: barbiturates, griseofulvin, penicillin, rifampin.

A

Interventions/Implications

Pretest
- Explain 24-hour urine collection procedure to the patient.
- Stress the importance of saving *all* urine in the 24-hour period. Instruct the patient to avoid contaminating the urine with toilet paper or feces.
- Inform the patient that there is no preservative in the collection bottle. It must be refrigerated during and after collection. The container should be wrapped in aluminum foil to protect the specimen from light.

Procedure
- Obtain the proper container from the laboratory.
- Begin the testing period in the morning after the patient's first voiding, which is discarded.
- Timing of the 24-hour period begins at the time the first voiding is discarded.
- *All* urine for the next 24 hours is collected in the container, which is to be kept refrigerated.
- If any urine is accidentally discarded during the 24-hour period, the test must be discontinued and a new test begun.
- The ending time of the 24-hour collection period should be posted in the patient's room.
- Gloves are worn whenever dealing with the specimen collection.

Posttest
- At the end of the 24-hour collection period, label and send the urine container on ice to the laboratory as soon as possible.
- Report abnormal findings to the primary care provider.

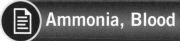

Ammonia, Blood

Test Description

Ammonia is a waste product that forms as a result of nitrogen breakdown during intestinal protein metabolism and from digestion of blood which may be in the gastrointestinal tract (such as from esophageal varices). Another major source of ammonia is from the synthesis and conversion of glutamine by the renal tubules. In the kidneys, ammonia serves as an important renal buffer.

Normally, ammonia is converted into urea by the liver and then excreted by the kidneys. If a physical disorder prevents this conversion from occurring, the ammonia accumulates in the bloodstream. Toxic levels of ammonia in the blood lead to a problem known as hepatic encephalopathy, in which brain function is affected by the high ammonia levels. Correlation between plasma ammonia and the degree of encephalopathy can be erratic. For example, an individual with very high blood ammonia may show minimal or no effect while another may be greatly affected. The test can be used to determine whether liver dysfunction is the cause of such symptoms as confusion, excessive sleepiness, coma, or hand tremor. It can also be used to monitor the effectiveness of treatment for liver disease, such as cirrhosis.

Normal Values

Adult: 15–45 mcg/dL (11–32 μmol/L SI units)
Children: 40–80 mcg/dL (28–57 μmol/L SI units)
Newborn: 90–150 mcg/dL (64–107 μmol/L SI units)

A

Possible Meanings of Abnormal Values

Increased	Decreased
Acute bronchitis	Essential hypertension
Azotemia	Malignant hypertension
Cirrhosis	
Cor pulmonale	
Gastrointestinal bleeding	
Heart failure	
Hemolytic disease of the newborn	
Hepatic encephalopathy	
Hepatic failure	
Hyperalimentation	
Leukemia	
Pericarditis	
Pulmonary emphysema	
Renal failure	
Reye's syndrome	

Contributing Factors to Abnormal Values

- Drugs that may *increase* blood ammonia levels: heparin, some diuretics (such as furosemide), acetazolamide, and valproic acid.
- Drugs that may *decrease* blood ammonia levels: neomycin, tetracycline, diphenhydramine, isocarboxazid, phenelzine, tranylcypromine, heparin, and lactulose.
- Smoking
- Strenuous exercise
- High-protein or low-protein diet

Interventions/Implications

Pretest
- Explain to the patient the purpose of the test and the need for a blood sample to be drawn.
- Instruct the patient to fast for 8 hours before the test. Water is permitted.
- Instruct the patient to avoid strenuous exercise and smoking just prior to the test.

Procedure
- A 5-mL blood sample is collected in an EDTA (lavender-top) tube. The tube should be kept on ice.
- Gloves are worn throughout the procedure.

Posttest
- Apply pressure at venipuncture site. Apply dressing, periodically assessing for continued bleeding.
- The sample is labeled, placed in ice, and transported to the laboratory immediately.
- Report abnormal results to the health-care provider.

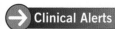

Clinical Alerts

- If the patient is symptomatic of a high ammonia level (such as confusion), treatment may include administration of lactulose, a laxative that works by reducing ammonia production in the intestines.

Amniocentesis (Amniotic Fluid Analysis)

Test Description

Amniocentesis is an invasive diagnostic procedure which involves the transabdominal needle aspiration of amniotic fluid. A 10 to 20 mL sample of the amniotic fluid is withdrawn for analysis. This test is useful in detecting chromosomal abnormalities such as Down syndrome and neural tube defects such as spina bifida, in determining fetal maturity, and in detecting hemolytic disease of the newborn due to Rh incompatibility. It can also be used for determining gender, although the test is not done with this purpose in mind unless there is question of an X-linked chromosomal abnormality. The timing of the procedure is based on the reason the procedure is being done. If it is to determine genetic abnormalities, it is usually performed after the fifteenth week of pregnancy, when the two layers of fetal membranes have fused sufficiently to allow safe withdrawal of the amniotic fluid sample. To determine fetal maturity, the procedure is more likely to be performed after the thirty sixth week of gestation.

The amniotic fluid is analyzed for the following: acetylcholinesterase, alpha-fetoprotein, bacteria, bilirubin, chromosomal karyotype, color, creatinine, glucose, lecithin-to-sphingomyelin (L/S) ratio, meconium, and phosphatidylglycerol (PG). Hemolytic disease of the newborn is indicated by high levels of bilirubin in the fluid. Meconium staining indicates possible fetal distress. Fetal pulmonary immaturity is demonstrated by a low L/S ratio and the absence of PG. A decreased creatinine level may also indicate fetal immaturity. Neural tube defects are suspected with increased levels of alpha-fetoprotein and acetylcholinesterase.

THE EVIDENCE FOR PRACTICE

Use of amniocentesis is recommended by the American College of Obstetricians and Gynecologists as follows (see: http://www.guideline.gov/summary/summary.aspx?doc_id=3976&nbr=003115&string=amniocentesis):

- Women pregnant with a single fetus who will be 35 years or older at delivery should be offered prenatal diagnosis for fetal aneuploidy.
- Counseling for amniocentesis in a twin pregnancy in women age 33 years is indicated because the midtrimester risk of fetal Down syndrome is approximately the same as for that of a single pregnancy at age 35 years.
- Patients with a high risk of fetal aneuploidy include women with a previous pregnancy complicated by a chromosomal abnormality, a major fetal structural defect identified by ultrasonography, either parent with a chromosome translocation, and carriers of a chromosomal abnormality.

Normal Values

Acetylcholinesterase: Absent
Alpha-fetoprotein: Varies with gestational age (peaks at 13–14 weeks)
Bacteria: Absent
Bilirubin: Absent at term
Chromosomes: Normal karyotype
Color: Colorless or light straw
Creatinine: >2 mg/100 mL when mature
Glucose: <45 mg/100 mL
L/S ratio: >2 indicates pulmonary maturity
Meconium: Absent
Phosphatidylglycerol: Present with pulmonary maturity

Possible Meanings of Abnormal Values

Chromosomal abnormalities (e.g., Down syndrome)
Fetal distress
Genetic aberrations (e.g., galactosemia)
Hereditary metabolic disorders (e.g., cystic fibrosis)
Neural tube defects (e.g., spina bifida)
Pulmonary immaturity
Rh isoimmunization
Sex-linked disorders (e.g., hemophilia)
Sickle cell anemia
Thalassemia

Contributing Factors to Abnormal Values

- Alpha-fetoprotein and acetylcholinesterase may be falsely elevated if the sample is contaminated with fetal blood.
- Bilirubin may be falsely elevated if the sample is contaminated with maternal hemoglobin or if meconium is present in the sample.
- Bilirubin may be falsely low if the sample is exposed to light.

Interventions/Implications

Pretest
- Explain to the patient the purpose of the test and procedure to be followed.
- No fasting is required prior to the test.
- Obtain a signed informed consent.
- If an ultrasound is to be performed just prior to the amniocentesis, the patient needs to be well-hydrated and have a full bladder. The bladder must then be emptied prior to the amniocentesis to avoid accidental puncture.

Procedure
- The patient is assisted to a supine position.
- The skin of the lower abdomen is cleansed with an antiseptic solution and draped.
- The skin overlying the chosen site is anesthetized with 1% lidocaine.
- A 20-gauge spinal needle is inserted into the amniotic cavity and the stylet is withdrawn. A 10-mL syringe is then attached to the needle.

- The fluid sample is aspirated and placed in an amber or foil-covered test tube. This will protect the sample from light and avoid breakdown of bilirubin in the sample.
- The needle is withdrawn, and a dressing is applied over the site.
- Gloves are worn throughout the procedure.

Posttest
- Monitor fetal heart rate and maternal vital signs every 15 minutes until stable.
- If the patient complains of nausea or feeling faint, assist her to lie on her left side. This will relieve uterine pressure on the vena cava.
- Observe the puncture site for drainage.
- Instruct the patient to notify the health-care provider immediately if any of the following occur: abdominal pain, cramping, chills, fever, vaginal bleeding, fetal hyperactivity, or unusual fetal lethargy.
- Protect the specimen from light, label it, and transport it to the laboratory immediately.
- Inform the patient that results may not be available for up to 3 weeks.
- Report abnormal findings to the primary care provider.

→ Clinical Alerts

- Possible complications include: amniotic fluid embolism, fetal injury, hemorrhage, infection, premature labor, Rh sensitization due to fetal bleeding into maternal circulation, and spontaneous abortion.
- It is possible for some fetal blood cells to enter the mother's bloodstream during the procedure. If the mother's blood is Rh negative and the fetus' is Rh positive, the mother may produce antibodies against the fetus. To avoid this, RhoGAM should be given to the mother.

CONTRAINDICATIONS!

- Patients with abruptio placentae, incompetent cervix, placenta previa
- Patients with a history of premature labor

Amylase, Serum

Test Description
Amylase is an enzyme found primarily in the pancreas and salivary glands and in minor amounts in the liver and fallopian tubes. Its function is to assist in the digestion of complex carbohydrates into simple sugars. Measurement of serum amylase is often performed to differentiate abdominal pain due to acute pancreatitis from other causes of abdominal pain that may require surgical treatment. The serum amylase begins to rise 3 to 6 hours after the onset of acute pancreatitis and peaks in approximately 24 hours. The values return to normal within 2 to 3 days after onset.

A

THE EVIDENCE FOR PRACTICE

Acute pancreatitis is suspected in patients presenting with epigastric upper abdominal pain that is acute in onset, rapidly increasing in severity, and persistent without relief. Serum amylase and/or lipase levels can be considered diagnostic when the reported value(s) is ≥3 times normal.

Normal Values

Adult: 53–123 U/L (0.88–2.05 nkat/L SI units)
Elderly: Slightly higher norms

Possible Meanings of Abnormal Values

Increased	Decreased
Acute pancreatitis	Cirrhosis of liver
Alcoholism	Hepatitis
Biliary obstruction	Pancreatic cancer
Cholelithiasis	Severe burns
Diabetic ketoacidosis	Severe thyrotoxicosis
Hyperlipidemia	
Hyperthyroidism	
Inflammation of salivary glands	
Mumps	
Perforated bowel	
Perforated peptic ulcer	
Pregnancy	
Ruptured tubal pregnancy	

Contributing Factors to Abnormal Values

- Hemolysis of the blood sample will alter test results.
- Contamination of the sample with saliva by talking over an uncovered blood sample may falsely increase test results.
- Drugs that may *increase* serum amylase levels: acetaminophen, antibiotics, aspirin, corticosteroids, estrogens, furosemide, NSAIDs, prednisone, salicylates, and thiazide diuretics.
- Drugs that may *decrease* serum amylase levels: citrates, glucose, oxalates.

Interventions/Implications

Pretest
- Explain to the patient the purpose of the test and the need for a blood sample to be drawn.
- No fasting is required before the test.

Procedure
- A 7-mL blood sample is drawn in a red-top collection tube.
- Gloves are worn throughout the procedure.

Posttest
- Apply pressure at venipuncture site. Apply dressing, periodically assessing for continued bleeding.
- Label the specimen and transport it to the laboratory.
- Report abnormal findings to the primary care provider.

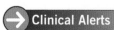

Clinical Alerts

- Serum amylase and lipase are typically both evaluated in suspected pancreatitis.
- In some patients, acute pancreatitis may be present in the absence of enzyme abnormalities.

 Amylase, Urine

Test Description

Amylase is an enzyme found primarily in the pancreas and salivary glands and in minor amounts in the liver and fallopian tubes. Whenever there is an inflammation of the pancreas or salivary glands, more amylase is released into the bloodstream and excreted by the kidneys. Amylase assists in the digestion of complex carbohydrates into simple sugars.

Amylase levels may be measured in the serum and in the urine. Whereas the serum amylase level begins to rise 3 to 6 hours after the onset of acute pancreatitis and returns to normal within 2 to 3 days after onset of acute pancreatitis, the urine amylase level is elevated for 7 to 10 days. Thus, testing for urine amylase is a useful way to demonstrate the presence of acute pancreatitis after serum amylase levels have returned to normal. The test may be conducted with a minimum of a 2-hour urine collection, a 24-hour urine collection, or a variety of other time periods.

Normal Values

0–375 U/L (0–6.25 μkat/L SI units)

Possible Meanings of Abnormal Values

Increased	Decreased
Acute pancreatitis	Cirrhosis of liver
Alcoholism	Hepatitis
Biliary obstruction	Pancreatic cancer
Cholelithiasis	Severe burns
Diabetic ketoacidosis	Severe thyrotoxicosis
Hyperlipidemia	Toxemia of pregnancy
Hyperthyroidism	
Inflammation of salivary glands	
Mumps	
Perforated bowel	
Perforated peptic ulcer	
Pregnancy	
Ruptured tubal pregnancy	

Contributing Factors to Abnormal Values

- Contamination of the sample with saliva by talking over an uncovered urine specimen may falsely increase test results.

- Drugs that may *increase* urine amylase levels: alcohol, aspirin, bethanechol, codeine, indomethacin, meperidine, morphine, pentazocine, thiazide diuretics.
- Drugs that may *decrease* urine amylase levels: fluorides, glucose.

Interventions/Implications

Pretest
- Explain 24-hour urine collection procedure to the patient. (Note: Shorter urine collection periods, such as 2 hours, may be ordered in place of a 24-hour collection.)
- Stress the importance of saving *all* urine in the 24-hour period. Instruct the patient to avoid contaminating the urine with toilet paper or feces.

Procedure
- Obtain the proper container containing no preservative from the laboratory.
- Begin the testing period in the morning after the patient's first voiding, which is discarded.
- Timing of the 24-hour period begins at the time the first voiding is discarded.
- *All* urine for the next 24 hours is collected in the container, which is to be kept refrigerated or on ice.
- If any urine is accidentally discarded during the 24-hour period, the test must be discontinued and a new test begun.
- The ending time of the 24-hour collection period should be posted in the patient's room.
- Gloves are worn whenever dealing with the specimen collection.

Posttest
- At the end of the 24-hour collection period, label and send the urine container to the laboratory as soon as possible.
- Report abnormal findings to the primary care provider.

 ## Androstenedione

Test Description
Androstenedione is one of the primary androgens produced in the ovaries of women, and, to a lesser degree, in the adrenal glands of both men and women. It is converted to estrone by adipose tissue and the liver. Estrone is a form of estrogen that is of relatively low potency, compared with estradiol. In premenopausal women, estrone levels are relatively small in comparison to estradiol levels. However, in children and postmenopausal women, estrone is a major estrogen source. If, for some reason, androstenedione production is increased, a child may experience premature sexual development. In postmenopausal woman, increased androstenedione production may result in bleeding, endometriosis, ovarian stimulation, and polycystic ovaries. Increased production in obesity may cause menstrual irregularities and, in men, such signs of feminization as gynecomastia. Owing to the results seen with androstenedione overproduction, this test is useful in the diagnosis of menstrual irregularities, premature sexual development, and postmenopausal irregularities.

Normal Values
80–300 ng/dL (3.8–6.6 nmol/L SI units)

A

Possible Meanings of Abnormal Values

Increased	Decreased
Adrenal tumor	Hypogonadism
Congenital adrenal hyperplasia	Menopause
Cushing's syndrome	
Ectopic ACTH-producing tumor	
Hirsutism	
Ovarian tumor	
Stein-Leventhal disease	
Testicular tumor	

Contributing Factors to Abnormal Values

- Radioactive dyes received within 1 week of the test will alter test results.
- Elevated results may be reduced to normal levels through the use of glucocorticoid therapy.

Interventions/Implications

Pretest
- Explain to the patient the purpose of the test and the need for a blood sample to be drawn.
- Fasting is required before the test.
- The blood sample is to be drawn 1 week before or after the menstrual period.
- The sample should be drawn when androstenedione is at its peak, which is approximately 7 A.M.

Procedure
- A 7-mL blood sample is drawn in a red-top collection tube.
- Gloves are worn throughout the procedure.

Posttest
- Apply pressure at venipuncture site. Apply dressing, periodically assessing for continued bleeding.
- Label the specimen and transport it to the laboratory.
- Report abnormal findings to the primary care provider.

→ Clinical Alerts

- Normal postmenopausal women have a 50% reduction in the serum androstenedione concentration as a result of decreased adrenal production.

Angiography (Vascular X-ray, Arteriography [Cerebral, Renal, Lower Extremity], Digital Subtraction Angiography)

Test Description

Angiography is a general term used to indicate visualization of any blood vessels, whether they be arteries or veins. The more precise term for visualization of the arteries is *arteriography*. Arteriograms are extremely valuable for observing the blood flow to a part of the body and to detect lesions that may be amenable to surgical treatment.

The purposes of *cerebral angiography* are to detect cerebrovascular abnormalities such as aneurysm or arteriovenous (A-V) malformation, to study vascular displacement due to such problems as tumor or hydrocephalus, and to evaluate the postoperative status of blood vessels. The test involves the introduction of a radiopaque catheter into either the femoral, carotid, or brachial artery, and injecting a contrast medium dye. The most commonly used site is the femoral artery.

The purposes of renal angiography are to visualize the renal parenchyma and renal vasculature, to evaluate chronic renal disease, renal failure, and transplant donors and recipients, and to conduct post-transplant evaluation of the kidney. This is accomplished by introducing a radiopaque catheter into the femoral artery and injecting a contrast media dye.

The primary purpose of *arteriography of the lower extremities* is to identify any occlusions within the femoral arteries and their branches. This is also accomplished by introducing a radiopaque catheter into the femoral artery and injecting a contrast media dye. This test is done for evaluation of peripheral vascular disease and in emergency situations in which blood flow to the extremity has suddenly stopped, as following some types of surgery.

Digital subtraction angiography is a special type of angiography in which the images are recorded in digital format through the computer. Images of nonvascular structures, such as bone, can be subtracted by the computer, leaving a clear image of only the blood vessels.

THE EVIDENCE FOR PRACTICE

Considering the availability of magnetic resonance and computerized tomography technology, it is recommended that conventional angiography should be reserved for confirmation and therapeutic reasons such as angioplasty and stent placement.

Normal Values

Normal vasculature without occlusion

Possible Meanings of Abnormal Values

Cerebral angiography
Arterial spasm
Arteriosclerosis
Arteriovenous malformations
Brain tumor
Cerebral aneurysm
Cerebral fistula
Cerebral occlusion
Cerebral thrombosis
Increased intracranial pressure

Renal angiography
Chronic pyelonephritis
Intrarenal hematoma

A

Renal abscess
Renal arteriovenous fistula
Renal artery aneurysms
Renal artery dysplasia
Renal artery stenosis
Renal cysts
Renal infarction
Renal parenchymal laceration
Renal tumor

Arteriography of the lower extremities
Aneurysm
Arterial disease (such as Buerger's disease)
Occlusion due to arteriosclerosis
Occlusion due to embolism
Occlusion due to neoplasm
Tumor neovascularity

Contributing Factors to Abnormal Values

- Any movement by the patient may alter quality of films taken.
- For renal angiography, bowel gas, stool, or retained barium from previous exam will hinder test results.

Interventions/Implications

Pretest

- Explain to the patient the purpose of the test. Provide any written teaching materials available on the subject. Note that discomfort involved with this test is primarily due to lying on a hard table for an extended period of time and the needle puncture. Explain that an intense hot flushing may be experienced for 15–30 seconds when the dye is injected.
- Check for allergies to iodine, shellfish, or contrast medium dye. Inform the radiologist of such possible allergy and obtain order for an antihistamine and steroid to be administered prior to the test.
- Baseline laboratory data (CBC, PT, PTT, creatinine) are obtained. Pregnancy test should be obtained on women of childbearing age.
- Note any medications, such as anticoagulants or aspirin, which may prolong bleeding.
- Patients receiving metformin (Glucophage) for Type 2 diabetes mellitus should discontinue the drug 2 days before angiographic exams. This is due to the possible occurrence of lactic acidosis, a potentially fatal complication of biguanide therapy.
- Fasting for at least 8 hours is required prior to the test.
- Obtain a signed informed consent.
- Administer any pretest sedation after consent form is signed.
- Assess and document patient's peripheral pulses bilaterally prior to the test.
- *For cerebral angiography:* Perform and document a baseline neurologic assessment.
- *For angiography using peripheral puncture sites:* Assess and document patient's peripheral pulses bilaterally prior to the test. Mark the location of the pulses with a marking pen.

Procedure

- The patient is assisted to a supine position on the examination table.
- A maintenance intravenous line is initiated.
- The area of the puncture site is shaved if necessary, cleansed, and then anesthetized.
- The needle puncture of the artery is made and a guide wire is placed through the needle.

- The catheter is then inserted over the wire and into the artery.
- The radiopaque catheter is advanced into the desired artery. Positioning is monitored via fluoroscopy.
- Once the catheter is in the correct position, contrast dye is injected through the catheter.
- Radiographic films are taken.
- After films of satisfactory quality are obtained, the catheter is removed and pressure held on the puncture site for at least 15 minutes.
- Gloves are worn throughout the procedure.

Posttest
- Most allergic reactions to radiopaque dye occur within 30 minutes of administration of the contrast medium. Observe the patient closely for: respiratory distress, hypotension, edema, hives, rash, tachycardia, and/or laryngeal stridor. Emergency resuscitation equipment must be readily accessible.
- A pressure dressing is applied to the puncture site. Check the dressing for bleeding and the area around the puncture site for swelling at frequent intervals.
- For *angiography using peripheral puncture sites:*
  - The patient is to remain on bedrest for 8–12 hours with the affected extremity immobilized.
  - Maintain pressure on the puncture site with a sandbag.
- Monitor vital signs every 15 minutes for one hour, then every 30 minutes for 2 hours, then every hour for 4 hours, and then every 4 hours.
  - For *cerebral angiography:* Monitor neurological status with each vital sign assessment.
- Monitor urinary output.
- Assess the color, movement, temperature, and sensation (CMTS) and the pulse(s) of the affected extremity with each vital sign check. Compare with the other extremity.
- Encourage fluid intake to promote dye excretion.
- Renal function should be assessed to be adequate before metformin is restarted.
- Report abnormal findings to the primary care provider.

→ Clinical Alerts

- Resuscitation and suctioning equipment should be available throughout the procedure.
- Possible complications include: Allergic reaction to dye, arterial embolism or stroke, arterial occlusion due to disruption of arteriosclerotic plaque or dissection of arterial lining, bleeding at the puncture site, infection at the puncture site, renal failure.

CONTRAINDICATIONS!

- Patients who are allergic to iodine, shellfish, or contrast medium dye
- Patients with bleeding disorders
- Pregnant women
  - Caution: A woman in her childbearing years should undergo radiography only during her menses or 12 to 14 days after its onset to avoid any exposure to a fetus.
- Patients who are unable to cooperate due to age, mental status, pain, or other factors
- Patients with renal failure or those susceptible to dye-induced renal failure (dehydrated patients)

Angiotensin-Converting Enzyme
(ACE, Serum Angiotensin-Converting Enzyme [SACE])

Test Description
Angiotensin-converting enzyme (ACE) is an enzyme found primarily in the epithelial cells of the lungs and in smaller concentrations in the blood vessels and kidneys. This enzyme is responsible for stimulating the conversion of angiotensin I to angiotensin II, a vasoconstricting agent, which, in turn, stimulates the adrenal cortex to produce aldosterone.

There has been found a high correlation between high ACE levels and patients with active sarcoidosis. Thus, this test is used in the diagnosis of sarcoidosis, as well as to monitor patient response to therapy for the disease. It can also be used in the diagnosis of Gaucher's disease.

Normal Values
<40 mcg/L (<670 nkat/L SI units)

Possible Meanings of Abnormal Values

Increased
Diabetes mellitus
Gaucher's disease
Hyperthyroidism
Leprosy
Liver disease
Sarcoidosis

Contributing Factors to Abnormal Values
- Drugs that may *decrease* ACE levels: ACE-inhibitors, prednisone.

Interventions/Implications

Pretest
- Explain to the patient the purpose of the test and the need for a blood sample to be drawn.
- No fasting is required before the test.

Procedure
- A 7-mL blood sample is drawn in a red-top collection tube.
- Gloves are worn throughout the procedure.

Posttest
- Apply pressure at venipuncture site. Apply dressing, periodically assessing for continued bleeding.
- Label the specimen and transport it to the laboratory.
- Report abnormal findings to the primary care provider.

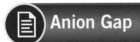 **Anion Gap**

Test Description

When electrolytes are evaluated, the substances being measured include two positive ions, called *cations,* and two negative ions, called *anions.* The cations are sodium (Na^+) and potassium (K^+), and the anions are chloride (Cl^-) and bicarbonate (HCO_3^-). When the total amount of cations and the total amount of anions are compared, there are normally more cations than anions, leading to what is known as the *anion gap.* This is because all of the possible anions are not measured. Those not measured include organic acids, phosphates, and sulfates.

Measurement of the anion gap assists the primary care provider in determining the potential causes of metabolic acidosis. Types of metabolic acidosis that have an increased anion gap include those associated with renal failure, diabetic ketoacidosis, and lactic acidosis.

The anion gap is calculated as follows:

$$(Na^+ + K^+) - (Cl^- + HCO_3^-) = \text{Anion Gap}$$

Normal Values

12 ± 4 mEq/L (12 ± 4 mmol/L SI units) if potassium not included
16 ± 4 mEq/L (16 ± 4 mmol/L SI units) if potassium is included

Possible Meanings of Abnormal Values

Increased	Decreased
Alcoholic ketoacidosis	Bromide intoxication
Dehydration	Hypercalcemia
Diabetic ketoacidosis	Hyperdilution
Hypocalcemia	Hypermagnesemia
Hypomagnesemia	Hypoalbuminemia
Lactic acidosis	Hyponatremia
Metabolic acidosis	Hypophosphatemia
Renal failure	Multiple myeloma
Salicylate toxicity	
Uremia	

Contributing Factors to Abnormal Values

- Hemolysis of the sample may alter test results.
- *False decreases* may occur owing to absorption of iodine from povidone-iodine packed wounds.
- Drugs that may *increase* the anion gap: acetazolamide, antihypertensives, carbenicillin, corticosteroids, dextrose in water, dimercaprol, ethacrynic acid, furosemide, methyl alcohol, nitrates, paraldehyde, penicillin, salicylates, sodium bicarbonate, thiazides.
- Drugs that may *decrease* the anion gap: antacids containing magnesium, boric acid, chlorpropamide, cholestyramine, cortisone acetate, corticotropin, iodide, lithium carbonate, phenylbutazone, polymyxin B, vasopressin.

Interventions/Implications

Pretest

- Explain to the patient the purpose of the test and the need for a blood sample to be drawn.
- No fasting is required before the test.

Procedure

- A 7-mL blood sample is drawn in a red-top collection tube for determination of the electrolytes.
- Gloves are worn throughout the procedure.

Posttest

- Apply pressure at venipuncture site. Apply dressing, periodically assessing for continued bleeding.
- Label the specimen and transport it to the laboratory.
- Report abnormal findings to the primary care provider.

Ankle-Brachial Index (ABI)

Test Description

Peripheral arterial occlusive disease (PAOD) affects approximately 18% of people over age 70. Typically the person presents with complaints of leg pain, which occurs with activity and resolves with rest. As the disease processes, leg ulcers often develop. The circulation can eventually become compromised to the point of requiring arterial reconstruction or amputation. It is important to be able to diagnose PAOD for more than treatment of the lower extremities. PAOD is also associated with the presence of coronary artery disease and carotid artery stenosis.

A simple but effective test for PAOD is the ankle-brachial index (ABI). The test measures the ratio of lower and upper extremity blood pressure. In addition to PAOD diagnosis, the ABI has also been found to be a significant predictor of cardiac events.

THE EVIDENCE FOR PRACTICE

One of the simplest and most useful parameters to objectively assess lower extremity arterial perfusion is the ankle-brachial index (ABI). The ABI helps to define the severity of the disease and successfully screens for hemodynamically significant disease. The Society of Interventional Radiology (SIR) recommends that all patients being evaluated for peripheral vascular disease should have their ABI measured.

Normal Values

ABI >0.95
Drop in Doppler pressure between segments ≤ 20 mm Hg.

Possible Meanings of Abnormal Values

ABI at rest or following exercise:
<0.95:   Abnormal

0.5–0.8:   Intermittent claudication
<0.5:   Severe arterial disease

Contributing Factors to Abnormal Values

- *False-negative* results may occur in patients with diabetes mellitus due to poorly compressible vessels.

Interventions/Implications

Pretest

- Explain to the patient the purpose of the test. Provide any written teaching materials available on the subject.
- The patient should not smoke or have caffeine intake for 2 hours prior to the test.

Procedure

- The patient lies supine on the examination table.
- Blood pressure is measured in both upper extremities.
- The highest systolic reading is recorded.
- The ankle systolic pressure is measured using the dorsalis pedis or posterior tibial arteries.
- The ABI is calculated by dividing the ankle pressure by the brachial systolic pressure.
- If the ABI is abnormal (<0.95), segmental arterial pressures and a pulse volume recording before and after exercising to the point of absolute claudication are done:
  - Blood pressure cuffs are placed on the proximal and distal thigh, below the knee and above the ankle
  - A continuous wave Doppler placed below the cuff provides recording of pulse-volume waveforms.
  - Pressures are recorded at each location in both lower extremities while at rest.
  - For the exercise portion of the test, the procedure is repeated after the patient has walked for 5 minutes on a treadmill.

Posttest

- Report abnormal findings to the primary care provider.

→ **Clinical Alerts**

- Patients with PAOD require education on risk factor management, exercise, and pharmacologic treatment:
  - Treatment of hyperlipidemia with a target LDL of <100 mg/dL
  - Cessation of smoking
  - Exercise, preferably walking
  - Use of antiplatelet agents
- If surgical intervention for PAOD is indicated, arteriography or magnetic resonance angiography is needed to determine the extent of the disease.
- Primary care providers should consider evaluation for carotid artery stenosis in patients newly diagnosed with PAOD.

A

Anticardiolipin Antibody (ACA, Cardiolipin Antibodies)

Test Description
Cardiolipin antibodies are the most common form of antiphospholipid antibodies. The antibodies play an important role in the blood clotting process. When autoantibodies (anticardiolipin antibodies, or ACA) are formed against cardiolipins, the patient has an increased risk of developing recurrent thrombosis. There are three types of cardiolipin antibodies: IgG, IgM, and IgA. ACA testing is used to determine the cause of thrombosis, thrombocytopenia, and recurrent fetal loss, and in the evaluation of patients with systemic lupus erythematosus.

Normal Values

IgG Cardiolipin Antibody
Negative: <10 GPL
Equivocal: 10–40 GPL
High Positive: >40 GPL

IgM Cardiolipin Antibody
Negative: <12 MPL
Equivocal: 12–40 MPL
High Positive: >40 MPL

IgA Cardiolipin Antibody
Negative: <12 APL
Equivocal: 12–40 APL
High Positive: >40 APL

Possible Meanings of Abnormal Values

Increased
Antiphospholipid syndrome
Idiopathic thrombocytopenic purpura
Psoriatic arthritis
Rheumatoid arthritis
Sjögren's syndrome
Systemic lupus erythematosus

Contributing Factors to Abnormal Values
- Current or past infection with syphilis may cause a *false-positive* ACA result.
- Drugs that may cause a *positive* ACA: anticonvulsants, antibiotics, hydralazine, oral contraceptives, phenothiazines, procainamide.

Interventions/Implications
Pretest
- Explain to the patient the purpose of the test and the need for a blood sample to be drawn.
- No fasting is required before the test.

Procedure
- A 7-mL blood sample is drawn in a gold-top (serum separator) collection tube.
- Gloves are worn throughout the procedure.

Posttest
- Apply pressure at venipuncture site. Apply dressing, periodically assessing for continued bleeding.
- Label the specimen and transport it to the laboratory.
- Report abnormal findings to the primary care provider.

 Clinical Alerts

- Patients with positive ACA should discuss the use of low-dose aspirin with their primary care provider.

Anticentromere Antibody Test

Test Description
CREST syndrome is a variant of scleroderma characterized by calcinosis, Raynaud's phenomenon, esophageal dysfunction, sclerodactyly, and telangiectasia. The anticentromere antibody has been found in most patients diagnosed with CREST syndrome.

Normal Values
Negative

Possible Meanings of Abnormal Values

Positive
CREST syndrome

Interventions/Implications
Pretest
- Explain to the patient the purpose of the test and the need for a blood sample to be drawn.
- No fasting is required before the test.

Procedure
- A 7-mL blood sample is drawn in a red-top collection tube.
- Gloves are worn throughout the procedure.

Posttest
- Apply pressure at venipuncture site. Apply dressing, periodically assessing for continued bleeding.
- Label the specimen and transport it to the laboratory.
- Report abnormal findings to the primary care provider.

A

Antideoxyribonuclease-B Titer (Anti-DNase B [ADB])

Test Description
Deoxyribonuclease B is an antigen produced by group A streptococci. When the body is confronted by this antigen, it produces antibodies against the antigen. The antideoxyribonuclease-B test is designed to detect these antibodies. If the antibodies are present, the person has had a streptococcal infection. The anti-DNase B level increases after the person has recovered from the infection. This test is considered more sensitive than the antistreptolysin-O (ASO) test. When both tests are consistently performed on blood samples, 95% of the streptococcal infections can be identified. The test is particularly useful in the diagnosis of rheumatic fever and post-streptococcal glomerulonephritis, both sequelae of infections involving group-A beta-hemolytic streptococci.

Normal Values
Adult:	<85 Todd U/mL
Child age 7 and older:	<170 Todd U/mL
Child younger than age 7:	<60 Todd U/mL

Possible Meanings of Abnormal Values

Increased
Acute rheumatic fever
Poststreptococcal glomerulonephritis
Pyodermic skin infection

Contributing Factors to Abnormal Values
- Hemolysis of the blood sample may alter test results.
- Drugs that may *decrease* results: antibiotics.

Interventions/Implications
Pretest
- Explain to the patient the purpose of the test and the need for a blood sample to be drawn.
- No fasting is required before the test.

Procedure
- A 7-mL blood sample is drawn in a red-top collection tube.
- Gloves are worn throughout the procedure.

Posttest
- Apply pressure at venipuncture site. Apply dressing, periodically assessing for continued bleeding.
- Label the specimen and transport it to the laboratory.
- Report abnormal findings to the primary care provider.

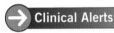

Clinical Alerts

- For the most reliable results, the Anti-DNase-B test should be performed in conjunction with the ASO test.

Antidiuretic Hormone (ADH, Arginine Vasopressin [AVP])

Test Description

Antidiuretic hormone (ADH), originally known as vasopressin, is a hormone produced by the hypothalamus. It is stored in the posterior pituitary and released when needed as indicated by serum osmolality levels. A high serum osmolality indicates that the serum is concentrated and that the amount of water is limited. When this occurs, ADH is released. ADH increases the permeability of the distal renal tubules and collecting ducts, resulting in water reabsorption. Conversely, a low serum osmolality indicates there is a water excess and that the serum is dilute. In this situation, ADH secretion is reduced, leading to increased excretion of water (diuresis).

Certain conditions can result in an abnormal secretion or lack of secretion of ADH, or in a lack of renal response to ADH secretion. In *diabetes insipidus*, there is either inadequate ADH secretion or the kidneys do not respond appropriately to ADH. Causes of diabetes insipidus include head trauma, brain tumor or inflammation, neurosurgical procedures, or primary renal diseases. In the *syndrome of inappropriate antidiuretic hormone secretion (SIADH)*, there is continuing release of ADH in the presence of low plasma osmolality. SIADH may be caused by ectopic ADH-producing tumors of the lung, thymus, pancreas, intestines, and urologic tract; by some pulmonary conditions; or by extreme stress.

Normal Values

1–5 pg/mL (1–5 ng/L SI units)

Possible Meanings of Abnormal Values

Increased	Decreased
Acute porphyria	Central (pituitary) diabetes insipidus
Addison's disease	Head trauma
Brain tumor	Hypervolemia
Bronchogenic cancer	Hypothalamic tumor
Circulatory shock	Metastatic disease
Ectopic ADH secretion	Neurosurgical procedures
Hemorrhage	Sarcoidosis
Hepatitis	Syphilis
Hypothyroidism	Viral infection
Hypovolemia	
Nephrogenic diabetes insipidus	
Pneumonia	
Stress	

A

Syndrome of inappropriate ADH secretion (SIADH)
Tuberculosis

Contributing Factors to Abnormal Values

- Test results can be altered by: physical and psychological stress, positive-pressure mechanical ventilation, use of glass tube for blood sample collection.
- Drugs that may *increase* ADH levels: acetaminophen, anesthetics, barbiturates, carbamazepine, chlorothiazide, chlorpropamide, cyclophosphamide, estrogens, lithium, morphine, nicotine, oxytocin, vincristine.
- Drugs that may *decrease* ADH levels: alcohol, phenytoin.

Interventions/Implications

Pretest

- Explain to the patient the purpose of the test and the need for a blood sample to be drawn.
- Fasting for 10 to 12 hours is required before the test. Physical activity and stress should be avoided during this time.

Procedure

- A 7-mL blood sample is drawn in a prechilled lavender top (EDTA) plastic collection tube. The patient should be in a sitting position.
- Gloves are worn throughout the procedure.

Posttest

- Apply pressure at venipuncture site. Apply dressing, periodically assessing for continued bleeding.
- Label the specimen and transport it immediately to the laboratory in an ice bath. The blood sample must be centrifuged within 10 minutes of collection.
- Report abnormal findings to the primary care provider.

 Anti-DNA Antibody Test (Anti-ds-DNA Antibody)

Test Description

The anti-DNA antibody test detects the presence of antibodies to native, or double-stranded DNA. Presence of these antibodies indicates the person has some type of autoimmune disease. The resultant antibody-antigen complexes which form play a major part in the tissue injury involved in autoimmune diseases. These antibodies are particularly prevalent in patients with systemic lupus erythematosus (SLE); thus, this test is useful in the diagnosis of SLE and for monitoring the course of SLE.

Normal Values

Immunofluorescence method:	Negative at 1:10 dilution
ELISA method:	Negative<50 IU/mL
	Borderline 50–60 IU/mL
	Positive>60 IU/mL

Enzyme immunoassay method: Negative<100 IU/mL
Borderline 100–300 IU/mL
Positive>300 IU/mL

Possible Meanings of Abnormal Values

Increased
Lupus nephritis
Myasthenia gravis
Rheumatoid arthritis
Sclerosis
Sjögren's syndrome
Systemic lupus erythematosus

Contributing Factors to Abnormal Values

- Hemolysis of the blood sample may alter test results.
- Drugs that may *increase* anti-DNA levels: hydralazine, procainamide.

Interventions/Implications

Pretest
- Explain to the patient the purpose of the test and the need for a blood sample to be drawn.
- Overnight fasting is preferred before the test.

Procedure
- A 7-mL blood sample is drawn in a red-top collection tube.
- Gloves are worn throughout the procedure.

Posttest
- Apply pressure at venipuncture site. Apply dressing, periodically assessing for continued bleeding.
- Label the specimen and transport it to the laboratory.
- Report abnormal findings to the primary care provider.

→ Clinical Alerts

- Risk of infection at venipuncture site due to immunocompromised state. Teach patient to notify health-care provider if drainage, redness, warmth, edema, or pain at the site or fever occur.

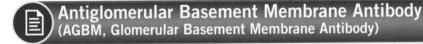

Antiglomerular Basement Membrane Antibody
(AGBM, Glomerular Basement Membrane Antibody)

Test Description
Goodpasture's syndrome is an autoimmune disease in which antibodies specific for renal structural components, such as the glomerular basement membrane in the kidney, and pulmonary structural components, such as the alveolar basement

membrane, are produced. These antibodies then bind to the tissue antigens, resulting in an immune response and the development of such problems as necrotizing glomerulonephritis and hemorrhagic pneumonitis. Because of the renal and pulmonary complications, kidney and lung biopsies may also be performed.

Normal Values

Negative: <20 units by ELISA

Possible Meanings of Abnormal Values

Increased
Antiglomerular glomerular nephritis
Goodpasture's syndrome
Systemic lupus erythematosus

Contributing Factors to Abnormal Values

- Drugs that may *decrease* test results: antibiotics

Interventions/Implications

Pretest
- Explain to the patient the purpose of the test and the need for a blood sample to be drawn.
- Fasting for 8 hours is required before the test.

Procedure
- A 7-mL blood sample is drawn in a red-top collection tube.
- Gloves are worn throughout the procedure.

Posttest
- Apply pressure at venipuncture site. Apply dressing, periodically assessing for continued bleeding.
- Label the specimen and transport it to the laboratory.
- Report abnormal findings to the primary care provider.

Anti-Insulin Antibody (Insulin Antibody Test)

Test Description
Insulin, whether beef, pork, or human type, contains insulin-related peptides, which may stimulate production of antibodies. With subsequent insulin injections, these antibodies join and neutralize the insulin so that it is no longer able to function appropriately. Larger doses of insulin are then required to attempt to meet the patient's needs, a phenomenon called insulin resistance. This is indicated by the presence of IgG and IgM anti-insulin antibodies. If the anti-insulin antibodies are found to be IgE, this indicates the body has developed an allergic response to the medication.

This allergy can result in minor allergy symptoms such as rash, or more severe responses. The insulin antibody test is performed when insulin is no longer controlling the patient's diabetes or if symptoms of allergy to the insulin are present.

Normal Values

Undetectable for antibodies

Possible Meanings of Abnormal Values

Increased

Allergy to insulin
Factitious hypoglycemia
Insulin resistance

Contributing Factors to Abnormal Values

- Radioactive scans within 7 days prior to the test will alter test results.

Interventions/Implications

Pretest
- Explain to the patient the purpose of the test and the need for a blood sample to be drawn.
- No fasting is required before the test.

Procedure
- A 7-mL blood sample is drawn in a red-top collection tube.
- Gloves are worn throughout the procedure.

Posttest
- Apply pressure at venipuncture site. Apply dressing, periodically assessing for continued bleeding.
- Label the specimen and transport it to the laboratory.
- Report abnormal findings to the primary care provider.

Anti-Liver/Kidney Microsomal Antibody
(LKM, Liver Kidney Microsomal Antibody)

Test Description
The presence of LKM antibodies is used in conjunction with clinical findings and other laboratory tests to aid in the diagnosis of autoimmune liver diseases such as autoimmune hepatitis type 2. Autoimmune hepatitis occurs primarily in women and is associated with very high transaminase levels and elevated gamma globulins, especially IgG. LKM antibodies are usually evaluated, along with anti-smooth muscle antibody and antinuclear antibody.

Normal Values

Negative: <20.1 Units

Possible Meanings of Abnormal Values

Positive
Autoimmune hepatitis type 2

Interventions/Implications
Pretest
- Explain to the patient the purpose of the test and the need for a blood sample to be drawn.
- No fasting is required before the test.

Procedure
- A 7-mL blood sample is drawn in a gold-top (serum separator) collection tube.
- Gloves are worn throughout the procedure.

Posttest
- Apply pressure at venipuncture site. Apply dressing, periodically assessing for continued bleeding.
- Label the specimen and transport it to the laboratory.
- Report abnormal findings to the primary care provider.

→ Clinical Alerts

- Diagnosis of autoimmune hepatitis usually requires liver biopsy.
- Once the diagnosis is confirmed, treatment involving corticosteroids is initiated.

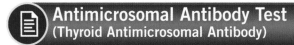

Antimicrosomal Antibody Test
(Thyroid Antimicrosomal Antibody)

Test Description
Microsomes are lipoproteins that are normally present within the epithelial cells of the thyroid. In some types of thyroid disorders, these microsomes escape from their normal locations. Once liberated, these substances appear as antigens to the body. In response, the body produces antibodies against the microsomes, leading to inflammation and destruction of the thyroid gland. Antimicrosomal antibodies are present in the majority of patients diagnosed with Hashimoto's thyroiditis. The most dilute serum in which antimicrosomal antibodies are detected is called the *titer*. This test is usually performed in conjunction with the antithyroglobulin antibody test.

Normal Values
Titer < 1:100

Possible Meanings of Abnormal Values

Increased
Autoimmune hemolytic anemias
Granulomatous thyroiditis

Hashimoto's thyroiditis
Juvenile lymphocytic thyroiditis
Myasthenia gravis
Myxedema
Nontoxic nodular goiter
Pernicious anemia
Primary hypothyroidism
Rheumatoid arthritis
Sjögren's syndrome
Systemic lupus erythematosus
Thyroid cancer

Contributing Factors to Abnormal Values

- Drugs that may *increase* antimicrosomal antibody titers: oral contraceptives.

Interventions/Implications

Pretest
- Explain to the patient the purpose of the test and the need for a blood sample to be drawn.
- No fasting is required before the test.

Procedure
- A 7-mL blood sample is drawn in a red-top collection tube.
- Gloves are worn throughout the procedure.

Posttest
- Apply pressure at venipuncture site. Apply dressing, periodically assessing for continued bleeding.
- Label the specimen and transport it to the laboratory.
- Report abnormal findings to the primary care provider.

 Clinical Alerts

- This test is usually performed in conjunction with the antithyroglobulin antibody test.

Antimitochondrial Antibody Test (AMA)

Test Description
The antimitochondrial antibody (AMA) test is used to detect the presence of autoimmune antibodies that have formed against a lipoprotein component of the mitochondrial membrane. These antibodies have a tendency to attack organs that expend a great deal of energy, such as those of the hepatobiliary system. The AMA test is used in the diagnosis of primary biliary cirrhosis.

Normal Values
Negative at 1:20 dilution

A

Possible Meanings of Abnormal Values

Increased

Cryptogenic cirrhosis
Drug-induced jaundice
Hepatic obstruction
Hepatitis
Primary biliary cirrhosis
Rheumatoid arthritis
Systemic lupus erythematosus

Contributing Factors to Abnormal Values

- Hemolysis of the blood sample may alter test results.

Interventions/Implications

Pretest
- Explain to the patient the purpose of the test and the need for a blood sample to be drawn.
- No fasting is required before the test.

Procedure
- A 7-mL blood sample is drawn in a red-top collection tube.
- Gloves are worn throughout the procedure.

Posttest
- Apply pressure at venipuncture site. Apply dressing, periodically assessing for continued bleeding.
- Label the specimen and transport it to the laboratory.
- Report abnormal findings to the primary care provider.

→ Clinical Alerts

- Prolonged bleeding from the venipuncture site due to vitamin K deficiency may occur secondary to liver dysfunction, as seen in severe hepatitis.
- The AMA test is usually performed in conjunction with the anti-smooth muscle antibody (ASMA) test.
- Interpretation of this test involves noting whether it is positive or negative; the level of titer does not correspond to severity of disease or response to treatment.

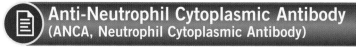

Anti-Neutrophil Cytoplasmic Antibody
(ANCA, Neutrophil Cytoplasmic Antibody)

Test Description

The anti-neutrophil cytoplasmic antibody test (ANCA) is used primarily in the diagnosis and monitoring of patients with Wegener's granulomatosis (WG). WG is an autoimmune disease, which is characterized by inflammation in many tissues of the body, including the upper and lower respiratory system, the kidneys, eyes, ears, and skin. The blood vessels in these areas become inflamed, a condition known as vasculitis, and granulomas develop. Once the diagnosis is confirmed, treatment with cytotoxic agents is usually needed.

Normal Values

ANCA by immunofluorescence: Negative
ANCA by EIA:　Negative:　　　<21 Units
　　　　　　　Weak Positive:　21–30 Units
　　　　　　　Positive:　　　　>30 Units

Possible Meanings of Abnormal Values

Increased
Glomerulonephritis
Inflammatory bowel disease
Polyarthritis nodosa
Systemic arthritis
Wegener's granulomatosis

Interventions/Implications

Pretest
- Explain to the patient the purpose of the test and the need for a blood sample to be drawn.
- No fasting is required before the test.

Procedure
- A 7-mL blood sample is drawn in a gold-top (serum separator) collection tube.
- Gloves are worn throughout the procedure.

Posttest
- Apply pressure at venipuncture site. Apply dressing, periodically assessing for continued bleeding.
- Label the specimen and transport it to the laboratory.
- Report abnormal findings to the primary care provider.

 Antinuclear Antibody Test (ANA, Fluorescent ANA [FANA])

Test Description
Antinuclear antibodies are antibodies the body produces against nuclear components of its own cells. This results in the development of an autoimmune disease. The antinuclear antibody (ANA) test is commonly used to rule out systemic lupus erythematosus (SLE) because 95% to 99% of SLE patients have positive ANA titers. A *titer* is the most dilute serum in which the ANA is detected. The ANA test uses an indirect immunofluorescent procedure, which results in several staining patterns: homogeneous, nucleolar, peripheral, and speckled patterns. These patterns assist in diagnosing the specific disease process affecting the individual.

A

Normal Values

Negative at 1:8 dilution

Possible Meanings of Abnormal Values

Positive
Bacterial endocarditis
Chronic autoimmune hepatitis
Cirrhosis
Connective tissue diseases
Dermatomyositis
Discoid lupus erythematosus
Drug-induced lupus
Infectious mononucleosis
Leukemia
Malignancy, especially lymphoma
Mixed connective tissue disease
Myasthenia gravis
Polymyositis
Raynaud's syndrome
Rheumatoid arthritis
Scleroderma
Sjögren's syndrome
Systemic lupus erythematosus
Tuberculosis

Contributing Factors to Abnormal Values

- Hemolysis of the blood sample may alter test results.
- Drugs that may cause a *false-positive* result due to a drug-induced syndrome similar to SLE: acetazolamide, carbidopa, chlorothiazide, chlorpromazine, clofibrate, ethosuximide, gold salts, griseofulvin, hydralazine, isoniazid, lithium, methyldopa, oral contraceptives, penicillin, phenylbutazone, phenytoin, primidone, procainamide, propylthiouracil, quinidine, reserpine, streptomycin, sulfonamides, tetracyclines, thiazide diuretics.
- Drugs that may cause a *false-negative* result: steroids.

Interventions/Implications

Pretest

- Explain to the patient the purpose of the test and the need for a blood sample to be drawn.
- No fasting is required before the test.

Procedure

- A 7-mL blood sample is drawn in a red-top collection tube.
- Gloves are worn throughout the procedure.

Posttest

- Apply pressure at venipuncture site. Apply dressing, periodically assessing for continued bleeding.
- Label the specimen and transport it to the laboratory.
- Report abnormal findings to the primary care provider.

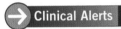

Clinical Alerts

- Positive ANA results can occur in people with no known autoimmune disease.
- Risk of infection at venipuncture site due to immunocompromised state. Teach patient to notify health-care provider if drainage, redness, warmth, edema, or pain at the site or fever occur.

Anti-Parietal Cell Antibody (APCA, Parietal Cell Antibody)

Test Description
The anti-parietal cell antibody test (APCA) measures the presence of antibodies against gastric parietal cells. When antibodies form against the parietal cells in the stomach, their production of intrinsic factor is disrupted. This results in pernicious anemia due to an autoimmune process. Thus the APCA test is used in the evaluation of pernicious anemia. It may be elevated in atrophic gastritis and in some other autoimmune processes.

Normal Values
Negative

Possible Meanings of Abnormal Values

Increased
Atrophic gastritis
Autoimmune pernicious anemia
Diabetes mellitus
Gastric cancer
Gastric ulcer
Thyroid disease

Interventions/Implications
Pretest
- Explain to the patient the purpose of the test and the need for a blood sample to be drawn.
- No fasting is required before the test.

Procedure
- A 7-mL blood sample is drawn in a gold-top (serum separator) collection tube.
- Gloves are worn throughout the procedure.

Posttest
- Apply pressure at venipuncture site. Apply dressing, periodically assessing for continued bleeding.
- Label the specimen and transport it to the laboratory.
- Report abnormal findings to the primary care provider.

A

Antiscleroderma Antibody (Scl-70 Antibody, Scleroderma Antibody)

Test Description
The antiscleroderma antibody is found in individuals with progressive systemic sclerosis (scleroderma) and individuals with CREST syndrome. CREST syndrome is characterized by calcinosis, Raynaud's phenomenon, esophageal dysfunction, sclerodactyly, and telangiectasia. Positive results with this test are considered highly diagnostic of scleroderma, because the antibody is found only rarely in diseases such as mixed connective tissue disease, rheumatoid arthritis, Sjögren's syndrome, and systemic lupus erythematosus.

Normal Values
Negative

Possible Meanings of Abnormal Values

Positive
CREST syndrome
Scleroderma

Contributing Factors to Abnormal Values
- Drugs that may *increase* antiscleroderma antibody levels: aminosalicylic acid, isoniazid, methyldopa, penicillin, propylthiouracil, streptomycin, tetracycline.

Interventions/Implications
Pretest
- Explain to the patient the purpose of the test and the need for a blood sample to be drawn.
- No fasting is required before the test.

Procedure
- A 7-mL blood sample is drawn in a red-top collection tube.
- Gloves are worn throughout the procedure.

Posttest
- Apply pressure at venipuncture site. Apply dressing, periodically assessing for continued bleeding.
- Label the specimen and transport it to the laboratory.
- Report abnormal findings to the primary care provider.

Anti-Smooth Muscle Antibody Test (ASMA)

Test Description
The anti-smooth muscle antibody (ASMA) test is used to detect the presence of autoimmune antibodies that have formed against smooth muscle. These antibodies

have a tendency to appear in chronic active hepatitis and other diseases in which there is liver damage. The ASMA test is used in the diagnosis of primary biliary cirrhosis and chronic active hepatitis

Normal Values

Negative at 1:20 dilution

Possible Meanings of Abnormal Values

Increased
Acute viral hepatitis
Chronic active hepatitis
Infectious mononucleosis
Intrinsic asthma
Malignancies
Primary biliary cirrhosis
Viral infection

Contributing Factors to Abnormal Values

- Hemolysis of the blood sample and the presence of antinuclear antibodies may alter test results.

Interventions/Implications

Pretest
- Explain to the patient the purpose of the test and the need for a blood sample to be drawn.
- No fasting is required before the test.

Procedure
- A 7-mL blood sample is drawn in a red-top collection tube.
- Gloves are worn throughout the procedure.

Posttest
- Apply pressure at venipuncture site. Apply dressing, periodically assessing for continued bleeding.
- Label the specimen and transport it to the laboratory.
- Report abnormal findings to the primary care provider.

→ Clinical Alerts

- Prolonged bleeding from the venipuncture site due to vitamin K deficiency may occur secondary to liver dysfunction, as seen in severe hepatitis.
- The ASMA test is usually performed in conjunction with the antimitochondrial antibody (AMA) test.

- Interpretation of this test involves noting whether it is positive or negative; the level of titer does not correspond to severity of disease or response to treatment.

Antisperm Antibody Test (Antispermatozoal Antibody)

Test Description
Antisperm antibodies may form in a male as a result of blocked efferent ducts in the testes. This blockage results in reabsorption of sperm, which can lead to the formation of autoantibodies to the sperm. Antisperm antibodies may also form in a female. Thus, this test may be performed on both males and females as one part of infertility screening.

Normal Values
Negative

Possible Meanings of Abnormal Values

Increased
Blocked efferent ducts in the testes
Infertility
Vasectomy

Interventions/Implications
Pretest
- Explain to the patient the purpose of the test and the specimen samples needed.
- No fasting is required before the test.
- If a semen sample is to be used, the male should avoid ejaculation for 3 days before the test.

Procedure
- The preferred specimen for a male is a semen sample. Provide a plastic container for the specimen collection.
- A 7-mL blood sample is drawn in a red-top collection tube from both the male and female.
- Although the blood sample is the preferred test for females, a 1-mL cervical mucus specimen may also be collected.
- Gloves are worn when handling any specimen.

Posttest
- Apply pressure at venipuncture site. Apply dressing, periodically assessing for continued bleeding.
- Semen samples collected elsewhere must be transported to the laboratory within 2 hours after collection.

- Label all specimens and transport it to the laboratory on dry ice.
- Report abnormal findings to the primary care provider.

Anti-SS-A (Ro) and Anti-SS-B (La) Antibody

Test Description
Anti-Ss-A (Ro) and anti-SS-B (La) are autoantibodies formed against ribonucleic acid (RNA) protein particles in the body. These antibodies are most often seen in Sjögren's syndrome, a disorder with symptoms similar to those of connective tissue disorders such as rheumatoid arthritis, systemic lupus erythematosus (SLE), or scleroderma. The syndrome is characterized by decreased secretion and eventual destruction of the exocrine glands, resulting in dryness of the mucosa and conjunctiva. The test is used in the differential diagnosis of Sjögren's syndrome, SLE, and mixed connective tissue disease.

Normal Values
Ro: Negative
La: Negative

Possible Meanings of Abnormal Values

Positive
ANA-negative lupus
Neonatal lupus
Scleroderma
Sjögren's syndrome

Interventions/Implications

Pretest
- Explain to the patient the purpose of the test and the need for a blood sample to be drawn.
- No fasting is required before the test.

Procedure
- A 7-mL blood sample is drawn in a red-top collection tube.
- Gloves are worn throughout the procedure.

Posttest
- Apply pressure at venipuncture site. Apply dressing, periodically assessing for continued bleeding.
- Label the specimen and transport it to the laboratory.
- Report abnormal findings to the primary care provider.

Clinical Alerts

- Infection at the venipuncture site may occur in immunocompromised individuals. Teach the patient to monitor the site and to report the occurrence of infection, including drainage, redness, warmth, edema, pain at the site, or fever.

Antistreptolysin-O Titer (ASO Titer, Streptococcal Antibody Test)

Test Description

Streptolysin-O is an enzyme produced by Group A beta-hemolytic streptococcal bacteria. When confronted by this foreign enzyme, the body produces antibodies against it. The antibodies appear 7 to 10 days after the acute streptococcal infection and continue to rise for 2 to 4 weeks. The ASO level will typically fall to preinfection levels with 6 to 12 months. The antistreptolysin-O (ASO) test is designed to detect these antibodies. If the antibodies are present, the person has had a streptococcal infection. Over 80% of patient with acute rheumatic fever and 95% of those with acute streptococcal glomerulonephritis have elevated ASO levels. ASO levels do not typically rise with cutaneous infections.

This test is considered less sensitive than the anti-DNase B test. When both tests are consistently performed on blood samples, 95% of the streptococcal infections can be identified. The test is particularly useful in determining whether such conditions as joint pain or glomerulonephritis are the result of a streptococcal infection.

Normal Values

Adult:	<160 Todd units/mL
Ages 5–12:	<170-33- Todd units/mL
Ages 2–5:	<160 Todd units/mL
Ages 0–2:	<50 Todd units/mL

Possible Meanings of Abnormal Values

Increased

Acute rheumatic fever
Poststreptococcal endocarditis
Poststreptococcal glomerulonephritis
Scarlet fever

Contributing Factors to Abnormal Values

- Hemolysis of the blood sample may alter test results.

- Drugs that may *decrease* ASO titers: antibiotics, corticosteroids.
- False-positive results may occur when blood sample has high lipid content.

A

Interventions/Implications

Pretest
- Explain to the patient the purpose of the test and the need for a blood sample to be drawn.
- No fasting is required before the test.

Procedure
- A 7-mL blood sample is drawn in a red-top collection tube.
- Gloves are worn throughout the procedure.

Posttest
- Apply pressure at venipuncture site. Apply dressing, periodically assessing for continued bleeding.
- Label the specimen and transport it to the laboratory.
- Report abnormal findings to the primary care provider.

Clinical Alerts

- For the most reliable results, the Anti-DNase-B test should be performed in conjunction with the ASO test.
- ASO titers are usually repeated in 10–14 days for comparison with initial results to determine if the antibody level is rising.
- The ASO test does not predict if complications will occur following a streptococcal infection, nor does it predict the severity of the disease.

Antithrombin III (AT-III, AT-III Activity, Heparin Cofactor)

Test Description

During hemostasis, a substance called thrombin stimulates the formation of fibrin from fibrinogen. This fibrin then forms a stable clot at the site of injury. Any excess amounts of clotting factors, which remain following hemostasis are inactivated by fibrin inhibitors which prevent clotting from occurring when it is not needed. One such substance is antithrombin III (AT-III).

AT-III is a naturally occurring protein immunoglobulin that is synthesized by the liver. The action of AT-III is catalyzed by heparin. Its role is to inactivate thrombin and other coagulation factors, thus inhibiting the coagulation process. The proper balance between thrombin and AT-III allows for appropriate hemostasis to occur. If, however, this balance is disrupted, problems can arise. For example, if there is a congenital deficiency of AT-III, coagulation will not be inhibited at an adequate level, resulting in a hypercoagulability state with a high risk of thrombosis.

A

THE EVIDENCE FOR PRACTICE

In women without a personal history of venous thromboembolism but with an underlying antithrombin deficiency that is identified through screening, hormone replacement therapy is not recommended.

Normal Values (Functional method)

Premature infant:	26–61%
Full-term infant:	44–76%
After 6 months:	80–120%

Possible Meanings of Abnormal Values

Increased	Decreased
Vitamin K deficiency	Cirrhosis
	Congenital AT-III deficiency
	Deep vein thrombosis
	Disseminated intravascular coagulation
	Hypercoagulation state
	Late pregnancy/early postpartum period
	Liver transplant
	Malnutrition
	Nephrotic syndrome
	Postoperative period
	Pulmonary embolism
	Septicemia

Contributing Factors to Abnormal Values

- Hemolysis of the blood sample and presence of lipemia may alter test results.
- Drugs that may *increase* AT-III levels: anabolic steroids, androgens, progesterone-containing oral contraceptives, warfarin.
- Drugs that may *decrease* AT-III levels: estrogen-containing oral contraceptives, fibrinolytics, heparin, L-asparaginase.

Interventions/Implications

Pretest
- Explain to the patient the purpose of the test and the need for a blood sample to be drawn.
- No fasting is required before the test.

Procedure
- A 7-mL blood sample is drawn in a light blue-top collection tube containing sodium citrate. The sample is mixed gently by inverting 3 to 4 times.
- Gloves are worn throughout the procedure.

Posttest
- Apply pressure at venipuncture site. Apply dressing, periodically assessing for continued bleeding.
- Label the specimen, place it on ice, and transport it to the laboratory immediately.
- Report abnormal findings to the primary care provider.

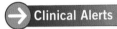

→ Clinical Alerts

- In adults, AT-III levels of 50 to 75% indicate a moderate risk for thrombosis; levels of <50% suggest a significant risk for thrombosis.

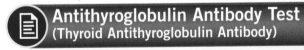

Antithyroglobulin Antibody Test
(Thyroid Antithyroglobulin Antibody)

Test Description

Thyroglobulin is a thyroid glycoprotein that has a role in the synthesis of triiodothyronine (T_3) and thyroxine (T_4). In some types of thyroid disorders, thyroglobulin may escape from the thyroid gland. Once liberated, these substances appear as antigens to the body. In response, the body produces antibodies against the thyroglobulin, leading to inflammation and destruction of the thyroid gland. Antithyroglobulin antibodies are present in the majority of patients diagnosed with Hashimoto's thyroiditis. The most dilute serum in which antithyroglobulin antibodies are detected is called the *titer*.

Normal Values

Titer <1:100

Possible Meanings of Abnormal Values

Increased

Autoimmune hemolytic anemia
Diabetes mellitus Type 1
Granulomatous thyroiditis
Hashimoto's thyroiditis
Hyperthyroidism
Juvenile lymphocytic thyroiditis
Myasthenia gravis
Myxedema
Nontoxic nodular goiter
Pernicious anemia
Primary hypothyroidism
Rheumatoid arthritis
Sjögren's syndrome
Systemic lupus erythematosus
Thyroid autoimmune diseases
Thyroid cancer
Thyrotoxicosis

Contributing Factors to Abnormal Values

- Drugs that may *increase* antithyroglobulin antibody titers: oral contraceptives.

Interventions/Implications

Pretest
- Explain to the patient the purpose of the test and the need for a blood sample to be drawn.
- No fasting is required before the test.

Procedure
- A 7-mL blood sample is drawn in a red-top collection tube.
- Gloves are worn throughout the procedure.

Posttest
- Apply pressure at venipuncture site. Apply dressing, periodically assessing for continued bleeding.
- Label the specimen and transport it to the laboratory.
- Report abnormal findings to the primary care provider.

Clinical Alerts

- This test is usually performed in conjunction with the antimicrosomal antibody test.
- If present in the mother, antithyroglobulin antibody can increase the risk of hypothyroidism or hyperthyroidism in the fetus or newborn.

Apolipoprotein A & B (Apo A-I, Apo B)

Test Description

Lipoproteins are important transporters of cholesterol. High-density lipoprotein (HDL or "good cholesterol") picks up cholesterol in the tissues and transports it back to the liver for either recycling or excretion in the bile. Since it works to get rid of excess cholesterol, high levels of HDL are preferred. Low-density lipoprotein (LDL, or "bad cholesterol") also transports excess cholesterol, however it has a tendency to transport it to the arteries, where it can result in the development of atherosclerosis. Thus, it is best to have low levels of LDL to decrease the risk of atherosclerotic disease.

Apolipoproteins (apo) are the protein components of lipoproteins. Two of the apolipoproteins, apo A and apo B, in particular serve important functions in control of cholesterol in the body. Apo A activates the enzymes that cause movement of cholesterol from the tissues into HDL and also causes HDL to be recognized by receptor sites in the liver where the cholesterol is deposited. There are two subtypes of apo A: apo A-I and apo A-II. Apo A-I is the more plentiful of the two and can be measured directly. Apo A-I tends to correlate with HDL levels and is thought to perhaps be better than HDL as an indicator of coronary artery disease (CAD) risk.

There are also two forms of apo B: apo B-100 and apo B-48. Apo B-48 is part of the structure of chylomicrons, the large lipoproteins that initially transport lipids to the liver. Once there, the lipids are combined with apo B-100 to form very low-density lipoproteins, which eventually become LDL. Apo B-100 levels correlate with LDL levels and can be measured directly. Apo B-100 is considered an indicator of CAD risk.

In addition to individual measurement of apo A-I and apo B-100, an apolipoprotein evaluation also includes calculation of the apo A/apo B ratio. The lower the ratio, the greater the risk of developing CAD. In addition to assessment of CAD risk, these apo tests can also be used to monitor patient response to treatment for hyperlipidemia.

Normal Values

Apolipoprotein A-1

Male:	Low risk:	> 123 mg/dL
	Borderline/High Risk:	109–123 mg/dL
	High Risk:	<109 mg/dL
Female:	Low risk:	> 140 mg/dL
	Borderline/High Risk:	123–140 mg/dL
	High Risk:	<123 mg/dL

Apolipoprotein B

Male:	Low risk:	52–110 mg/dL
	Borderline/High Risk:	111–127 mg/dL
	High Risk:	> 127 mg/dL
Female:	Low risk:	49–103 mg/dL
	Borderline/High Risk:	104–127 mg/dL
	High Risk:	> 127 mg/dL

Apolipoprotein A-1/B Ratio

Male:	Low risk:	> 1.11
	Borderline/High Risk:	0.86–1.11
	High Risk:	< 0.86
Female:	Low risk:	> 1.35
	Borderline/High Risk:	0.97–1.35
	High Risk:	< 0.97

Possible Meanings of Abnormal Values

Apo A-I

Increased	Decreased
Familial hyperalphalipoproteinemia	Coronary artery disease
Pregnancy	Diabetes mellitus
Weight loss	Hepatocellular disease
	Hypertriglyceridemia
	Nephrotic syndrome
	Renal failure
	Tangier disease

Apo B

Increased	Decreased
Biliary obstruction	Chronic anemia
Cigarette smoking	Chronic pulmonary disease

A

Cushing's syndrome	Hyperlipidemia (Type I)
Diabetes mellitus	Hyperthyroidism
Hemodialysis	Inflammation
Hepatic disease	Malnutrition
Hyperlipoproteinemia	Reye's syndrome
(Types II, III, V)	Tangier disease
Hypothyroidism	Weight loss
Increased risk of CAD	
Nephrotic syndrome	
Porphyria	
Pregnancy	
Renal failure	

Contributing Factors to Abnormal Values

- Apo levels may be affected by unstable weight and dietary habits.
- Apo levels should not be drawn for at least 3 months following surgery or myocardial infarction.
- Drugs that may *increase* apo A-I levels: carbamazepine, cholesterol lowering agents, estrogens, ethanol, oral contraceptives, and phenobarbital.
- Drugs that may *decrease* apo A-I levels: androgens, beta-blockers, diuretics, and progestins.
- Drugs that may *increase* apo B-100 levels: beta-blockers, corticosteroids, cyclosporine, diuretics.
- Drugs that may *decrease* apo B-100 levels: cholesterol lowering agents, estrogens, indapamide.

Interventions/Implications

Pretest
- Explain to the patient the purpose of the test and the need for a blood sample to be drawn.
- Fasting for 12 hours is required before the test. Water is permitted.
- No smoking is allowed for at least 12 hours before the test.

Procedure
- A 7-mL blood sample is drawn in a gold-top (serum separator) collection tube.
- Gloves are worn throughout the procedure.

Posttest
- Apply pressure at venipuncture site. Apply dressing, periodically assessing for continued bleeding.
- Label the specimen and transport it to the laboratory.
- Report abnormal findings to the primary care provider.

→ Clinical Alerts

- Increased risk of CAD occurs with *decreased* apo A-I levels and *increased* apo B levels.

Apt Test for Swallowed Blood

Test Description

The Apt test for swallowed blood is a test to determine if blood in an infant's stool or vomitus is from the mother or from the infant. The test is based on the fact that a newborn's blood contains primarily fetal hemoglobin (Hb F). The mother's blood, unless she has thalassemia major, is primarily Hb A. When blood is seen in a newborn's stool or vomitus, it must be tested to ensure that the newborn is not having internal bleeding. If bleeding is occurring, immediate treatment is needed.

To differentiate the type of hemoglobin in the sample of bloody stool or vomitus, the sample is first mixed with water and then centrifuged, producing a pink solution. This solution is then tested with sodium hydroxide. If the blood is maternal blood, the solution will turn brownish yellow, due to the presence of hematin, a product of the breakdown of Hb A. If the blood is fetal blood, the solution will remain pink. This is because Hb F is resistant to breakdown by alkali such as sodium hydroxide.

Normal Values

Negative for Hb F fetal bleeding (pink solution)
Positive for Hb A maternal blood (brown/yellow solution)

Possible Meanings of Abnormal Values

Fetal gastrointestinal hemorrhage (pink solution)
Swallowed maternal blood (brown/yellow solution)

Contributing Factors to Abnormal Values

- Sample must have visible blood present. Black tarry stool is not acceptable since the hemoglobin has already broken down into hematin.
- *False-positive* results may occur if the mother has thalassemia major, since in this condition, up to 90% of the mother's blood is Hb F.

Interventions/Implications

Pretest
- Explain to the parent(s) the purpose of the test. Provide any written teaching materials available on the subject.

Procedure
- Obtain a sample of grossly bloody stool or vomitus.
- Gloves are worn during specimen collection.

Posttest
- Label the specimen and transport to the laboratory.
- Report abnormal findings to the primary care provider.

→ **Clinical Alerts**

- If the Apt test is positive for fetal hemoglobin, further evaluation of the infant will be needed to determine the source of bleeding. Close monitoring of the infant is essential.

 ## Arterial Blood Gases (ABGs, Blood Gases)

Test Description

Arterial blood gases (ABGs) are performed when information is needed regarding the acid-base status of the patient. The acid-base balance of the body is controlled via three mechanisms: the buffering system, the respiratory system, and the renal system.

The buffering system assists with maintaining acid-base balance through the retention or loss of hydrogen ions (H^+). There are also minor buffers in the blood in the form of phosphates and proteins.

The effect of the respiratory system occurs through the *carbonic acid-bicarbonate* buffer system. In order for the pH of the blood to be within the normal range, these two substances need to be in a 20:1 ratio—20 parts bicarbonate for every 1 part carbonic acid (H_2CO_3). The breakdown of carbonic acid forms carbon dioxide and water, thus the carbonic acid level can be measured indirectly with the PCO_2 level. The PCO_2 level is controlled by the lungs. The lungs are able to respond relatively quickly to changes in the acid-base balance of the body through the amount of CO_2 retained. The more CO_2 retained, the more carbonic acid in the body, which leads to a state known as *acidosis*. When less CO_2 is retained, the result is less carbonic acid in the body, or *alkalosis*.

Although the lungs are capable of making rapid changes in the acid-base balance of the body, they are only approximately 80% efficient since they must continue to be the site of oxygen exchange. In order to bring the body into a normal acid-base balance once again, another mechanism must be involved. This mechanism involves the kidneys. The kidneys make changes in the acid-base balance at a slower rate than the lungs, taking several days for their effect to be fully noted. The kidneys regulate the pH of the blood through the excretion or retention of H^+ ions, bicarbonate (HCO_3^-), sodium, potassium, and chloride.

Unlike the lungs, the kidneys are 100% efficient; that is, they will continue to work on the acid-base problem until either the pH of the blood returns to the normal range, a state known as *full compensation*, or the condition worsens. If all of the compensatory mechanisms (buffering system, lungs, and kidneys) are unsuccessful in bringing the acid-base imbalance under control, the problem progresses. Severe acidotic states lead to coma and death, due to depression of the central nervous system. Alkalotic states stimulate the central nervous system, leading to irritability, tetany, and possibly death. Acidotic states are generally considered more life-threatening than alkalotic states.

In patients with known chronic obstructive pulmonary disease (COPD), it is recommended that arterial blood gases be obtained with O_2 saturation of less than 88%, positive history of hypercapnia, questionable accuracy of oximetry, somnolence, or other evidence of impending respiratory failure (e.g., respiratory rate greater than 40 breaths per minute).

pH

The pH of the blood is the negative logarithm of the H^+ ion concentration in the blood. For example, if the H^+ ion concentration is 1×10^{-7}, the pH is 7; if the H^+ ion concentration is 1×10^{-6}, the pH is 6. Thus, the pH of 6 has a higher H^+ ion concentration and is more acidic. A blood pH of normal range is needed for many of the chemical reactions in the body to take place. The normal range of pH for arterial blood is 7.35 to 7.45. Blood pH less than 7.35 is considered acidemia or *acidosis*. Blood pH greater than 7.45 is considered alkalemia or *alkalosis*.

Normal Values

7.35–7.45

Contributing Factors to Abnormal Values

- Drugs which may *increase* the blood pH (more alkaline): sodium bicarbonate.

PARTIAL PRESSURE OF CARBON DIOXIDE (PCO$_2$, PACO$_2$)

The partial pressure of carbon dioxide in the arterial blood, designated as $PaCO_2$, is the amount of pressure exerted by CO_2 dissolved in the blood. It is measured in millimeters of mercury (mm Hg) or torr (1 torr = 1 mm Hg). The normal range for $PaCO_2$ is 35 to 45 torr, but lower values are normal at higher altitudes where the atmospheric pressure is decreased.

When the lungs retain CO_2, the level of CO_2 in the blood increases. This is known as *hypercarbia* or *hypercapnia*, which is an acidotic state. This problem is exhibited in clinical signs and symptoms of headache, dizziness, and decreasing levels of consciousness. When the lungs expire more CO_2 than normal, the level of CO_2 in the blood decreases, an alkalotic state known as h*ypocarbia* or *hypocapnia*. This results in the patient complaining of tingling of the fingers, muscle twitching, lightheadedness, and dizziness.

Normal Values

35–45 torr (mm Hg)

Contributing Factors to Abnormal Values

- Failure to expel all air from the syringe will result in a falsely low $PaCO_2$ value.
- Drugs which may *increase* $PaCO_2$: aldosterone, ethacrynic acid, hydrocortisone, metolazone, prednisone, sodium bicarbonate, thiazides.
- Drugs which may *decrease* $PaCO_2$: acetazolamide, dimercaprol, methicillin, nitrofurantoin, tetracycline, triamterene.

BICARBONATE (HCO$_3^-$)

As discussed previously, bicarbonate works with carbonic acid to help regulate the pH of the blood. There are two ways in which bicarbonate may be measured. The first is through

A

direct measurement of the bicarbonate level. The second is an indirect measurement using the values for total CO_2 content and $PaCO_2$ in the following formula: $HCO_3^- = Total\ CO_2 - (0.03 \times PaCO_2)$. When the bicarbonate level is less than 22, the value is considered acidotic; greater than 26, alkalotic.

Normal Values

22–26 mEq/L (22–26 mmol/L)

Contributing Factors to Abnormal Values

- Drugs which may *increase* bicarbonate: alkaline salts, diuretics.
- Drugs which may *decrease* bicarbonate: acid salts.

BASE EXCESS/DEFICIT

Determination of the base excess/deficit provides information about the total buffer anions (bicarbonate, hemoglobin, phosphates, and plasma proteins) and whether changes in acid-base balance are respiratory or nonrespiratory (metabolic) in nature. Values below −2 mEq/L indicate a base deficit, which correlates to a decrease in bicarbonate level. Values greater than +2 mEq/L indicate a base excess. This information assists in the planning of appropriate treatment for the patient.

Normal Values

−2 to +2 mEq/L

ANALYSIS OF ARTERIAL BLOOD GASES

Following these steps should simplify the analysis of ABG results:
1. Determine whether the pH is acidotic (<7.35) or alkalotic (>7.45). (Note: If the pH is normal and the PCO_2 and HCO_3^- are abnormal, see step #6.)
2. Determine whether the PCO_2 is acidotic (>45) or alkalotic (<35).
3. Determine whether the HCO_3^- is acidotic (<22) or alkalotic (>26).
4. Compare the above 3 values and find the two, which "match" in terms of acidity/alkalinity to determine the underlying acid-base imbalance. This step is summarized in Table A-1.

Table A-1	Determining Acid-Base Imbalances		
pH	**PCO₂** Respiratory Component	**HCO₃⁻** Metabolic (Renal) Component	**Acid-Base Imbalance**
Acidotic	Acidotic		Respiratory acidosis
Alkalotic	Alkalotic		Respiratory alkalosis
Acidotic		Acidotic	Metabolic acidosis
Alkalotic		Alkalotic	Metabolic alkalosis

5. If the third value (the one, which did not "match" in acidity/alkalinity) is: *Normal*: the imbalance is *uncompensated*; *Abnormal*: The imbalance is *partially compensated*. For example, if the pH and PCO_2 are both acidotic and the HCO_3^- is alkalotic, the analysis is a "partially compensated respiratory acidosis."

6. If the pH is normal, but the PCO_2 and HCO_3^- are abnormal, the imbalance is considered *fully compensated*. To determine the underlying, or initial imbalance, look at the base excess, shown as BE on a laboratory report. If the base excess is normal when the pH is normal, the underlying problem was *metabolic*. The HCO_3^- value, which is considered the metabolic component, is then referred to in order to determine whether the problem was acidotic or alkalotic.

The above steps are summarized in Table A-2: ABG Analysis.

Table A-2	ABG Analysis				
pH **(7.35–7.45)**	**PCO₂** **(35–45)**	**HCO₃⁻** **(22–26)**	**Base Excess** **(–/+ 2)**	**Acid-Base Imbalance**	
Acidotic (<7.35)	Acidotic (>45)	Normal		Respiratory acidosis with no compensation	
Acidotic (<7.35)	Acidotic (>45)	Alkalotic (>26)		Respiratory acidosis with partial compensation	
Normal	Acidotic (>45)	Alkalotic (>26)	Abnormal	Respiratory acidosis with full compensation	
Acidotic (<7.35)	Normal	Acidotic (<22)		Metabolic acidosis with no compensation	
Acidotic (<7.35)	Alkalotic (<35)	Acidotic (<22)		Metabolic acidosis with partial compensation	
Normal	Alkalotic (<35)	Acidotic (<22)	Normal	Metabolic acidosis with full compensation	
Alkalotic (>7.45)	Alkalotic (<35)	Normal		Respiratory alkalosis with no compensation	
Alkalotic (>7.45)	Alkalotic (<35)	Acidotic (<22)		Respiratory alkalosis with partial compensation	
Normal	Alkalotic (<35)	Acidotic (<22)	Abnormal	Respiratory alkalosis with full compensation	
Alkalotic (>7.45)	Normal	Alkalotic (>26)		Metabolic alkalosis with no compensation	
Alkalotic (>7.45)	Acidotic (>45)	Alkalotic (>26)		Metabolic alkalosis with partial compensation	
Normal	Acidotic (>45)	Alkalotic (>26)	Normal	Metabolic alkalosis with full compensation	

Possible Meanings of Abnormal Values

Respiratory Acidosis: (increased PCO_2 due to hypoventilation)
Anesthesia/drugs
Asthma
Cardiac arrest
Chronic bronchitis
Congestive heart failure
Emphysema
Head trauma
Neuromuscular depression
Obesity

A

Pickwickian syndrome
Pneumonia
Pulmonary edema
Respiratory failure

Respiratory Alkalosis: (decreased PCO_2 due to hyperventilation)
Adult cystic fibrosis
Anemia
Anxiety
Carbon monoxide poisoning
Cerebral hemorrhage
Fever
Heart failure
Hypoxia
Improperly set ventilator
Myocardial infarction
Pain
Pregnancy (third trimester)
Pulmonary emboli

Metabolic Acidosis: (decreased HCO_3^- due to either excess acid production or loss of bicarbonate)
Cardiac arrest (lactic acidosis)
Diabetic ketoacidosis
Diarrhea
Renal failure
Renal tubular acidosis
Starvation (ketoacidosis)

Metabolic Alkalosis: (increased HCO_3^- due to either excessive intake of bicarbonate or lactate, or increased loss of chloride, hydrogen, and potassium ions)
Diuretics
Hypochloremia
Hypokalemia
Ingestion of sodium bicarbonate, antacids
Nasogastric suctioning
Sodium bicarbonate infusion
Vomiting

PARTIAL PRESSURE OF OXYGEN (PAO$_2$, PO$_2$)

The partial pressure of oxygen in the arterial blood, designated as PaO_2, is the amount of pressure exerted by O_2 dissolved in the blood. It is measured in millimeters of mercury (mm Hg) or torr (1 torr = 1 mm Hg). The PaO_2 is used to measure how effective the lungs are in oxygenating the blood. When the value is below normal, the patient is said to be **hypoxic**. The PaO_2 is directly influenced by the amount of oxygen inhaled; thus, it can also be used to assess the effectiveness of oxygen therapy.

Normal Values

75–100 torr (mm Hg)—on room, or ambient air
Elderly: value decreases with age

Possible Meanings of Abnormal Values

Increased	Decreased
High doses of oxygen	Anemia
Polycythemia	Atelectasis
	Cardiac decompensation
	Emphysema
	Hypoventilation
	Insufficient atmospheric oxygen
	Pneumonia
	Pulmonary edema
	Pulmonary embolism

Contributing Factors to Abnormal Values

- Falsely-elevated PaO$_2$ levels may occur due to failure to expel all air from the syringe when drawing the arterial blood sample.

OXYGEN CONTENT (O$_2$, O$_2$CT)

The amount of oxygen, which the blood can contain is based upon the amount of oxygen carried by the hemoglobin and upon the amount of oxygen contained in the plasma. One gram of hemoglobin can carry up to 1.34 mL of oxygen. In addition, up to 0.3 mL of oxygen can be carried in 100 mL of blood plasma.

The oxygen content is a measurement of the actual amount of oxygen being carried in the blood. This value is determined through the following formula:

$$O_2 \text{ Content} = \frac{SaO_2\%}{100\%} \times Hgb \times 1.34 + (PaO_2 \times 0.003)$$

Normal Values

Arterial: 15–22 mL/100 mL of blood (15–22%)
Venous: 11–16 mL/100 mL of blood (11–16%)

Possible Meanings of Abnormal Values

Decreased

Asthma
Chronic bronchitis
Emphysema
Flail chest
Hypoventilation
Kyphoscoliosis
Neuromuscular impairment
Obesity
Postoperative respiratory complications

OXYGEN SATURATION (SAO$_2$, SO$_2$, O$_2$ SAT)

The oxygen saturation value is a comparison of the actual amount of oxygen carried by the hemoglobin compared to the amount of oxygen which the hemoglobin is capable of carrying. Thus, if the hemoglobin is carrying the amount of oxygen it is capable of carrying, the oxygen saturation is approximately 100%. Oxygen saturation may be measured with arterial blood gases or through pulse oximetry, a noninvasive procedure. (See "Oximetry.")

Normal Values

95–100%

Possible Meanings of Abnormal Values

Increased	Decreased
Adequate oxygen therapy	Carbon monoxide poisoning
	Hypoxia

Contributing Factors to Abnormal Values

- The oxygen saturation is affected by the partial pressure of oxygen in the blood, by the body temperature, by the pH of the blood, and by the structure of the hemoglobin.

Interventions/Implications

Pretest
- Explain to the patient the purpose of the test, noting that the puncture is momentarily painful. (Note: Some institutions allow for anesthetizing the area with 1% Xylocaine.)
- Perform the Allen's test to assess for adequate collateral circulation in the ulnar artery. This collateral circulation is important should the radial artery become obstructed by a thrombus following the arterial puncture.
  - To perform the Allen's test, apply pressure to both the radial and ulnar pulses of one of the patient's wrists until the pulses are obliterated. The hand will blanch (pale) due to lack of circulation to the hand. Release the pressure on the ulnar artery. If the hand returns to normal color immediately, the test is considered positive, and the arterial puncture may be done in that wrist. If the hand remains pale, the ulnar circulation is inadequate. The test is considered negative and the other arm should be tested for adequacy. Should both arms be found to inappropriate sites, the use of the femoral artery may need to be explored.
- No fasting is required prior to the test.

Procedure
- The area over the radial artery in the wrist is anesthetized with 1% Xylocaine, if allowed per institutional policy.
- An airtight syringe containing 0.2 mL of heparin is used to draw a 3 to 5 mL arterial blood sample. (Note: Venous blood can be used if arterial blood is unaccessible; however, venous is useful only for evaluating pH, $PaCO_2$, and base excess.)
- All air bubbles are expelled from the syringe. The syringe is capped to prevent loss of gases from the sample.
- The syringe is labeled, placed in ice, and taken to the laboratory immediately for analysis.
- Gloves are worn throughout the procedure.

Posttest
- Apply continuous pressure on the radial site for at least 5 minutes, 10 minutes if the femoral site was used.

- Apply dressing, periodically assessing for continued bleeding, especially if the patient has bleeding problems or is receiving anticoagulant therapy.
- Assess the extremity for signs of circulatory impairment: changes in the color, movement, temperature, sensation, and, if femoral site, pulses distal to the puncture site.
- Note on the laboratory slip whether the patient was breathing ambient (room) air or, if receiving supplemental oxygen, the oxygen flow.
- Report abnormal findings to the primary care provider.

Clinical Alerts

- Possible complications: Circulatory impairment due to arterial occlusion, nerve damage during arterial puncture.

CONTRAINDICATIONS!

- No palpable pulse in the extremity
- Negative Allen's test in the extremity
- Any skin infection in the area of the proposed arterial puncture
- Any arteriovenous (AV) shunt in area of proposed arterial puncture
- Severe coagulopathies

Arthrocentesis (Synovial Fluid Analysis)

Test Description

An arthrocentesis is the insertion of a sterile needle into a joint space to obtain a sample of synovial fluid for analysis. Although the procedure may be performed on any joint, the knee is the most common site. Arthrocentesis is used to assist in the differential diagnosis of arthritis, to investigate joint effusion, and to remove excess fluid from the joint, which may be causing pain for the patient. If indicated, corticosteroids may be injected into the joint following fluid sample acquisition.

Normal Values

Synovial fluid is clear to straw colored with 0–200 white blood cells/μL, no crystals, and a good mucin clot. Values for protein, glucose, and uric acid are similar to serum values.

Possible Meanings of Abnormal Values

Gout
Osteoarthritis
Pseudogout
Rheumatic fever
Rheumatoid arthritis

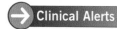

Septic arthritis
Systemic lupus erythematosus
Traumatic arthritis
Tuberculous arthritis

Interventions/Implications

Pretest
- Explain to the patient the purpose of the test. Provide any written teaching materials available on the subject. Note that minimal discomfort during the test is due to the injection of the local anesthetic.
- Obtain a signed informed consent.
- No fasting is required prior to the test.

Procedure
- The patient is assisted to a supine position.
- The skin is cleansed with an antiseptic, and the skin overlying the puncture site is anesthetized.
- A needle is inserted into the joint space. A minimum of 10 mL of fluid is aspirated for analysis.
- If indicated, the needle is left in place, and a syringe containing a steroid is attached.
- After the steroid is injected, the needle is withdrawn.
- Pressure is applied to the puncture site, followed by a sterile dressing.
- Gloves are worn throughout the procedure.

Posttest
- The patient may experience discomfort after the procedure. The patient is instructed to rest the joint for 12 hours after the test. Elastic wraps, ice applications, and mild analgesics may be used. Strenuous activity should be avoided until approved by the primary care provider.
- Assess the joint for redness, swelling, and tenderness.
- Report abnormal findings to the primary care provider.

Clinical Alerts

- Possible complications include hemarthrosis and joint infection

CONTRAINDICATIONS!

- Patients with joint infection or skin infection near proposed site of arthrocentesis

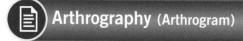

Arthrography (Arthrogram)

Test Description
Arthrography is the examination of the joint after injection of a radiopaque dye and/or air into a joint. Performed using local anesthesia, the arthrogram assists in the evaluation of joint damage, such as possible cartilage tears, by outlining the soft

tissue structures and contour of the joint. Radiographs are taken as the joint is manipulated. This test is used primarily for persistent unexplained joint discomfort. If surgical intervention is anticipated, arthroscopy may be performed in place of the arthrogram.

Normal Values

Normal muscle, ligament, cartilage, synovial, and tendon structures of the joints

Possible Meanings of Abnormal Values

Arthritis
Baker cyst
Cartilaginous abnormalities
Chondromalacia patellae
Disruption of the collateral ligaments
Disruption of the joint capsule
Meniscal tears/lacerations
Osteochondral fractures
Osteochondritis dissecans
Synovial abnormalities
Synovitis
Tears of the cruciate ligaments

Interventions/Implications

Pretest
- Explain to the patient the purpose of the test. Provide any written teaching materials available on the subject. Note that minimal discomfort during the test is due to the injection of the local anesthetic. Pressure or tingling may be felt during injection of the dye.
- Check for allergies to iodine, shellfish, or contrast medium dye. Inform the radiologist of such possible allergy and obtain order for an antihistamine and steroid to be administered prior to the test.
- Obtain a signed informed consent.
- No fasting is required prior to the test.

Procedure
- The patient is assisted to a supine position.
- The skin is cleansed with an antiseptic, and the skin overlying the puncture site is anesthetized.
- A needle is inserted into the joint space. Fluid is usually aspirated for analysis.
- Leaving the needle in place, the radiopaque contrast dye is injected into the joint. Occasionally air is used in place of, or in addition to, the dye.
- The needle is removed and the joint is manipulated to spread the dye around the knee joints.
- Radiographs are taken with the joint in various positions.
- Gloves are worn throughout the procedure.

Posttest

- Most allergic reactions to radiopaque dye occur within 30 minutes of administration of the contrast medium. Observe the patient closely for: respiratory distress, hypotension, edema, hives, rash, tachycardia, and/or laryngeal stridor. Emergency resuscitation equipment must be readily accessible.
- The patient may experience discomfort after the procedure. The patient is instructed to rest the joint for 12 hours after the test. Elastic wraps, ice applications, and mild analgesics may be used. Strenuous activity should be avoided until approved by the primary care provider.
- Teach the patient to monitor the site and to notify the health-care provider if signs or symptoms of infection occur, such as drainage, redness, warmth, edema, pain at the site, or fever.
- Report abnormal findings to the primary care provider.

→ Clinical Alerts

- Resuscitation equipment must be available throughout the procedure.
- Possible complications include: Allergic reaction to the dye, infection, persistent joint crepitus, and thrombophlebitis.

CONTRAINDICATIONS!

- Pregnant women
    - Caution: A woman in her childbearing years should undergo radiography only during her menses or 12 to 14 days after its onset to avoid any exposure to a fetus.
- Patients who are allergic to iodine, shellfish, or contrast medium dye
- Patients with active arthritis
- Patients with joint infection

Arthroscopy

Test Description

Arthroscopy allows direct visualization of a joint through use of a fiberoptic endoscope. A camera is attached to the scope to allow a clear view of the joint's interior. In addition to providing direct visualization of the joint structures, this endoscopic procedure also allows the performance of biopsy and simple repairs to the joint, such as removal of loose bodies. Although this procedure might be performed on any joint, the knee is the most frequent site. The procedure is usually performed under general or spinal anesthesia. Diagnostic arthroscopy is often done when pain and functional limitations continue despite conservative care (medications or physical therapy) and imaging is inconclusive.

Normal Values

Normal muscle, ligament, cartilage, synovial, and tendon structures of the joints

Possible Meanings of Abnormal Values

Chondromalacia
Cysts
Degenerative joint changes
Fracture
Joint tumors
Meniscal disease
Osteoarthritis
Osteochondritis
Rheumatoid arthritis
Synovitis
Torn cartilage
Torn ligament
Trapped synovium

Contributing Factors to Abnormal Values

- If an arthrogram was recently performed on the joint, residual contrast media and inflammation may affect the arthroscopy.

Interventions/Implications

Pretest

- Explain to the patient the purpose of the test. Provide any written teaching materials available on the subject. Note that discomfort during the test is due to the injection of the local anesthetic and penetration of the synovium with a blunt instrument. Pressure may be felt during the use of the arthroscope.
- Obtain a signed informed consent.
- The patient is kept NPO after midnight prior to the test.
- The area 5 to 6 inches above and below the joint is shaved.
- Administer a preprocedure sedative as ordered.

Procedure

- The patient is assisted to a supine position.
- A maintenance intravenous line is initiated. Anesthesia is administered.
- The extremity is scrubbed, elevated, and wrapped with an elastic bandage from the distal portion of the extremity to the proximal portion, to drain as much blood from the limb as possible.
- A pneumatic tourniquet placed around the proximal portion of the limb is inflated and the elastic bandage is removed.
  - Note: If a tourniquet is not used, a normal saline solution containing 1% lidocaine and epinephrine is instilled into the joint to distend it and help reduce bleeding.
- The joint is bent to a 45° angle.
- A small incision is made in the skin in the lateral or medial aspect of the joint. An opening is made through the synovia using a blunt instrument.
- The arthroscope is then inserted into the joint spaces. The joint is manipulated as it is visualized. Additional puncture sites may be needed to provide full view of the joint.

A

- Any biopsy or needed treatment can be performed at this time.
- The joint is irrigated and the arthroscope is removed. Manual pressure is applied to the joint to remove remaining irrigating solution.
- The incision sites are sutured and a pressure dressing is applied.
- Sterile technique is maintained throughout the procedure.

Posttest

- Assess the patient's vital signs, neurologic status, and neurovascular status to the extremity.
- Ice is maintained to the knee.
- Instruct the patient to observe the incision site for redness, swelling, and tenderness.
- Strenuous activity involving the joint should be avoided until approved by the surgeon.
- Crutches are often used postoperatively to decrease weight-bearing on the affected extremity.
- Inform the patient regarding proper use of pain medication.
- Report abnormal findings to the primary care provider.

→ Clinical Alerts

- Possible complications include: hemarthrosis, infection, infrapatellar anesthesia, joint injury, synovial rupture, and thrombophlebitis.
- The patient will need a follow-up appointment for suture removal.

CONTRAINDICATIONS!

- Patients with fibrous ankylosis of the joint, which prevents effective use of the arthroscope in the joint
- Patients with joint infection or skin infection near the proposed arthroscopic site.

Aspartate Aminotransferase (AST, Serum Glutamic Oxaloacetic Transaminase [SGOT])

Test Description

Aspartate aminotransferase (AST) is an enzyme found primarily in the heart, liver, and muscle. It is released into the circulation after injury or death of cells. AST levels usually increase within 12 hours of the injury and remain elevated for 5 days. Thus, this test is one of several that are performed when there has been damage to the heart muscle, as in myocardial infarction, and in assessing liver damage. Other cardiac enzymes also assessed are the creatine kinase (CK) isoenzymes, lactic dehydrogenase (LDH, LD), and troponin.

AST is assessed along with alanine aminotransferase (ALT) in monitoring liver damage. These two values normally exist in an approximately 1:1 ratio. The AST is greater than the ALT in alcohol-induced hepatitis, cirrhosis, and metastatic cancer of the liver. ALT is greater than AST in the case of viral or drug-induced hepatitis and hepatic obstruction due to causes other than malignancy.

The degree of increase in these enzyme levels provides information as to the possible source of the problem. A twofold increase is suggestive of an obstructive problem, often requiring surgical intervention. A 10-fold increase of ALT and AST indicates a probable medical problem such as hepatitis.

THE EVIDENCE FOR PRACTICE

In managing abnormal lipids, statin medications are commonly used. One major side effect of statin use is liver toxicity, although the likelihood of liver transaminase elevations >3 times the upper limit of normal is small. Liver transaminases (ALT and AST) are obtained 6 to 12 weeks after statin therapy is initiated. (Full text of guidelines available at http://circ.ahajournals.org/cgi/content/full/112/20/3184.)

Normal Values

Female:	9–25 U/L (0.15–0.42 µkat/L SI units)
Male:	10–40 U/L (0.17–0.67 µkat/L SI units)
Elderly:	Slightly higher norms
Newborn:	Norms two to three times higher

Possible Meanings of Abnormal Values

Increased	Decreased
Acute renal disease	Beriberi
Biliary obstruction	Diabetic ketoacidosis
Bone metastases	Hemodialysis
Brain trauma	Pregnancy
Cancer of the prostate	Uremia
Cirrhosis	
Eclampsia	
Gangrene	
Hemolytic disease	
Hepatitis	
Infectious mononucleosis	
Liver cancer	
Liver metastases	
Liver necrosis	
Malignant hyperthermia	
Muscle inflammation	
Myocardial infarction	
Pancreatitis	
Progressive muscular dystrophy	
Pulmonary infarction	
Reye's syndrome	
Shock	
Severe burns	
Trauma	

Contributing Factors to Abnormal Values

- Drugs that may *increase* AST levels: acetaminophen, allopurinal, antibiotics, ascorbic acid, chlorpropamide, cholestyramine, cholinergics, clofibrate, codeine, HMG-CoA reductase inhibitors, hydralazine, isoniazid, meperidine, methyldopa, morphine, oral contraceptives, phenothiazines, procainamide, pyridoxine, salicylates, sulfonamides, verapamil, vitamin A.
- Drugs that may *decrease* AST levels: metronidazole, trifluoperazine.

Interventions/Implications

Pretest
- Explain to the patient the purpose of the test and the need for a blood sample to be drawn.
- When assessing for myocardial infarction, this test is often performed on 3 consecutive days, and again in 1 week, necessitating multiple venipunctures.
- No fasting is required before the test.

Procedure
- A 7-mL blood sample is drawn in a red-top collection tube.
- Gloves are worn throughout the procedure.

Posttest
- Apply pressure 3–5 minutes at venipuncture site. Apply dressing, periodically assessing for continued bleeding.
- Teach the patient to monitor the site. If the site begins to bleed, the patient should apply direct pressure and, if unable to control the bleeding, return to the laboratory.
- Label the specimen and transport it to the laboratory.
- Report abnormal findings to the primary care providers.

 Clinical Alerts

- Patients with liver dysfunction may have prolonged clotting time.
- Liver enzymes, including ALT and AST, are routinely monitored in patients who take HMG-CoEnzyme A reductase inhibitors ("statin" medications).

Barium Enema (Large Bowel Study, Lower GI Series, Colon X-Ray, Air Contrast Barium Enema)

Test Description
The barium enema is the fluoroscopic examination of the large intestine after instillation of barium sulfate into the rectum. If a "double contrast" or "air contrast" study is being used, air is also instilled. During this procedure, a fluoroscopic screen is positioned over the intestines. These structures are then projected onto the fluoroscopic screen. The image remains on the monitor for continuous observation; therefore, as the barium is instilled, the flow of barium can be monitored on the screen. The patient's position is changed throughout the exam to allow visualization of the structures and their function, including peristalsis. This test is especially

useful in the evaluation of patients experiencing lower abdominal pain, changes in their bowel habits, or the passage of stools containing blood or mucus, and for visualizing polyps, diverticula, and tumors. Videotaping of the fluoroscopic procedure enables the movements to be studied at later times.

THE EVIDENCE FOR PRACTICE

According to the American Cancer Society, if colonoscopy is unavailable, not feasible, or not desired by the patient, double contrast barium enema (DCBE) alone, or the combination of flexible sigmoidoscopy and DCBE are acceptable alternatives. Adding flexible sigmoidoscopy to DCBE may provide a more comprehensive diagnostic evaluation than DCBE alone in finding significant lesions. These procedures should be done every 5 years.

Normal Values

Normal size, shape, position, and functioning of the large intestine

Possible Meanings of Abnormal Values

Appendicitis
Carcinoma
Crohn's disease
Diverticulitis
Diverticulosis
Fistulas
Gastroenteritis
Granulomatous colitis
Hirschsprung's disease
Intussusception
Irritable bowel syndrome
Perforation of the colon
Polyps
Sigmoid torsion
Sigmoid volvulus
Telescoping of the bowel
Tumors
Ulcerative colitis

Contributing Factors to Abnormal Values

- Under- or overexposure of the film may alter film quality.
- When patients are unable to hold still, due to pain or mental status, the quality of the film may be affected.
- Barium retained from other exams and inadequate bowel preparation will interfere with the procedure.

Interventions/Implications

Pretest
- Explain to the patient the purpose of the test and the benefits and risks associated with the test. Provide any written teaching materials available on the subject. Explain to the

patient that instillation of the barium and/or air may cause cramping and the urge to defecate. Reassure the patient that there is a balloon on the tube which will prevent leakage
of the barium from the rectum.

- Explain to the patient the importance of all aspects of the preparation to ensure complete emptying of the intestinal tract. If fecal material has been retained, the test must be repeated at another time.
- Preparation of the patient includes:
    - a liquid diet with no dairy products for 24 hours prior to the exam
    - intake of at least 1200 cc of fluids the day prior to the exam
    - stool softeners, laxatives, and enemas as per institutional policy the evening before and the morning of the exam (Note: Enemas may occasionally be ordered "until clear". This means that enemas are given until the solution returned is clear and colorless.)
    - being NPO (nothing by mouth) after midnight before the exam
- The patient should be monitored throughout the bowel preparation for fatigue and fluid and electrolyte imbalance.
- Instruct the patient to remove all objects containing metal, such as jewelry or undergarments, as these will show on the film.

Procedure

- The patient is first assisted to a supine position on the exam table, and a preliminary film is taken. This provides verification that no stool remains in the large intestine. If preparation is adequate, the test may continue.
- The patient is then turned to the side (Sims' position) and a lubricated rectal tube is inserted.
- The barium is allowed to flow slowly into the intestine until the entire intestine up to the ileocecal valve is filled. During this time, the flow of barium is observed on the fluoroscopic screen and periodic films are taken.
- Once the intestine is filled, the rectal tube is removed. The patient is assisted to the restroom, or provided a bedpan, and is instructed to expel as much barium as possible.
- After expulsion of the barium, an additional film is taken of the intestine.
- If a double-contrast barium enema has been ordered, air is then instilled in the intestine and additional films taken.
- The procedure takes 45 minutes to 1 1/4 hours.

Posttest

- Resume the patient's diet and medications as taken prior to the test. Encourage fluid intake.
- Instruct the patient on the need to evacuate all of the barium. Administer a cathartic or enema as ordered. Check all stools for presence of barium, explaining to the patient that the stools will be white initially and return to normal color following passage of all of the barium.
- Instruct the patient to report any abdominal pain, fever, or weakness.
- Notify the primary care provider if the barium is not expelled within 2 to 3 days.
- Report abnormal findings to the primary care provider.

→ Clinical Alerts

- If a barium swallow or an upper gastrointestinal and small-bowel series test is ordered, these should be completed after the barium enema is performed. Otherwise the barium sulfate ingested during the other exams may obscure the films made during the barium enema.

- If an intestinal perforation is suspected, a water-soluble contrast medium (Gastrografin) is used. No bowel preparation is performed.
- Possible complications include: perforation of the colon, fluid and electrolyte imbalance, and fecal impaction due to retention of barium.

B

CONTRAINDICATIONS!

- Pregnant women
  - Caution: A woman in her childbearing years should undergo radiography only during her menses or 12 to 14 days after its onset to avoid any exposure to a fetus.
- Patients with tachycardia.
- Patients with severe active ulcerative colitis accompanied by systemic toxicity and megacolon.
- Patients with suspected intestinal perforation.
- Patients who are unable to cooperate in retaining the barium due to age, mental status, pain, or other factors.

Barium Swallow (Esophageal Radiography, Esophagography)

Test Description
The barium swallow, which is usually included as a part of the upper gastrointestinal series, is the fluoroscopic examination of the pharynx and the esophagus after ingestion of barium sulfate mixtures. During this procedure, a fluoroscopic screen is positioned over the heart, lungs, and abdomen. These structures are then projected on the fluoroscopic screen. The image remains on the monitor for continuous observation; therefore, as the patient swallows barium, the flow of barium can be monitored on the screen. The patient's position is changed throughout the exam to allow visualization of the entire esophagus and to assess for such problems as gastric reflux. This test is especially useful in the evaluation of patients experiencing dysphagia and regurgitation. Videotaping of the fluoroscopic procedure enables the movements to be studied at later times.

THE EVIDENCE FOR PRACTICE
Abnormalities of the mid or distal esophagus or even the uppermost part of the stomach may cause referred dysphagia to the upper chest or pharynx, whereas abnormalities of the pharynx rarely cause referred dysphagia to the lower chest. The esophagus and upper stomach should therefore be evaluated in patients with pharyngeal symptoms, particularly if no abnormalities are found in the pharynx to explain these symptoms.

Normal Values
Normal size, shape, position, and functioning of the esophagus

Possible Meanings of Abnormal Values

Achalasia
Cancer of the esophagus
Cancer of the stomach invading the esophagus
Chalasia
Congenital abnormalities
Diverticula
Esophageal motility disorders, such as spasms
Esophageal ulcers
Esophageal varices
Esophagitis
Hiatal hernia
Perforation of the esophagus
Polyps
Strictures

Contributing Factors to Abnormal Values

- Under- or overexposure of the film may alter film quality.
- When patients are unable to hold still, due to pain or mental status, the quality of the film may be affected.

Interventions/Implications

Pretest

- Explain to the patient the purpose of the test and the benefits and risks associated with the test. Provide any written teaching materials available on the subject. Note that no discomfort is associated with this procedure. The barium, although in a milkshake-type solution, may taste chalky.
- Fasting for 8 hours is required prior to the test.
- Instruct the patient to remove all objects containing metal, such as jewelry or undergarments, as these will show on the film.

Procedure

- The patient is placed in an upright position for the first part of the procedure.
- The fluoroscopic screen is placed in front of the patient and the heart, lungs, and abdomen are viewed.
- The patient is instructed to take one swallow of a thick barium mixture while the videotape is made of the pharyngeal action.
- As the patient then continues to drink the barium mixture, in addition to the fluoroscopic viewing, spot films are made of the esophageal area from a variety of angles.
- The patient is then placed in different positions and instructed to drink more of the barium. This allows for evaluation of the patient for such problems as gastric reflux.
- The test takes approximately 30 minutes to 1 hour.

Posttest

- Resume the patient's diet and medications as taken prior to the test. Encourage fluid intake.
- Instruct the patient on the need to evacuate all of the barium. Administer a cathartic as ordered. Check all stools for the presence of barium, explaining to the patient that the stools will be white initially and will return to normal color following passage of all of the barium.

- Notify the primary care provider if the barium is not expelled within 2 to 3 days.
- Report abnormal findings to the primary care provider.

B

Clinical Alerts

- If cholangiography and/or a barium enema test are ordered, these should be completed *before* the barium swallow is performed. Otherwise the barium sulfate ingested during the barium swallow may obscure the films made during the other exams.
- Possible complication of procedure: fecal impaction due to retention of barium.

CONTRAINDICATIONS!

- Pregnant women.
  - Caution: A woman in her childbearing years should undergo radiography only during her menses or 12 to 14 days after its onset to avoid any exposure to a fetus.
- Patients with intestinal obstruction.
- Patients with a perforated esophagus. (Gastrografin, a water-soluble contrast medium, would be used in place of barium.)
- Patients who are unable to cooperate due to age, mental status, pain, or other factors.
- Patients with unstable vital signs.

Bence Jones Protein (Immunoglobulin Light Chains)

Test Description
Individuals with such conditions as multiple myeloma and amyloidosis often have an increased production of a single homogeneous immunoglobulin or immunoglobulin fragment (i.e., kappa or lambda light chains). These immunoglobulin light chains, called Bence Jones proteins, are small and easily cleared by the kidney. Hence, they will be present in the urine and are usually absent in the plasma. Historically, the detection of light chains in urine was based on their unique solubility characteristics related to temperature. On heating a urine sample, these proteins will precipitate out of solution when at 40°C to 60°C, redissolve at 100°C, and reappear on cooling. This "heat precipitation test" is insensitive and nonspecific. Today, sensitive and specific detection of Bence Jones protein is obtained using the immunoelectrophoresis process.

Normal Values
Absence of Bence Jones protein in the urine

Possible Meanings of Abnormal Values

B

Increased
Adult Fanconi's syndrome
Amyloidosis
Benign monoclonal gammopathy
Chronic lymphocytic leukemia
Chronic renal insufficiency
Cryoglobulinemia
Hyperparathyroidism
Lymphoma
Metastases
Multiple myeloma
Rheumatoid arthritis
Systemic lupus erythematosus
Waldenström's macroglobulinemia

Contributing Factors to Abnormal Values

- *False-negative* test results may occur with dilute urine or in the presence of severe urinary tract infection.

Interventions/Implications

Pretest
- Explain the procedure to the patient, stressing the importance of not contaminating the specimen.
- No fasting is required before the test.

Procedure
- A minimum of 50 mL of urine is needed for the test. Collection of an early morning specimen is best.
- Use of clean-catch midstream technique is recommended to prevent contamination of the specimen.
    - A clean-catch kit containing cleansing materials and a sterile specimen container is given to the patient.
    - Male patients should cleanse the urinary meatus with the materials provided or with soap and water, void a small amount into the toilet, and then void directly into the specimen container.
    - Female patients should cleanse the labia minora and urinary meatus, cleansing from front to back. While keeping the labia separated, the female should void a small amount into the toilet and then void directly into the specimen container.
    - Instruct patients to avoid touching the inside of the specimen container and lid.
- A 24-hour urine collection may be needed to detect trace amounts of protein. If so, refrigerate specimen throughout the collection.
- Gloves are worn by the health-care worker when dealing with the specimen.

Posttest
- Label the specimen. The specimen must be transported to the laboratory immediately or refrigerated to prevent bacterial growth that can lead to a breakdown of proteins.
- Report abnormal findings to the primary care provider.

📄 Bilirubin, Blood (Direct, Indirect, Total)

Test Description
Bilirubin, which is one of the components of bile, is formed in the liver, spleen, and bone marrow. It is also formed as a result of hemoglobin breakdown, as in the destruction of red blood cells. There are three types of bilirubin: total, direct (conjugated), and indirect (unconjugated). *Total bilirubin* is composed of the direct bilirubin plus the indirect bilirubin. The total bilirubin level increases with any type of jaundice.

Normally, *direct* or *conjugated, bilirubin* is excreted by the gastrointestinal (GI) tract, with only minimal amounts entering the bloodstream. It was originally named "direct" bilirubin because this water-soluble type of bilirubin reacts directly with the reagents added to the blood sample. Its level rises in the blood when obstructive jaundice (as from gallstones) or hepatic jaundice occurs, because the bilirubin is unable to reach the intestines for excretion and instead, enter the bloodstream for excretion by the kidneys. Direct bilirubin is the only type of bilirubin able to cross the glomerular filter; thus it is the only type of bilirubin that can be found in the urine.

Indirect bilirubin, also known as *free* or *unconjugated bilirubin*, is normally found in the bloodstream. Its name comes from the fact that this non-water-soluble bilirubin does not directly react with reagents added to a blood sample. Alcohol must be added for the reaction to occur. Indirect bilirubin rises in cases of hemolytic jaundice, in which the breakdown of hemoglobin results in a higher than normal level of indirect bilirubin being present in the bloodstream. This is the type of bilirubin elevated in cases of hepatocellular dysfunction, such as hepatitis.

Typically, only the total bilirubin is reported. If the total bilirubin is abnormal, further testing is done to differentiate the level of direct and indirect bilirubin.

THE EVIDENCE FOR PRACTICE
Initial evaluations should determine whether the elevated serum bilirubin is conjugated (direct) or unconjugated (indirect). Asymptomatic adult patients with an isolated, mild unconjugated hyperbilirubinemia should be evaluated for Gilbert's syndrome, hemolysis, and medication-induced hyperbilirubinemia. If conjugated hyperbilirubinemia is present, the presence of concomitant alkaline phosphatase elevations must be assessed and biliary obstruction should be excluded. (AGAI guidelines at http://www.gastrojournal.org/article/PIIS0016508502002408/fulltext)

Normal Values
Total bilirubin: 0.3–1.0 mg/dL (5–17 μmol/L SI units)
Direct (conjugated) bilirubin: 0.0–0.4 mg/dL (0–7 μmol/L SI units)
Indirect (unconjugated) bilirubin: 0.1–1.0 mg/dL (1–17 μmol/L SI units)

Possible Meanings of Abnormal Values

Increased Direct (Conjugated) Bilirubin
Biliary obstruction
Cancer of the head of the pancreas

B

Choledocholithiasis
Cirrhosis
Dubin-Johnson syndrome
Hepatitis
Obstructive jaundice
Pregnancy

Increased Indirect (Unconjugated) Bilirubin

Autoimmune hemolysis
Cirrhosis
Crigler-Najjer syndrome
Erythroblastosis fetalis
Gilbert's syndrome
Hemolytic transfusion reaction
Hepatitis
Malaria
Myocardial infarction
Pernicious anemia
Septicemia
Sickle cell disease
Tissue hemorrhage

Contributing Factors to Abnormal Values

- Hemolysis of the blood sample will alter test results.
- Exposure of the blood sample to sunlight or artificial light for 1 hour or more will decrease the bilirubin content of the sample.
- Testing with contrast media within 24 hours will alter test results.
- Drugs that may *increase* total bilirubin: allopurinal, anabolic steroids, antimalarials, ascorbic acid, azathioprine, chlorpropamide, cholinergics, codeine, dextran, diuretics, epinephrine, isoproterenol, levodopa, MAO inhibitors, meperidine, methyldopa, methotrexate, morphine, oral contraceptives, phenazopyridine, phenothiazines, quinidine, rifampin, streptomycin, theophylline, tyrosine, vitamin A.
- Drugs that may *decrease* total bilirubin: barbiturates, caffeine, chlorine, citrate, corticosteroids, ethanol, penicillin, protein, salicylates, sulfonamides, urea.

Interventions/Implications

Pretest

- Explain to the patient the purpose of the test and the need for a blood sample to be drawn.
- Fasting for 4 to 8 hours is required before the test. Water is permitted.

Procedure

- A 7-mL blood sample is drawn in a lavender-top collection tube.
- Gloves are worn throughout the procedure.

Posttest

- Apply pressure at venipuncture site. Apply dressing, periodically assessing for continued bleeding.
- Protect the specimen from bright light by wrapping the sample tube in foil or placing in a refrigerator.
- Label the specimen and transport it to the laboratory.
- Report abnormal findings to the primary care provider.

Bioterrorism Infectious Agents Testing (Anthrax, Botulism, Plague, Smallpox, Tularemia, Viral Hemorrhagic Fevers [VHFs])

B

Test Description

Among the health protection goals of the Centers for Disease Control and Prevention (CDC) is to prepare people for emerging health threats, including those of bioterrorism. The CDC website (http://www.bt.cdc.gov/bioterrorism/) provides access to information on many biological agents. Biological agents are classified according to three priority levels. The highest priority is Category A. According to the CDC, higher priority agents include organisms that pose a risk to national security because they:

- can be easily disseminated or transmitted from person to person;
- result in high mortality rates and have the potential for major public health impact;
- might cause public panic and social disruption; and
- require special action for public health preparedness.

Currently, the agents classified as Category A include:

- Anthrax (*Bacillus anthracis*)
- Botulism (*Clostridium botulinum* toxin)
- Plague (*Yersinia pestis*)
- Smallpox (variola major)
- Tularemia (*Francisella tularensis*)
- Viral hemorrhagic fevers (filoviruses [e.g., Ebola, Marburg] and arenaviruses [e.g., Lassa, Machupo])

Following is a compilation of information on the Category A agents, including a description of the agent and how it is diagnosed.

Anthrax

Anthrax is caused by *Bacillus anthracis*, a bacterium that forms spores. People can become infected through handling or breathing in the anthrax spores, or from ingesting undercooked meat from infected animals. There are three types of anthrax: cutaneous, gastrointestinal (GI), and inhalation. The cutaneous form begins with a papule resembling an insect bite, which then progresses to development of a central vesicle. This vesicle becomes a painless, necrotic ulcer. Lesions may be solitary or multiple and are accompanied by regional lymphadenopathy, fatigue, fever, and/or chills. Even without treatment, 80% of people with cutaneous anthrax survive. GI anthrax is more serious, with 25% to 50% mortality. Symptoms include nausea, loss of appetite, bloody diarrhea, fever, and abdominal pain. The most serious form is inhalation anthrax. It first appears with cold or flu-like symptoms which progress to more severe respiratory difficulty. Death can occur in 50% of the cases. Treatment involves antibiotic therapy (ciprofloxacin or doxycycline) for 60 days. Survival depends on the type of anthrax and how soon treatment is initiated.

Diagnostic Testing: Testing method depends on the type of anthrax suspected.

Cutaneous anthrax:
- Swabs of lesion for Gram stain, culture, and polymerase chain reaction (PCR)
- Biopsies for PCR
- Blood testing: acute and convalescent titers, blood culture

Gastrointestinal anthrax:
- Stool specimen

Inhalation anthrax:
- Blood for Gram stain, culture, and PCR.
- If pleural effusion present, pleural fluid can be obtained for Gram stain, culture, and PCR.
- Blood testing: acute and convalescent titers.
- If possible meningitis, cerebrospinal fluid (CSF) can be used for Gram stain, culture, and PCR.

Botulism

Botulism is a neuroparalytic illness caused by a toxin made by the bacterium *Clostridium botulinum*. The disease is caused by ingestion of the toxin in food including vegetables, meat, poultry, and milk products. Symptoms include dysphagia, dysarthria, progressive weakness with paralysis, double vision, nausea, vomiting, abdominal pain, dry mouth, and respiratory distress leading to possible respiratory failure. Treatment, involving respiratory support and administration of botulinus antitoxin, is begun prior to laboratory results being available.

Diagnostic Testing: Because botulism involves paralysis, it can easily be misdiagnosed as Guillain-Barre, myasthenia gravis, or stroke. A normal Tensilon test can rule out myasthenia gravis; normal neuroimaging studies rule out stroke. Confirmation of botulism is made through identifying the toxin in serum, stool, or food or by culturing the bacterium from stool, a wound, or food.

Plague

Plague is caused by the bacterium *Yersinia pestis*. It is usually transmitted by the bites of infected fleas. However, it can also be spread through the handling of infected animals, direct contact with contaminated tissue, or through inhalation of infectious droplets from another person infected with plague pneumonia. Plague usually first appears as a tender lymph gland ("bubo") in the groin, axilla, or neck, followed by development of fever, chills, headache, and fatigue. Pneumonic plague, characterized by fever, cough, hemoptysis, and dyspnea, can also occur. Since the symptoms are not unlike many other illnesses, a thorough history is needed to assess for exposure to infected animals or fleas. Without treatment 50% to 60% of the patients die; mortality is 14% with treatment. Treatment with antibiotics (streptomycin, tetracyclines, or chloramphenicol) should begin immediately after laboratory specimens are obtained.

Diagnostic Testing: Testing involves blood cultures for plague bacteria and microscopic examination and culture of lymph gland, blood, and sputum samples, or bronchial washings.

Smallpox

Smallpox is caused by the variola virus, usually the variola major virus. There are four types of variola major including ordinary (most frequent type), modified, flat, and hemorrhagic. Overall, the four types have a 30% mortality rate; however, the flat and hemorrhagic types are usually fatal. Symptoms include high fever and a rash. During the prodromal stage, fever, malaise, headache, body aches, and possibly vomiting occur. The rash begins as red spots in the mouth and on the tongue which develop into lesions that break open. At the same time, a rash appears on the skin, covering the body in 24 hours. Over the next 3 to 5 days, the rash progresses through becoming raised, umbilicating, becoming pustular, crusting, scabbing, and then falling off, leaving pitted scars. There is no treatment for smallpox; it is prevented through vaccination against the virus. There have been no cases of smallpox in the world since 1977, however, since there are laboratory stockpiles of the virus, the potential use for bioterrorism exists.

Diagnostic Testing: Diagnosis is confirmed through a viral culture conducted on the contents of a skin vesicle.

Tularemia

Tularemia is caused by a coccobacillus, *Francisella tularensis.* This is one of the most infectious pathogenic bacteria known because it takes so few (<10) of the organisms to infect someone with the disease. Infection can occur through bites from infected insects (tick, deerfly), handling of infected animal carcasses, eating or drinking contaminated food or water, or through breathing in the bacteria (most likely route in the case of a bioterrorism attack). Symptoms begin abruptly with fever, headache, chills, body aches, coryza, sore throat, cough, and chest pain/tightness. If untreated, the bacilli multiply in the skin or mucous membranes, spread to regional lymph nodes, and may disseminate to organs throughout the body. With inhalational exposure, hemorrhagic inflammation of the airways may progress to bronchopneumonia. Treatment involves antibiotics, typically parenteral streptomycin or intravenous gentamicin. However, ciprofloxacin or doxycycline would be used in case of a mass casualty situation.

Diagnostic Testing: The bacteria may be identified through direct examination of secretions, exudates, or biopsy specimens using special staining techniques. Cultures can be done on pharyngeal washings or sputum. There is also a blood test available to check for the presence of Tularemia antibody formation.

Viral Hemorrhagic Fevers

Viral hemorrhagic fevers (VHFs) include illnesses caused by certain families of viruses which typically cause multisystem damage. Symptoms vary, but may include high fever, fatigue, dizziness, muscle aches, weakness, and exhaustion. Hemorrhage may occur in the skin, in internal organs, or from body orifices. Death occurs in those who are severely ill from shock, renal failure, and nervous system dysfunction, leading to delirium, seizures, and coma. The various VHFs are similar in that humans are not the natural reservoir for these viruses. Hosts include rats, mice, and other field rodents. Ticks and mosquitoes may carry the virus from host to victim. Humans are infected when they come into contact with infected hosts. However, with some of the viruses (such as Ebola), after accidental transmission from the host, humans can transmit the virus to one another. Treatment is quite limited at this time. It is preferable to prevent VHFs through controlling rodent populations. If human infection does occur, it is essential that strict infection control techniques be used when caring for the infected individual.

Diagnostic Testing: Testing can occur through serologic testing for viral antigens and culture of biopsy material (lung, bone marrow) for virus isolation.

Normal Values

Negative for infectious agent

Possible Meanings of Abnormal Values

Presence of infectious agent

Interventions/Implications

Pretest
- Explain to the patient the purpose of the test. Provide any written teaching materials available on the subject.

Procedure
- See discussions of individual biological agents for type of testing to be done, and type of sample required.
- Appropriate personal protection is used throughout sample collection and delivery of specimen to testing facility.

Posttest
- Label the specimen and transport to laboratory as soon as possible.
- Notify the laboratory of suspected diagnosis so that special precautions can be taken when handling the specimen(s), and to assist in determining the type of procedure/staining to be used in the testing procedure.
- Gloves are worn when handling any specimen.
- Report abnormal findings to the primary care provider.

→ Clinical Alerts

- Confirmed cases of any of the above illnesses must be reported to local and state authorities, as well as the CDC.

Bleeding Time (Ivy Bleeding Time, Template Bleeding Time)

Test Description

Bleeding time measures the duration of bleeding after a standardized skin incision has been made. Commercially manufactured bleeding template devices predominate in the performance of bleeding times because of the standardization of testing that only they can provide. In addition, they are cost effective, sterile, and disposable, and reduce scarring. With the template method, one or two standardized incisions are made on the volar surface of the forearm and the time required for bleeding to stop is determined—this is the "bleeding time." The Ivy method requires three small punctures.

Bleeding time is a screening test for detecting disorders involving platelet function and for vascular (i.e., capillary) defects that interfere with the clotting process.

B

Prolonged bleeding time in the absence of a low platelet count indicates that a qualitative platelet disorder exists. The test is indicated when there is a personal or family history of bleeding tendencies and as a screening test for preoperative patients when a hemostatic defect is suspected.

Normal Values

1–9 minutes (Ivy method)

Possible Meanings of Abnormal Values

Increased (Prolonged)

Anemia due to folic acid deficiency
Aplastic anemia
Aspirin ingestion
Bone marrow disorder
Collagen vascular disease
Cushing's disease
Disseminated intravascular coagulation (DIC)
Factor VI, VII, XI deficiencies
Fibrinogen defects
Heat stroke
Hypocalcemia
Leukemia
Pernicious anemia
Renal failure
Severe liver disease
Thrombocytopenia
Uremia
Vascular abnormalities
Von Willebrand's disease

Contributing Factors to Abnormal Values

- Many variables influence the result, including skin thickness, temperature, location of incision, and presence of edema.
- Platelet counts <100,000 mm^3 and low hematocrit can alter the test result.
- Drugs that may *prolong* the bleeding time: alcohol, antibiotics, anticoagulants, antineoplastics, nitroglycerin, nonsteroidal anti-inflammatory drugs (NSAIDs), salicylates, thiazides, thrombolytics.

Interventions/Implications

Pretest

- Obtain medication history. Aspirin, anticoagulants, NSAIDs, and over-the-counter cold medications should be avoided for 7 days before the test.
- Explain the procedure to the patient.
- No fasting is required before the test.

- Advise the patient to abstain from drinking alcoholic beverages for 24 hours before the test.
- Inform the patient that scar formation may occur, especially in those patients with a history of keloid formation.

Procedure
- The volar surface of the patient's forearm should be extended and inspected for superficial veins, scarring, bruises, and swelling. The muscular portion below the elbow fold is the site of choice. If visually satisfactory, the site is cleansed with an antiseptic and allowed to air dry completely.
- A blood pressure cuff is placed on the patient's arm and inflated to 40 mm Hg. This pressure should be maintained throughout the procedure.
- The commercially manufactured bleeding template device is placed in the prepared area on the forearm. Only enough pressure is applied to ensure that the entire device is touching the skin. Too much pressure will result in an incision that is too deep.
- Activate the device and start a stopwatch.
- As drops of blood form, they (not the wound) are blotted every 30 seconds with filter paper. Care must be taken not to touch the wound at any time during testing.
- When bleeding ceases, the watch is stopped and the blood pressure cuff is released.
- If two incisions are made, they must be in the same orientation, either parallel or perpendicular to the elbow, and the individual times obtained are averaged.
- If bleeding does not stop within 15 minutes, the test should be discontinued.
- Gloves are worn throughout the procedure.

Posttest
- Butterfly bandages are placed over each cut. These should remain in place for 48 hours to minimize scarring. Assess periodically for continued bleeding.
- If the patient has bleeding tendencies, apply a pressure dressing over the butterfly bandages. The pressure dressing can be removed after 12 hours, leaving the butterfly bandages in place.
- Teach the patient to monitor the site. If the site begins to bleed, the patient should apply direct pressure and, if unable to control the bleeding, return to the laboratory or notify the primary care provider.
- Teach the patient to report if signs or symptoms of infection occur, such as drainage, redness, warmth, edema, pain at the site, or fever.
- Report abnormal findings to the primary care provider.

Clinical Alerts

- Possible complications include bleeding, scar formation, and skin infection at site of testing.

CONTRAINDICATIONS!

- Patients with platelet counts <75,000/mm^3
- Patients with edematous arms, such as postmastectomy
- Patients who are unable to cooperate during the test

Blood Culture and Sensitivity

Test Description

A blood culture is performed to detect infection in the blood. Such infections may be bacterial in origin (as with meningitis, osteomyelitis, or sepsis) or fungal (yeast). Bacteria may enter the bloodstream in a variety of ways, including invasion by bacteria through the lymphatic system from infections of the kidneys, bowel, or gallbladder; through indwelling venous or arterial catheters; or from bacterial endocarditis associated with prosthetic heart valves. When bacteria enter the bloodstream, chills and fever may occur. It is usually at this point that a blood culture is performed to confirm the presence of bacteria in the blood, a condition called *bacteremia*. Bacteria tested may include aerobic organisms such as *Staphylococcus pneumoniae*, or anaerobic, such as *Clostridium difficile*.

Once the blood sample is obtained, the blood is cultured, during which time the organisms are allowed to grow in special culture media. In 48 to 72 hours, the organism is usually identified, although fungal cultures can take up to 30 days for final results to be reported. If bacteria are found in the culture, additional sensitivity testing is done to determine the antibiotic that is most effective at killing the bacteria. The culture is considered negative for bacteria if no growth is observed after one week.

THE EVIDENCE FOR PRACTICE

Initial empirical anti-infective therapy should include one or more drugs that have activity against the likely pathogens (bacterial or fungal). Other factors to consider are the location of the presumed source of the infection and the patterns of antibiotic resistance in the institution and community. Once a causative pathogen is identified, there is no evidence that combination therapy is more effective than monotherapy. However, treatment should be guided by clinical response.

Normal Values

Negative culture (no bacteria or fungus are found)

Possible Meanings of Abnormal Values

Positive

Bacteremia

Contributing Factors to Abnormal Values

- False negatives or delayed growth may occur if antimicrobials are given prior to the specimen collection.
- Contamination of the specimen, whether from inadequate skin preparation or from drawing the blood from an intravenous line.

Interventions/Implications

Pretest

- Explain to the patient the purpose of the test and the need for a blood sample to be drawn.

- Some institutions require two samples to be drawn, each from a different site. This provides a verification of whether positive cultures are the result of contamination during sample collection or the actual presence of bacteria. Contamination will generally be cultured in one bottle, whereas pathogens will be found in both bottles.
- Sometimes two sets of blood cultures will be drawn 45 to 60 minutes apart. Additional sets may be drawn in 24 to 48 hours.
- No fasting is required for the test.
- Whenever possible, blood cultures should be obtained prior to initiating antimicrobial therapy.

Procedure
- The venipuncture site is cleansed, starting at the center and moving outward in a circular pattern. Most institutions cleanse the site with povidone-iodine (Betadine) if the patient has no allergy to this. The skin is allowed to air dry.
- The stoppers of the culture bottles are cleansed with Betadine, allowed to air dry, and then cleansed with 70% alcohol.
- A 10- to 20-mL blood sample is collected into a 20-mL syringe from each site. Institution policy should be followed for transfer of the blood from the syringe to the culture bottle. (Some institutions require a change of needle before the transfer; others use the original needle for the transfer to prevent an accidental needle stick.)
- If two culture bottles are to be inoculated, one for anaerobic and one for aerobic organisms, the anaerobic bottle is inoculated first.
- Mix the bottle(s) gently.
- Gloves are worn throughout the procedure.

Posttest
- Apply pressure at venipuncture site. Cleanse the site with alcohol to remove Betadine. Apply dressing, periodically assessing for continued bleeding.
- Label the specimens, noting whether the patient is currently taking an antimicrobial, and transport to the laboratory.

→ Clinical Alerts

- Once the specimen is obtained, the patient may be given a broad-spectrum antibiotic known to be effective against the suspected bacteria.
- The final culture and sensitivity report will note the type of organism and provide a list of antibiotics to which the organism is susceptible or resistant.
- The antibiotic the patient may be taking may need to be changed based on the sensitivity report.

Blood Smear (Peripheral Blood Smear, RBC Smear, Red Blood Cell Smear)

Test Description
There are many quantitative blood tests available to the health-care provider that provide an enormous amount of information about the various blood components. However, the blood smear, a qualitative measure, is viewed as being equally, if not more, informative.

The test involves the preparation of a smear of peripheral blood on a slide. The smear is then microscopically examined to note the appearance of the red blood cells, white blood cells, and platelets. Red blood cells are examined in terms of size, shape, color, and structure. Examination of the white blood cells provides data regarding total quantity and differential count (see "White Blood Cell Count and Differential"). Platelets are also examined for number and the presence of abnormal appearance, or thrombocytopathy.

Normal Values

Normal quantity and appearance of red blood cells, white blood cells, and platelets

Possible Meanings of Abnormal Values

White Blood Cells: See White Blood Cell Count and Differential

Platelets: See Platelet Count

Red Blood Cell Abnormalities:

Abnormal colors
Hyperchromic (highly colored due to concentrated hemoglobin) as seen in dehydration
Hypochromic (pale cells due to low hemoglobin content) as seen in anemia

Abnormal sizes
Anisocytes (vary in size): Seen in anemia
Macrocytes (large): Seen in macrocytic anemias such as pernicious anemia and folic acid deficiency, increased erythropoiesis, and postsplenectomy anemia
Microcytes (small): Seen in microcytic anemias such as iron deficiency and thalassemia major

Abnormal shapes
Ovalocytes/elliptocytes (oval or elliptical shaped cells): Seen in microcytic anemias (iron deficiency, thalassemia), megaloblastic anemia and hemoglobinopathies
Poikilocytes (irregular in shape): Seen in anemia
Schistocytes (fragmented cells noted for their unusual shapes [helmet, spirals, triangles]): Seen in hemolytic anemia, prosthetic heart valves, severe valvular heart disease, and severe burns
Sickle cells (crescent-shaped due to abnormal hemoglobin [Hb S]): Seen in sickle cell anemia
Spherocytes (small and round cells, instead of normal biconcave shape): Seen in hereditary spherocytosis and immunohemolytic anemia
Target cells (thin cells, with less hemoglobin present): Seen in hemoglobin C disease/trait, thalassemia minor, iron deficiency anemia, liver disease, and postsplenectomy

Other RBC abnormalities
Basophilic stippling (dark spots caused by abnormal hemoglobin synthesis): Seen in thalassemia and lead or heavy-metal poisoning
Heinz-Ehrlich bodies (particles of denatured hemoglobin attached to the cell membrane): Seen in congenital glucose-6-phosphate dehydrogenase deficiency, induced hemolytic anemias, and unstable hemoglobin disorders after splen

B

Howell-Jolly bodies (dark purple spherical bodies [remnants of nuclear material]): Occasionally seen in severe hemolytic anemias, pernicious anemia, leukemia, thalassemia, myelodysplasias, and in postsplenectomy

Rouleaux formation (RBCs stick to one another): Seen in cryoglobulinemia, giant cell arteritis, macroglobulinemia, and multiple myeloma

Stomatocytes (one or more slitlike areas of central pallor are present, producing a mouth-like appearance): Seen in acute alcoholism, congenital stomatocytosis, with drugs such as phenothiazines, and with neoplastic, cardiovascular, and hepatobiliary diseases

Contributing Factors to Abnormal Values

- The quality of the microscopic examination is highly dependent on the knowledge and experience of the individual performing the examination.
- Hemolysis of specimen may alter test results.

Interventions/Implications

Pretest
- Explain to the patient the purpose of the test and the need for a blood sample to be drawn.
- No fasting is required before the test.

Procedure
- The blood smear may be prepared from blood obtained from a finger or heel stick (in infant) or from venipuncture.
- If a venipuncture is used, blood is drawn in a lavender-top collection tube containing EDTA.
- Gloves are worn throughout the procedure.

Posttest
- Apply pressure at venipuncture site. Apply dressing, periodically assessing for continued bleeding.
- Report abnormal findings to the primary care provider.

→ **Clinical Alerts**

- If blood smear is found to be abnormal, follow-up testing via bone marrow aspiration or biopsy may be done.

Blood Typing (ABO Typing, ABO Red Cell Groups, Blood Groups, Rh-Typing, Type and Crossmatch, T & C, Type and Screen)

Test Description

The foundation of blood typing is the detection of ABO and Rh antigens on the red blood cells of an individual's blood. Each person has one blood type (A, B, AB, or O) which is genetically determined. These blood type designations specify the antigen present on the person's red blood cells. For example, a person with type B blood has the B antigen on the red blood cells, and someone with type O blood has no antigens.

Another important aspect of blood typing is understanding the presence of antibodies in the blood and what they mean to blood transfusion therapy. In order for someone to receive blood from a donor with a minimum of risk for a transfusion reaction, the donor's blood must have no antibodies against the recipient's red blood cells, and the recipient's blood must have no antibodies against the donor's red blood cells. For example, a person with type AB blood has no antibodies present and can therefore theoretically receive blood of any of the four blood types (A, B, AB, or O). Thus a person with type AB blood is often called the "universal recipient". A person with type O blood, on the other hand, has both anti-A and anti-B antibodies and can therefore receive only type O blood, the only type with no antigen on its red blood cells. Individuals with type O blood are referred as "universal donors", because their blood, which has no antigens present on the red blood cells, will theoretically cause no reaction when administered to any of the four blood types.

The blood types with their associated antigens and antibodies, and a synopsis of donor and recipient blood types is summarized in Table B-1. Please note that although several blood types may be listed as being appropriate for use in a transfusion for a particular blood type, this applies to small volumes of blood being received. However, when large volumes of whole blood are transfused, ABO matching is essential.

Table B-1	Blood Types			
Blood Type	**O**	**A**	**B**	**AB**
Antigen(s) present on red blood cells	None	A	B	A and B
Antibodies present	Anti-A Anti-B	Anti-B	Anti-A	None
May receive what type blood	O	A, O	B, O	A, B, AB, O
May donate blood to people of what type	A, B, AB, O	A, AB	B, AB	AB

Another component of blood typing is that of Rh-typing. *Rh factor*, also known as D factor, was so named because the rhesus monkey was used in the initial investigations into this factor. An individual is either Rh-positive or Rh-negative. The Rh-positive individual has the Rh antigen present on the red blood cells and no antibodies against the Rh factor. The Rh-negative individual has no antigens present on the red blood cells and has anti-Rh antibodies *if* previously sensitized by Rh-positive blood. In Rh-negative males, this sensitization would have occurred through transfusion with Rh-positive blood. In Rh-negative females, the sensitization could have occurred either through transfusion with Rh-positive blood, or through pregnancy in which the fetus was Rh-positive.

B

Determination of the Rh-factor is crucial for pregnant women. If the woman is Rh-negative and her partner's blood is Rh-positive, the fetus is Rh-positive. If the woman is Rh-negative, an indirect Coombs' test, which screens for Rh antibodies, is ordered. If the test is positive, Rh antibodies are present and Rh antibody titers are then obtained. If the antibody test is negative both initially and again late in the pregnancy, there is no risk to the fetus. If, however, the test is positive, the Rh-negative mother is producing antibodies against the red blood cells of the Rh-positive fetus. These antibodies may cross the placenta and cause destruction of fetal red blood cells before or during birth. This results in a hemolytic disease known as *hemolytic disease of the newborn* or *erythroblastosis fetalis*. This disease can be prevented by administering an anti-Rh antibody preparation (RhoGAM) in the third trimester of pregnancy to women at risk.

RhoGAM acts to suppress the mother's production of antibodies in response to receiving the Rh-positive antigen. RhoGAM should be given to all Rh-negative women whenever there is a possibility of fetal-maternal transplacental hemorrhage, no matter how minor. Such hemorrhage may occur as a result of chorionic villus sampling, amniocentesis, spontaneous or therapeutic abortion, or delivery.

When a person receives an incompatible type of blood, that person's antibodies attack the antigens present on the red blood cells of the donor blood. For example, a person with Type A blood has anti-B antibodies present in the blood. If this person is given type B blood, which has B antigens on the red blood cells, the recipient's anti-B antibodies will attack the donor's B antigens, resulting in a *hemolytic, or transfusion reaction*. Such a reaction can result in renal failure and death of the recipient. To avoid the occurrence of transfusion reactions, testing of both the recipient's blood and the donor's blood is done in order to ensure compatibility. Two tests which are conducted are the "type and crossmatch" and the "type and screen".

The *type and crossmatch* testing includes several components which take approximately an hour to complete. First, the ABO group and Rh-type of the recipient are determined. Next, from the donated blood supply available, donor blood of the same ABO group and Rh-type is chosen for compatibility testing. Indirect Coombs' testing, which is a general screening for antibodies, is performed on both the recipient and donor blood. More specific antibody testing may be required to identify unusual antibodies. Once these tests are completed, samples of the recipient's blood and the donor's blood are combined (crossmatched). If no antigen-antibody reaction occurs, the donor blood is considered to be compatible, and thus acceptable for transfusion into the recipient.

Type and screen testing includes only testing to determine the ABO group and Rh-type and the indirect Coombs' test. Actual crossmatching with donor blood is not performed. Type and screen testing is conducted in situations in which there is only a slight chance of the person requiring blood, or in emergency situations.

THE EVIDENCE FOR PRACTICE

The U.S. Preventive Services Task Force (USPSTF) strongly recommends Rh(D) blood typing and antibody testing for all pregnant women during their first visit for pregnancy-related care. The USPSTF found good evidence that Rh(D) blood typing, anti-Rh(D) antibody testing, and intervention with Rh(D) immunoglobulin, as appropriate, prevents maternal sensitization and improves outcomes for newborns.

Normal Values

Compatible (no antigen-antibody reactions between donor and recipient blood samples)

Contributing Factors to Abnormal Values

- Hemolysis of the blood sample may alter test results.
- Administration of Dextran or IV contrast media prior to the test may alter test results.

Interventions/Implications

Pretest
- Explain to the patient the purpose of the test and the need for a blood sample to be drawn.
- No fasting is required prior to the test.
- The blood sample should be drawn before administration of Dextran, a plasma volume expander.

Procedure
- A 10-mL blood sample is drawn in a lavender-top (EDTA) collection tube.
- Gloves are worn throughout the procedure.

Posttest
- Apply pressure at venipuncture site. Apply dressing, periodically assessing for continued bleeding.
- Label the specimen and transport it to the laboratory.
- Report ABO group and Rh type to the primary care provider.

→ Clinical Alerts

- Avoidance of errors is essential. Typically when blood is drawn for a type and cross-match, a blood bank identification band is applied to the patient's wrist. This band can be compared to blood products to be administered to the patient.
- Follow institutional policy regarding identification of the patient prior to blood administration. Typically two health-care providers must verify that the blood group and Rh type of the recipient and donor are compatible and that the proper unit of blood is being used prior to blood administration.

 ## Bone Marrow Biopsy (Bone Marrow Aspiration)

Test Description

Bone marrow is the soft, sponge-like material contained in the medullary canals of the long bones and within the spaces between trabeculae of cancellous bone. The primary function of the bone marrow is the production of erythrocytes, leukocytes, and platelets. When abnormal types or numbers of cells are found in a complete blood count or the health-care provider needs to evaluate whether there might be a systemic disease present in the bone marrow, a bone marrow biopsy and/or aspiration is performed. In this procedure, a sample of the bone marrow is removed via a needle inserted through the cortex of the bone and into the bone marrow. An aspiration of liquid bone marrow may also be performed. The preferred site for the bone marrow biopsy/aspiration is the iliac crest, although the sternum is also occasionally used.

THE EVIDENCE FOR PRACTICE

Bone marrow biopsy should be performed on patients with an abnormal complete blood count, general symptoms such as fever, night sweats, weight loss, fatigue, and appetite loss, elevated alkaline phosphatase, or symptoms of bone pain.

Normal Values

Red marrow contains connective tissue, fat cells, and hematopoietic cells. Yellow marrow contains connective tissue and fat cells.

Possible Meanings of Abnormal Values

Agranulocytosis
Amyloidosis
Cancer
Depressed hematopoiesis
Granuloma
Infection
Infectious mononucleosis
Iron deficiency anemia
Leukemia
Lymphoma
Multiple myeloma
Myelodysplastic syndrome
Myelofibrosis
Platelet dysfunction
Polycythemia vera
Sideroblastic anemia
Thalassemia

Interventions/Implications

Pretest
- Explain to the patient the purpose of the test. Provide any written teaching materials available on the subject. Note that discomfort during the test is due to the injection of the local anesthetic and removal of the marrow sample. Pressure may be felt during insertion of the biopsy needle.
- Obtain baseline data regarding coagulation, such as prothrombin time, partial thromboplastin time, and platelet count.
- No fasting is required prior to the test.
- Obtain a signed informed consent.
- Administer a sedative prior to the procedure, if ordered.

Procedure
- The procedure is usually done at the bedside with the patient in the prone or lateral position.
- The skin overlying the proposed site of the aspiration is cleansed and draped. A local anesthetic is administered to the area. A very small incision may be made.
- A large-bore needle is slowly advanced through the incision, subcutaneous tissue, and the cortex of the bone. Once inside the marrow, the stylet is removed from the needle, and a syringe is attached.
- A sample of 0.5 to 2 mL of liquid bone marrow is aspirated and slide preparation is completed.
- The biopsy needle is then advanced and rotated in both directions, forcing a sample of the bone marrow into the needle.
- The needle is then withdrawn, with pressure applied to the site for 10 to 15 minutes. The sample is forced out of the needle and into a specimen jar containing fixative.
- A sterile dressing is applied to the biopsy site.
- Gloves are worn throughout the procedure.

Posttest
- Observe the puncture site for bleeding.
- Assess for signs of infection: tenderness and erythema at the site, fever.
- Assess for signs of hemorrhage: increased pulse rate, decreased blood pressure, pain.
- Ideally, the patient should maintain bedrest for at least 1 hour. However, this procedure is now often done in clinic settings where this is not practical.
- Label the specimen and transport it to the laboratory immediately.
- Report abnormal findings to the primary care provider.

→ Clinical Alerts

- Possible complications include: Hemorrhage from the puncture site and infection at the site.

CONTRAINDICATIONS!

- Patients with bleeding disorders
- Patients unable to cooperate with the examination

Bone Mineral Density (BMD, Bone Densitometry)

Test Description
Osteoporosis and osteopenia (low bone mass) involve bone loss, placing the individual at risk of fracture. Oftentimes, testing is done after a fracture has occurred. However, diagnosis of osteoporosis should be made before the first fracture occurs, so that preventive measures such as lifestyle changes and pharmacologic treatment

B

can be initiated. Women who are over 65 years of age, with a history of bone fracture after age 40, family history of osteoporosis, with low estrogen levels (or early menopause before age 45), low body weight, and who smoke are at higher risk of osteoporosis. Men can also have osteoporosis and have increased risk with alcoholism, steroid therapy, low testosterone levels, and smoking.

The only way to diagnose osteoporosis is through measurement of bone mineral density (BMD). This is most commonly done through use of dual-energy x-ray absorptiometry (DEXA). DEXA uses x-ray at two energy levels to determine the bone mineral content. Less precise BMD testing techniques include peripheral DXA (assessing the radius or calcaneus), quantitative computer tomography (QCT) which requires high doses of radiation, and ultrasonometry which assesses the heel, fingers, and tibia. The scanner software then calculates the bone mineral density, by dividing the bone mineral content by the area of the region of interest. The areas typically measured are the first four lumbar vertebrae and the proximal femur (femoral neck and trochanteric areas). The results are expressed in T-scores and Z-scores. The T-score is the number of standard deviations above or below the mean value for young adult reference data. This is considered the reference for "peak bone mass." The Z-score is the number of standard deviations between the mean for an age-matched population. The World Health Organization (WHO) uses T-scores to define normal bone mass, low bone mass (or osteopenia), and osteoporosis. (See "Normal Values.") T-scores are expressed in standard deviations (SD); the more negative the number, the greater the risk of fracture. Each SD represents a 10% to 12% bone loss.

In addition to suggested screening for women aged 65 or older, BMD testing is recommended for the following clinical indications:
- Estrogen deficiency
- Prolonged glucocorticoid therapy
- Osteopenia
- Fracture
- Primary hyperparathyroidism
- Monitoring antiresorptive therapy

THE EVIDENCE FOR PRACTICE

The U.S. Preventive Services Task Force (USPSTF) recommends that women aged 65 and older be screened routinely for osteoporosis. The USPSTF recommends that routine screening begin at age 60 for women at increased risk for osteoporotic fractures.
- Lower body weight (weight<70 kg) is the single best predictor of low bone mineral density. Low weight and no current use of estrogen therapy are incorporated with age into the 3-item Osteoporosis Risk Assessment Instrument (ORAI). There is less evidence to support the use of other individual risk factors (for example, smoking, weight loss, family history, decreased physical activity, alcohol or caffeine use, or low calcium and vitamin D intake) as a basis for identifying high-risk women under age 65. At any given age, African American women on average have higher bone mineral density (BMD) than white women and are thus less likely to benefit from screening.

Normal Values

WHO guidelines state:

Normal bone mass	T score of −1.0 through +1.0 SDs
Osteopenia	T score of −2.5 through −1.0 SDs
Osteoporosis	T score of −4.0 through −2.5 SDs

Possible Meanings of Abnormal Values

Demineralization due to immobilization
Estrogen deficiency
Hyperparathyroidism
Inadequate calcium intake
Long-term corticosteroid therapy
Malabsorption
Osteopenia
Osteoporosis
Renal insufficiency

Contributing Factors to Abnormal Values

- BMD results may be affected by nuclear scans within previous 3 days or barium studies within previous 7 to 10 days.
- Metallic implants may affect the BMD imaging.
- Absence of normal structures, such as after laminectomy, can affect BMD results

Interventions/Implications

Pretest
- Explain to the patient the purpose of the test. Provide any written teaching materials available on the subject.
- The patient must remain still while the scan is being performed.
- No fasting is required before the test.

Procedure
- The patient is assisted to a supine position on the examination table.
- A positioning pillow is used to hold the legs in position for the testing. The leg must be somewhat internally rotated to provide the best image of the femoral area.
- The testing takes approximately 10 minutes.

Posttest
- A computer printout of the images, along with T-scores, Z-scores, and interpretation are provided.
- Report abnormal findings to the primary care provider.

→ Clinical Alerts

- To help prevent osteoporosis, all adults should obtain adequate amounts of calcium (1200 mg/day) and vitamin D (400 to 800 IU/day), engage in regular weight-bearing exercise, and avoid tobacco smoking or alcohol abuse.
- Follow-up BMD testing is recommended every 2 years.

B

Bone Scan (Bone Scintigraphy)

Test Description

The primary purpose for performing a bone scan is to detect metastatic cancer of the bone. It is also used to monitor the progression of degenerative bone disorders. Another use of a bone scan is to detect fractures in patients who continue to have pain, even though x-rays have proven negative. Further testing is warranted when abnormal findings are discovered in a bone scan, since the test is not specific. That is, all abnormalities are shown by increased radionuclide uptake, but the type of abnormality is not differentiated by the scan.

During a bone scan, the patient is given a radionuclide compound, usually a radiopharmaceutical such as technetium-99m, via an IV injection. One to three hours later, a scintillation camera is used to take a radioactivity reading from the bone. These readings are fed into a computer, which translates these readings into a two-dimensional gray scale picture. Normally the bone has a fairly consistent uptake of the radionuclide, with the exception of areas of growing bone (epiphyseal plate). Such areas show as very dark spots on the scintigram and are called **hot spots** because more of the radionuclide was deposited in that spot. Hot spots may be caused by such abnormalities as arthritis, fractures, osteomyelitis, and tumors. Spots without radionuclide uptake are known as **cold spots**.

Normal Values

Normal patterns of bone uptake of the radionuclide

Possible Meanings of Abnormal Values

Bone necrosis
Bone tumors
Degenerative arthritis
Fracture
Metastatic bone neoplasm
Osteomyelitis
Paget's disease
Primary bone malignancy
Renal osteodystrophy
Rheumatoid arthritis

Contributing Factors to Abnormal Values

- Any movement by the patient may alter quality of films taken.

Interventions/Implications

Pretest

- Explain to the patient the purpose of the test. Provide any written teaching materials available on the subject. Note that discomfort involved with this test is primarily due to lying on a hard table for an extended period of time and the needle puncture. Reassure the patient that only trace amounts of the radionuclide are involved in the test.
- The patient must remain still while the scan is being performed.
- No fasting is required prior to the test.
- Obtain a signed informed consent.

Procedure

- A radionuclide such as ^{99m}Tc is administered by IV injection into a peripheral vein.
- The patient is to drink 4 to 6 glasses of water during the time between receiving the injection and undergoing the scan. This will help clear the body of excess radionuclide which the bone will not take up.
- Depending on the reason for the test, images may be taken shortly after the radionuclide is administered and again 3 to 4 hours later (if evaluating for infection) or only 3 to 4 hours after the radionuclide administration.
- The patient is to urinate just prior to the examination.
- The patient is assisted to a supine position on the examination table.
- A scintillation camera is positioned over the patient's body. This camera takes a radioactivity reading from the body. This information is transformed into a two-dimensional picture of the skeleton.
- Depending on the area of interest needing to be scanned, the patient may be placed in the prone and/or lateral positions for additional pictures to be taken.
- Gloves are worn during the radionuclide injection.

Posttest

- Check the injection site for redness or swelling.
- Although the amount of diagnostic radionuclide excreted in the urine is low, the urine should not be used for any laboratory tests for the time period indicated by the Nuclear Medicine Department.
- Encourage fluid intake by the patient to enhance excretion of the radionuclide.
- Report abnormal findings to the primary care provider.

→ Clinical Alerts

- Reactions to the radionuclide are rare. However, the patient should be monitored for rash, swelling, or anaphylaxis.
- If a woman who is lactating *must* have a nuclear scan, she should not breast-feed the infant until the radionuclide has been eliminated, possibly for 3 days.
- No other radionuclide tests should be scheduled for 24 to 48 hours.

CONTRAINDICATIONS!

- Pregnant women
  - Caution: A woman in her childbearing years should undergo radiography only during her menses or 12 to 14 days after its onset to avoid any exposure to a fetus.

B

- Patients who are lactating
- Patients who are unable to cooperate due to age, mental status, pain, or other factors

 Brain Scan (Cerebral Blood Flow)

Test Description

Normally, there is an impediment to blood coming in contact with the brain tissue. This hindrance is known as the **blood-brain barrier**. It is this barrier which normally prevents radionuclides from being taken up by the brain. However, in pathologic conditions, the blood-brain barrier is interrupted, allowing the radionuclide to become concentrated in the abnormal areas of the brain.

The primary use of the brain scan is to assess for brain abscesses, tumors, contusions, hematomas, and cerebral vascular accidents. An immediate scan after the injection of the radionuclide will show differences in the cerebral blood flow between the two sides of the brain. Allowing some time between the injection and the scanning will show pathogenic tissue. Such tissue will appear as a **hot spot** because more of the radionuclide will be deposited in that spot. Although a commonly used diagnostic test in the past, the brain scan is steadily being replaced with computed tomography and magnetic resonance imaging. However, it is still a useful test for determining brain death.

Normal Values

Normal cerebral blood flow
Normal distribution of radionuclide within the brain

Possible Meanings of Abnormal Values

Alzheimer's disease
Aneurysm
AV malformation
Brain abscess
Brain death
Brain tumor
Cerebral hemorrhage
Cerebral thrombosis
Cerebral vascular accident
Cerebrospinal spinal fluid leak
Contusion of the brain
Dementia
Hematoma
Huntington's disease
Metastatic cancer of the brain
Parkinson's disease
Seizure disorders

Contributing Factors to Abnormal Values

- Any movement by the patient may alter quality of films taken.

Interventions/Implications

Pretest

- Explain to the patient or family the purpose of the test. Provide any written teaching materials available on the subject. Note that discomfort involved with this test is primarily due to lying on a hard table for an extended period of time and the needle puncture. Reassure the patient that only trace amounts of the radionuclide are involved in the test.
- The patient must remain still while the scan is being performed.
- No fasting is required prior to the test.
- Obtain a signed informed consent.
- Depending on the type of radionuclide to be used for the test, potassium chloride, a blocking agent, may be administered by mouth 2 hours prior to the test to prevent an unusually high level of radionuclide uptake by the choroid plexus, which would mimic a pathologic condition in the brain.

Procedure

- The patient is assisted to a supine position on the examination table, with the scintillation camera positioned over the patient's head. This camera takes a radioactivity reading from the body. This information is transformed into a two-dimensional picture of the brain.
- A radionuclide such as ^{99m}Tc is administered by IV injection into a peripheral vein.
- The scan is started immediately to provide a study of the cerebral blood flow.
- The scan is repeated 1 hour later to detect the presence of pathogenic tissue.
- Gloves are worn during the radionuclide injection.

Posttest

- Check the injection site for redness or swelling.
- Although the amount of diagnostic radionuclide excreted in the urine is low, the urine should not be used for any laboratory tests for the time period indicated by the Nuclear Medicine Department.
- Encourage fluid intake by the patient to enhance excretion of the radionuclide.
- Report abnormal findings to the primary care provider.

→ Clinical Alerts

- If a woman who is lactating *must* have a nuclear scan, she should not breast-feed the infant until the radionuclide has been eliminated, possibly for 3 days.
- No other radionuclide tests should be scheduled for 24 to 48 hours.

CONTRAINDICATIONS!

- Pregnant women
  - Caution: A woman in her childbearing years should undergo radiography only during her menses or 12 to 14 days after its onset to avoid any exposure to a fetus.
- Patients who are lactating
- Patients who are unable to cooperate due to age, mental status, pain, or other factors

B

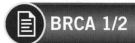 **BRCA 1/2**

Test Description

Among all cases of breast cancer in women, approximately 5% to 10% involve a hereditary form of the disease. Most of these hereditary cases are due to mutations in breast cancer (BRCA 1 or BRCA 2) genes. There is a higher risk of these mutations in Eastern European Jewish women. These mutations are also associated with increased risk of ovarian cancer in women and breast cancer in men. Women with altered BRCA 1 or 2 genes have a lifetime risk for developing breast cancer of up to 85% (compared to 13% for women without BRCA mutations). Ovarian cancer risk is up to 60% compared to 2% in the general population.

BRCA genes are present in all cells of the body. Proteins of the BRCA genes affect only breast and ovarian tissue. The test involves checking a sample of DNA from white blood cells for the presence of BRCA mutations. Individuals considering undergoing this test should not do so lightly. Counseling should be offered regarding what test results will mean, what options are available for prevention of cancer, and the ramifications of having the test information in the medical record. However, the testing should be considered for women with close male/female relatives with breast cancer or female relatives with ovarian cancer. This is especially important if the cancer was diagnosed before age 50. Some individuals with positive test results may choose to have prophylactic surgery, although this does not guarantee that the cancer will not appear in remaining tissue. Due to the high risk of breast cancer in these women, consideration might be given to adding breast magnetic resonance imaging (MRI) to mammography for cancer screening; however, risk-benefit, and cost analysis is needed.

THE EVIDENCE FOR PRACTICE

- The USPSTF recommends against routine referral for genetic counseling or routine *breast cancer susceptibility genes (BRCA)* testing for women whose family history is not associated with an increased risk for deleterious mutations in *breast cancer susceptibility gene 1 (BRCA1)* or *breast cancer susceptibility gene 2 (BRCA2)*.
- The USPSTF recommends that women whose family history is associated with an increased risk for deleterious mutations in *BRCA1* or *BRCA2* genes be referred for genetic counseling and evaluation for *BRCA* testing.

Normal Values

Normal BRCA genes

Possible Meanings of Abnormal Values

Positive	Negative
Increased risk of developing breast and/or ovarian cancer	Not at risk for hereditary breast cancer due to BRCA mutations (can develop other types)

Interventions/Implications

Pretest
- Explain to the patient the purpose of the test and the need for a blood sample to be drawn.
- No fasting is required before the test.

Procedure
- A 7-mL blood sample is drawn in a red-top collection tube.
- Gloves are worn throughout the procedure.

Posttest
- Apply pressure at venipuncture site. Apply dressing, periodically assessing for continued bleeding.
- Label the specimen and transport it to the laboratory.
- Report abnormal findings to the primary care provider.

→ Clinical Alerts

- Patients considering BRCA testing should receive pretest counseling to discuss the possible ramifications of having genetic information in their medical record.
- Individuals with positive BRCA mutations should receive counseling regarding surveillance and risk avoidance.

Breast Biopsy (Core Needle Biopsy, Fine Needle Aspiration)

Test Description
Several diagnostic tests, including mammography and sonography, are used in the evaluation of breast masses. However, determination of whether a mass is malignant can only be made by obtaining a biopsy of the tissue. The tissue sample may be obtained via needle aspiration, by core biopsy, or by open incision. Breast biopsy is also used when there has been an observable change in the breast, such as skin ulceration or nipple drainage.

THE EVIDENCE FOR PRACTICE
Large core imaging-guided breast biopsy is now the technique of choice in many institutions in the United States for biopsy of nonpalpable breast masses and abnormal calcifications. Either stereotactic or ultrasound-guided breast biopsy may be used for reliable diagnosis of breast cancer.

Normal Values
No abnormal cells or tissue present

Possible Meanings of Abnormal Values
Adenofibroma
Breast cancer

B

Fibrocystic disease
Inflammatory breast cancer
Intraductal papilloma
Mammary fat necrosis
Plasma cell mastitis

Interventions/Implications

Pretest

- Explain to the patient the purpose of the test and the procedure to be done.
- The biopsy is usually obtained using a local anesthetic, although general anesthesia is an option.
- No fasting is required prior to the test, unless general anesthesia is to be used.
- Obtain a signed informed consent.

Procedure

- The patient is assisted to a supine position.
- The skin is cleansed with an antiseptic and draped.
- A local anesthetic is typically administered.
- Gloves are worn throughout the procedure.

For a needle biopsy

- For a fine needle aspiration biopsy, a needle is inserted into the mass, and a sample of tissue or fluid is aspirated into the syringe. A slide of the aspirate is made for cytology review. A sterile dressing is applied.
- For a core needle biopsy, a very small incision is made and multiple samples are taken of the lesion using a commercially available device. This device is spring-loaded and allows the health-care provider to obtain samples which fill the needle core. The tissue specimens are placed in a specimen container with normal saline solution or formaldehyde. Steri-strips and a sterile pressure dressing are applied to the incision.

For an open biopsy

- An incision is made in the breast to expose the mass.
- The mass is then excised in entirety if it is smaller than 2 cm in size. If the mass is larger or appears malignant, a portion of the mass is excised.
- The tissue specimen is placed in a specimen container with normal saline solution or formaldehyde.
- If the mass appears malignant, the tissue sample is sent for frozen section and receptor assays. Do *not* place tissue for receptor assay testing in formaldehyde.
- The wound is sutured, and a sterile dressing is applied.

Posttest

- For biopsy under local anesthesia, check vital signs after the procedure. If general anesthesia was used, check vital signs every 15 minutes for the first hour, every 30 minutes for the next hour after that, every hour for 4 additional hours, and then every 4 hours.
- Check the dressing for drainage.
- Teach the patient to monitor the site and to notify the health-care provider if signs or symptoms of infection occur, such as drainage, redness, warmth, edema, pain at the site, or fever.
- Administer analgesics as needed.
- Provide emotional support as the patient awaits test results.
- Report abnormal findings to the primary care provider.

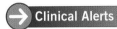

Clinical Alerts

- The finding of an abnormality in the breast and then waiting for test results can be quite anxiety-producing for the patient. If possible, schedule testing (mammography and sonography) on the same day and at a time when a specially-trained radiologist would be available to perform a needle biopsy, if warranted.
- Potential complication of the procedure is infection.

CONTRAINDICATIONS!

- Patients unable to cooperate with the examination

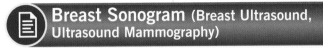

Breast Sonogram (Breast Ultrasound, Ultrasound Mammography)

Test Description

Ultrasonography is a noninvasive method of diagnostic testing in which ultrasound waves are sent into the body with a small transducer pressed against the skin. The transducer then receives any returning sound waves, which are deflected back as they bounce off various structures. The transducer converts the returning sound waves into electric signals that are then transformed by a computer into a visual display on a monitor.

In this particular type of ultrasonography, the transducer is passed over all of the skin of each breast. The purpose is to detect and measure breast cysts and tumors. It is especially useful for screenings of young women with a family history of breast cancer, for screenings when mammography is not available, for use in pregnant women and in others who must avoid radiation, in women who refuse mammography for a variety of reasons, and in women who have silicone breast implants. It is also helpful in the assessment of women with very dense breast tissue and in those with fibrocystic breast disease. The sonogram is often used in conjunction with mammography when there is a palpable mass on physical examination, if something abnormal is noted on the mammogram, or if the patient is complaining of pain, redness, or swelling of the breast. It is also used to guide breast biopsies and fine needle aspirations of cysts. In women with fibrocystic breast disease, the water path method of ultrasonography may be used.

THE EVIDENCE FOR PRACTICE

Using magnification mammography and ultrasound, patients with tumors suitable for breast conservation can be identified with at least 95% certainty preoperatively.

Normal Values

Normal breast tissue

B

Possible Meanings of Abnormal Values

Breast cancer
Cyst
Fibroadenoma
Fibrocystic breast disease
Hematoma
Infection/abscess

Contributing Factors to Abnormal Values

- The transducer must be in good contact with the skin as it is being moved.

Interventions/Implications

Pretest

- Explain to the patient the purpose of the test. Provide any written teaching materials available on the subject. Note that there is no discomfort involved with this test unless there is an underlying infection or if there is premenstrual breast tenderness.
- No fasting is required before the test.
- Inform patient of need to remove clothes above the waist during the procedure.
- The patient should use no deodorants, powders, or lotions during the days of the procedure, especially if a mammogram is also being performed that day.

Procedure

- The patient is assisted to a supine position on the ultrasonography table. Some minor position changes may be needed during the exam in order to provide the best view of the breast tissue.
- A coupling agent, such as a water-based gel, is applied to the area to be evaluated.
- A transducer is placed on the skin and moved as needed to provide good visualization of the breast tissue.
- The sound waves are transformed into a visual display on the monitor. Printed copies of this display are made.
- For the water path method, the patient is positioned prone on a special bed with the breast suspended into heated water. The scanning is performed through the water by a transducer located at the bottom of the water tank.

Posttest

- Cleanse the patient's skin of remaining coupling agent, if used.
- Report abnormal findings to the primary care provider.

→ Clinical Alerts

- Palpation of a mass in the breast can cause the patient to be quite anxious regarding the possible outcome of diagnostic testing.
- Whenever possible, schedule all of the testing on one day. In some facilities, a radiologist may be available to aspirate cysts or perform biopsies of solid masses while the patient remains in the ultrasound area.

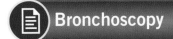

Bronchoscopy

B

Test Description

Bronchoscopy is the direct visualization of the larynx, trachea, and bronchi through use of either a rigid bronchoscope (which requires general anesthesia) or, more frequently, a flexible fiberoptic bronchoscope (using local anesthesia). The scope is less than $1/2$ inch in diameter and approximately 2 feet long. This procedure is used diagnostically to visually examine abnormalities found on x-ray and to obtain sputum specimens for bacteriologic and cytologic examination. Tissue biopsy may also be done. Therapeutically, the procedure can be used to control tracheobronchial bleeding, to remove foreign bodies, to conduct endobronchial radiation therapy, to obliterate neoplastic obstruction through use of a laser, and to place a stent in the airway.

THE EVIDENCE FOR PRACTICE

In patients suspected of having small cell lung cancer based on the radiographic and clinical findings, the diagnosis should be obtained by whatever method is easiest (i.e., sputum cytology, fine needle aspiration, and bronchoscopy), as dictated by the patient's presentation.

Normal Values

Normal larynx, trachea, bronchi, and alveoli

Possible Meanings of Abnormal Values

Carcinoma
Foreign body
Hemorrhage
Infection
Inflammation
Lung abscess
Sarcoidosis
Strictures
Superior vena cava obstruction
Tracheal stenosis
Tuberculosis

Interventions/Implications

Pretest

- Explain to the patient the purpose of the test. Provide any written teaching materials available on the subject. Note that a local anesthetic will be used in the throat. Reassure the patient that breathing will not be obstructed during the procedure.
- Obtain a signed informed consent.
- Fasting for 8 to 12 hours is required prior to the test.

B

- Administer preprocedure medications as ordered. An anticholinergic such as atropine may be used to decrease bronchial secretions. A medication such as midazolam may be used for sedation and relief of anxiety.
- Dentures are removed.
- Resuscitation and suctioning equipment should be readily available.

Procedure
- The patient is assisted to either a sitting or supine position.
- A local anesthetic is sprayed into the patient's throat.
- The bronchoscope is then introduced through the patient's mouth or nose. When it is located just above the vocal cords, more local anesthetic is sprayed into the trachea to anesthetize deeper areas and to inhibit the cough reflex.
- The anatomy of the trachea and bronchi is inspected. Biopsy forceps may be used to remove a tissue specimen, or a bronchial brush may be used to obtain cells from the surface of a lesion.
- Lavage of the lungs may also be done. This involved instilling saline solution through the scope into the lungs, which is then removed, providing samples of lung cells, fluids, and any other materials inside the lungs.
- Removal of foreign bodies or mucous plugs is accomplished, if needed.
- Gloves are worn throughout the procedure.

Posttest
- Monitor vital signs until stable.
- Withhold fluids and food until the gag reflex returns (approximately 2 hours).
- Provide an emesis basis for the patient. Instruct the patient to spit out saliva rather than swallow it until the gag reflex returns. Observe the sputum for frank bleeding.
- Observe for and immediately report indications of respiratory dysfunction: laryngeal stridor, dyspnea, cyanosis, diminished breath sounds, and wheezing. Assess for presence of subcutaneous crepitus around the face and neck, which would indicate tracheal or bronchial perforation.
- Inform the patient that normal temporary consequences of the procedure include hoarseness, loss of voice, and sore throat.
- Label the specimen and transport it to the laboratory immediately.
- Report abnormal findings to the primary care provider.

→ Clinical Alerts

- Possible complications of the procedure include: aspiration, bacteremia, bronchial or tracheal perforation, bronchospasm, cardiac arrhythmias, fever, hemorrhage from biopsy site, hypoxemia, laryngospasm, pneumonia, and pneumothorax.

CONTRAINDICATIONS!

- Patients with severe respiratory failure
- Patients who cannot tolerate interruption of high-flow oxygen

CA 15-3 (Cancer Antigen 15-3, CA 15-3 Tumor Marker)

Test Description

A tumor marker is a substance produced by body cells in response to the presence of cancer. Cancer antigen 15-3 (CA 15-3) is a glycoprotein that has been found in benign and malignant disease of the breast, as well as breast carcinoma that has metastasized to the liver or bone. Highest CA 15-3 values are found in metastatic breast disease. Testing for CA 15-3 is useful in the diagnosis of metastatic breast cancer and for the monitoring of patient response to breast cancer treatment. Because CA 15-3 values may not increase in early malignancy of the breast, it is not useful as a screening test. Elevated CA 15-3 levels have also been found in patients without cancer and in patients with other cancers such as liver, lung, and ovarian cancer.

The higher the CA 15-3 level, the more advanced the breast cancer and greater likelihood of metastasis. Mild to moderate elevation of this marker can also be seen in some noncancerous conditions, such as cirrhosis.

THE EVIDENCE FOR PRACTICE

According to the American Society of Clinical Oncology, present data are insufficient to recommend CA 15-3 or CA 27.29 for screening, diagnosis, staging, or surveillance following primary treatment.

Normal Values

<22 U/mL (<22 kU/L SI units)

Possible Meanings of Abnormal Values

Increased

Breast cancer
Chronic hepatitis
Cirrhosis
Colorectal cancer
Fibrocystic breast disease
Liver cancer
Lung cancer
Metastatic breast cancer
Ovarian cancer
Pancreatic cancer
Sarcoidosis
Systemic lupus erythematosus

Interventions/Implications

Pretest

- Explain to the patient the purpose of the test and the need for a blood sample to be drawn.
- No fasting is required before the test.

Procedure
- A 5-mL blood sample is collected in a red-top tube.
- Gloves are worn throughout the procedure.

Posttest
- Apply pressure at venipuncture site. Apply dressing, periodically assessing for continued bleeding.
- The sample is labeled and transported to the laboratory.
- Report abnormal findings to the primary care provider.

→ Clinical Alerts

- CA 15-3 levels in noncancerous conditions have a tendency to remain stable over time, whereas in metastatic breast cancer, the levels continue to rise.
- Normal CA 15-3 values may occur early in breast cancer.

📄 CA 19-9 (Cancer Antigen 19-9, CA 19-9 Tumor Marker)

Test Description
A tumor marker is a substance produced by body cells in response to the presence of cancer. Cancer antigen 19-9 (CA 19-9) is an antigen that has been found elevated in patients with tumors of the gastrointestinal tract. This test is especially useful in the diagnosis of pancreatic cancer. CA 19-9 is neither sensitive nor specific enough to be used for cancer screening. However, monitoring the CA 19-9 levels can be useful in assessing the effectiveness of treatment for pancreatic cancer and watching for cancer recurrence. The highest levels of CA 19-9 are seen in excretory ductal pancreatic cancer. Unfortunately, by the time symptoms are present and the CA 19-9 is elevated, the pancreatic cancer may be quite advanced.

THE EVIDENCE FOR PRACTICE
The U.S. Preventive Services Task Force (USPSTF) recommends against routine screening for pancreatic cancer in asymptomatic adults using abdominal palpation, ultrasonography, or serologic markers.

Normal Values
<37 U/mL (<37 kU/L SI units)

Possible Meanings of Abnormal Values

Increased

Cholecystitis
Cholelithiasis
Cirrhosis
Colorectal cancer

Cystic fibrosis
Gall bladder cancer
Gastric cancer
Hepatobiliary cancer
Liver disease
Lung cancer
Pancreatic cancer
Pancreatitis

Interventions/Implications

Pretest
- Explain to the patient the purpose of the test and the need for a blood sample to be drawn.
- No fasting is required before the test.

Procedure
- A 5-mL blood sample is collected in a red-top tube.
- Gloves are worn throughout the procedure.

Posttest
- Apply pressure at venipuncture site. Apply dressing, periodically assessing for continued bleeding.
- The sample is labeled and transported to the laboratory.
- Report abnormal findings to the primary care provider.

Clinical Alerts

- Further diagnostic testing may include CT (computed tomographic) scan, ultrasound, MRI (magnetic resonance imaging), ERCP (endoscopic retrograde cholangiopancreatography), and/or biopsy.

CA-125 (Cancer Antigen 125, CA-125 Tumor Marker)

Test Description
A tumor marker is a substance produced by body cells in response to the presence of cancer. Cancer antigen-125 (CA-125) is a glycoprotein normally present in endometrial tissue and in uterine fluid. It is *not* normally found in the bloodstream. It is only when there has been destruction of such tissue, as through endometrial or ovarian cancer, that CA-125 is detectible in the blood. There is a high incidence of false results with this test, making it inappropriate for use as a screening tool. The test is used to monitor response to treatment for ovarian cancer and to detect recurrence of the cancer. It is also sometimes used to monitor high-risk women who have a family history of ovarian cancer but do not yet have the disease.

THE EVIDENCE FOR PRACTICE
There is no existing evidence that any screening test, including CA-125, ultrasound, or pelvic examination, reduces mortality from ovarian cancer. Furthermore, existing evidence

that screening can detect early-stage ovarian cancer is insufficient to indicate that this earlier diagnosis will reduce mortality.

Normal Values

<35 U/mL (<35 kU/L SI units)

Possible Meanings of Abnormal Values

Increased
Acute pancreatitis
Breast cancer
Cirrhosis
Colon neoplasm
Endometrial cancer
Endometriosis
Fallopian tube cancer
Liver cancer
Lung cancer
Menstruation
Ovarian cancer
Pancreatic cancer
Pancreatitis
Pelvic inflammatory disease
Peritonitis
Pregnancy
Uterine cancer

Interventions/Implications

Pretest
- Explain to the patient the purpose of the test and the need for a blood sample to be drawn.
- No fasting is required before the test.

Procedure
- A 5-mL blood sample is collected in a red-top tube.
- Gloves are worn throughout the procedure.

Posttest
- Apply pressure at venipuncture site. Apply dressing, periodically assessing for continued bleeding.
- The sample is labeled and transported to the laboratory.
- Report abnormal findings to the primary care provider.

Clinical Alerts

- Patients at risk for ovarian cancer include those of low parity, decreased fertility, and delayed childbearing, with incidence increasing with age. The strongest predictor for ovarian cancer is familial evidence of ovarian cancer.

Calcitonin (Thyrocalcitonin)

C

Test Description

Calcitonin, a polypeptide hormone secreted by the C cells of the thyroid, assists in the regulation of serum calcium and phosphorus levels. When an elevated level of calcium is present in the blood (hypercalcemia), calcitonin is secreted. This results in inhibition of calcium absorption from the gastrointestinal tract, inhibition of calcium resorption from the bone by osteoclasts and osteocytes, and increased excretion of calcium by the kidneys. These actions are antagonistic to parathyroid hormone and result in lower serum calcium levels. The test is used primarily to evaluate suspected medullary carcinoma of the thyroid (MTC), which is characterized by hypersecretion of calcitonin in the presence of normal serum calcium levels. In some patients who have medullary cancer of the thyroid, the fasting level of calcitonin is normal. If this occurs, a provocative testing involving intravenous pentagastrin or calcium administration is used.

THE EVIDENCE FOR PRACTICE

Although studies have suggested that, in the evaluation of a thyroid nodule, the routine measurement of serum calcitonin is a cost-effective and important technique to avoid missing medullary thyroid cancer, not all clinicians agree that screening calcitonin is useful.

Normal Values

Basal:
     Female: <14 pg/mL (<14 ng/L SI units)
     Male: <19 pg/mL (<19 ng/L SI units)
Postcalcium infusion (administered at 2.4 mg/kg):
     Female: <130 pg/mL (<130 ng/L SI units)
     Male: <190 pg/mL (<190 ng/L SI units)
Postpentagastrin injection (administered at 0.5 mcg/kg):
     Female: <35 pg/mL (<35 ng/L SI units)
     Male: <110 pg/mL (<110 ng/L SI units)

Possible Meanings of Abnormal Values

Increased

Alcoholic cirrhosis
Breast cancer
C-cell hyperplasia
Chronic renal failure
Cushing's disease
Ectopic calcitonin production (as with pancreatic cancer)
Hypercalcemia
Islet cell tumors
Lung cancer (oat cell)

Medullary thyroid cancer
Parathyroid adenoma
Parathyroid hyperplasia
Pernicious anemia
Pheochromocytoma
Thyroiditis
Uremia
Zollinger-Ellison syndrome

Contributing Factors to Abnormal Values

- Drugs that may *increase* calcitonin levels: calcium, epinephrine, glucagon, oral contraceptives, pentagastrin.
- Hemolysis of the blood sample may alter test results.

Interventions/Implications

Pretest

- Explain to the patient the purpose of the test and the need for a blood sample to be drawn.
- Overnight fasting is preferred. Water is permitted.

Procedure

- A 1-mL serum sample is collected in red-top (no gel) tube and placed on ice.
- Stimulation tests are more sensitive than calcitonin measurements alone. This involves collecting a baseline sample, then giving the patient an injection of intravenous calcium or pentagastrin to stimulate calcitonin production. Several more blood samples are then collected over the next few minutes to gauge the effect of the stimulation. Patients with early C-cell hyperplasia and/or MTC will usually have very significant increases in their levels of calcitonin during this test.
- Gloves are worn throughout the procedure.

Posttest

- Apply pressure at venipuncture site. Apply dressing, periodically assessing for continued bleeding.
- The sample is labeled and transported to the laboratory.
- Report results to the primary care provider.

→ Clinical Alerts

- If the patient is found to have medullary thyroid cancer and surgery is performed, follow-up calcitonin levels are checked periodically to ensure that levels return to normal. If levels remain elevated, some calcitonin-producing tissue remains. If levels lower after surgery and later rise, the cancer may have returned.
- It is suggested that family members of patients with medullary cancer of the thyroid be screened via the calcitonin test.

Calcium, Blood

Test Description

Calcium (Ca^{++}) is present in the blood in two forms. Approximately 50% is present in a free state, and the other 50% is bound to plasma protein, primarily to albumin. The calcium which is circulating in the free state is biologically active. Its functions include important roles in muscle contraction, heart function, transmission of nerve impulses, and clotting of the blood.

The amount of calcium in the blood is minute compared to the 98% to 99% present in the teeth and bones. The storage of calcium in the bones provides an excellent reservoir which is readily available for release into the bloodstream to assist in maintaining a normal level of calcium in the blood.

Two hormones work together to control serum calcium levels. *Calcitonin*, which is secreted by the thyroid gland, causes calcium to be excreted by the kidneys, thus preventing a calcium excess in the blood. *Parathyroid hormone* (PTH) works directly on the bones to release calcium into the bloodstream when needed and also increases absorption of calcium by the intestines and kidneys. There is an inverse relationship between calcium and phosphorus: as serum calcium levels increase, serum phosphorus levels decrease.

This laboratory test measures the *total* calcium present in the blood. This provides information regarding parathyroid gland function and the metabolism of calcium. It is also used to evaluate malignancies, since cancer cells release calcium, often resulting in high calcium levels in the blood (*hypercalcemia*).

Since much of the circulating calcium is bound to albumin, calcium levels in the blood must be interpreted in relation to serum albumin levels. As serum albumin decreases 1 g, the total serum calcium decreases approximately 0.8 mg due to the decrease in the bound calcium; the amount of free calcium would not change.

Patients with hypercalcemia may have deep bone pain, renal calculi, and muscle hypotonicity. Patients with *hypocalcemia*, or decreased serum calcium levels, may experience numbness and tingling in the hands, feet, and around the mouth, muscle twitching, cardiac arrhythmias, and possibly convulsions. These patients may also demonstrate Chvostek's sign and Trousseau's sign.

Normal Values

8.5–10.5 mg/dL (2.1–2.6 mmol/L SI units)
Elderly: Decreased

Possible Meanings of Abnormal Values

Increased	Decreased
Acromegaly	Acute pancreatitis
Addison's disease	Alcoholism
Antacid abuse	Chronic renal disease
Dehydration	Diarrhea
Hodgkin's disease	Early neonatal hypocalcemia
Hyperparathyroidism	Hyperphosphatemia
Hyperthyroidism	Hypoparathyroidism

C

Prolonged immobilization
Leukemia
Lung cancer
Metastatic bone cancer
Multiple myeloma
Paget's disease
Parathyroid tumor
Renal cancer
Respiratory acidosis
Sarcoidosis
Vitamin D intoxication
Williams syndrome

Low albumin level
Malabsorption
Massive blood transfusions
Metabolic alkalosis
Osteomalacia
Renal failure
Rickets
Severe malnutrition
Vitamin D deficiency

Contributing Factors to Abnormal Values

- Use of a tourniquet during the acquisition of the blood sample causes venous stasis. This may alter test results.
- Drugs which may *increase* blood calcium levels: anabolic steroids, androgens, antacids, calcium carbonate, calcium gluconate, calcium salts, ergocalciferol, estrogens, hydralazine, indomethacin, lithium, parathyroid hormone, progesterone, tamoxifen, theophylline, thiazide diuretics, thyroid hormones, vitamin A, vitamin D.
- Drugs which may *decrease* blood calcium levels: acetazolamide, antacids, anticonvulsants, asparaginase, aspirin, barbiturates, calcitonin, cisplatin, corticosteroids, cholestyramine, furosemide, gastrin, gentamicin, glucagon, glucose, heparin, hydrocortisone, insulin, iron, laxatives, loop diuretics, magnesium salts, mercurial diuretics, methicillin, phenobarbital, phenytoin, sulfonamides.

Interventions/Implications

Pretest
- Explain to the patient the purpose of the test and the need for a blood sample to be drawn.
- No fasting is usually required prior to the test, although some laboratories do require a fast with water permitted.

Procedure
- A 7-mL blood sample is drawn in a red-top collection tube. Use of a tourniquet is avoided, if possible.
- Gloves are worn throughout the procedure.

Posttest
- Apply pressure at venipuncture site. Apply dressing, periodically assessing for continued bleeding.
- Label the specimen and transport it to the laboratory.
- Report abnormal findings to the primary care provider.

→ Clinical Alerts

- Patients with low calcium levels should be informed of dietary sources of calcium: milk, cheese, turnip greens, collard greens, white beans, and lentils.
- Infants with Williams syndrome can have critically high calcium levels due to idiopathic hypercalcemia. This tends to resolve as the child gets older, but may necessitate use of calcium-free formula during infancy and early childhood.

Calcium, Urine

Test Description

Calcium (Ca⁺⁺) plays important roles in muscle contraction, heart function, transmission of nerve impulses, and clotting of the blood. Only 1% to 2% of the calcium is in the blood; the remaining 98% to 99% is stored in the teeth and bones, which can be released as needed to maintain normal serum calcium levels. Most of the calcium excreted from the body is lost in stool; 99% of the calcium filtered by the kidneys is reabsorbed. When increased levels of urinary calcium do exist, it is usually due to elevated serum calcium levels. Urinary calcium is used primarily to evaluate parathyroid function and the effects of Vitamin D.

Normal Values

0–300 mg/day (0–7.5 mmol/day SI units)

Possible Meanings of Abnormal Values

Increased	Decreased
Breast cancer	Hypoparathyroidism
Cushing's syndrome	Malabsorption
Fanconi syndrome	Renal osteodystrophy
Glucocorticoid excess	Vitamin D deficiency
Hyperthyroidism	
Hyperparathyroidism	
Lung cancer	
Metastatic cancer	
Milk-alkali syndrome	
Multiple myeloma	
Osteoporosis	
Paget's disease	
Renal tubular acidosis	
Sarcoidosis	
Vitamin D intoxication	
Wilson's disease	

Contributing Factors to Abnormal Values

- Urinary calcium levels are higher immediately after meals.
- False-negative results may occur with alkaline urine.
- Drugs which may *increase* urinary calcium levels: ammonium chloride, androgens, anabolic steroids, antacids, anticonvulsants, cholestyramine, furosemide, mercurial diuretics, parathyroid hormone, phosphates, vitamin D.
- Drugs which may *decrease* urinary calcium levels: corticosteroids, aspirin, indomethacin, oral contraceptives, thiazide diuretics.

Interventions/Implications

Pretest
- Explain 24-hour urine collection procedure to the patient.

- Stress the importance of saving *all* urine in the 24-hour period. Instruct the patient to avoid contaminating the urine with toilet paper or feces.
- Inform the patient of the presence of a preservative in the collection bottle.

Procedure
- Obtain the proper container containing HCl as preservative from the laboratory.
- Begin the testing period in the morning after the patient's first voiding, which is discarded.
- Timing of the 24-hour period begins at the time the first voiding is discarded.
- *All* urine for the next 24 hours is collected in the container, which is to be kept refrigerated or on ice.
- If any urine is accidentally discarded during the 24-hour period, the test must be discontinued and a new test begun.
- The ending time of the 24-hour collection period should be posted in the patient's room.
- Gloves are worn whenever dealing with the specimen collection.

Posttest
- At the end of the 24-hour collection period, label and send the urine container to the laboratory as soon as possible.
- Report abnormal findings to the primary care provider.

Candida Antibody Test

Test Description
Candidiasis, also known as moniliasis and thrush, is caused by the organism *Candida albicans*. It affects the mucous membranes, skin, and nails. The organism is a yeast-like fungus which is normally present in vaginal secretions. Under certain circumstances, rapid growth of the organism occurs. Such circumstances include: long-term antibiotic therapy, corticosteroid therapy, pregnancy, oral contraceptives, diabetes, wearing nonventilated undergarments, and immunocompromised patients. Oral candidiasis is often noted as the first sign of AIDS. The serologic test for the *Candida* antibody is used in conjunction with histologic study and culture to confirm the diagnosis and is especially useful if the other tests are inconclusive.

Normal Values
Negative for *Candida* antibodies

Abnormal Values
Titer >1:8 indicates systemic infection
A fourfold increase in titers drawn 10 to 14 days apart indicates an acute infection.

Possible Meanings of Abnormal Values

Increased
Candida infection

Contributing Factors to Abnormal Values

- False positive results occur in about 25% of the population.
- Positive results can occur in patients with severe candidiasis of the skin/mucous membranes.
- False negative results may occur in immunocompromised patients due to their inability to produce antibodies.
- Hemolysis due to excessive agitation of the blood sample or contamination of the sample may alter test results.

Interventions/Implications

Pretest
- Explain to the patient the purpose of the test and the need for a blood sample to be drawn.
- The patient is to be NPO for 12 hours prior to the test

Procedure
- A 7-mL blood sample is drawn in a red-top collection tube with no gel.
- Gloves are worn throughout the procedure.

Posttest
- Apply pressure at venipuncture site. Apply dressing, periodically assessing for continued bleeding.
- Label the specimen and transport it to the laboratory.
- Report abnormal findings to the primary care provider.

Clinical Alerts

- Inform the patient of the possible need for a second blood sample, should a comparison of titers be desired.

Carboxyhemoglobin (Carbon Monoxide [CO])

Test Description
Carbon monoxide (CO) is a colorless, odorless, gaseous substance found in tobacco smoke, automobile exhaust, fires burning with poor ventilation, improperly functioning furnaces, and defective gas-burning appliances such as stoves. When the hemoglobin of the blood is exposed to CO through inhalation, carboxyhemoglobin is formed. The affinity of hemoglobin for CO is over 200 times greater than for oxygen. Thus, hemoglobin is prevented from combining with, and transporting, oxygen to such tissues as the brain. This results in a lack of oxygen being released in the tissues of the body, a condition known as *hypoxia*.

Symptoms of CO poisoning vary with the carboxyhemoglobin level. Levels of 20% to 30% cause headache, dizziness, nausea, vomiting, and impaired judgment. Levels of 30% to 40% result in confusion, muscle weakness, hyperpnea, hypotension, and tachycardia. When levels reach 50% to 60%, there is a loss of consciousness and possible seizures, and with values greater than 60%, respiratory arrest and death may occur.

THE EVIDENCE FOR PRACTICE

- CO poisoning must be evaluated through testing for CO.
- Arterial blood gases cannot be used to diagnose carbon monoxide (CO) overexposure. CO does not affect the amount of oxygen dissolved in the serum, only what is attached to hemoglobin. Thus, PO_2 and oxygen saturation will be normal.
- Pulse oximetry monitoring will provide a false normal reading, because the probe will read the carboxyhemoglobin saturation as oxyhemoglobin.

Normal Values

Nonsmoker:	<3% of total hemoglobin
Smoker:	2–10% of total hemoglobin
Newborn:	10–12% of total hemoglobin

Possible Meanings of Abnormal Values

Increased
Carbon monoxide poisoning

Contributing Factors to Abnormal Values

- Contamination of the blood sample with room air will alter test results.

Interventions/Implications

Pretest
- Explain to the patient the purpose of the test and the need for a blood sample to be drawn.
- No fasting is required before the test.
- No smoking is allowed prior to the test.
- Specimen should be drawn as soon as possible after exposure.

Procedure
- A blood sample is collected to fill an EDTA (lavender-top) tube.
- Gloves are worn throughout the procedure.

Posttest
- Apply pressure at venipuncture site. Apply dressing, periodically assessing for continued bleeding.
- The sample is labeled and transported to the laboratory.
- Provide high concentration oxygen to the patient as ordered by the primary care provider.
- Report results to the primary care provider.

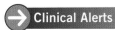

Clinical Alerts

- A person who may have carbon monoxide poisoning should be removed from the place of likely exposure and given oxygen before being tested.
- Women and children may have more severe symptoms of CO poisoning at lower CO levels than men because of the fewer number of red blood cells normally available to carry oxygen.

C

 # Carcinoembryonic Antigen (CEA)

Test Description
Carcinoembryonic antigen (CEA) is a glycoprotein that is normally produced by the fetus and secreted by gastrointestinal cells. In adults, it is normally found in trace amounts. However, CEA tends to increase in the case of malignancies. It is primarily nonspecific and thus is not used alone in cancer diagnosis. This test has been found to be effective in the early detection of colorectal cancer, with CEA levels rising several months before clinical symptoms appear. Smaller tumors found early in development will have low or normal CEA levels, whereas advanced or metastatic conditions are likely to have higher CEA levels. Measurement of CEA levels can also be helpful monitoring the response of the patient to cancer treatment, and for monitoring the patient for recurrence of cancer.

THE EVIDENCE FOR PRACTICE
- Drawing a CEA level has been recommended before and every 3 months for the first 2 years after resection of colorectal cancer.
  - Postoperative return to normal of an elevated preoperative CEA is associated with complete tumor resection, whereas persistently elevated values indicate the presence of residual disease.
  - Elevated preoperative CEA levels have been found to be an independent predictor of poor outcome.

Normal Values
Nonsmoker: <3 ng/mL (<3 mcg/L SI units)
Smoker: <5 ng/mL (<5 mcg/L SI units)

Possible Meanings of Abnormal Values

Increased
Acute pancreatitis
Acute renal failure
Bacterial pneumonia
Breast cancer
Cholecystitis
Chronic obstructive pulmonary disease
Cirrhosis

Colorectal cancer
Crohn's disease
Diverticulitis
Hypothyroidism
Leukemia
Lung cancer
Neuroblastoma
Ovarian cancer
Pancreatic cancer
Peptic ulcer disease
Pulmonary emphysema
Radiation therapy
Smoking
Ulcerative colitis

Contributing Factors to Abnormal Values

- Smoking may *increase* CEA levels.
- Drugs that may *increase* CEA levels: antineoplastic agents, hepatotoxic drugs.

Interventions/Implications

Pretest
- Explain to the patient the purpose of the test and the need for a blood sample to be drawn.
- No fasting is required before the test.

Procedure
- A 5-mL blood sample is collected in an EDTA (lavender-top) tube.
- Gloves are worn throughout the procedure.

Posttest
- Apply pressure at venipuncture site. Apply dressing, periodically assessing for continued bleeding.
- The sample is labeled and transported to the laboratory.
- Report abnormal results to the primary care provider.

Clinical Alerts

- When cancer metastasizes to other organs, CEA levels rise and may be present in other body fluids, such as cerebrospinal fluid.

Cardiac Catheterization (Angiocardiography, Coronary Angiography, Coronary Arteriography, Heart Catheterization)

Test Description
Angiography is a general term used to indicate visualization of any blood vessels, whether they be arteries or veins. The more precise term for visualization of the arteries is *arteriography*. Arteriograms are extremely valuable for observing the

blood flow to a part of the body and to detect lesions that may be amenable to surgical treatment.

The purposes of cardiac catheterization are to investigate congenital disorders of the heart and great vessels, to evaluate the coronary arteries, to evaluate cardiac muscle function, and to assess valvular function. This procedure allows for determination of pressure readings within the heart chambers, for collection of blood samples, and for recording pictures of the cardiac structure and movement. The test involves the introduction of a radiopaque catheter into the femoral artery or the brachial artery and injecting a contrast medium dye. Left heart catheterization, in which the catheter is advanced retrograde through the aorta into the left ventricle, is used to evaluate patency of the coronary arteries, mitral and aortic valve function, and left ventricular function. Right heart catheterization, used to evaluate tricuspid and pulmonary valve function and to measure pulmonary artery pressures, involves advancing the catheter through the vena cava, right atrium and ventricle, and into the pulmonary artery.

While performing a cardiac catheterization, the *interventional cardiologist* is able to perform a variety of treatments for structural heart diseases. These include:

- Angioplasty, or Percutaneous Transluminal Coronary Angioplasty (PTCA)—This involves inserting a balloon into the area of narrowing in the coronary artery and then inflating the balloon to open the narrowing.
- Stenting—This procedure can be done during angioplasty. A metal mesh tube (stent) is placed over the balloon catheter. When the balloon is inflated during angioplasty, the stent expands, locks in place, and holds the artery open. Over 70% of coronary angioplasty procedures now include stenting.
- Valvuloplasty—This involves dilation of narrowed cardiac valves.

THE EVIDENCE FOR PRACTICE

Cardiac catheterization with coronary angiography is the "gold standard" for demonstrating coronary pathology. This is usually the final diagnostic test in defining heart disease, although MDCT (multi detector chest CT) has recently shown promise as an accurate non-invasive alternative, particularly if the diagnosis is in question.

Normal Values

Normal heart size, structure, movement, and wall thickness
Normal blood flow and valve motion
Normal coronary vasculature

Possible Meanings of Abnormal Values

Aneurysm
Cardiomyopathy
Congenital anomalies
Coronary artery disease
Intracardiac tumors
Pulmonary emboli
Pulmonary hypertension
Septal defects
Valvular heart disease

Contributing Factors to Abnormal Values

- Any movement by the patient may alter quality of films taken.

C Interventions/Implications

Pretest

- Explain to the patient the purpose of the test. Provide any written teaching materials available on the subject. Note that discomfort involved with this test is primarily due to lying on a hard table for an extended period of time and the needle puncture. Explain that an intense hot flushing may be experienced for 15 to 30 seconds when the dye is injected.
- Check for allergies to iodine, shellfish, or contrast medium dye. Inform the cardiologist of such possible allergy and obtain order for an antihistamine and steroid to be administered prior to the test.
- Baseline laboratory data (CBC, PT, PTT) is obtained.
- Note any medications, such as anticoagulants or aspirin, which may prolong bleeding.
- Patients receiving metformin (Glucophage) for Type 2 diabetes mellitus should discontinue the drug 2 days before elective surgery or angiographic exams. This is due to the possible occurrence of lactic acidosis, a potentially fatal complication of biguanide therapy.
- Fasting for at least 8 hours is required prior to the test.
- Obtain a signed informed consent.
- Administer any pretest sedation after consent form is signed.
- Assess and document patient's peripheral pulses bilaterally prior to the test. Mark the location of the pulses with a marking pen.
- Perform and document a baseline neurologic assessment.

Procedure

- The patient is assisted to a supine position on the examination table.
- A maintenance IV line is initiated.
- Cardiac monitoring is initiated.
- Resuscitation and suctioning equipment should be readily available.
- The area of the puncture site is shaved, cleansed, and then anesthetized.
- The needle puncture of the artery is made and a guide wire is placed through the needle. The catheter is then inserted over the wire and into the artery.
- The radiopaque catheter is advanced into the desired artery. Positioning is monitored via fluoroscopy.
- Once the catheter is in the correct position, contrast dye is injected through the catheter.
- Radiographic films are taken.
- After films of satisfactory quality are obtained, several options may occur: (1) the catheter may be removed and pressure held on the puncture site for at least 15 minutes; (2) another procedure such as angioplasty with/without stenting may be done after which the sheath that guides the treatment catheter into and out of the artery is left in place for 4 hours and removed by the nurse; or (3) the guiding sheath is removed immediately after the coronary procedure and a metal clip is positioned against the outside arterial wall at the puncture site and released, causing it to fold inward and sealing the puncture.
- Gloves are worn throughout the procedure.

Posttest

- Most allergic reactions to radiopaque dye occur within 30 minutes of administration of the contrast medium. Observe the patient closely for: respiratory distress, hypotension, edema, hives, rash, tachycardia, and/or laryngeal stridor. Emergency resuscitation equipment must be readily accessible.
- A pressure dressing is applied to the puncture site. Check the dressing for bleeding and the area around the puncture site for swelling at frequent intervals.
- The patient is to remain on bedrest for 8 to 12 hours with the affected extremity immobilized.
- Maintain pressure on the puncture site with a sandbag.
- Note: If the puncture site is sealed with a metal clip, patients can usually ambulate after 1 hour. No pressure is needed to be maintained on the puncture site.
- Monitor vital signs and neurological status every 15 minutes for 1 hour, then every 30 minutes for 2 hours, then every hour for 4 hours, and then every 4 hours.
- Monitor urinary output.
- Assess the color, movement, temperature, and sensation (CMTS) and the pulse(s) of the affected extremity with each vital sign check. Compare with the other extremity.
- Encourage fluid intake to promote dye excretion.
- Renal function should be assessed before metformin is restarted.
- Report abnormal findings to the primary care provider.

C

Clinical Alerts

- Possible complications include: allergic reaction to dye, arterial occlusion resulting in embolic stroke or myocardial infarction, bleeding at puncture site, cardiac arrhythmias, infection at the puncture site, perforation of the myocardium, pneumothorax, renal failure.
- Patients found to have coronary artery disease should receive education regarding treatment protocols, including medication, exercise, diet, and weight loss.
- Patients receiving stent placement are placed on clopidogrel for up to 12 months and on lifetime low-dose aspirin.

CONTRAINDICATIONS!

- Patients who are allergic to iodine, shellfish, or contrast medium dye
- Patients with bleeding disorders
- Pregnant women
  - Caution: A woman in her childbearing years should undergo radiography only during her menses or 12 to 14 days after its onset to avoid any exposure to a fetus.
- Patients who are unable to cooperate due to age, mental status, pain, or other factors
- Patients with renal failure or those susceptible to dye-induced renal failure (dehydrated patients)
- Patients who would refuse surgery if a surgically correctable problem was found during the procedure

Cardiac Nuclear Scan (Cardiac Flow Studies, Gated Blood Pool Scan, Heart Scan, Myocardial Perfusion Imaging [MPI], MUGA Scan, PYP Scan, Thallium Scan)

C

Test Description

The heart scan is a noninvasive procedure which involves the intravenous injection of a radiopharmaceutical followed by nuclear imaging. There are several types of heart scan.

The *PYP scan* is also known as "hot spot myocardial imaging". It involves the injection of technetium-99m stannous pyrophosphate, which is thought to combine with calcium present in damaged myocardial cells. These hot spots appear within 12 hours of infarction and are most prominent 48 to 72 hours postinfarction. This test is used to determine the occurrence, extent, and prognosis of myocardial infarction. The PYP scan is especially useful when the electrocardiogram (ECG) and the cardiac enzyme studies are inconclusive.

The *thallium scan* involves the injection of thallium-201, which is absorbed in *healthy* tissue. Ischemic tissue eventually absorbs the radionuclide, but infarcted tissue never does. This results in what is known as "cold spots" on the scan. This scan is used to show myocardial perfusion, to demonstrate the location and extent of acute or chronic myocardial infarction, to diagnose coronary artery disease, and to monitor the effectiveness of angioplasty, coronary artery grafts, and antianginal therapy. In some patients, no evidence of myocardial ischemia occurs during a resting state. For this type of patient, the thallium is injected during exercise stress testing. The thallium accumulates in the myocardium in direct proportion to the perfusion to the area. Normal myocardial muscle will have a higher thallium concentration than ischemic heart muscle. The heart is scanned shortly after the exercise to show blood flow to the myocardium during exercise and again 2 to 3 hours later to show its blood flow during rest. This type of testing is known as *thallium stress testing*. Similar type procedure is followed for the scan using other radioisotopes, such as technetium-99m sestamibi (Cardiolite), or technetium-99m tetrofosmin (Myoview),

The *MUGA scan* stands for "multigated acquisition scan". It is also called the *gated blood pool scan*. This test is performed by attaching technetium 99 to red blood cells (RBCs) and then injecting the RBCs into the patient's bloodstream. The gamma camera is able to detect the low-level radiation being given off by the RBCs as they fill the cardiac chambers. The test can be used to determine the location and extent of any damage. It is most useful and highly accurate in determining left ventricular ejection fraction

Single-photon emission computed tomography (SPECT) is now being used to provide a three-dimensional image of the functioning heart. This test provides excellent resolution and allows areas of myocardial ischemia to be quantified.

Normal Values

Normal ejection fraction (>50%)
No evidence of myocardial ischemia or infarction

Possible Meanings of Abnormal Values

Aneurysm
Cardiomyopathy
Coronary artery disease
Myocardial infarction
Myocardial ischemia
Myocardial necrosis
Myocarditis

Contributing Factors to Abnormal Values

- Any movement by the patient may alter quality of films taken.
- Test results may be altered by myocardial trauma, recent nuclear scans, and drugs such as long-acting nitrates.

Interventions/Implications

Pretest

- Explain to the patient the purpose of the test. Provide any written teaching materials available on the subject. Note that discomfort involved with this test is primarily due to lying on a hard table for an extended period of time and the venipuncture. Reassure the patient that only trace amounts of the radionuclide are involved in the test.
- The patient must remain still while the scan is being performed.
- Fasting for 6 hours prior to the test is required. Water is permitted.
- There should be no caffeine intake for 24 hours prior to the test. This includes coffee, tea, soda, chocolate, sports drinks, and some over-the-counter and prescription medications.
- The patient should not smoke or chew tobacco for 6 hours prior to the test.
- Obtain a signed informed consent.
- Resuscitation and suctioning equipment should be readily available.

Procedure

- The selected radionuclide is administered by IV injection in a peripheral vein.
- PYP scan: Injection 2 to 3 hours prior to the scan.
- Thallium scan: Scanning begins 5 minutes after injection.
- MUGA scan: Scanning begins 1 minute after injection.
- The patient is assisted to a supine position on the examination table.
- A gamma scintillation camera is positioned over the patient's chest. This camera takes a radioactivity reading from the body. This information is transformed into a two-dimensional picture of the heart.
- Gloves are worn during the radionuclide injection.

Posttest

- Check the injection site for redness or swelling.
- If a woman who is lactating *must* have a nuclear scan, she should not breast feed the infant until the radionuclide has been eliminated, possibly for 3 days.
- Although the amount of diagnostic radionuclide excreted in the urine is low, the urine should not be used for any laboratory tests for the time period indicated by the Nuclear Medicine Department.
- Gloves are worn whenever dealing with the urine.
- No other radionuclide tests should be scheduled for 24 to 48 hours.

- Encourage fluid intake by the patient to enhance excretion of the radionuclide.
- Report abnormal findings to the primary care provider.

C

→ **Clinical Alerts**

- Myocardial perfusion imaging, when done in conjunction with exercise stress testing, may be scheduled on 1 or 2 days.

CONTRAINDICATIONS!

- Pregnant women
  - Caution: A woman in her childbearing years should undergo radiography only during her menses or 12 to 14 days after its onset to avoid any exposure to a fetus.
- Patients who are lactating
- Patients who are unable to cooperate due to age, mental status, pain, or other factors

 Carotid Artery Duplex Scan (Carotid Ultrasound)

Test Description

Ultrasonography is a noninvasive method of diagnostic testing in which ultrasound waves are sent into the body with a small transducer pressed against the skin. The transducer then receives any returning sound waves, which are deflected back as they bounce off various structures. The transducer converts the returning sound waves into electric signals that are then transformed by a computer into audible sounds (Doppler method) which can be graphed. A visual image of the carotid artery can be seen on the monitor, as well as in a printed copy of the image.

In this particular type of ultrasonography, the blood flow through the carotid arteries is studied. The movement of blood cells causes a change in pitch of the reflected sound waves, a phenomenon known as the Doppler effect. The sound pitch does not change if there is no blood flow through the artery. This provides a noninvasive method of assessing bruits during systole and diastole. Sounds emitted during the examination change when turbulent blood flow caused by plaque, stenosis, or partial occlusion of the artery is encountered. Such testing is often used in the evaluation of patients diagnosed with syncope, transient ischemic attack (TIA), and stroke.

There are two types of Doppler ultrasound typically used for evaluating the carotid artery. *Duplex Doppler* ultrasound uses standard ultrasound methods to produce pictures of the blood vessel and surrounding organizations. *Color Doppler* ultrasound provides the same information as the Duplex Doppler but with the addition of colors to the blood vessel to represent the speed and direction of blood flow through the vessel.

THE EVIDENCE FOR PRACTICE

Carotid endarterectomy (CE) is established as effective for recently symptomatic (within previous 6 months) patients with 70% to 99% internal carotid artery (ICA) angiographic stenosis.

C

Normal Values

Normal carotid artery blood flow

Possible Meanings of Abnormal Values

Aneurysm
Carotid artery occlusive disease

Contributing Factors to Abnormal Values

- The transducer must be in good contact with the skin as it is being moved.
- Use of nicotine in any form within 2 hours of the test will cause vasoconstriction and possibly false results.

Interventions/Implications

Pretest
- Explain to the patient the purpose of the test. Provide any written teaching materials available on the subject. Note that there is no discomfort involved with this test.
- No fasting is required before the test

Procedure
- The patient is assisted to a supine position on the ultrasonography table, with the head turned slightly to one side.
- The patient must remain very still during the exam.
- A coupling agent, such as a water-based gel, is applied to the area to be evaluated.
- A transducer is placed on the skin and moved as needed to provide clearly emitted sounds.
- The sound waves are transformed into audible sounds which are then printed in graphic form.

Posttest
- Cleanse the patient's skin of remaining coupling agent.
- Report abnormal findings to the primary care provider.

→ Clinical Alerts

- Unless contraindicated, aspirin therapy should be considered for symptomatic and asymptomatic patients undergoing CE prior to surgery and for at least 3 months following surgery to reduce the combined endpoint of stroke, myocardial infarction, and death.

Ceruloplasmin

C

Test Description

Ceruloplasmin is an alpha$_2$-globulin protein that transports copper. It also regulates iron uptake by transferrin. Testing for ceruloplasmin gives direct information regarding the amount of copper in the blood serum. Ceruloplasmin levels increase during times of stress, infection, and pregnancy.

This test is used to aid in the diagnosis of Wilson's disease, a hereditary syndrome in which decreased levels of ceruloplasmin are manufactured by the liver. Without ceruloplasmin to transport it, copper accumulates in the tissues of the brain, eye, kidney, and liver. One of the hallmarks of this disease is the presence of copper deposits around the iris of the eye, known as Kayser-Fleischer rings.

THE EVIDENCE FOR PRACTICE

Serum ceruloplasmin should be routinely measured during the evaluation of unexplained hepatic, neurologic, or psychiatric abnormalities in children and adults through middle age.

Normal Values

23–43 mg/dL (230–430 mg/L SI units)

Possible Meanings of Abnormal Values

Increased	Decreased
Cancer	Hypocupremia due to hyperalimentation
Cirrhosis	Kwashiorkor
Infection	Malabsorption
Inflammation (rheumatoid arthritis)	Menkes' kinky hair syndrome
Pregnancy	Nephrotic syndrome
Primary sclerosing cholangitis	Normal infants (under 6 months)
Stress	Sprue
Thyrotoxicosis	Wilson disease

Contributing Factors to Abnormal Values

- Drugs that may *increase* ceruloplasmin levels: estrogen, methadone, oral contraceptives, phenytoin.
- Hemolysis of the blood sample will alter test results.

Interventions/Implications

Pretest
- Explain to the patient the purpose of the test and the need for a blood sample to be drawn.
- No fasting is required before the test.

Procedure
- A 7-mL blood sample is drawn in a collection tube containing no additives.
- Gloves are worn throughout the procedure.

Posttest
- Apply pressure at venipuncture site. Apply dressing, periodically assessing for continued bleeding.
- The sample is labeled and transported to the laboratory.
- Report abnormal findings to the primary care provider.

→ Clinical Alerts

- First-degree relatives of any patient newly diagnosed with Wilson disease must be screened for the disease.

Cervical Biopsy (Punch Biopsy, Endocervical Curettage, Cone Biopsy, Cervical Conization, Loop Electrosurgical Excision Procedure)

Test Description

Cervical biopsy involves taking samples of tissue from the cervix for examination. Biopsy typically follows a Pap smear which has indicated *significant* abnormalities or when an abnormal area is noted on the cervix during a pelvic examination. Minor cell changes are usually monitored through frequent Pap testing. There are several types of cervical biopsies:

- *Punch biopsy* involves removing a small amount of tissue from an area using a small, round instrument. Multiple punch biopsies may be done. The punch biopsy is typically done in conjunction with a colposcopy.
- *Endocervical curettage (ECC)* involves the curettage, or scraping of the endocervical canal lining. This is tissue which is not visible from the external cervical os.
- *Cone biopsy or cervical conization* involves removal of a large cone-shaped section of tissue from the cervix. Cone biopsy may be done using the cold knife cone biopsy procedure (using a laser or surgical scalpel) or through use of LEEP. Regional or general anesthesia is needed for cone biopsy.
  - *Loop Electrosurgical Excision Procedure (LEEP)* uses an electrical current through a fine wire loop to cut away a thin layer of abnormal tissue. The amount of tissue removed depends on the whether it is done for biopsy only or to remove the abnormal tissue to allow healthy tissue to grow. LEEP is not usually done unless another type of biopsy has shown cervical intraepithelial neoplasia (CIN).

Due to the risk of scarring in the cervix from removal of tissue and possible future problems with infertility or miscarriage, the patient needs to discuss with the gynecologist the advantages and disadvantages of each type of procedure. It is important to find the best procedure for the patient's particular problem.

Normal Values

No abnormal cells

Possible Meanings of Abnormal Values

Cervical intraepithelial neoplasia
Cervical polyps
Genital warts
Invasive carcinoma

Interventions/Implications

Pretest

- Explain to the patient the purpose of the test. Provide any written teaching materials available on the subject. Note that cramping may occur during the procedure.
  - Use of an analgesic 30 minutes before the procedure may be ordered.
  - Review deep breathing exercises to encourage relaxation during the procedure.
- The patient must remain still during the procedure.
- No fasting is required before the test (unless general anesthesia is to be used).
- No douching, use of tampons or vaginal creams, or sexual intercourse for 24 hours prior to the procedure.
- Pregnancy testing may be done.
- Obtain a signed informed consent.
- If the procedure is done in an outpatient clinic under anesthesia, the patient will need to have someone drive her home after the procedure.

Procedure

- The procedure may be performed with or without anesthesia.
- The patient is instructed to empty the bladder prior to the procedure.
- The patient is assisted into a lithotomy position.
- A speculum is inserted into the vagina.
- The cervix is visualized using a colposcope.
- The cervix is cleaned and covered with acetic acid solution. This causes abnormal tissues to turn white and become more visible.
- The area to be biopsied may be given local anesthetic.
- The biopsy is performed using one of the procedures described previously.
  - If LEEP is performed, a tenaculum (forceps) may be used to the grasp and hold the cervix steady during the procedure.
- Bleeding from the biopsy site may be treated with a paste-like topical medication. Electrocauterization or sutures may be needed.
- If a cone biopsy is done, the cervix may be packed with a pressure dressing to be removed by the patient after a specified period of time.

Posttest

- The specimen is placed in preservative, labeled, and transported to the laboratory.
- A sanitary pad will need to be worn for bleeding. The discharge will be dark/black for several days.
- An analgesic will be prescribed for discomfort. Over-the-counter pain relievers should not be taken without checking with the health-care provider due to the risk of bleeding with some such preparations.
- The patient should avoid sexual intercourse, douching, or using tampons for a week to allow the cervix to heal. If a cone biopsy was done, this time will be extended to several weeks. No strenuous activity or heavy lifting is allowed.
- Report abnormal findings to the primary care provider.

Clinical Alerts

- Possible complications include: bleeding, infection, and changes or scarring in the cervix from removal of tissue with possibility of future infertility or miscarriage.
- Instruct the patient to report any signs of infection (fever, foul odor, or discharge), or if bleeding continues for more than 2 weeks. Severe lower abdominal pain needs to be reported immediately.
- Following a positive biopsy and treatment for carcinoma, Pap testing is done frequently (every 3 to 4 months) to ensure no abnormal tissue remains or returns. Colposcopy may also be done.

CONTRAINDICATIONS!

- Pregnancy
- Current menstruation
- Patients with clotting disorders
- Patients with acute pelvic inflammatory disease
- Patients with acute inflammation of the cervix

Chest X-ray (CXR, Chest Radiography)

Test Description

Radiography is the use of radiation (roentgen rays, or "x-rays") to cause some substances to fluoresce and affect photographic plates. X-rays penetrate air easily; therefore, areas filled with air, such as the lungs, appear very dark on the film. Conversely, bones appear almost white on the film because the x-rays cannot penetrate them to reach the x-ray film. Organs and tissues such as the heart appear as shades of gray because they have more mass than air but not as much as bone.

Chest radiographs are used to identify abnormalities of the lungs and other structures in the thorax, including the heart, ribs, and diaphragm. Common pulmonary disorders detected are pneumonia, atelectasis, and pneumothorax. The chest x-ray may be performed in the radiology department or through use of a portable x-ray machine. When taken in the radiology department, the chest x-ray is a posteroanterior (PA) view, since the patient is positioned with the anterior part of the body next to the film. Portable x-rays are done with the film behind the person, resulting in an anteroposterior (AP) view. Other views such as lateral, oblique, supine, and lateral decubitus positions may also be obtained. Ideally, the part of the body which needs to be studied should be next to the film.

Normal Values

Normal lungs and other thoracic structures

Possible Meanings of Abnormal Values

Asthma
Atelectasis
Atherosclerosis
Bronchitis
Cardiomyopathy
Congestive heart failure
Cor pulmonale
Diaphragmatic hernia
Emphysema
Enlarged lymph nodes
Foreign body
Fractures of sternum, ribs, or vertebrae
Kyphosis
Lung cancer
Mediastinal tumor
Pericardial effusion
Pericarditis
Phrenic nerve paresis
Pleural effusion
Pleurisy
Pneumonia
Pneumothorax
Pulmonary abscess
Pulmonary fibrosis
Pulmonary infiltrates
Scoliosis
Tuberculosis

Contributing Factors to Abnormal Values

- Portable chest x-rays are less reliable than those taken in the radiology department
- Under- or overexposure of the film may alter film quality
- When patients are unable to hold a deep breath due to pain or mental status, the quality of the film may be affected
- Obesity

Interventions/Implications

Pretest

- Explain to the patient the purpose of the test and the benefits and risks associated with the test. Provide any written teaching materials available on the subject. Note that no discomfort is associated with this procedure.
- No fasting is required prior to the test.
- Instruct the patient to remove all objects containing metal, such as jewelry or undergarments, as these will show on the film.

Procedure

- The patient's reproductive organs should be covered with a lead apron to prevent unnecessary exposure to radiation.

- Position the patient as ordered. If able, the patient stands during the procedure. The patient is instructed to take a deep breath and to hold it while the films are taken.

Posttest
- No special physical posttest nursing care is needed.
- Report abnormal findings to the primary care provider.

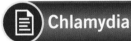

Clinical Alerts

- If the chest x-ray is positive for pneumonia, it is suggested that a follow-up chest x-ray be done in 4 weeks to check for resolution of the infection.

CONTRAINDICATIONS!

- Pregnant women
    - Caution: A woman in her childbearing years should undergo radiography only during her menses or 12 to 14 days after its onset to avoid any exposure to a fetus.

Chlamydia

Test Description

Chlamydia trachomatis is the most common cause of sexually transmitted disease in the United States. It is also responsible for trachoma, a serious eye infection. *Chlamydia* can cause cervicitis, urethritis, epididymitis, and proctitis. Mode of transmission for this bacterium includes direct contact through sexual activity or direct contact of the infant with the mother's cervix during birth. Although prevalent, the disease is often unrecognized. Many women with chlamydial infections are asymptomatic. However, the consequences of untreated chlamydial infection in women include the development of pelvic inflammatory disease, resulting in possible infertility. Thus, testing for the organism is very important. This is accomplished through either a culture of the cervix or eye, or through detection of the antigen by enzyme-linked immunosorbent assay (ELISA) technique. DNA testing using polymerase chain reaction (PCR) methodology is the newest method of testing for *Chlamydia*. This is done on female endocervical swabs, male urethral swabs, or on urine specimens.

THE EVIDENCE FOR PRACTICE

The Centers for Disease Control recommend testing in the following cases:
- All sexually active females under 20 years of age (test at least annually).
- Women ages 20 and older who have one or more risk factors (test annually).
    - Risk factors include having new or multiple sex partners, having sex with someone who has other partners, and not using barrier contraceptives, such as condoms.
- All women with an infection of the cervix.

- All pregnant women.
- Men with painful and frequent urination (dysuria), penile discharge, infection of the prostate (prostatitis), or inflammation involving the anus and rectum (proctitis).

Normal Values

Culture:	Negative
Antibody testing:	Negative

Possible Meanings of Abnormal Values

Positive
Chlamydia infection

Contributing Factors to Abnormal Values

- Drugs which may cause *false-negative* results: antibiotics, immunosuppressive drugs.

Interventions/Implications

Pretest
- Explain to the patient the purpose of the test and the need for a specimen to be collected.
- No fasting is required prior to the test.

Procedure

For antibody testing
- A 7-mL blood sample is drawn in a red-top collection tube.
- Gloves are worn for this procedure.

For eye culture
- Cleanse any mucus from the eye with a dry cotton swab.
- Use a sterile swab to swab the inner canthus or lower conjunctiva.
- Place the swab in the medium required by the reference laboratory.
- Gloves are worn for this procedure.

For cervical culture
- The female patient is assisted into the lithotomy position, draped, and encouraged to relax through deep breathing techniques.
- A vaginal speculum lubricated with warm water is inserted.
- Cervical mucus is removed using a large cotton swab.
- A dry, sterile cotton swab is then inserted into the endocervical canal and rotated from side to side.
- Place the swab in the medium required by the reference laboratory.
- Gloves are worn throughout this procedure.

For a urethral culture
- The male patient is assisted into a supine position. This position is recommended to avoid falling if vasovagal syncope occurs during the procedure. Such a reaction would be characterized by profound hypotension, bradycardia, pallor, and diaphoresis.
- The urethral meatus is cleansed with sterile gauze.

- A calcium alginate swab or a sterile bacteriologic wire loop is inserted 2 to 3 cm into the urethra and rotated from side to side.

For urine testing
- Instruct the patient not to urinate for 1 hour prior to collection.
- The patient should collect the first 15 to 50 mL of voided urine (the first part of the stream) in a plastic, preservative-free, sterile urine collection cup.
- Gloves are worn when handling urine specimen.

Posttest
- Apply pressure at venipuncture site. Apply dressing, periodically assessing for continued bleeding.
- Refrigerate any urine specimen immediately at 2 to 8°C.
- Label any specimen and transport it to the laboratory as soon as possible.
- Report abnormal findings to the primary care provider.

→ **Clinical Alerts**

- Patients with positive test results should have their sexual partners examined.
- Remind female patients that use of oral contraceptives *do not* protect against sexually transmitted diseases.

 Chloride, Blood

Test Description

Chloride (Cl⁻) is the major anion of the extracellular fluid. Chloride levels have an inverse relationship with those of bicarbonate; thus, they reflect acid-base status. Chloride has several functions, including maintaining electrical neutrality by counterbalancing cations such as sodium (NaCl, HCl), acting as one component of the buffering system, aiding in digestion, and helping to maintain osmotic pressure and water balance. Because chloride is most often seen in combination with sodium, shifts in sodium levels result in corresponding shifts in chloride levels.

Patients with elevated serum chloride levels (*hyperchloremia*) may experience weakness, deep rapid breathing, lethargy, and stupor, which may progress to coma. Patients with *hypochloremia*, or decreased serum chloride levels may exhibit hypertonicity of the muscles, tetany, and shallow breathing.

Blood chloride testing is often evaluated as part of screening laboratory tests. It may also be ordered to evaluate patients complaining of prolonged vomiting or diarrhea or weakness.

Normal Values

96–106 mEq/L (96–106 mmol/L SI units)

Possible Meanings of Abnormal Values

Increased (Hyperchloremia)	Decreased (Hypochloremia)
Acute renal failure	Acute infections
Alcoholism	Addison's disease
Anemia	Adrenal cortical insufficiency
Cardiac decompensation	Burns
Cushing's syndrome	Chronic renal failure
Dehydration	Congestive heart failure
Diabetes insipidus	Diabetic acidosis
Eclampsia	Diarrhea
Excessive saline infusion	Diaphoresis
Hyperparathyroidism	Heat exhaustion
Hyperventilation	Hypokalemia
Metabolic acidosis	Hyponatremia
Multiple myeloma	Metabolic alkalosis
Renal tubular acidosis	Nasogastric suctioning
Respiratory alkalosis	Primary aldosteronism
Salicylate intoxication	Pulmonary emphysema
	Pyloric obstruction
	Ulcerative colitis
	Vomiting

Contributing Factors to Abnormal Values

- Hemolysis of the blood sample may alter test results.
- Use of a tourniquet during acquisition of the blood sample may alter test results.
- Drugs which may *increase* serum chloride levels: acetazolamide, ammonium chloride, androgens, boric acid, cholestyramine, cyclosporine, estrogens, glucocorticoids, imipenem-cilastatin, methyldopa, nonsteroidal anti-inflammatory drugs, phenylbutazone, sodium bromide, sodium chloride, spironolactone, thiazide diuretics
- Drugs which may *decrease* serum chloride levels: aldosterone, amiloride, bumetanide, corticosteroids, corticotropin, dextrose infusions, ethacrynic acid, furosemide, loop diuretics, mercurial diuretics, prednisolone, sodium bicarbonate, spironolactone, triamterene, thiazide diuretics.

Interventions/Implications

Pretest
- Explain to the patient the purpose of the test and the need for a blood sample to be drawn.
- No fasting is required before the test.

Procedure
- A 7-mL blood sample is drawn in a green-top collection tube, avoiding use of a tourniquet, if possible.
- Gloves are worn throughout the procedure.

Posttest
- Apply pressure at venipuncture site. Apply dressing, periodically assessing for continued bleeding.
- Label the specimen and transport it to the laboratory.
- Report abnormal findings to the primary care provider.

Chloride, Urine

C

Test Description

Chloride (Cl-) is the major anion of the extracellular fluid. Chloride levels have an inverse relationship with those of bicarbonate; thus, they reflect acid-base status. In individuals with too much base, urine chloride measurements help differentiate the cause of the problem: loss of salt through dehydration, vomiting, or use of diuretics (urinary chloride would be very low) or excess hormones such as cortisol or aldosterone (urinary chloride would be very high).

Chloride has several functions, including maintaining electrical neutrality by counterbalancing cations such as sodium (NaCl, HCl), acting as one component of the buffering system, aiding in digestion, and helping to maintain osmotic pressure and water balance. The amount of chloride excreted by the kidneys in a 24-hour period is an indication of the patient's electrolyte balance and mirror the dietary intake of chloride and of sodium.

Normal Values

110–250 mEq/L (110–250 mmol/L SI units)

Possible Meanings of Abnormal Values

Increased	Decreased
Cushing's syndrome	Addison's disease
Dehydration	Congestive heart failure
Excessive salt intake	Diarrhea
Salicylate intoxication	Diaphoresis
Syndrome of inappropriate	Emphysema
ADH secretion (SIADH)	Low-sodium diet
Starvation	Malabsorption
	Nasogastric suctioning
	Pyloric obstruction
	Renal damage

Contributing Factors to Abnormal Values

- Drugs which may *increase* urinary chloride levels: bromides, mercurial diuretics, thiazide diuretics

Interventions/Implications

Pretest
- Explain 24-hour urine collection procedure to the patient.
- Stress the importance of saving *all* urine in the 24-hour period. Instruct the patient to avoid contaminating the urine with toilet paper or feces.

Procedure
- Obtain the proper container containing no preservative from the laboratory.
- Begin the testing period in the morning following the patient's first voiding, which is discarded.

- Timing of the 24-hour period begins at the time the first voiding is discarded.
- *All* urine for the next 24 hours is collected in the container, which is to be kept refrigerated or on ice.
- If any urine is accidentally discarded during the 24-hour period, the test must be discontinued and a new test begun.
- The ending time of the 24-hour collection period should be posted in the patient's room.
- Gloves are to be worn whenever dealing with the specimen collection.

Posttest

- At the end of the 24-hour collection period, label and send the urine container to the laboratory as soon as possible.
- Report abnormal findings to the primary care provider.

→ Clinical Alerts

- If urine creatinine is ordered along with chloride, the urine should be kept refrigerated during collection.

Cholangiography (Bile Duct A-ray, Percutaneous Transhepatic Cholangiogram, Operative Cholangiogram, T-Tube Cholangiogram)

Test Description

Cholangiography involves visualizing the bile ducts through use of a contrast medium. In this section, three techniques will be discussed: percutaneous transhepatic cholangiography, operative cholangiography, and T-tube cholangiography.

Percutaneous transhepatic cholangiography is the fluoroscopic examination of the biliary ducts using an iodine-based contrast dye which is injected directly into the bile duct. This test is performed in jaundiced patients since, in these patients, the cells of the liver are unable to transport the dye if administered orally or by intravenous infusion. With this procedure, the cystic, hepatic, and common bile ducts can be visualized and their diameter and filling evaluated. This allows differential diagnosis of obstructive jaundice and nonobstructive jaundice. If the ducts are found to be of normal size and intrahepatic cholestasis is indicated, further testing, such as a biopsy of the liver, is needed to distinguish among other problems such as cirrhosis or hepatitis. Percutaneous transhepatic cholangiography may be performed when a diagnostic endoscopic retrograde cholangiopancreatography (ERCP) cannot be performed or has failed in the past.

Because this is an invasive procedure, there is the chance of complications such as bleeding and peritonitis occurring. However, for patients who are jaundiced, this procedure and ERCP are the only methods available for visualization of the biliary tree. Thus, benefits and risks to the patient must be weighed. Currently, ERCP is more commonly performed due its lower complication rate.

In *operative cholangiography*, the procedure occurs while the patient is undergoing a cholecystectomy. Common bile duct (CBD) stones are discovered in about 15% of patients with acute cholecystitis. For this reason, an intraoperative cholangiogram is usually done during surgery and common bile duct exploration is performed if necessary. If a stone is discovered near the distal part of the CBD, ERCP may be used to perform a sphincterotomy and stone extraction.

When a patient undergoes a cholecystectomy with an exploration of the CBD, a rubber T-tube is usually inserted into the duct to facilitate bile drainage. Every effort is made to find and remove any obstructions, such as stones, from within the duct. Approximately 7 to 10 days after surgery, the patient is taken to the radiology department for a *T-tube*, or *postoperative*, *cholangiogram*. This test involves the injection of contrast dye through the T-tube into the biliary ducts. The flow of the dye is observed with the fluoroscope, allowing for the verification of patency of the CBD prior to removal of the T-tube.

Normal Values

Normal diameter and filling of the cystic, hepatic, and common bile ducts
No calculi, strictures, or obstructions present
Normal flow of dye into the duodenum

Possible Meanings of Abnormal Values

Biliary sclerosis
Biliary tract carcinoma
Carcinoma of the papilla of Vater
Carcinoma of the pancreas
Choledocholithiasis
Cholelithiasis
Sclerosing cholangitis
Strictures of the ducts

Contributing Factors to Abnormal Values

- Under- or overexposure of the film may alter film quality.
- When patients are unable to hold still, due to pain or mental status, the quality of the film may be affected.
- Retained barium from other exams will affect test results.

Interventions/Implications

Pretest

For all cholangiograms

- Inform the radiologist of any potential allergy to the contrast dye and obtain order for antihistamine and steroid to be given prior to the procedure.
- Patients receiving metformin (Glucophage) for Type 2 diabetes mellitus should discontinue the drug 2 days before elective surgery or angiographic exams. This is due to the

possible occurrence of lactic acidosis, a potentially fatal complication of biguanide therapy.
- Baseline BUN and creatinine should be obtained.

For percutaneous transhepatic cholangiogram
- Explain to the patient the purpose of the test and the benefits and risks associated with the test. Provide any written teaching materials available on the subject. Explain that the patient will experience discomfort when the injection site is anesthetized and as the dye is injected.
- Obtain a signed informed consent from the patient.
- The patient is given a low-fat or fat-free diet for 1 day, prior to the test.
- Obtain baseline laboratory tests to assess for coagulopathy (clotting time, platelet count, and prothrombin time).
- The patient is to be NPO after midnight prior to the test.
- Additional aspects of the preparation *may* include:
    - type and crossmatch of blood in case of bleeding during the procedure
    - administration of IV antibiotics 24 to 48 hours prior to the procedure
    - administration of a sedative prior to the procedure.
- Instruct the patient to remove all objects containing metal, such as jewelry or undergarments, as these will show on the film.

For T-tube cholangiogram
- Explain to the patient the purpose of the test and the benefits and risks associated with the test. Provide any written teaching materials available on the subject.
- Obtain a signed informed consent from the patient.
- The patient is to be fasting for 4 to 6 hours before the test.
- Clamp the T-tube the day before the procedure, if ordered.

Procedure

For percutaneous transhepatic cholangiogram
- The patient is in a supine position on the examination table.
- The skin of the right upper quadrant is cleansed, draped, and anesthetized with Xylocaine.
- Conscious sedation may be used.
- The patient is instructed to inhale and exhale several times and then to hold the breath after a full expiration. A long, flexible needle is inserted into the liver and advanced under fluoroscopy until bile is aspirated from the duct. Placement of the needle is checked by injecting a small amount of the dye. If visualization by fluoroscopy verifies correct placement, the remaining dye is injected. As the flow of the dye is observed, films are periodically taken.
- When the films are found to be satisfactory for diagnostic purposes, the needle is removed, and a sterile dressing is applied.

For operative cholangiogram
- Contrast medium is injected into the cystic duct and common bile duct during cholecystectomy.
- X-rays are taken and reviewed.
- If x-rays are negative, the surgery can be completed without need for CBD exploration.

For T-tube cholangiogram
- The patient is placed in a supine position on the examination table.
- The T-tube is cleansed with povidone-iodine and contrast medium is injected.

- Films are taken as the contrast medium flows through the ducts and into the duodenum.

Posttest
- Most allergic reactions to radiopaque dye occur within 30 minutes of administration of the contrast medium. Observe the patient closely for: respiratory distress, hypotension, edema, hives, rash, tachycardia, and/or laryngeal stridor. Emergency resuscitation equipment must be readily accessible.

For percutaneous transhepatic cholangiogram
- Assess the patient's vital signs until stable. Observe for signs of respiratory distress, hemorrhage, and peritonitis (chills, fever, abdominal pain, distention, and tenderness).
- Check the puncture site for bleeding, swelling, and tenderness often.
- Assist the patient to a right side lying position, which is to be maintained for 6 hours.

For All Cholangiograms
- Resume the patient's diet and medications as taken prior to the test. Encourage fluid intake.
- Renal function should be assessed before metformin is restarted.
- Report abnormal findings to the primary care provider.

Clinical Alerts

- Possible complications include: adverse reaction or allergy to dye, peritonitis caused by bile extravasation from the liver after needle removal, hemorrhage, and tension pneumothorax.
- If a barium swallow or an upper gastrointestinal and small-bowel series test is ordered, these should be completed *after* the cholangiography is performed, otherwise the barium sulfate ingested during the other exams may obscure the films made of the ducts.

CONTRAINDICATIONS!

- Pregnant women
  - Caution: A woman in her childbearing years should undergo radiography only during her menses or 12 to 14 days after its onset to avoid any exposure to a fetus.
- Patients with hypersensitivity to iodine, seafood, or contrast media
- Patients with cholangitis, since injection of the dye will increase biliary pressure and cause bacteremia
- Patients with massive ascites
- Patients with uncontrolled coagulopathy (platelet count <50,000/mm^3, prolonged bleeding time)
- Patients who are unable to cooperate due to age, mental status, pain, or other factors

Cholecystography (Gallbladder Radiography, Gallbladder [GB] Series, Oral Cholecystogram)

C

Test Description

The oral cholecystogram is used when a patient is experiencing symptoms of biliary tract disease, such as right upper quadrant pain, fat intolerance, and jaundice, and is suspected of having gallbladder disease. This test is used to study the gallbladder after ingestion of a contrast medium, in this case, a radiopaque, iodinated dye. The dye is processed by the liver, excreted in the bile, and then accumulates in the gallbladder. The peak concentration of the dye in the gallbladder occurs 12 to 14 hours after ingestion, at which time films are taken. This test often performed in conjunction with an ultrasound examination of the gallbladder.

Normal Values

Normal functioning of the gallbladder
No stones in gallbladder or ducts

Possible Meanings of Abnormal Values

Benign tumor
Cancer of the gallbladder
Cholecystitis
Cholesterol polyps
Cystic duct obstruction
Duct defects
Gallstones

Contributing Factors to Abnormal Values

- Under- or overexposure of the film may alter film quality.
- When patients are unable to hold still, due to pain or mental status, the quality of the film may be affected.
- Retained barium for other exams, vomiting, and diarrhea will affect test results.

Interventions/Implications

Pretest

- Explain to the patient the purpose of the test and the benefits and risks associated with the test. Provide any written teaching materials available on the subject. Note that no discomfort is associated with this procedure.
- The patient is given a low-fat or fat-free diet the evening before the test.
- Two hours after the meal and after assessing for allergy to the dye, the patient is given six tablets (3 g) of iopanoic acid. These should be taken at 5 minute intervals with at least 2 ounces of water each time.
- Fasting is required from the time of dye ingestion until the time of the test.
- Most allergic reactions to radiopaque dye occur within 30 minutes of administration of the contrast medium. Observe the patient closely for: respiratory distress, hypotension, edema, hives, rash, tachycardia, and/or laryngeal stridor. Emergency resuscitation equipment must be readily accessible.

- Instruct the patient to remove all objects containing metal, such as jewelry or undergarments, as these will show on the film.

Procedure
- Films are taken of the right upper quadrant area with the patient in prone, left lateral decubitus, and erect positions.
- Occasionally, the patient is given a high-fat meal or a synthetic fat-containing agent to stimulate and test for gallbladder contractility. Films are taken 1 to 2 hours after this fat stimulus.

Posttest
- Resume the patient's diet and medications as taken prior to the test. Encourage fluid intake to enhance excretion of the dye.
- Inform the patient that the dye is excreted in the urine and may cause mild dysuria.
- If the gallbladder does not visualize, the test may be repeated following ingestion of a double dose of the dye tablets.
- Report abnormal findings to the primary care provider.

→ Clinical Alerts

- If a barium swallow or an upper gastrointestinal and small-bowel series test is ordered, these should be completed *after* the cholecystography is performed, otherwise the barium sulfate ingested during the other exams may obscure the films made of the gallbladder.
- Possible Complication: Allergic reaction to dye

CONTRAINDICATIONS!

- Pregnant women
    - Caution: A woman in her childbearing years should undergo radiography only during her menses or 12 to 14 days after its onset to avoid any exposure to a fetus.
- Patients with renal or hepatic failure
- Patients with hypersensitivity to iodine, seafood, or contrast media
- Patients with bilirubin of >2 mg/dL (gallbladder will not be visualized by the dye)
- Patients who are unable to cooperate due to age, mental status, pain, or other factors

Cholesterol (Total)

Test Description
Cholesterol is synthesized in the liver from dietary fats. Its functions include being used in the production of bile salts and several of the steroid hormones, and as a part of cell membranes. Cholesterol is transported in the blood by the low density lipoproteins (LDLs, or "bad" cholesterol) and high density lipoproteins (HDLs, or

"good" cholesterol). A great deal of research has focused on the role of cholesterol in heart disease. High levels of cholesterol in the blood (*hypercholesterolemia*), especially in combination with low levels of HDL, have been found to increase the person's risk of atherosclerosis and heart disease. This test allows evaluation of this risk potential, assists in determining treatment options, and is used to monitor effectiveness of treatment.

THE EVIDENCE FOR PRACTICE

According to the Third Report of the National Cholesterol Education Program (NCEP) Expert Panel on Detection, Evaluation, and Treatment of High Blood Cholesterol in adults (http://www.nhlbi.nih.gov/guidelines/cholesterol/atp3_rpt.htm):

- In all adults aged 20 years or older, a fasting lipoprotein profile (total cholesterol, LDL cholesterol, HDL cholesterol, and triglycerides) should be obtained once every 5 years. If the testing opportunity is nonfasting, only the values for total cholesterol and HDL cholesterol will be usable. In such a case, if total cholesterol is ≥200 mg/dL or HDL is <40 mg/dL, a follow-up lipoprotein profile is needed for appropriate management based on LDL.

Normal Values

Desirable: <200 mg/dL (<5.18 mmol/L SI units)

Abnormal Values

Borderline High: 200–239 mg/dL (5.18–6.19 mmol/L SI units)
High: >239 mg/dL (>6.20 mmol/L SI units)

Possible Meanings of Abnormal Values

Increased	Decreased
Atherosclerosis	AIDS
Biliary cirrhosis	Chronic anemia
Cardiovascular disease	Hemolytic anemia
Hypercholesterolemia	Hyperthyroidism
Hyperlipidemia	Hypolipoproteinemia
Hypertriglyceridemia	Liver disease
Hypothyroidism	Malabsorption
Liver disease/biliary obstruction	Malnutrition
Nephrotic syndrome	Pernicious anemia
Obesity	Sepsis
Pancreatic dysfunction	Severe infections
Preeclampsia	Stress
Pregnancy	
Uncontrolled diabetes mellitus	
Xanthomatosis	

Contributing Factors to Abnormal Values

- Drugs which may *increase* cholesterol levels: atypical antipsychotics, beta-blockers, corticosteroids, disulfiram, lansoprazole, levodopa, lithium, oral contraceptives, pergolide, phenobarbital, phenytoin, sulfonamides, testosterone, thiazide diuretics, ticlopidine, venlafaxine.

- Drugs which may *decrease* cholesterol levels: ACE-inhibitors, allopurinol, androgens, cholesterol lowering agents, erythromycin, estrogens, filgrastim, levothyroxine, metformin, phenytoin, prazosin, tamoxifen, terazosin.

C

Interventions/Implications

Pretest
- Explain to the patient the purpose of the test and the need for a blood sample to be drawn.
- Fasting for 12 hours is required prior to the test. Water is permitted.
- No alcohol is allowed for 24 hours prior to the test.

Procedure
- A 7-mL blood sample is drawn in a red-top collection tube.
- Gloves are worn throughout the procedure.

Posttest
- Apply pressure at venipuncture site. Apply dressing, periodically assessing for continued bleeding.
- Label the specimen and transport it to the laboratory.
- Report abnormal findings to the primary care provider.

→ Clinical Alerts

- If the test result is >200 mg/dL, patient education is needed regarding:
  - reduced intake of saturated fat and cholesterol
  - increased physical activity
  - weight control
- Depending on levels of other lipoproteins and the degree of hypercholesterolemia present, cholesterol-lowering medication may be initiated, along with lifestyle modifications.

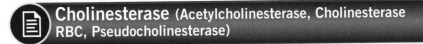

Cholinesterase (Acetylcholinesterase, Cholinesterase RBC, Pseudocholinesterase)

Test Description
There are two enzymes which hydrolyze acetylcholine (ACh): acetylcholinesterase, or true cholinesterase, and pseudocholinesterase, or serum cholinesterase. *Acetylcholinesterase*, which is present in nerve tissue, the spleen, and the gray matter of the brain, helps with the transmission of impulses across nerve endings to muscle fibers. *Pseudocholinesterase*, produced mainly in the liver, appears in small amounts in the pancreas, intestine, heart, and white matter of the brain.

C

Two groups of anticholinesterase chemicals, organophosphates and muscle relaxants, either affect or are affected by these enzymes. Organophosphates, which inactivate acetylcholinesterase, are found in many insecticides and nerve gas. Muscle relaxants, such as succinylcholine, are normally destroyed by pseudocholinesterase. If, however, there is a lack of pseudocholinesterase, the patient may experience a prolonged period of apnea if given muscle relaxants during surgery. Thus, patients who are to receive such drugs during surgery should be pretested for cholinesterase.

Normal Values

7–19 U/mL 7–19 kU/L (SI units)

Possible Meanings of Abnormal Values

Decreased

Acute infections
Anemia
Chronic malnutrition
Cirrhosis with jaundice
Dermatomyositis
Hepatitis
Inability to hydrolyze muscle relaxants in surgery
Infectious mononucleosis
Metastasis
Myocardial infarction
Poisoning from organic phosphate insecticides
Tuberculosis
Uremia

Contributing Factors to Abnormal Values

- Hemolysis of the blood sample will alter test results.
- Due to medications used during surgery, cholinesterase levels should not be checked in the recovery room.
- Drugs which may *decrease* cholinesterase levels: atropine, caffeine, chloroquine hydrochloride, codeine, cyclophosphamide, estrogens, folic acid, MAO-inhibitors, morphine sulfate, neostigmine, oral contraceptives, phenothiazines, physostigmine, phospholine iodine, pyridostigmine bromide, quinidine, quinine sulfate, succinylcholine, theophylline, vitamin K.

Interventions/Implications

Pretest
- Explain to the patient the purpose of the test and the need for a blood sample to be drawn.
- No fasting is required before the test.
- Medications which might affect the cholinesterase level should be held for 24 hours before the sample is drawn.
- If surgery is planned, the blood should be drawn at least 2 days prior to surgery.

Procedure
- A 5-mL blood sample is drawn in a lavender-top (EDTA) tube and 2 mL in a red-top collection tube (no gel).
- Gloves are worn throughout the procedure.

C

Posttest
- Apply pressure at venipuncture site. Apply dressing, periodically assessing for continued bleeding.
- Label the specimen and transport it to the laboratory.
- Report abnormal findings to the primary care provider.

 Chorionic Villus Sampling (CVS, Chorionic Villus Biopsy)

Test Description

The chorionic villi are finger-like projections that surround the embryonic membrane. These projections establish a connection with the endometrium, leading to the development of the placenta. Chorionic villi sampling (CVS) is a test used for the detection of genetic and biochemical disorders. CVS may be performed in situations where there is increased risk of birth defects, including maternal age over 35 years, previous child or pregnancy with a birth defect, or family medical history indicating increased risk of inheriting a genetic disorder.

It is performed during the first trimester of pregnancy, usually between the tenth and twelfth weeks of gestation. The test may be performed via transabdominal or transcervical approaches; however, the transcervical is most commonly used. The transabdominal approach is suggested if the uterus is retroverted, since there is an increased risk of spontaneous abortion when the transcervical approach is used in this situation.

The sample obtained through the procedure is used to study the DNA, chromosomes, and enzymes of the fetus. Advantages of this procedure versus amniocentesis are that it can be performed earlier in the pregnancy and provides diagnostic information much sooner. However, CVS does not detect neural tube defects. If neural tube defects or Rh incompatibility are a concern, an amniocentesis is needed.

Normal Values

Absence of genetic or biochemical disorders

Possible Meanings of Abnormal Values

Biochemical disorder
Genetic disorder

Interventions/Implications

Pretest
- Explain to the patient the purpose of the test. Note that some mild discomfort may be felt during insertion of the cannula through the cervix.
- No fasting is required prior to the test.

- The morning of the procedure, the patient is to drink at least 16 ounces of fluid and refrain from urinating to fill the bladder. This allows for better visualization during the procedure.
- Obtain a signed written consent.
- An ultrasound is performed to determine the position of the uterus, the size of the gestational sac, and the position of the placenta within the uterus.

Procedure
- The patient is placed in the lithotomy position with her legs supported in the stirrups. Privacy is maintained with proper draping.
- The external genitalia are cleansed and a vaginal speculum is inserted.
- The cervix is swabbed with an antiseptic solution.
- Under ultrasound guidance, the catheter is inserted through the cervix into the uterine cavity, and rotated to the site of the developing placenta.
- Suction is applied to the catheter by a syringe to obtain a tissue sample from the villi.
- The sample is prepared per institutional policy.
- Gloves are worn throughout the procedure.

Posttest
- Monitor the vital signs after the procedure and assess for vaginal bleeding.
- An ultrasound is done after the procedure is completed.
- Inform the patient that mild cramping and vaginal discomfort may occur following the procedure. Instruct the patient to report immediately any excessive pain, cramping, or bleeding.
- Label the specimen and transport it to the laboratory immediately.
- Report abnormal findings to the primary care provider.

→ Clinical Alerts

- Possible complications include: bleeding, infection, and spontaneous abortion.
- Due to the possibility of mixing of fetal and maternal blood cells during the procedure, if the woman's blood is Rh-negative, RhoGAM may be administered to avoid Rh incompatibility.
- An ultrasound of the fetus is usually performed 2 to 4 days following the chorionic villi sampling to assess continued fetal viability.

CONTRAINDICATIONS!

- Cervical infections with *Chlamydia* or herpes are contraindications to transcervical CVS.
- CVS is usually not recommended if a woman has bleeding or spotting during the pregnancy.

Chromosome Analysis (Chromosome Karyotype)

Test Description
Chromosome analysis involves the study of an individual's chromosomal makeup, or karyotype. Both chromosomal number and structure are studied. The test is used to determine chromosomal abnormalities and to identify the child's sex in the case

of ambiguous genitalia or prior to delivery. This test is considered part of the workup done for amenorrhea, infertility, and frequent miscarriages. It is also used in genetic counseling for individuals with a family history of genetic disease. Chromosome analysis usually involves a culture of leukocytes from peripheral blood. However, karyotyping may also be completed on other tissues, including amniotic fluid, bone marrow, buccal smear, chorionic villus, placental tissue, skin, and tumor cells.

C

Normal Values

Female: 44 autosomes, plus 2 X chromosomes; Karyotype: 46, XX
Male: 44 autosomes, plus 1X, 1Y chromosome; Karyotype: 46, XY

Possible Meanings of Abnormal Values

Ambiguous genitalia
Down syndrome
Hyperploidy (>46 chromosomes)
Hypogonadism
Hypoploidy (<46 chromosomes)
Kleinfelter's syndrome
Mental retardation
Physical retardation
Trisomy 18
Turner's syndrome

Contributing Factors to Abnormal Values

• Hemolysis of the blood sample will alter test results.

Interventions/Implications

Pretest
• Explain to the patient the purpose of the test and the need for a blood sample to be drawn.
• No fasting is required before the test.

Procedure
• A 7-mL blood sample is drawn in a green-top (heparinized) collection tube.
• Gloves are worn throughout the procedure.

Posttest
• Apply pressure at venipuncture site. Apply dressing, periodically assessing for continued bleeding.
• Label the specimen and transport it to the laboratory.
• Report abnormal findings to the primary care provider.

Clinical Alerts

• Provide emotional support throughout the test and during the period of time spent waiting for results (time varies depending on type of tissue to be analyzed).
• Make appropriate referrals for genetic counseling, as needed.

Clostridium difficile Toxin Assay (*C. difficile,* Clostridial Toxin Assay)

C

Test Description

Clostridium difficile is a gram-positive bacterium that is normally present in the large intestine. When patients are taking broad-spectrum antibiotics, especially ampicillin, cepalosporins, or clindamycin, the normal flora of the intestine are diminished. However, *C. difficile* is resistant to these antibiotics, so its presence actually increases under these circumstances. Its presence can also increase in immunocompromised patients.

  C. difficile releases two necrotizing toxins (A and B), one of which causes necrosis of the lining of the colon. This results in the development of *Pseudomembranous colitis*, a potentially fatal condition, 4 to 10 days after the antibiotic therapy is initiated. Symptoms include complaints of abdominal cramping, fever, and copious amounts of watery diarrhea. Leukocytosis is also present. Through testing for this bacterial infection, treatment can be initiated, including discontinuance of the broad-spectrum antibiotics, administration of metronidazole or vancomycin, and, if needed, intravenous infusion of fluids.

THE EVIDENCE FOR PRACTICE

Any illness involving diarrhea that persists for greater than 7 days, especially in an immunocompromised patient, should prompt further testing of stool specimens.

Normal Values

  Negative

Possible Meanings of Abnormal Values

Increased

- Antibiotic-related pseudomembranous enterocolitis
- *C. difficile* colitis

Contributing Factors to Abnormal Values

- False negative may result if sample was not processed promptly or stored correctly prior to processing.
- False positive may occur with grossly (visibly) bloody stool samples.

Interventions/Implications

Pretest
- Explain to the patient the purpose of the test and the need for a stool sample to be collected.
- Instruct the patient to avoid contaminating the stool with toilet paper or urine. This can be done through use of a plastic collection receptacle in the toilet.
- No fasting is required before the test.

Procedure
- Obtain a 5-mL stool specimen in a plastic screw-cap container.

- The specimen should be placed on ice or refrigerated.
- Gloves are worn when dealing with the specimen collection.

Posttest
- The sample is labeled and transported to the laboratory as soon as possible after collection of the specimen.
- Report abnormal findings to the primary care provider.

Clinical Alerts

- Due to the effect of the toxin on the colon lining, patients should be monitored for signs/symptoms of colon perforation.
- Endoscopic evaluation of the colon may be useful for diagnosis.
- Due to its high cost, use of vancomycin may require preauthorization from the patient's insurance carrier for medication coverage.

Coagulation Factor Assay (Factor Assay, Clotting Factors)

Test Description
Whenever there is tissue injury or injury to blood vessels, platelets aggregate at the area of the injury. These platelets release factors which begin the clotting process (hemostasis). The original type of injury dictates the pathway by which the process is initiated.

The *intrinsic pathway* is involved when there is damage to the blood or the blood is exposed to collagen in the walls of traumatized blood vessels. The intrinsic pathway requires the sequential activation of several coagulation factors: factor XII (Hageman factor), factor XI (plasma thromboplastin antecedent), factor IX (Christmas factor), and factor VIII (antihemophilic globulin).

The *extrinsic pathway* is launched when there is injury to tissue or to the vascular wall. In this pathway, clotting is triggered by the release of tissue thromboplastin (factor III) from the damaged vascular or tissue cells. When this substance encounters factor VII (stable factor), the extrinsic pathway is stimulated.

Both pathways ultimately lead to the activation of coagulation factor X (Stuart-Prower factor). This leads to the next step, in which prothrombin (factor II) is converted to thrombin (factor IIa [activated]). Thrombin then stimulates the formation of fibrin (factor Ia) from fibrinogen (factor I). This fibrin, with the addition of fibrin stabilizing factor (XIII), forms a stable fibrin clot at the site of injury. Once the fibrin clot is no longer needed, it is dissolved by fibrinolytic agents such as plasmin, resulting in fibrin degradation products.

Any excess amounts of clotting factors which remain following hemostasis are inactivated by fibrin inhibitors, such as antiplasmin, antithrombin III, and protein C. This prevents clotting from occurring indiscriminately.

The coagulation factor assay is conducted to determine whether a congenital or acquired deficiency of any blood clotting factor is present. This test is useful in diagnosing hemophilia and/or coagulation disorders. In the test, the patient's blood is mixed with either normal serum or a prepared serum with a known specific deficiency. The coagulation factor assay is performed after the review of other test results which may indicate the factor which is possibly deficient.

Normal Values

50%–150% (Refer to reference laboratory for normal values for specific factor)

Possible Meanings of Abnormal Values

Factor I (Fibrinogen)

Decreased

Congenital deficiency
Disseminated intravascular coagulation
Fibrinolysis
Liver disease

Factor II (Prothrombin)

Decreased

Congenital deficiency
Liver disease
Vitamin K deficiency

Factor V (Labile factor/Proaccelerin)

Decreased

Congenital deficiency
Deep venous thrombosis
Disseminated intravascular coagulation
Fibrinolysis
Liver disease
Pulmonary embolism

Factor VII (Stable factor/Proconvertin)

Decreased

Congenital deficiency
Hemorrhagic disease of the newborn
Kwashiorkor
Liver disease
Vitamin K deficiency

Factor VIII (Antihemophilic globulin)

Increased	**Decreased**
Coronary artery disease	Autoimmune disease
Cushing's syndrome	Congenital deficiency
Hyperthyroidism	Disseminated intravascular coagulation
Hypoglycemia	Fibrinolysis

Inflammation
Late pregnancy
Macroglobulinemia
Myeloma
Postoperative period
Progesterone use
Rebound activity after sudden
  cessation of warfarin
Thromboembolic conditions

Hemophilia A
von Willebrand's disease

Factor IX (Christmas factor)

Decreased

Cirrhosis
Congenital deficiency
Disseminated intravascular coagulation
Hemophilia B (Christmas disease)
Hemorrhagic disease of newborn
Liver disease
Nephrotic syndrome
Normal newborn
Vitamin K deficiency

Factor X (Stuart-Prower factor)

Increased	Decreased
Pregnancy	Congenital deficiency
	Disseminated intravascular coagulation
	Liver disease
	Vitamin K deficiency

Factor XI (Plasma thromboplastin antecedent)

Decreased

Congenital deficiency
Congenital heart disease
Hemophilia C
Intestinal malabsorption of vitamin K
Liver disease
Normal newborn
Stress
Vitamin K deficiency

Factor XII (Hageman factor)

Increased	Decreased
Exercise	Congenital deficiency
	Nephrotic syndrome
	Normal newborn
	Pregnancy

Factor XIII (Fibrin stabilizing factor)

Decreased

Agammaglobulinemia
Hyperfibrinogenemia

Lead poisoning
Liver disease
Myeloma
Pernicious anemia
Postoperative period

C

Contributing Factors to Abnormal Values

- Hemolysis of the blood sample may alter test results.
- Drugs which may alter values on the coagulation factor assay: anticoagulants.

Interventions/Implications

Pretest

- Explain to the patient the purpose of the test and the need for a blood sample to be drawn.
- No fasting is required before the test.
- If possible, the patient should receive no warfarin sodium for 2 weeks or heparin for 2 days, prior to the test. Check with the primary care provider regarding the appropriateness of withholding these medications from the patient.

Procedure

- A 7-mL blood sample is drawn in a light blue-top collection tube and immediately placed on ice.
- Gloves are worn throughout the procedure.

Posttest

- Apply pressure 3 to 5 minutes at venipuncture site. Apply dressing, periodically assessing for continued bleeding.
- Label the specimen and immediately transport it on ice to the laboratory.
- Teach the patient to monitor the site. If the site begins to bleed, the patient should apply direct pressure and, if unable to control the bleeding, return to the laboratory or notify the primary care provider.
- Resume any medications as taken prior to the test, if appropriate.
- Report abnormal findings to the primary care provider.

→ Clinical Alerts

- Possible complication: hematoma at site due to prolonged bleeding time.
- The prothrombin time and partial thromboplastin time can be analyzed to assist with determining what particular factor(s) may be deficient:
  - If the prothrombin time (PT) and activated partial thromboplastin time (APTT) are both abnormally prolonged, the deficiency is likely to involve factors II, V, or X.
  - If the PT is abnormal, but the APTT is normal, factor VII may be deficient.
  - If the PT is normal, but the APTT is abnormal, the deficient factor(s) may be from among those in the intrinsic pathway (VIII, IX, XI, XII).

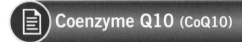

Coenzyme Q10 (CoQ10)

C

Test Description

Coenzyme Q10 (CoQ10) is an enzyme essential to mitochondrial ATP generation and antioxidant function in lipid and mitochondrial membranes. According to the American Association of Clinical Endocrinologists (2003), it has been found to have beneficial effects for mitochondrial disorders, congestive heart failure (CHF), and ischemia-reperfusion injury. In cases of insufficient CoQ10, electron transfer activity of the mitochondria decreases. This results in an energy production inadequate for cell operation. This can be especially stressful for tissues with very high energy demand such as the heart muscle.

The role of CoQ10 in myopathy associated with statin use is also being studied. Statins have been shown to create a CoQ10 deficiency, especially in the elderly, since the enzyme typically decreases with age and in those with congestive heart failure. The use of CoQ10 supplementation for statin-associated myopathy is starting to gain support, since dietary sources of the enzyme are insufficient. Prophylactic therapy may be considered with initiation of statin therapy. It may also be considered for use with patients complaining of statin-associated myalgias who do not have laboratory evidence of myositis or rhabdomyolysis, such as elevated creatine kinase levels.

Normal Values

Therapeutic range for cardiovascular disease >2.5 mg/L

Possible Meanings of Abnormal Values

Decreased
CoQ10 deficiency

Interventions/Implications

Pretest
- Explain to the patient the purpose of the test and the need for a blood sample to be drawn.
- No fasting is required before the test.

Procedure
- A 7-mL blood sample is drawn in a red-top collection tube.
- Gloves are worn throughout the procedure.

Posttest
- Apply pressure at venipuncture site. Apply dressing, periodically assessing for continued bleeding.
- Label the specimen and transport it to the laboratory.
- Report abnormal findings to the primary care provider.

Clinical Alerts

- CoQ10 is best absorbed when taken with a balanced meal.
- Providers should investigate CoQ10 benefits and side effects prior to considering its use with patients.

Cold/Febrile Agglutinins

C

Test Description

Agglutinins are antibodies which cause red blood cells to aggregate, or clump. These antibodies can cause hemolytic anemia. It is important to know which type of agglutinin is causing the hemolytic anemia so that appropriate therapy can be initiated.

Cold agglutinins are active at low temperatures. These antibodies, which are primarily of the IgM type, are most active at temperatures below 37°C, thus the term "cold" is used. This test is often used to diagnose primary atypical pneumonia caused by *Mycoplasma pneumoniae*. Cold agglutinins usually rise within 8 to 10 days after the onset of atypical pneumonia, peak in 12 to 25 days, and decrease 30 days after onset.

Febrile agglutinins are those which are associated with diseases which cause fever. Such infectious diseases include *Brucellosis*, rickettsial infections such as Rocky Mountain spotted fever and typhus, salmonellosis, and tularemia. To test for febrile agglutinins, a sample of the patient's serum is mixed with a few drops of prepared antigens on a slide. If agglutination occurs, antigen is added to serial dilutions of the patient's serum until agglutination is no longer noted.

Normal Values

Cold Agglutinins:	No agglutination with titers ≤1:16
Febrile Agglutinins:	No agglutination with titers ≤1:80

Possible Meanings of Abnormal Values

Increased Cold Agglutinins

Hemolytic anemia
Hodgkin's disease
Infectious mononucleosis
Lymphoma
Malaria
Multiple myeloma
Mycoplasma pneumoniae
Primary atypical pneumonia
Scleroderma
Syphilitic cirrhosis
Viral pneumonia

Increased Febrile Agglutinins

Brucellosis
Rickettsial diseases
Rocky Mountain spotted fever
Salmonellosis
Tularemia
Typhus

Contributing Factors to Abnormal Values
- Hemolysis of the blood sample may alter test results.
- Drugs which may interfere with the development of cold/febrile agglutinins: antibiotics.

Interventions/Implications
Pretest
- Explain to the patient the purpose of the test and the need for a blood sample to be drawn. Inform the patient that additional blood samples may be needed in 12 to 25 days and again in 30 days if checking for cold agglutinins and every 3 to 5 days if checking for febrile agglutinins.
- No fasting is required prior to the test.

Procedure
- A 7-mL blood sample is drawn in a red-top collection tube. The tube is prewarmed to 37°C if checking cold agglutinins and cooled if checking for febrile agglutinins.
- Gloves are worn throughout the procedure.

Posttest
- Apply pressure at venipuncture site. Apply dressing, periodically assessing for continued bleeding.
- Label the specimen and transport it to the laboratory *immediately.*
- Report abnormal findings to the primary care provider.

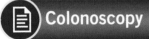

Colonoscopy

Test Description
Colonoscopy is the direct visualization of the large intestine through the use of a flexible fiberoptic endoscope. This endoscope is a multilumen instrument which allows viewing of the organ linings, insufflation of air, aspiration of fluid, removal of foreign objects, obtaining of tissue biopsies, and passage of a laser beam for obliteration of abnormal tissue or control of bleeding. This procedure is performed when the patient has experienced lower gastrointestinal bleeding or a change in bowel habits and when the patient is at high risk for colon cancer due to having polyps, ulcerative colitis, or previous colon cancer. As a screening test, it is recommended as a part of preventive health maintenance.

THE EVIDENCE FOR PRACTICE
According to American Gastroenterological Association Institute (AGAI) guidelines (http://www.gastrojournal.org/article/PIIS0016508502158951/fulltext), men and women at average risk should be offered screening with one of the following options beginning at age 50 years: yearly fecal occult blood testing (FOBT), flexible sigmoidoscopy every 5 years, combined FOBT and flexible sigmoidoscopy, colonoscopy every 10 years, or double-contrast barium enema every 5 years.

People with a first-degree relative (parent, sibling, or child) with colon cancer or adenomatous polyps diagnosed at age <60 years or 2 first-degree relatives diagnosed with colorectal cancer at any age should be advised to have screening colonoscopy starting at age 40 years or 10 years younger than the earliest diagnosis in their family, whichever comes first, and repeated every 5 years.

C

Normal Values

Normal colon

Possible Meanings of Abnormal Values

Benign lesions
Colon cancer
Crohn's disease
Diverticulosis
Granulomatous colitis
Hemorrhoids
Polyps
Proctitis
Pseudomembranous colitis
Ulcerative colitis

Contributing Factors to Abnormal Values

- Retention of barium following previous tests, inadequate preparation of the colon resulting in retained feces, and active gastrointestinal bleeding hinders successful completion of this test.

Interventions/Implications

Pretest

- Explain to the patient the purpose of the test. Provide any written teaching materials available on the subject. Inform the patient that pressure in the colon may be experienced during movement of the endoscope and during insufflation with air or carbon dioxide.
- Obtain a signed informed consent.
- The colon is prepared for the examination as follows:
  - clear liquid diet for 2 days prior to the test
  - either a strong cathartic is given the evening before the test, followed by an enema the morning of the test, *or* the patient drinks a large volume of a bowel prep solution such as Colyte (polyethylene glycol/electrolyte solution) the day before the test
- Monitor the patient for dehydration.
- Fasting for 8 to 12 hours is required prior to the test.
- Resuscitation and suctioning equipment should be readily available.
- Administer preprocedure medications as ordered. An anticholinergic such as atropine and a medication such as midazolam may be used for sedation and relief of anxiety.

Procedure
- The patient is assisted into the left lateral decubitus position on the endoscopy table.
- Baseline vital signs are obtained. Periodic vital sign assessment is performed during the procedure.
- A maintenance IV infusion is initiated.
- The endoscope is inserted through the anus and advanced through the rectum into the sigmoid colon and continuing to the cecum. The patient may need to be assisted to change positions to aid in advancement of the endoscope.
- During the procedure, insufflation of the bowel with air is used for better visualization.
- Encourage the patient to take slow, deep breaths to induce relaxation and to minimize the urge to defecate.
- Biopsy forceps may be used to remove a tissue specimen, or a cytology brush may be used to obtain cells from the surface of a lesion. Removal of foreign bodies or polyps is accomplished, if needed.
- Videotaping of the procedure is often done via a camera attached to the endoscope.
- Gloves are worn throughout the procedure.

Posttest
- Monitor vital signs every 15 minutes until stable.
- Observe the patient for indications of bowel perforation: rectal bleeding, abdominal pain and distention, fever.
- Oversedation of the patient may require administration of a narcotic antagonist, such as naloxone.
- Once fully awake, fluids and food may be resumed.
- Inform the patient that passage of a large amount of flatus is normal after this procedure.
- Report abnormal findings to the primary care provider.

→ Clinical Alerts

- Possible complications of the procedure include: Bleeding, perforation of the bowel, and oversedation.
- The patient may be drowsy due to the medications administered during the procedure. Someone else will need to drive the patient home and plan to stay with the patient until fully recovered.
- Findings of the colonoscopy determine recommended follow-up. For example, if the test is normal, the recommended subsequent colonoscopy is in 10 years. If polyps are found, recommended follow-up ranges from 1 to 5 years.

CONTRAINDICATIONS!

- Patients with acute diverticulitis, peritonitis, ischemic bowel disease, or fulminant ulcerative colitis
- Patients with suspected perforation of the colon
- Patients who are medically unstable
- Patients unable to cooperate with the examination

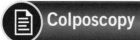
Colposcopy

C

Test Description
Colposcopy is the direct visualization of the cervix and vagina via a colposcope, which is an instrument containing a magnifying lens and a light. This magnification is 10 to 40 times normal. When a patient has had abnormal cervical Pap results, this procedure is used to identify the area of cellular dysplasia. Any suspicious lesions which are found can then be accurately biopsied.

THE EVIDENCE FOR PRACTICE
Referral for colposcopy is recommended for all immunosuppressed patients with ASC-US. This includes all women infected with human immunodeficiency virus (HIV), irrespective of CD4 cell count, HIV viral load, or antiretroviral therapy.

Normal Values
Normal vagina and cervix

Possible Meanings of Abnormal Values
Atrophic changes
Cervical neoplasia
Condyloma
Erosion
Human papilloma virus (HPV)
Infection
Inflammation
Invasive carcinoma
Precancerous cervical changes

Contributing Factors to Abnormal Values
- Scarring of the cervix and failure to thoroughly remove secretions from the cervix during the procedure may limit visualization of the cervix.

Interventions/Implications
Pretest
- Explain to the patient the purpose of the test.
- No fasting is required prior to the test.
- Instruct the patient to avoid douching and sexual intercourse for 24 hours prior to the exam.
- Obtain a signed written consent.

Procedure
- The patient should empty her bladder prior to the exam.
- The patient is placed in the lithotomy position with her legs supported in the stirrups. Privacy is maintained with proper draping.
- The external genitalia are cleansed and a vaginal speculum is inserted.
- Endocervical curettage is performed to prevent epithelial cells dislodged during the colposcopy from interfering with the test results.

- The cervix is then swabbed with 3% acetic acid solution to remove secretions and medications, and to highlight abnormal areas.
- The colposcope is placed at the vaginal opening and its light is focused on the cervix.
- The cervix is examined and a biopsy is taken of any suspicious lesions.
- The vagina is rinsed with sterile saline or water to remove the acetic acid, which can cause a burning sensation.
- Gloves are worn throughout the procedure

Posttest
- Cleanse the perineal area and assist the patient to a position of comfort. A sanitary pad may be used in case of vaginal bleeding.
- Inform the patient that mild cramping, vaginal discomfort, and vaginal discharge may occur following the procedure. Note that the discharge may continue for 1 week.
- Instruct the patient to avoid strenuous exercise for 24 hours and that use of tampons, douching and intercourse should be avoided for 2 weeks.
- Instruct the patient to report any abdominal pain, fever, or frank vaginal bleeding, or if the bleeding lasts longer than 2 weeks.
- Report abnormal findings to the primary care provider.

Clinical Alerts

- Possible complication: Vaginal bleeding.
- If warranted based on colposcopy results, additional procedures may be needed including cone biopsy and LEEP procedure.

CONTRAINDICATIONS!

- Patients with heavy menstrual flow
- Patients unable to cooperate with the examination

Complement Assay (C$_3$ and C$_4$ Complement)

Test Description
The term *complement* refers to the 20 serum beta-globulin protein enzymes which are a part of the immune system response to antigen-antibody reactions. The complement system is necessary for phagocytosis, destruction of foreign bacteria, and mediation of the overall inflammatory response. Activation of the complement cascade may occur by way of the *classic pathway*, in which activation is stimulated by an antigen-antibody response, or by the *alternate pathway*, in which polysaccharides, endotoxins, or immunoglobulins are the stimulating forces. Regardless of the stimulus, the final product of the complement cascade's work is a complex protein capable of destroying the cell membrane of the antigen.

To assess the functioning of the complement system and to determine whether deficiencies of these proteins are contributing to increased infections or increased

C

autoimmune activity, two of the components are typically measured. C_3 is involved in both the classic and alternate pathways and composes about 70% of the total complement protein. C_4 is involved in only the classic pathway. Individuals found to be deficient in C_4 have a lowered resistance to infection.

Normal Values

C_3:   83–177 mg/dL (0.83–1.77 g/L SI units)
C_4:   15–45 mg/dL (0.15–0.45 g/L SI units)

Possible Meanings of Abnormal Values

C_3 Complement

Increased	Decreased
Infection	Anemia
Inflammatory	Acute glomerulonephritis
Malignancy with metastasis	Anorexia nervosa
Necrotizing disorders	Arthralgias
Rheumatic fever	Celiac disease
Rheumatoid arthritis	Chronic active hepatitis
	Chronic liver disease
	Cirrhosis
	Congenital C_3 deficiency
	Disseminated intravascular coagulation
	Immune complex disease
	Malnutrition
	Multiple myeloma
	Multiple sclerosis
	Renal transplant rejection
	Septicemia
	Serum sickness
	Subacute bacterial endocarditis
	Systemic lupus erythematosus
	Uremia

C_4 Complement

Increased	Decreased
Cancer	Chronic active hepatitis
Juvenile rheumatoid arthritis	Congenital C_4 deficiency
Rheumatoid spondylitis	Cryoglobulinemia
	Glomerulonephritis
	Hereditary angioedema
	Immune complex disease
	Lupus nephritis
	Renal transplant rejection
	Serum sickness
	Subacute bacterial endocarditis
	Systemic lupus erythematosus

Contributing Factors to Abnormal Values

- Hemolysis of the sample may alter test results.

Interventions/Implications

Pretest
- Explain to the patient the purpose of the test and the need for a blood sample to be drawn.
- No fasting is required before the test.

C

Procedure
- A 7-mL blood sample is drawn in a red-top collection tube.
- Gloves are worn throughout the procedure.

Posttest
- Apply pressure at venipuncture site. Apply dressing, periodically assessing for continued bleeding.
- Label the specimen and transport it to the laboratory.
- Report abnormal findings to the primary care provider.

→ Clinical Alerts

- Risk of infection at venipuncture site due to possible immunocompromised state. Teach patient to notify health-care provider if drainage, redness, warmth, edema, or pain at the site or fever occur.

Complete Blood Count with Differential
(CBC with Differential)

Test Description

The complete blood count (CBC) with differential is one of the most commonly performed tests in health care. This is due to the vast amount of data obtained through the various components of this test. The test actually consists of several tests, which are discussed individually in this text.

If appropriate, the tests may be ordered individually. For example, a patient undergoing a total joint replacement has a complete blood count with differential drawn preoperatively. Postoperatively, the surgeon may choose to order a repeat testing of only the hemoglobin and hematocrit to determine the extent of blood loss which may have occurred during surgery.

Please refer to the following pages for these test descriptions:
- **Blood smear**, page 100
- **Hematocrit**, page 306
- **Hemoglobin**, page 308
- **Platelet count**, page 439
- **Red blood cell count**, page 488
- **Red blood cell indices** (includes mean corpuscular volume [MCV], mean corpuscular hemoglobin [MCH], and mean corpuscular hemoglobin concentration [MCHC]), page 491
- **White blood cell count and differential**, page 612

Computed Tomography (CT Scan, Computerized Axial Tomography [CAT], CT of Abdomen/Brain/Chest, Electron Beam Computed Tomographic Coronary Calcium Scanning [EBCT])

C

Test Description

Computed tomography (CT) is considered a radiographic procedure. X-rays are projected along the lines of the area of the body being assessed. An x-ray detector records the intensity of the x-rays as they are transmitted through the tissue. Different types of tissue cause differences in how the tissue decreases the x-ray beam as it passes through the tissue (tissue attenuation). This leads to an assignment of a *density coefficient* to the various tissues. The information is compiled and results in a visual display. The image may be enhanced by repeating the procedure after IV administration of iodine-based contrast dye.

CT of the abdomen is performed to diagnose pathologic conditions of the abdominal organs. Such conditions include inflammation, cysts, and tumors of the liver, gallbladder, pancreas, spleen, kidneys, and pelvic organs. Unenhanced helical (spiral) CT can accurately detect acute appendicitis, thereby avoiding possible allergic reactions and cost associated with contrast enhancement. The recent introduction of 64-slice CT is providing a possible future alternative to more invasive procedures by providing a "virtual colonoscopy."

CT of the brain is particularly sensitive to the presence of blood. It is especially useful after trauma and when neurologic symptoms suggest a stroke and/or hemorrhage due to embolus, arteriovenous malformation (AVM), angioma, or aneurysm. Noncontrast CT of the brain is currently the examination of choice for initial imaging of suspected acute stroke. Contrast-enhanced CTs do not consistently visualize low-grade tumors or the full extent of infiltrative neoplasms and associated edema as well as magnetic resonance imaging does.

CT of the chest is performed to diagnose pathologic conditions of the organs contained within the chest. Such conditions include inflammation, cysts, and tumors of the lungs, esophagus, and lymph nodes. Spiral (or helical) CT of the chest captures images of the chest from many angles, making it very useful in the evaluation of suspected pulmonary embolism.

CT of the kidneys/ureters is considered by most radiologists and urologists as the new gold standard for detecting urinary calculi in the acute setting due to its sensitivity of 95% to 96% and specificity of 98%. This is compared to ultrasonography with a sensitivity of 44%, intravenous urography, 64%, and KUB x-ray, 45%.

CT of the heart is improving with each new generation of scanner. The newest type of heart CT is the 64-slice CT which can produce "motion-free" images of the beating heart and coronary arteries due to its faster scan times. This type of CT has been found to be highly reliable in ruling out the presence of a significant coronary stenosis and may eventually be regarded as a suitable alternative to invasive coronary angiography.

Electron beam computed tomographic coronary calcium scanning (EBCT) uses both a stationary source-detector and a rotating electron beam to produce images which are synchronous with the cardiac cycle. The scan depicts areas of calcium in the coronary arteries. The Agatston calcium scoring algorithm is used to provide calcium scores for the various coronary arteries and a composite score. These scores are then compared with those of the same gender and age. The higher the calcium score, the greater the need for risk factor modification, including pharmacologic treatment with aspirin and statin medications. Exercise testing and myocardial perfusion imaging may be needed.

C

Other types of CT scans are those for the cervical, thoracic, or lumbosacral spine, neck, sinuses, and pelvis.

THE EVIDENCE FOR PRACTICE

A recent study (Henschke, 2006) noted approximately 80% of deaths from lung cancer could be prevented by spiral CT scanning in high-risk populations, since such screening detects lung cancer at its earliest stage, when it is curable.

Normal Values

No abnormalities

Possible Meanings of Abnormal Values

CT of Abdomen
Abdominal aortic aneurysm
Abscesses
Appendicitis
Bile duct dilation
Cysts
Diverticulitis
Gallstones
Hemorrhage
Infection
Laceration of spleen
Prostatic hypertrophy
Tumors

CT of Brain
Abscess
Arteriovenous malformation
Cerebral aneurysms
Cerebral infarction
Hemorrhage/hematoma
Hydrocephalus
Meningiomas
Multiple sclerosis
Neoplasms
Ventricular displacement
Ventricular enlargement

CT of Chest
Aortic aneurysm
Cyst
Enlarged lymph nodes

Esophageal tumors
Granuloma
Hiatal hernia
Inflammation
Mediastinal tumors
Metastatic tumors
Pleural effusion
Pneumonitis
Pulmonary embolism
Pulmonary tumor

Contributing Factors to Abnormal Values

- Any movement by the patient may alter quality of films taken.
- For CT of abdomen: retained barium, gas, or stool in the intestines may result in poor quality films.

Interventions/Implications

Pretest

- Explain to the patient the purpose of the test. Provide any written teaching materials available on the subject. Note that minimal discomfort during the test is due to the venipuncture, and that during injection of the dye, transient sensations including warmth, flushing, a salty taste, and nausea may be experienced. Explain that no movement is allowed during the procedure.
- Check for allergies to iodine, shellfish, or contrast medium dye. Inform the radiologist of such possible allergy and obtain order for an antihistamine and steroid to be administered prior to the test.
- Patients receiving metformin (Glucophage) for Type 2 diabetes mellitus should discontinue the drug 2 days before elective surgery or angiographic exams. This is due to the possible occurrence of lactic acidosis, a potentially fatal complication of biguanide therapy.
- Baseline BUN and creatinine levels are obtained.
- Fasting for at least 4 hours is required prior to the test if contrast dye is to be administered. The patient should be well hydrated prior to the beginning of the fasting period.
- For CT of abdomen: the patient will need to drink a contrast agent, such as barium sulfate, the evening prior to the test and again 1 hour before the test.
- Obtain a signed informed consent.
- For CT of brain, instruct the patient to remove any metal items from the hair or mouth prior to the procedure.

Procedure

- The patient is assisted to a supine position on the CT scan table.
- A maintenance IV line is initiated.
- The contrast dye is administered by IV injection. Resuscitation and suctioning equipment should be readily available.
- The patient is then placed in the CT scanner.
- Films are made, during which the patient may be asked to hold his or her breath.

Posttest

- Most allergic reactions to radiopaque dye occur within 30 minutes of administration of the contrast medium. Observe the patient closely for: respiratory distress, hypotension, edema, hives, rash, tachycardia, and/or laryngeal stridor. Emergency resuscitation equipment must be readily accessible.

- Observe for allergic reaction to the dye for 24 hours.
- Discontinue the IV infusion. Apply pressure at venipuncture site. Apply dressing, periodically assessing for continued bleeding.
- Resume the patient's diet. Encourage fluid intake of at least three glasses of liquid to speed the excretion of the dye from the body.
- Monitor urinary output.
- Inform the patient that if oral contrast dye was ingested, diarrhea may occur.
- Renal function should be assessed before metformin is restarted.
- Report abnormal findings to the primary care provider.

→ Clinical Alerts

- Possible complications include: allergic reaction to dye and acute renal failure from dye.
- Patients who are claustrophobic may require sedation prior to the CT exam.

CONTRAINDICATIONS!

- Patients who are allergic to iodine, shellfish, or contrast medium dye.
- Pregnant women.
    - Caution: A woman in her childbearing years should undergo radiography only during her menses or 12 to 14 days after its onset to avoid any exposure to a fetus.
- Patients who are morbidly obese or claustrophobic.
- Patients whose vital signs are unstable.
- Patients who are unable to cooperate due to age, mental status, pain, or other factors.
- Patients with renal failure or those susceptible to dye-induced renal failure (dehydrated patients).

Contraction Stress Test (CST, Contraction Challenge Test, Oxytocin Challenge Test, OCT)

Test Description

The contraction stress test (CST) is used to evaluate the ability of the fetus to withstand the contractions of labor. It is usually administered to those patients whose nonstress test (NST) was nonreactive. The CST mimics labor, in that uterine contractions are stimulated either through nipple stimulation which stimulates endogenous release of oxytocin or through the administration of exogenous oxytocin. During normal labor, uterine contractions cause a decrease in the placental blood flow. It is important to know that the fetus will be able to withstand this decrease in placental blood flow, otherwise the fetus is at risk of intrauterine asphyxia.

A negative CST is considered the norm. In this case, the placental reserve is adequate, resulting in a normal fetal heart rate (FHR) during uterine contraction. The test can be repeated weekly until the onset of labor.

C

A CST is considered positive when the uterine contraction results in late deceleration of the FHR. This indicates intrauterine hypoxia due to inadequate placental reserve. There must be late deceleration with two or more uterine contractions in order for the test to be considered positive. Due to the possibility of false-positive results, a positive CST should be considered in conjunction with other test results, such as that of an amniocentesis, before the fetus is delivered prior to the anticipated due date.

The CST is used in high-risk pregnancies in which the fetus may be threatened. These include maternal diabetes mellitus or hypertension, preeclampsia, intrauterine growth retardation, postmaturity syndrome, and Rh isoimmunization.

Normal Values

Negative (no late deceleration in the FHR following uterine contraction)

Possible Meanings of Abnormal Values

Inadequate placental reserve

Contributing Factors to Abnormal Values

- Maternal hypotension may cause a false-positive test result.

Interventions/Implications

Pretest

- Explain to the patient the purpose of the test and the procedure to be done. Note that discomfort associated with the test is due to mild labor contractions.
- Fasting for 4 to 8 hours is usually ordered in case premature labor occurs.
- Obtain a signed informed consent.

Procedure

- The patient is instructed to void.
- The patient is assisted into a semi-Fowler's, semi-side-lying position.
- An external fetal monitor is applied to the patient's abdomen, which will provide a graph of FHR and uterine contractions.
- Obtain baseline blood pressure. The blood pressure is monitored every 10 minutes during the procedure.
- Obtain a 20-minute baseline recording of the FHR. Assess for any uterine contractions.
- If uterine contractions are present, withhold oxytocin and monitor fetal response to the spontaneous contractions.
- If no uterine contractions are present, the nipples are stimulated for 15 minutes.
- If no uterine contractions occur with nipple stimulation, oxytocin is administered IV by electronic infusion pump.
- The oxytocin is increased in rate until the patient is having 3 contractions per 10 minutes. The oxytocin is then discontinued while the FHR and uterine contractions continue to be monitored for 30 minutes. (Note: It usually takes 20 to 25 minutes for the body to metabolize the oxytocin.)

Posttest

- Monitor the patient's blood pressure and the FHR until all uterine contractions have ceased.

- Discontinue the IV and apply a dressing to the venipuncture site. Check the dressing periodically for continued bleeding.
- Report abnormal findings to the primary care provider.

C

→ **Clinical Alerts**

- Possible complication: Premature labor
  - It is recommended that the contraction stress test not be done until at least the thirty-fourth week of gestation to improve chances of fetal survival should delivery occur prematurely.

CONTRAINDICATIONS!

- Patients with multiple fetuses
- Patients with premature ruptured membranes
- Patients with placenta previa or abruptio placentae
- Patients with previous classic or low transverse cesarean sections
- Patients with pregnancies of less than 32 weeks
- Patients with a history of premature labor or incompetent cervix

Coombs' Test, Direct (Direct Antiglobulin Test, RBC Antibody Screen)

Test Description

In some types of diseases, such as infectious mononucleosis and systemic lupus erythematosus, and in sensitizations such as to the Rh factor, the red blood cells become coated with antibodies. The direct Coombs' test serves as a screening test to determine whether such antibodies are attached to the patient's red blood cells.

In this test a sample of the patient's blood is mixed with Coombs' antihuman globulin serum. This serum is actually a rabbit serum which contains antibodies against human globulins. When the patient's blood is mixed with the rabbit serum, *clumping* or *agglutination* occurs if antibodies are present on the patient's red blood cells. A common cause of a positive direct Coombs' test is autoimmune hemolytic anemia in which the person has antibodies against his own red blood cells.

The test has multiple purposes. It is used to screen blood during type and cross-match procedures. It can also be used to detect red blood cell sensitization to drugs or blood transfusions, as in the testing for the occurrence of a hemolytic transfusion reaction. In cases of suspected erythroblastosis fetalis, the test can be used to determine the presence of antibodies to the newborn's red blood cells.

Normal Values

Negative

Possible Meanings of Abnormal Values

Positive	Negative
Elderly	Hemolytic anemia
Erythroblastosis fetalis	(nonautoimmune, non-drug-induced)
Hemolytic anemia (autoimmune,	Normal finding
drug-induced)	
Infectious mononucleosis	
Lymphomas	
Neoplasms	
Renal disorders	
Rheumatoid arthritis	
Systemic lupus erythematosus	
Transfusion reaction	

Contributing Factors to Abnormal Values

- Hemolysis of the blood sample may alter test results.
- Drugs which may cause a *positive* direct Coombs' test: ampicillin, captopril, cephalosporins, chlorpromazine, chlorpropamide, ethosuximide, hydralazine, indomethacin, insulin, isoniazid, levodopa, mefenamic acid, melphalan, methyldopa, para-aminosalicylic acid, penicillin, phenylbutazone, phenytoin, procainamide, quinidine, quinine sulfate, rifampin, streptomycin, sulfonamides, tetracyclines.

Interventions/Implications

Pretest
- Explain to the patient the purpose of the test and the need for a blood sample to be drawn.
- No fasting is required before the test.

Procedure
- A 7-mL blood sample is drawn in a lavender-top (EDTA) collection tube.
- For newborns, a 5-mL umbilical cord blood sample is sufficient.
- Gloves are worn throughout the procedure.

Posttest
- Apply pressure at venipuncture site. Apply dressing, periodically assessing for continued bleeding.
- Label the specimen and transport it to the laboratory.
- Report abnormal findings to the primary care provider.

Coombs' Test, Indirect (Antibody Screening Test)

Test Description
The indirect Coombs' test is used to detect unexpected circulating antibodies in the patient's serum which may react against transfused red blood cells. These antibodies are ones other than those of the A, B, and O blood groups. This is different from the direct Coombs' test, which detects antibodies already attached to the red blood cells.

In this test, the patient's serum is considered the antibody and the donor red blood cells as the antigen. The serum and antigenic red blood cells are brought together to allow any antibodies to attach to the red blood cells. Antihuman globulin is then added. If the patient's serum contains an antibody that reacted with and attached to the donor red blood cells, agglutination will occur and the test is considered positive. If no agglutination occurs, no antigen-antibody reaction has taken place. The serum may contain an antibody, but the donor red blood cells do not have the antigen against which the antibody would respond. Positive tests are followed with additional testing to identify the specific antibody present.

Normal Values

Negative

Possible Meanings of Abnormal Values

Positive

Erythroblastosis fetalis
Hemolytic anemia (drug-induced)
Incompatible crossmatch
Maternal-fetal Rh incompatibility
Prior transfusion reaction

Contributing Factors to Abnormal Values

- Hemolysis of the blood sample may alter test results.
- Administration of dextran or IV contrast media prior to the test may alter test results.
- Drugs which may cause a *positive* indirect Coombs' test: cephalosporins, chlorpromazine, insulin, isoniazid, levodopa, mefenamic acid, methyldopa, penicillin, phenytoin, procainamide, quinidine, sulfonamides, tetracyclines.

Interventions/Implications

Pretest
- Explain to the patient the purpose of the test and the need for a blood sample to be drawn.
- No fasting is required before the test.

Procedure
- A 7-mL blood sample is drawn in a red-top collection tube.
- Gloves are worn throughout the procedure.

Posttest
- Apply pressure at venipuncture site. Apply dressing, periodically assessing for continued bleeding.
- Label the specimen and transport it to the laboratory.
- Report abnormal findings to the primary care provider.

Clinical Alerts

- Positive indirect Coombs' tests indicate the need for antibody identification testing.

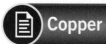 Copper

C

Test Description
Copper is an essential trace element needed in the synthesis of hemoglobin and oxidation reduction. Normally urine contains a very small amount of free copper, since most copper in the plasma is bound to ceruloplasmin, an alpha$_2$-globulin protein. Testing for urine copper content is used to aid in the diagnosis of *Wilson's disease*, a hereditary syndrome transmitted as an autosomal recessive trait. In this condition, decreased levels of ceruloplasmin are manufactured by the liver, serum copper levels are low, and urine copper levels are high. Without ceruloplasmin to transport the copper, Wilson's disease leads to an accumulation of copper in the tissue of the brain, eye, kidney, and liver. One of the hallmarks of this disease is the presence of Kayser-Fleischer rings around the iris of the eye, which are caused by copper deposits. Wilson's disease can be treated with penicillamine, an anticopper drug, which promotes the renal excretion of excess copper.

Normal Values
0–60 mcg/24 hours (0–0.96 μmol/day SI units)
Elderly: Increased

Possible Meanings of Abnormal Values

Increased
Alzheimer's disease
Biliary cirrhosis
Chronic, active hepatitis
Hypoceruloplasminemia
Nephrotic syndrome
Pellagra
Proteinuria
Wilson's disease

Interventions/Implications
Pretest
- Instruct the patient to refrain from taking vitamins, minerals, or herbal supplements for at least 1 week prior to the urine collection.
- Explain 24-hour urine collection procedure to the patient.
- Stress the importance of saving *all* urine in the 24-hour period. Instruct the patient to avoid contaminating the urine with toilet paper or feces.
- Inform the patient of the presence of a preservative in the collection bottle.

Procedure
- Obtain the proper container containing the appropriate preservative from the laboratory.
- Begin the testing period in the morning following the patient's first voiding, which is discarded.
- Timing of the 24-hour period begins at the time the first voiding is discarded.

- *All* urine for the next 24 hours is collected in the container, which is to be kept refrigerated or on ice.
- If any urine is accidentally discarded during the 24-hour period, the test must be discontinued and a new test begun.
- The ending time of the 24-hour collection period should be posted in the patient's room.
- Gloves are to be worn whenever dealing with the specimen collection.

Posttest
- Label the container and transport it on ice to the laboratory as soon as possible following the end of the 24-hour collection period.
- Report abnormal findings to the primary care provider.

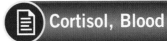
Cortisol, Blood

Test Description
In response to a stimulus such as stress, the hypothalamus secretes corticotropin-releasing hormone. This hormone stimulates the secretion of adrenocorticotropic hormone (ACTH) by the anterior pituitary gland. ACTH, in turn, causes the adrenal cortex to release the glucocorticoid hormone, *cortisol*. Cortisol has several functions, including:

- stimulation of glucose formation (gluconeogenesis)
- stimulation of stored energy molecular breakdown (fats, proteins, carbohydrates)
- promotion of sympathetic responses to stressors
- reduction of inflammation and immune function
- stimulation of gastric acid secretion

Cortisol levels in the blood provide valuable information regarding the functioning of the adrenal cortex. Cortisol is normally secreted in a diurnal pattern, with the peak or highest levels being between 6 and 8 a.m. and trough, or lowest, levels being at midnight.

Normal Values

8 a.m.–12 noon	5.0–25.0 mcg/dL (138–690 nmol/L SI units)
12 noon–8 p.m.	5.0–15.0 mcg/dL (138–410 nmol/L SI units)
8 p.m.–8 a.m.	0.0–10.0 mcg/dL (0–276 nmol/L SI units)

Possible Meanings of Abnormal Values

Increased	Decreased
Adrenal adenoma	Addison's disease
Burns	Adrenal insufficiency
Cushing's disease	Hypoglycemia
Cushing's syndrome	Hypopituitarism
Eclampsia	Hypothyroidism
Ectopic ACTH-producing tumors	Liver disease
Exercise	Postpartum pituitary necrosis

Hyperpituitarism
Hypertension
Hyperthyroidism
Infectious disease
Obesity
Pancreatitis (acute)
Pregnancy
Shock
Stress
Surgery

Contributing Factors to Abnormal Values

- Levels of cortisol may vary with exercise, sleep, and stress.
- Hemolysis of the sample may alter test results.
- Drugs which may *increase* cortisol levels include: amphetamines, estrogens, ethyl alcohol, lithium carbonate, methadone, nicotine, oral contraceptives, spironolactone, synthetic glucocorticoids (prednisone, prednisolone).
- Drugs which may *decrease* cortisol levels include: androgens, barbiturates, dexamethasone, levodopa, phenytoin.

Interventions/Implications

Pretest
- Explain to the patient the purpose of the test and the need for a blood sample to be drawn.
- Fasting and limited physical activity for 10 to 12 hours is required prior to the test.

Procedure
- A 7-mL blood sample is drawn in a red-top collection tube at 8 AM and again at 4 p.m.
- Gloves are worn throughout the procedure.

Posttest
- Apply pressure at venipuncture site. Apply dressing, periodically assessing for continued bleeding.
- Label the specimen and transport it to the laboratory. Include the time when the sample was obtained and any medications which might affect the test results.
- Report abnormal findings to the primary care provider.

 Cortisol, Urine (Free Cortisol)

Test Description

In response to a stimulus such as stress, the hypothalamus secretes corticotropin-releasing hormone. This hormone stimulates the secretion of *adrenocorticotropic hormone* (ACTH) by the anterior pituitary gland. ACTH, in turn, causes the adrenal cortex to release the glucocorticoid hormone, *cortisol*. Cortisol has several functions, including:

- stimulation of glucose formation (gluconeogenesis)
- stimulation of stored energy molecular breakdown (fats, proteins, carbohydrates)

- promotion of sympathetic responses to stressors
- reduction of inflammation and immune function
- stimulation of gastric acid secretion

Most of the cortisol present in the body is bound to cortisol-binding globulin and albumin. Five to ten percent is "free" or unconjugated, and is thus filtered by the kidneys into the urine. It is the free urinary cortisol which is measured by this test, which is used to evaluate adrenal function, especially hyperfunction. Generally, the urinary cortisol level will increase when the plasma cortisol level increases, and will decrease when the plasma cortisol level decreases. The creatinine level in the 24-hour urine specimen is usually measured along with the urinary cortisol level to confirm that the urine volume is adequate.

Normal Values

10–100 mcg/24 hour (27.6–276 nmol/day SI units)

Possible Meanings of Abnormal Values

Increased	Decreased
Amenorrhea	Addison's disease
Cushing's syndrome	Hypopituitarism
Hyperthyroidism	Hypothyroidism
Lung cancer	Renal glomerular dysfunction
Pituitary tumor	
Pregnancy	
Stress	

Contributing Factors to Abnormal Values

- Exercise and stress can affect cortisol levels.
- Drugs which may *increase* urinary cortisol levels: amphetamines, corticotropin, estrogens, nicotine, oral contraceptives, spironolactone, synthetic glucocorticoids (prednisone, prednisolone).
- The drug dexamethasone may *decrease* urinary cortisol levels.

Interventions/Implications

Pretest
- Explain 24-hour urine collection procedure to the patient.
- Stress the importance of saving *all* urine in the 24-hour period. Instruct the patient to avoid contaminating the urine with toilet paper or feces.
- Inform the patient of the presence of a preservative in the collection bottle.

Procedure
- Obtain the proper container containing 10 g of boric acid as preservative from the laboratory.
- Begin the testing period in the morning after the patient's first voiding, which is discarded.
- Timing of the 24-hour period begins at the time the first voiding is discarded.

- *All* urine for the next 24 hours is collected in the container, which is to be kept refrigerated or on ice.
- If any urine is accidentally discarded during the 24-hour period, the test must be discontinued and a new test begun.
- The ending time of the 24-hour collection period should be posted in the patient's room.
- Gloves are worn whenever dealing with the specimen collection.

Posttest

- At the end of the 24-hour collection period, label and send the urine container on ice to the laboratory as soon as possible.
- Report abnormal findings to the primary care provider.

➡ Clinical Alerts

- It is not recommended for this test to be performed if the patient is on prednisone/prednisolone therapy due to a cross-reactivity with the antibody used in this assay.

C-Peptide (Connecting Peptide, Insulin C-Peptide)

Test Description

Proinsulin is converted to insulin in the beta-cells of the pancreas. A by-product of this conversion is C-peptide, an inactive amino acid. C-peptide levels usually correlate with endogenous insulin levels and are not affected by exogenous insulin administration. Measurement of C-peptide levels is useful in:

- determining endogenous insulin levels, since the C-peptide level is not affected by exogenous insulin administration;
- determining whether hypoglycemia is being caused by nontherapeutic insulin injections (factitious hypoglycemia), in which case the C-peptide level will be low while insulin levels are elevated;
- determining presence of an insulinoma, which can be indicated by elevation of both insulin and C-peptide levels; and
- monitoring for recurrence of insulinoma, indicated by increasing C-peptide levels.

Normal Values

0.5–2.0 ng/mL (0.17–0.67 nmol/L SI units)

Possible Meanings of Abnormal Values

Increased	Decreased
Insulinoma	Diabetes mellitus
Islet cell tumor	Hypoglycemia due to insulin
Pancreas transplants	insulin overdose/abuse
Renal failure	Pancreatectomy

Contributing Factors to Abnormal Values

- Hemolysis of the blood sample may alter test results.
- C-peptide levels may not correlate with endogenous insulin levels in the presence of obesity or islet cell tumors.
- Drugs which may *increase* C-peptide levels: sulfonylureas.

C

Interventions/Implications

Pretest

- Explain to the patient the purpose of the test and the need for a blood sample to be drawn.
- Fasting for 8 to 10 hours is required prior to the test. Water is permitted.

Procedure

- A 7-mL blood sample is drawn in a red-top collection tube.
- Gloves are worn throughout the procedure.

Posttest

- Apply pressure at venipuncture site. Apply dressing, periodically assessing for continued bleeding.
- Label the specimen and transport it to the laboratory.
- Report abnormal findings to the primary care provider.

 C-Reactive Protein (CRP, hs-CRP)

Test Description

C-reactive protein (CRP) is a glycoprotein produced by the liver, which is normally absent from the blood. The presence of acute inflammation with tissue destruction within the body stimulates its production. Therefore, a positive CRP indicates the presence of an inflammatory process. When the acute inflammation is no longer present, the CRP rapidly dissipates from the body. The CRP typically rises within 6 hours of the start of inflammation, allowing the inflammation to be confirmed much sooner than through the use of the erythrocyte sedimentation rate (ESR), which usually increases about a week after inflammation begins.

There are two types of CRP which can be measured. The standard CRP is used to assess how active inflammation is in such chronic problems as inflammatory bowel disease, arthritis, and autoimmune diseases; to assess for a new infection such as in appendicitis and postoperative conditions; and to monitor response to treatment of these conditions. The other type of CRP is high-sensitivity CRP (hs-CRP). This substance is considered a marker of low-grade vascular inflammation, which is a key factor in the development and rupture of atheromatous plaque. Elevated CRP levels predict future coronary events, stroke, peripheral vascular disease, and type 2 diabetes mellitus. Thus this test is used to assess risk of cardiovascular problems in conjunction with other testing, such as measuring cholesterol levels.

THE EVIDENCE FOR PRACTICE

When dealing with such problems as rheumatoid arthritis, skin infections, and pelvic inflammatory disease, laboratory tests include the acute phase reactants (APRs), erythrocyte sedimentation rate (ESR), and C-reactive protein (CRP). These two APRs are good indicators of the inflammatory activity of such diseases.

Measurement of serum CRP concentration may be helpful in determining use of antibiotics in patients with CSF findings consistent with meningitis, but for whom the Gram stain result is negative. This recommendation is based on data showing that a normal CRP has a high negative predictive value in the diagnosis of bacterial meningitis

Current research is continuing to look at the utility of hs-CRP in cardiovascular risk prediction, especially in women and in those with metabolic syndrome, to predict risk for colon cancer development, and as a marker for lung lesion progression.

Normal Values

CRP: 0–1.0 mg/dL or <10 mg/L (SI units)
hs-CRP (assessing risk of CV disease):
    <1.0 mg/L   = Lowest risk
    1.0–3.0 mg/L = Average risk
    >3.0 mg/L   = Highest risk

Possible Meanings of Abnormal Values

Increased CRP	Increased hs-CRP
Acute pancreatitis	Increased risk of cardiovascular disease
Appendicitis	
Bacterial infection	
Burns	
Increased risk of colon cancer development	
Inflammatory bowel disease	
Lupus	
Lymphoma	
Myocardial infarction	
Pelvic inflammatory disease	
Polymyalgia rheumatica	
Rheumatoid arthritis	
Sepsis	
Surgery (first 3 post-op days)	
Tuberculosis	

Contributing Factors to Abnormal Values

- False-negative: medications including nonsteroidal anti-inflammatory drugs (NSAIDs), aspirin, corticosteroids, statins, beta blockers
- False-positive: medications including hormone replacement therapy, oral contraceptives
- Use of an intrauterine device (IUD)
- Vigorous exercise
- Pregnancy
- Obesity

Interventions/Implications

Pretest
- Explain to the patient the purpose of the test and the need for a blood sample to be drawn.

- Laboratories may vary in preparation for the test: some require no preparation while others require fasting for 4 to 12 hours before the test. Water is allowed.

Procedure
- A 5-mL blood sample is drawn in a green-top collection tube
- Gloves are worn throughout the procedure

Posttest
- Apply pressure at venipuncture site, periodically assessing for continued bleeding, apply dressing.
- Label specimen and transport to the laboratory immediately.
- Report abnormal findings to the primary care provider.

> **Clinical Alerts**

- The patient with elevated hs-CRP levels should be counseled on ways to reduce cardiovascular disease risk, and may require additional diagnostic testing to determine the presence of beginning cardiovascular disease.
- Elevated CRP levels should be correlated with other diagnostic results, such as elevated white blood count, to further narrow the list of possible causes of the abnormal finding.

Creatine Kinase and Isoenzymes
(CK, Creatine Phosphokinase [CPK])

Test Description

Creatine kinase (CK) is an enzyme found primarily in the heart and skeletal muscles, and in smaller amounts in the brain. When the total CK level is substantially elevated, it usually indicates injury or stress to one or more of these areas. When a muscle is damaged, CK leaks into the bloodstream. Determining which isoenzyme (specific form of CK) is elevated will help determine which tissue has been damaged.

CK can be measured as the total enzyme in the serum, or each of its three isoenzymes may be measured. The isoenzymes include:

CK_1 **(CPK-BB):** produced primarily by brain tissue and smooth muscle of the lungs
CK_2 **(CPK-MB):** produced primarily by heart tissue
CK_3 **(CPK-MM):** produced primarily by skeletal muscle

CK, along with asparate aminotransferase (AST) and troponin, is assessed in the case of suspected myocardial infarction. It typically appears in the bloodstream within 3 to 6 hours of the tissue injury, with peak values occurring 18 to 24 hours postinjury. CK levels are usually elevated for approximately 2 to 3 days. Thus, CK is one of the first cardiac enzymes to become elevated following a myocardial infarction.

THE EVIDENCE FOR PRACTICE

The Third Report of the Adult Treatment Panel III (ATP III) recommends that baseline CK levels be checked upon initiating statin therapy, the rationale being that asymptomatic CK elevations are relatively common. Determining the patient's pretreatment CK levels will prevent inappropriately attributing CK elevation to statin therapy in the event of muscle complaints later and assuming the presence of rhabdomyolysis.

C

Normal Values

Total CK
Female: 40–150 U/L (0.67–2.50 µkat/L SI units)
Male: 38–174 U/L (0.63–2.90 µkat/L SI units)

Isoenzymes
CK_1 (CPK-BB):   0–1%
CK_2 (CPK-MB):   <3%
CK_3 (CPK-MM):   95–100%

Possible Meanings of Abnormal Values

Increased Total CK
Acute cerebrovascular disease
Acute psychosis
Alcoholism
Brain trauma
Cardiac defibrillation
Cardiac surgery
Convulsions
Delirium tremens
Dermatomyositis
Electrical shock
Hypokalemia
Hypothyroidism
IM injections
Muscle inflammation
Myocardial infarction
Myxedema
Polymyositis
Progressive muscular dystrophy
Pulmonary infarction
Rhabdomyolysis

Decreased Total CK
Addison's disease
Anterior pituitary hyposecretion
Connective tissue disease
Early pregnancy
Hepatic disease
Low muscle mass
Metastatic neoplasia

Increased CK_1 (CPK-BB) Isoenzyme
Brain tissue injury
Brain tumors
Cancer of breast, lung, prostate
Cerebrovascular accident
Pulmonary infarction
Seizure
Shock

Increased CK_2 (CPK-MB) Isoenzyme
Acute myocardial infarction
Cardiac defibrillation

Congestive heart failure
Electrical injuries
Malignant hyperthermia
Myocarditis
Reye's syndrome
Trauma to heart

Increased CK$_3$ (CPK-MM) Isoenzyme

Hypokalemia
Hypothyroidism
IM injections
Myocardial infarction
Muscle inflammation
Muscle necrosis
Muscular dystrophy
Myositis
Polymyositis
Postoperative period
Rhabdomyolysis
Shock
Strenuous exercise

Contributing Factors to Abnormal Values

- Hemolysis of the blood sample or strenuous exercise prior to the test will alter test results.
- Factors that may affect test results include cardiac catheterization, intramuscular injections, trauma to muscles, recent surgery, and prolonged exercise.
- Drugs which may *increase* total CK: amphotericin B, ampicillin, anticoagulants, aspirin, clofibrate, cocaine, dexamethasone, ethanol, furosemide, lithium, morphine, and some anesthetics.

Interventions/Implications

Pretest
- Explain to the patient the purpose of the test and the need for a blood sample to be drawn.
- Inform the patient that this test is often performed on three consecutive days, and again in one week, necessitating multiple venipunctures.
- No fasting is required prior to the test.
- Do not administer any intramuscular injections for 1 hour prior to the test.

Procedure
- A 7-mL blood sample is drawn in a red-top collection tube.
- Gloves are worn throughout the procedure.

Posttest
- Apply pressure at venipuncture site. Apply dressing, periodically assessing for continued bleeding.
- Label the specimen and transport it to the laboratory.
- Report abnormal findings to the primary care provider.

Creatinine, Blood (Serum Creatinine)

Test Description

Creatinine is the waste product of creatine phosphate, a compound found in the skeletal muscle tissue. It is excreted entirely by the kidneys. The creatinine level is affected primarily by renal dysfunction and is thus very useful in evaluating renal function. Increased levels of creatinine indicate a slowing of the glomerular filtration rate. Since creatinine levels normally remain constant, even with aging, this test is particularly useful in evaluating renal dysfunction in which a large number of nephrons have been destroyed. The creatinine level is usually determined in conjunction with the blood urea nitrogen (BUN) in assessing renal function. The normal ratio of BUN to creatinine ranges from 6:1 to 20:1. Testing of the creatinine level in the blood is also used to monitor patients on drugs known to be nephrotoxic, such as aminoglycosides.

Normal Values

Female:	0.6–1.2 mg/dL (53–106 μmol/L SI units)
Male:	0.8–1.4 mg/dL (70–123 μmol/L SI units)
Children:	0.2–1.0 mg/dL (18–88 μmol/L SI units)

Possible Meanings of Abnormal Values

Increased	Decreased
Congestive heart failure	Atrophy of muscle tissue
Dehydration	Pregnancy
Diabetes mellitus	
Glomerulonephritis	
Gout	
Hyperthyroidism	
Multiple myeloma	
Nephritis	
Pyelonephritis	
Renal failure	
Rheumatoid arthritis	
Shock	
Subacute bacterial endocarditis	
Systemic lupus erythematosus	
Uremia	
Urinary obstruction	

Contributing Factors to Abnormal Values

- Creatinine levels are 20% to 40% higher in the late afternoon than in the morning.
- Test results may be altered by hemolysis of the blood sample and by ingestion of a high meat diet.
- Drugs which may *increase* creatinine levels: amphotericin B, androgens, arginine, ascorbic acid, barbiturates, captopril, cephalosporins, chlorthalidone, cimetidine,

clofibrate, clonidine, corticosteroids, dextran, disopyramide, doxycycline, fructose, gentamicin, glucose, hydralazine, hydroxyurea, kanamycin, levodopa, lithium, mannitol, meclofenamate, methicillin, methyldopa, metoprolol, minoxidil, nitrofurantoin, propranolol, protein, pyruvate, sulfonamides, streptokinase, testosterone, triamterene, trimethoprim.

- Drugs which may *decrease* creatinine levels: cefoxitin, cimetidine, chlorpromazine, marijuana, thiazide diuretics, vancomycin.

Interventions/Implications

Pretest
- Explain to the patient the purpose of the test and the need for a blood sample to be drawn.
- No fasting is required before the test.

Procedure
- A 7-mL blood sample is drawn in a red-top collection tube.
- Gloves are worn throughout the procedure.

Posttest
- Apply pressure at venipuncture site. Apply dressing, periodically assessing for continued bleeding.
- Label the specimen and transport it to the laboratory.
- Report abnormal findings to the primary care provider.

→ Clinical Alerts

- Both BUN and creatinine should be assessed prior to administration of any nephrotoxic drug.
- Monitor creatinine at baseline and at least every 12 months for patients taking metformin for diabetes mellitus Type 2. The drug can accumulate and potentially cause lactic acidosis in patients with renal insufficiency.

Creatinine Clearance

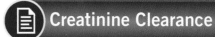

Test Description

Creatinine is the waste product of creatine phosphate, a compound found in the skeletal muscle tissue. It is excreted entirely by the kidneys. Increased levels of creatinine indicate a slowing of the glomerular filtration rate. The creatinine clearance test consists of two components: a 24-hour urine collection and a blood sample. Conducting both urine and blood testing allows for the comparison of the serum creatinine level with the amount of creatinine excreted in the urine. This is a more sensitive indicator of kidney function than serum creatinine alone. The creatinine clearance normally decreases with aging due to a decline in the glomerular filtration rate.

C

Since "clearance" means the amount of blood cleared of creatinine in 1 minute, a monitoring of the creatinine clearance rate provides valuable information regarding the progression of renal disease. A minimum creatinine clearance of 10 mL/minute is necessary to maintain life without the use of hemodialysis or peritoneal dialysis. The creatinine clearance rate is calculated by the following formula:

$$\frac{\text{Urine creatinine} \times \text{urine volume}}{\text{Creatinine in serum}} = \frac{\text{Creatinine clearance rate (expressed in}}{\text{mL} / \text{min} / 1.73\,\text{m}^2 \text{ of body surface)}}$$

Normal Values

Female:	85–125 mL/min (0.8–1.2 mL/sec SI units)
Male:	95–135 mL/min (0.9–1.3 mL/sec SI units)
Pregnancy:	Increased
Elderly:	Decreased
Children:	Decreased

Possible Meanings of Abnormal Values

Increased	Decreased
Exercise	Acute tubular necrosis
Pregnancy	Congestive heart failure
	Dehydration
	Glomerulonephritis
	Obstruction of renal artery
	Polycystic kidney disease
	Preeclampsia
	Pyelonephritis
	Renal malignancy
	Renal tuberculosis
	Shock

Contributing Factors to Abnormal Values

- Test results may be altered if urine collection is not kept on ice.
- Drugs which may *increase* creatinine clearance rate: aminoglycosides, anabolic steroids, androgens, cefoxitin, chlorpromazine, cimetidine, cisplatin, marijuana, thiazide diuretics, vancomycin.

Interventions/Implications

Pretest
- Explain 24-hour urine collection procedure to the patient.
- Stress the importance of saving all urine in the 24-hour period. Instruct the patient to avoid contaminating the urine with toilet paper or feces.
- Explain that a blood sample will also need to be drawn during the period of the urine collection.
- Instruct the patient to avoid excessive exercise for 8 hours prior to the test.

Procedure
- Although a 2-hour, 6-hour, or 12-hour urine collection can be used, a 24-hour urine collection is preferred.
- Obtain the proper container from the laboratory.
- Begin the testing period in the morning following the patient's first voiding, which is discarded.
- Timing of the 24-hour period begins at the time the first voiding is discarded.
- *All* urine for the next 24 hours is collected in the container and kept on ice.
- If any urine is accidentally discarded during the 24-hour period, the test must be discontinued and a new test begun.
- The ending time of the 24-hour collection period should be posted in the patient's room.
- A 7-ml blood sample is drawn in a red-top collection tube anytime during the test period, usually at the beginning of the collection period.
- Gloves are worn throughout the procedure.

Posttest
- Label the urine container and transport it on ice to the laboratory as soon as possible following the end of the 24-hour collection period.
- Apply pressure at venipuncture site. Apply dressing, periodically assessing for continued bleeding.
- Label the blood sample and transport it to the laboratory.
- Report abnormal findings to the primary care provider.

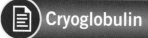

Cryoglobulin

Test Description

Cryoglobulins are abnormal serum proteins which precipitate at low laboratory temperatures and redissolve after being warmed. When patients with cryoglobulins present in their blood are subjected to cold, they may experience vascular problems of their extremities, with Raynaud-like symptoms such as pain, cyanosis, and coldness of the fingers and toes due to the formed complexes blocking small blood vessels. The presence of cryoglobulins in the blood (cryoglobulinemia) is usually associated with immunologic disease.

The test is conducted by refrigerating a serum sample at 4°C for at least 72 hours and observing for the formation of a precipitate. The reversibility of the reaction is verified by rewarming the serum sample. If the presence of cryoglobulins is thus shown, further study is done to identify the cryoglobulin components.

THE EVIDENCE FOR PRACTICE

Evidence of renal disease in hepatitis C virus-positive individuals requires early nephrologic consultation. Renal disease may exist in the absence of active hepatitis. The most common renal disease found in these patients is membrane proliferative glomerulonephritis, which may be associated with cryoglobulinemia. Testing for complement levels and the presence of cryoglobulins may be initiated prior to referral.

C

Normal Values

Negative

Possible Meanings of Abnormal Values

Positive

Chronic infection
Chronic lymphocytic leukemia
Cytomegalovirus infection
Hepatitis C
Hodgkin's disease
Infectious mononucleosis
Infective endocarditis
Leprosy
Lymphoma
Mixed essential cryoglobulinemia
Multiple myeloma
Polymyalgia rheumatica
Poststreptococcal glomerulonephritis
Primary biliary cirrhosis
Raynaud's disease
Rheumatoid arthritis
Scleroderma
Sjögren's syndrome
Systemic lupus erythematosus
Tropical splenomegaly syndrome
Viral infection
Waldenström's macroglobulinemia

Interventions/Implications

Pretest
- Explain to the patient the purpose of the test and the need for a blood sample to be drawn.
- Fasting for 8 hours is required prior to the test.

Procedure
- A 10-mL blood sample is drawn in a collection tube containing a silicone gel prewarmed to 37°C.
- Gloves are worn throughout the procedure.

Posttest
- Apply pressure at venipuncture site. Apply dressing, periodically assessing for continued bleeding.
- Label the specimen and transport it to the laboratory.
- Report abnormal findings to the primary care provider.

Cutaneous Immunofluorescence Biopsy (Skin Biopsy)

C

Test Description
Immunofluorescence is a histological technique in which fluorescent dyes are attached to antibody molecules. When viewed under an ultraviolet microscope, these antibody molecules appear as a colored fluorescence when they have become joined with an antigen to form antibody-antigen complexes. This technique is used when performing a biopsy of the skin. This test is indicated in the evaluation of skin disorders such as lupus erythematosus and blistering diseases such as pemphigus and pemphigoid.

Normal Values
Normal skin histology
Absence of antibody/antigen complexes

Possible Meanings of Abnormal Values
Bullous pemphigoid
Dermatitis herpetiformis
Discoid lupus erythematosus
Pemphigus
Systemic lupus erythematosus

Interventions/Implications

Pretest
- Explain to the patient the purpose of the test and the need for a skin sample to be obtained.
- No fasting is required prior to the test.
- Obtain a signed informed consent.

Procedure
- A punch or shave biopsy or tissue excision specimen of skin is obtained.
- Pressure is applied to the site to control bleeding. With punch biopsies and tissue excision procedures, suturing of the area may be necessary.
- Gloves are worn throughout the procedure.

Posttest
- Label the specimen and transport it on ice to the laboratory immediately to be quick frozen in liquid nitrogen.
- Apply a sterile dressing to the biopsy site.
- Teach the patient to monitor the site and to notify the health-care provider if signs or symptoms of infection occur, such as drainage, redness, warmth, edema, pain at the site, or fever.
- Test results will not be available for 3 days.
- Report abnormal findings to the primary care provider.

> **→ Clinical Alerts**
>
> - Potential complications include: bleeding from the biopsy site, infection, and keloid formation.
> - If suturing is done, instruct the patient on when sutures are to be removed.

CONTRAINDICATIONS!

- Patients who are unable to cooperate during the procedure.
- Patients who are on anticoagulant therapy.

Cystometrography/Cystourethrography
(CMG, Urethral Pressure Profile)

Test Description

Cystometrography (CMG), also known as *cystometry* is used to evaluate detrusor muscle function and tone and to determine the cause of bladder dysfunction. The test involves the instillation of fluid and/or air into the patient's bladder. Assessments are made of the patient's neurologic sensations and muscular responses to this filling of the bladder. The patient's voiding is also assessed for abnormalities. The results of this test are considered in conjunction with those of other urinary diagnostic tests, such as excretory urography and cystourethrography.

Cystourethrography involves the instillation of a contrast medium into the bladder through a urethral catheter. As the bladder fills, x-ray films are taken. The catheter is then removed and additional films are taken as the patient voids. This test is often used to evaluate patients who suffer from chronic urinary tract infections.

Normal Values

CMG: Normal filling pattern of the bladder and ability to distinguish temperature of solution instilled
Residual urine: <30 mL
First urge to void: 150–200 mL   Bladder capacity: 400–500 mL

Cystourethrogram: Normal structure and function of the bladder and urethra

Possible Meanings of Abnormal Values

Bladder hypertonicity
Bladder infection
Bladder obstruction
Diminished bladder capacity
Neurogenic bladder
Prostatic enlargement
Ureterocele
Urethral diverticula
Urethral stricture

Urethral valve
Vesical diverticula
Vesicoureteral reflux

Interventions/Implications

Pretest
- Explain to the patient the purpose of the test and the procedure to be done. Explain that even though a catheter will be in place during the procedure, the patient will feel the urge to void as fluid or gas fills the bladder.
- Obtain a signed informed consent.
- No fasting is required prior to the test.

Procedure

For cystometrogram
- The patient is asked to void to empty the bladder.
- The patient is assisted into the supine position.
- A Foley catheter is inserted into the bladder, and the residual urine volume is measured.
- Thermal sensation is assessed by instilling 30 mL of room temperature sterile saline or water into the bladder, followed by 30 mL of warm fluid. Any sensations reported by the patient are recorded.
- The fluid is drained from the bladder, and a cystometer is connected to the catheter. This instrument graphically displays pressures and volumes within the bladder.
- Sterile saline or water or a gas, such as carbon dioxide, is slowly introduced into the bladder.
- Notations are made on the cystometrogram printout as to the point when the patient first feels an urge to void, and again when the patient feels that the bladder is completely full and that he or she must void.
- The patient is then requested to urinate around the catheter, which permits recording of the maximal intravesical voiding pressure.
- If cystourethrography is *not* being done, the bladder is then drained and the catheter is removed.
- Other testing may involve repeating the above procedure with the patient in a standing or sitting position or after administration of a bladder tone stimulant such as bethanechol chloride.

For cystourethrogram
- The contrast medium is instilled through the catheter until the bladder is filled, then the catheter is clamped.
- X-ray films are taken with the patient in various positions.
- The catheter is removed, and the patient is assisted into the right oblique position.
- Additional films are taken as the patient voids.

Posttest
- Assess the patient for complaints of burning on urination, frequency of urination, and bladder spasms.
- Assess vital signs.
- Encourage the patient to increase fluid intake.
- Administer analgesics as ordered.
- Administer antibiotics as ordered.
- Warm tub baths may aid in comfort.
- Monitor intake and output for 24 hours. Observe urine for frank bleeding.
- Report abnormal findings to the primary care provider.

Clinical Alerts

- Possible complications: Urinary tract infection

C

CONTRAINDICATIONS!

For CMG/Cystourethrogram
- Patients with acute urinary tract infection
- Patients with urinary tract obstruction

For Cystourethrogram
- Pregnant women
    - Caution: A woman in her childbearing years should undergo radiography only during her menses or 12 to 14 days after its onset to avoid any exposure to a fetus.
- Patients who are allergic to radiographic dye

Cystoscopy (Cystourethroscopy)

Test Description
Cystoscopy involves the insertion of a well-lubricated sheath into the urethra. During the procedure, a cystoscope is inserted through the sheath for direct visualization of the bladder. A urethroscope is used for examination of the bladder neck and the urethra. With the sheath in place, other instruments may be interchanged, allowing the physician to obtain tissue for biopsy, to resect lesions, to collect calculi, and to pass a ureteral catheter to the renal pelvis for pyelography. Indications for performing cystoscopy include recurrent urinary tract infections, dysuria with no known cause, hematuria, and bladder tumors.

THE EVIDENCE FOR PRACTICE
For asymptomatic microscopic hematuria patients without risk factors for transitional cell carcinoma, urinary cytology or cystoscopy may be used. If cytology is chosen and malignant or atypical/suspicious cells are identified, cystoscopy is required since the presence of hematuria is a significant risk factor for malignancy in such patients.

Normal Values
Normal bladder and urethra

Possible Meanings of Abnormal Values
Calculi
Congenital anomalies
Diverticula
Polyps
Prostatic hypertrophy
Prostatitis
Tumors

Ulcers
Urethral stricture

Interventions/Implications

Pretest

- Explain to the patient the purpose of the test and the procedure to be done. If the patient is to have local anesthesia only, explain that a burning sensation may be felt as the sheath is inserted into the urethra, and that the urge to void may be felt during the procedure.
- Obtain a signed informed consent.
- No fasting is required prior to the test if a local anesthetic is to be used. If a general anesthetic is planned, the patient must fast for 8 hours prior to the procedure.
- Instruct the patient to void prior to the procedure.
- Administer preprocedure sedation, as ordered.

Procedure

- The patient is assisted into the lithotomy position with the feet supported in stirrups.
- The external genitalia are cleansed with antiseptic and draped.
- A local anesthetic is instilled into the urethra.
- The urethroscope is inserted into the well-lubricated sheath, and both are then inserted into the urethra.
- The urethroscope is then exchanged with the cystoscope to allow for examination of the bladder lining.
- A urine sample for routine analysis is obtained.
- The cystoscope is then replaced with the urethroscope to allow visualization of the urethra as the scope and the sheath are slowly removed.
- Gloves are worn throughout the procedure.

Posttest

- Monitor the vital signs until stable. Note indications of infection and bladder perforation, such as elevated temperature, elevated pulse, and decreased blood pressure.
- Assess the patient for complaints of burning on urination, frequency of urination, and bladder spasms.
- Encourage the patient to increase fluid intake.
- Administer analgesics as ordered (antispasmodic medication, such as B and O suppository, may also be ordered).
- Administer antibiotics as ordered.
- Warm tub baths may aid in comfort.
- Monitor intake and output for 24 hours. Observe urine for frank bleeding.
- Report abnormal findings to the primary care provider.

→ **Clinical Alerts**

- Possible complications include: Hematuria, infection, leading to sepsis, perforation of the bladder, and urinary retention.

CONTRAINDICATIONS!

- Patients with acute cystitis, prostatitis, or urethritis.

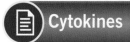 Cytokines

C

Test Description

Cytokines are proteins—chemicals produced by the cells of the immune system in order to mediate and regulate immunity, inflammation, and hematopoiesis. Cytokines are able to act on other immune cells, especially cells nearby. For example, when stimulated by cytokines, monocytes move out of the circulation and become macrophages in the tissues.

Cytokines have several interesting characteristics. The same cytokine may be made by several different cells. The same cytokine may have different effects in different situations, and different cytokines may have the same effect. Cytokines can work together synergistically or as antagonists.

Examples of cytokines include granulocyte-monocyte colony stimulating factor, interleukin, interferon, tumor growth factor, and tumor necrosis factor. Measurement of cytokines determines immune function and response, potential appropriate treatments, and treatment response. In addition to blood sampling, cytokines can be studied in other types of specimens including cerebrospinal fluid, synovial fluid, stool, and urine.

Normal Values

Values vary with the reference laboratory.

Possible Meanings of Abnormal Values

AIDS
Immune deficiency
Malignancies
Rheumatoid arthritis

Contributing Factors to Abnormal Values

- Cytokines can still be produced or can degrade in the collection container.

Interventions/Implications

Pretest
- Explain to the patient the purpose of the test and the need for a blood sample to be drawn.
- No fasting is required before the test.

Procedure
- A 7-mL blood sample is drawn in a red-top collection tube.
- Gloves are worn throughout the procedure.

Posttest
- Apply pressure at venipuncture site. Apply dressing, periodically assessing for continued bleeding.
- Label the specimen and transport it to the laboratory.
- Report abnormal findings to the primary care provider.

Cytomegalovirus (CMV)

Test Description

Cytomegalovirus (CMV) is a member of the herpes virus family. It is a very common virus in that it is estimated that depending on the area, 40% to 100% of a population may be infected. In most people, the virus remains latent and causes no symptoms. In those who are immunocompromised, however, CMV can have devastating effects. In patients with AIDS, CMV infection can cause pneumonitis, esophagitis, colitis, encephalitis, hepatitis, and retinitis leading to blindness. In organ transplant patients, CMV is considered a major complication, often resulting in death. Infection with CMV during pregnancy can cause mental retardation and microencephaly in the newborn.

CMV is found in all body secretions. Pregnant health-care workers should be cautioned about the potential risk of acquiring CMV. Since it is impossible to eliminate from a health-care worker's caseload all patients who might be carrying CMV, it is essential that careful handwashing and strict adherence to universal precautions be a consistent part of patient care.

If the test is being used to diagnose acute infection with CMV, an initial blood sample, called the "acute titer" is obtained. A second sample, the "convalescent titer" is drawn 10 to 14 days later. A diagnosis of CMV is made when a fourfold increase between the acute titer and the convalescent titer occurs.

Normal Values

Negative or titer <1:5: No past infection

Abnormal Values

Positive for antibodies: Past infection

Possible Meanings of Abnormal Values

Increased	Decreased
CMV infection	Susceptible to CMV

Contributing Factors to Abnormal Values

- *False-positive* results have occurred in individuals with rheumatoid factor present in their blood, and in those exposed to Epstein-Barr virus.

Interventions/Implications

Pretest
- Explain to the patient the purpose of the test and the need for one or two blood samples to be drawn.
- No fasting is required before the test.

Procedure
- A 7-mL blood sample is drawn in a red-top collection tube.
- If the test is being done to determine presence of antibodies to CMV, only one sample is needed.
- Gloves are worn throughout the procedure.

Posttest

- Apply pressure at venipuncture site. Apply dressing, periodically assessing for continued bleeding.
- Label the specimen and transport it to the laboratory.
- Report abnormal findings to the primary care provider.
- If a convalescent titer will be needed, remind the patient of the date to return for the blood to be drawn.

Clinical Alerts

- Blood and organ transplants given to immunosuppressed patients who are found to have no antibodies to CMV should be from donors who are also seronegative.
- Risk of infection at venipuncture site due to immunocompromised state. Teach patient to notify health-care provider if drainage, redness, warmth, edema, or pain at the site or fever occur.

Dexamethasone Suppression Test
(DST, ACTH Suppression Test, Cortisol Suppression Test)

Test Description

In response to a stimulus such as stress, the hypothalamus secretes corticotropin-releasing hormone. This hormone stimulates the secretion of *adrenocorticotropic hormone* (ACTH) by the anterior pituitary gland. ACTH, in turn, causes the adrenal cortex to release the glucocorticoid hormone, *cortisol*. As levels of cortisol in the blood rise, the pituitary gland is stimulated to decrease ACTH production, via a negative feedback mechanism.

During the dexamethasone suppression test, a corticosteroid (dexamethasone) is given. Normally, this substance decreases the formation of ACTH due to suppression of the pituitary gland. However, in patients with hyperfunctioning of the adrenal cortex (Cushing's syndrome), pituitary suppression does not prevent the hyperactive adrenal cortex from continuing to produce large amounts of cortisol. This test is used to diagnose Cushing's syndrome.

Normal Values

<5 µg/dL (140 nmol/L SI units)

Possible Meanings of Abnormal Values

No suppression
Adrenal adenoma
Adrenal carcinoma
Ectopic ACTH-producing tumor

Suppression occurs
Adrenal hyperfunction (Cushing's syndrome)
Clinical depression

Contributing Factors to Abnormal Values

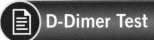

- *False-positive* test results may occur with acute illnesses, alcoholism, anorexia nervosa, dehydration, diabetes mellitus, fever, malnutrition, nausea, obesity, pregnancy, severe stress, and with the following drugs: aldactone, barbiturates, caffeine, carbamazepine, diethylstilbestrol, estrogens, glutethimide, meprobamate, oral contraceptives, phenytoin, reserpine, tetracycline.
- *False-negative* test results may occur with Addison's disease, hypopituitarism, and with the following drugs: benzodiazepines, corticosteroids, cyproheptadine.

Interventions/Implications

Pretest
- Explain to the patient the purpose of the test and the need for a blood sample to be drawn.
- No fasting is required before the test.
- The patient should avoid caffeine after midnight, the night before the test.
- The patient should stop taking medications which might interfere with the test for 24 to 48 hours before the test.

Procedure
- Administer dexamethasone 1 mg orally at 11 p.m.
- The next morning at 8 a.m., a 5-mL blood sample is drawn in a red-top collection tube.
- Additional blood samples may be drawn at 4 p.m. and 11 p.m.
- Gloves are worn throughout the procedure.

Posttest
- Apply pressure at venipuncture site. Apply dressing, periodically assessing for continued bleeding.
- Label the specimen and transport it to the laboratory.
- Report abnormal findings to the primary care provider.

D-Dimer Test

Test Description
During hemostasis, thrombin stimulates the formation of fibrin from fibrinogen. This fibrin, with the addition of fibrin stabilizing factor, forms a stable fibrin clot at the site of injury. Once the fibrin clot is no longer needed, it is dissolved by fibrinolytic agents such as plasmin, resulting in fibrin degradation products. D-dimer is one of the measurable by-products of the fibrinolytic system.

Measurement of D-dimer assesses fibrinolytic activation and intravascular thrombosis. It is very useful to help *exclude* acute venous thromboembolic disease, such as deep venous thrombosis (DVT) or pulmonary embolism, as the cause of a patient's symptoms. It is also measured, along with other tests, to diagnose disseminated intravascular coagulation (DIC). Current research is investigating use of D-dimer in guiding the duration of anticoagulation therapy.

D

THE EVIDENCE FOR PRACTICE

In patients with low clinical probability for lower-extremity DVT, the following test results can be used to exclude DVT:

1. A negative quantitative D-dimer assay result (turbidimetric or enzyme-linked immunosorbent assay [ELISA]) for exclusion of proximal (DVT from the knee to the inguinal ligament) and distal (DVT isolated to the calf) lower-extremity DVT.
2. A negative whole blood D-dimer assay result in conjunction with the Wells et al scoring system for exclusion of proximal and distal DVT.
3. A negative whole blood D-dimer assay result for exclusion of proximal lower-extremity DVT.

Patients with a moderate-to-high risk of lower-extremity DVT cannot have DVT excluded by a single negative D-dimer test.

Normal Values

<250 µg/L (<1.37 nmol/L SI units)

Possible Meanings of Abnormal Values

Increased

Arterial thrombosis
Disseminated intravascular coagulation (DIC)
Eclampsia
Fibrinolysis
Heart disease
Infection
Late pregnancy
Liver disease
Malignancy
Postoperative period
Pulmonary embolism
Trauma
Venous thrombosis

Contributing Factors to Abnormal Values

- Drugs which *increase* test results: thrombolytic agents.
- *False-positive* results may occur in the presence of high rheumatoid factor (RF) titers.

Interventions/Implications

Pretest

- Explain to the patient the purpose of the test and the need for a blood sample to be drawn.
- No fasting is required before the test.

Procedure
- A 7-mL blood sample is drawn in a light blue-top collection tube.
- Gloves are worn throughout the procedure.

Posttest
- Apply pressure 3 to 5 minutes at venipuncture site. Apply dressing, periodically assessing for continued bleeding.
- Teach the patient to monitor the site. If the site begins to bleed, the patient should apply direct pressure and, if unable to control the bleeding, return to the laboratory or notify the primary care provider.
- Report abnormal findings to the primary care provider.

Clinical Alerts

- Possible complication: hematoma at site due to prolonged bleeding time.
- A positive D-dimer indicates the presence of an abnormally high level of fibrin degradation products. This means there has been significant thrombus formation and fibrinolysis in the body. Other testing is needed to find the location or cause.
- A normal D-dimer test means that it is most likely that no acute condition is present to cause abnormal clot formation and breakdown.

2,3-Diphosphoglycerate (2,3-DPG)

Test Description
2,3-Diphosphoglycerate (2,3-DPG) is the most abundant intracellular organic phosphate in the red blood cells. It is involved with oxygen transport to the tissues and binds to specific amino acid sites on proteins. The oxygen affinity of red blood cells is inversely proportional to 2,3-DPG levels. When hemoglobin levels are decreased, as in anemia, 2,3-DPG levels increase and cause decreased oxygen binding of hemoglobin. This results in increased amounts of oxygen being released to the tissues at lower oxygen tensions. Deficiency of 2,3-DPG results in defects in the release of oxygen to the tissues.

Normal Values

Female:	4.5–6.1 µmol/mL of packed cells
	8.4–18.8 µmol/g of hemoglobin
Male:	4.2–5.4 µmol/mL of packed cells
	9.2–17.4 µmol/g of hemoglobin

Possible Meanings of Abnormal Values

Increased	Decreased
Anemia	Acidosis
Cardiac disease	2,3-DPG deficiency

Chronic renal failure
Cirrhosis
Cystic fibrosis
Hyperthyroidism
Lung disease
Pyruvate kinase deficiency
Thyrotoxicosis
Uremia

Polycythemia
Respiratory distress syndrome

D

Contributing Factors to Abnormal Values

- Factors which may *increase* 2,3-DPG levels: high altitudes, strenuous exercise.
- Factors which may *decrease* 2,3-DPG levels: acidosis, receipt of banked blood.

Interventions/Implications

Pretest
- Explain to the patient the purpose of the test and the need for a blood sample to be drawn.
- No fasting is required before the test.

Procedure
- A 7-mL blood sample is drawn in a red-top collection tube.
- Gloves are worn throughout the procedure.

Posttest
- Apply pressure at venipuncture site. Apply dressing, periodically assessing for continued bleeding.
- Label the specimen and transport it on ice to the laboratory.
- Report abnormal findings to the primary care provider.

Disseminated Intravascular Coagulation Screening (DIC Screening)

Test Description
Disseminated intravascular coagulation (DIC) is a paradoxical, often fatal, condition in which both clotting and bleeding occur at abnormally high levels. DIC can be triggered by a variety of conditions, including amniotic fluid embolism, extensive surgery, hemolytic transfusion reactions, massive tissue trauma, metastatic malignancies, premature separation of the placenta in pregnancy, retained dead fetus, septicemia, severe burns, and shock. When the process is triggered, widespread clotting occurs in small vessels of the body, causing clotting factors and platelets to be used up. As a result, the patient develops a bleeding disorder due to lack of needed clotting factors. Patients with DIC may exhibit bleeding ranging from minimal bleeding from venipuncture sites or mucous membranes to profuse hemorrhage from all orifices. Patients may develop organ dysfunction, such as renal failure and pulmonary and multifocal central nervous system (CNS) infarctions due to microvascular occlusion and anoxic injury in the affected organs.

Several tests are used in the diagnosis of DIC. Each of these tests is described in detail elsewhere in this text. The expected results of these tests in the patient with DIC are:

- Antithrombin III: Decreased
- Bleeding time: Prolonged
- Coagulation factors: Decreased
- D-dimer: Increased
- Fibrin degradation products: Increased
- Fibrinogen: Decreased
- Fibrinopeptide A: Increased
- Partial thromboplastin time: Prolonged
- Platelet count: Decreased
- Prothrombin time: Prolonged
- Thrombin time: Increased

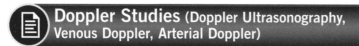

Doppler Studies (Doppler Ultrasonography, Venous Doppler, Arterial Doppler)

Test Description

Ultrasonography is a noninvasive method of diagnostic testing in which ultrasound waves are sent into the body with a small transducer pressed against the skin. The transducer not only sends the sound waves into the body but also receives any returning sound waves, which are deflected back as they bounce off various structures. The transducer converts the returning sound waves into electric signals that are then transformed by a computer into audible sounds (Doppler method).

This particular form of ultrasonography is used to evaluate blood flow in the major veins and arteries of the arms and legs. The sound waves strike moving red blood cells and are reflected back to that transducer. The sound which is emitted by the transducer corresponds to the velocity of the blood flow through the vessel. This provides valuable information used in the diagnosis of chronic venous insufficiency, venous thromboses, peripheral artery disease, arterial occlusion, and arterial trauma. It can also be used to monitor patients following arterial reconstruction and bypass graft surgery. Similar testing can be done on the carotid arteries. (See "Carotid Artery Duplex Scan.")

THE EVIDENCE FOR PRACTICE

In patients with low clinical probability for lower-extremity deep vein thrombosis, negative findings on a single venous ultrasound in symptomatic patients excludes proximal (DVT from the knee to the inguinal ligament) lower-extremity DVT and clinically significant distal (DVT isolated to calf) lower-extremity DVT.

In patients with moderate to high pretest probability of lower-extremity DVT, serial ultrasonographic examinations need to be performed, meaning a follow-up ultrasound within 5 to 7 days to rule out DVT.

Normal Values

Normal Doppler signal with no evidence of vessel occlusion

Possible Meanings of Abnormal Values

Arterial occlusion
Arterial stenosis
Arteriosclerosis
Deep vein thrombosis
Peripheral arterial disease
Venous disease
Venous occlusion

Contributing Factors to Abnormal Values

- The transducer must be in good contact with the skin as it is being moved. A lubricant, such as mineral oil, glycerin, or a water-based jelly, is used to ensure good contact with the skin.
- Cigarette smoking may alter test results due to vasoconstriction.

Interventions/Implications

Pretest

- Explain to the patient the purpose of the test. Provide any written teaching materials available on the subject. Note that there is no discomfort involved with this test.
- Explain the importance of limiting movement during the test to ensure accurate measurements.
- No fasting is required prior to the test.

Procedure

- The patient is assisted to a supine position on the ultrasonography table.

For peripheral arterial studies

- A blood pressure cuff is wrapped about the extremity, pressure readings are taken, and waveforms are recorded for the arteries distal to the cuff location. The cuff application sites and the arteries assessed include:
  - calf: dorsalis pedis, posterior tibial arteries
  - thigh: popliteal artery
  - forearm: radial and ulnar arteries
  - upper arm: brachial artery

For peripheral venous studies

- The transducer is placed over the appropriate vein and waveforms are recorded. Variations in the waveforms due to respiratory influences are noted.
- Veins to be tested include: popliteal, superficial femoral, common femoral, posterior tibial vein, brachial, axillary, subclavian, and jugular.

Posttest

- Cleanse the patient's skin of remaining coupling agent.
- Report abnormal findings to the primary care provider.

D-Xylose Absorption Test (Xylose Tolerance Test)

Test Description
D-Xylose is a monosaccharide which is normally absorbed in the small intestine and excreted by the kidneys. It is not metabolized by the body, meaning its serum levels are direct reflections of intestinal absorption of the substance. Adequate intestinal absorption is indicated by high serum and urinary levels of the substance. Malabsorptive disorders affecting the proximal small intestine, such as celiac disease/sprue, result in decreased levels of D-Xylose in the blood and urine.

This test is used to differentiate between patients with diarrhea due to maldigestion from pancreatic and biliary dysfunction and those with diarrhea due to malabsorption such as Crohn's disease. It involves ingestion of D-Xylose and collection of both blood and urine samples.

Normal Values
Adult
> Serum: >25 mg/dL (>1.67 mmol/L SI units) 2 hours after D-Xylose ingestion
> Urine: >4 g of D-Xylose excreted in 5 hours

Child
> Serum: >20 mg/dL (>1.3 mmol/L SI units) 1 hour after D-Xylose ingestion
> Urine: 16–33% excreted in 5 hours

Possible Meanings of Abnormal Values

Decreased
Bacterial overgrowth
Celiac disease/sprue
Crohn's disease
Intestinal malabsorption
Mesenteric ischemia
Non-Hodgkin's lymphoma
Tropical sprue
Viral gastroenteritis
Whipple's disease

Normal
Malabsorption due to pancreatic insufficiency

Contributing Factors to Abnormal Values
- Physical activity will alter test results.
- Drugs which will *decrease* test results: aspirin, atropine, colchicine, diuretics, glipizide, indomethacin, neomycin.

Interventions/Implications
Pretest
- Explain to the patient the purpose of the test and the need for collection of both blood and urine samples.

- Fasting overnight prior to the test and during the test is required.
- There are no water restrictions, in fact, patient should be encouraged to drink during the fasting period and during test.
- Withhold medications which may alter the test results for 24 hours prior to the test.
- The patient should avoid food containing pentose for 24 hours prior to the test. Such foods include fruits, jams, jellies, and pastries.
- Explain 5 hour urine collection procedure to the patient.
- Stress the importance of saving *all* urine in the 5-hour period. Instruct the patient to avoid contaminating the urine with toilet paper or feces.
- Obtain patient's weight.
- Obtain urine collection bottle containing preservative. Inform the patient of the presence of a preservative in the collection bottle.

Procedure

- Remind the patient to remain at rest and nothing by mouth (NPO) throughout the testing period, with the exception of the D-Xylose ingestion and water.
- Instruct patient to void completely. Discard this urine.
- A 10-mL blood sample is drawn in a red-top collection tube.
- Send the blood sample to the laboratory immediately.
- Administer D-Xylose dissolved in 250 mL of water, followed by an additional 250 mL of water. Dosage of D-Xylose is weight-based: 0.5 g/kg body weight up to a maximum of 25 g. Typical adult dose is 25 g; 5 g for child younger than 12 years.
- Have the patient drink another 250 mL of water after 1 hour.
- Draw an additional blood sample in 2 hours in an adult patient; in 1 hour in a child. Use a 10-mL red-top collection tube.
- *All* urine for the next 5 hours is collected in the proper container, which is to be kept refrigerated or on ice.
- Gloves are to be worn whenever dealing with the specimen collection.

Posttest

- Apply pressure at venipuncture sites. Apply dressing, periodically assessing for continued bleeding.
- Label the blood specimen and transport it to the laboratory.
- Label the urine container, noting total volume of urine, and transport it on ice to the laboratory as soon as possible following the end of the 5-hour collection period.
- Resume diet and medications as taken prior to the test.
- Report abnormal findings to the primary care provider.

→ Clinical Alerts

- Possible complication: D-Xylose ingestion may cause abdominal discomfort or mild diarrhea.

CONTRAINDICATIONS!

- Patients who are dehydrated
- Patients with kidney dysfunction

Echocardiography

Test Description

Ultrasonography is a noninvasive method of diagnostic testing in which ultrasound waves are sent into the body with a small transducer pressed against the skin. The transducer then receives any returning sound waves, which are deflected back as they bounce off various structures. The transducer converts the returning sound waves into electric signals that are then transformed by a computer into a visual display on a monitor.

Echocardiography is a particular type of ultrasonography in which the transducer is placed at an area of the chest where bone and lung tissue are absent, so that the sound waves can be directed toward cardiac structures. This is normally in the third or fourth intercostal space to the left of the sternum.

Two techniques are used in echocardiography. In M-mode, or motion-mode, echocardiography, a single ultrasound beam is used which records the motion and dimensions of intracardiac structures in a linear tracing. In two-dimensional, or cross-sectional, echocardiography, the ultrasound beam sweeps through an arc, giving a cross-sectional view of the heart. This information is converted to images shown on the oscilloscope that are videotaped for review by a cardiologist. In addition to evaluating the functioning of the heart muscle and valves, the echocardiogram allows calculation of the ejection fraction of the heart, which is normally 60% to 70%.

THE EVIDENCE FOR PRACTICE

Echocardiography is an essential tool for the evaluation of the functional and structural changes underlying or associated with acute heart failure as well as in the assessment of acute coronary syndromes.

Normal Values

No abnormalities of the heart chambers, valves, blood flow, or muscle

Possible Meanings of Abnormal Values

- Cardiac tumor
- Cardiomyopathy
- Congenital heart disease (patent ductus arteriosus, transposition of the great vessels)
- Heart chamber problems (atrial septal defect, ventricular septal defect)
- Infectious processes (endocarditis, pericarditis, subacute bacterial endocarditis)
- Marfan's syndrome
- Myocardial infarction
- Pericardial effusion
- Valvular problems (stenosis, regurgitation, or rupture of the aortic, pulmonic, mitral, and tricuspid valves, mitral valve prolapse)

Contributing Factors to Abnormal Values

- The transducer must be in good contact with the skin as it is being moved. A water-based gel is used to ensure good contact with the skin.

- Quality of the test results may be hindered in the presence of patient movement, chest wall abnormalities, chronic obstructive lung disease, and obesity.

Interventions/Implementation

Pretest

- Explain to the patient the purpose of the test. Provide any written teaching materials available on the subject. Note that there is no discomfort involved with this test.
- Explain the importance of limiting movement during the test to ensure accurate images.
- No fasting is required before the test.

Procedure
- The patient is assisted to a supine position on the ultrasonography table.
- A coupling agent, such as a water-based gel, is applied to the chest wall.
- A transducer is placed on the skin and moved as needed to provide good visualization of the cardiac structures.
- The sound waves are transformed into a visual display on the monitor. A videotaped copy of this display is made.
- The patient is also usually turned on to the left side to obtain additional views of the heart. This position moves the heart closer to the chest wall.

Posttest
- Cleanse the patient's skin of any lubricant.
- Report abnormal findings to the primary care provider.

Clinical Alerts

- Patients who are unable to cooperate owing to age, mental status, pain, or other factors may not be able to have an echocardiogram, since movement during the test may limit clear views of the heart.

Electrocardiography (ECG, EKG, Electrocardiogram)

Test Description
Electrocardiography is the recording of the electrical current generated by the heart. Electrical impulses, generated by the heart during its depolarization and repolarization, are detected by monitoring electrodes placed on the body. The graphic depiction of this electrical activity is called an electrocardiogram (ECG or EKG). The standard type of electrocardiogram performed is the 12-lead EKG, which measures the electrical activity by way of 12 leads: three standard limb leads, three augmented limb leads, and six chest leads. The ECG is recorded on special paper on which each marking represents 0.04 second. This standardized marking allows measurement of the duration of the various ECG components.

The ECG is composed of several waveforms, including the P wave, the QRS complex, the T wave, the ST segment, the PR interval, and possibly a U wave. Each of the waveforms represents different aspects of cardiac depolarization and repolarization.

The *P wave* represents atrial muscle depolarization. This wave is 0.11 second or less in duration. The *QRS complex*, which includes the time from the beginning of the Q wave to the end of the S wave, represents ventricular muscle depolarization. The QRS complex is 0.04 to 0.10 second in duration. The *T wave*, which follows the QRS complex, represents ventricular muscle repolarization. The *U wave* is occasionally seen in patients with hypokalemia. It follows the T wave and is sometimes mistaken for an extra P wave. The *PR interval*, measured from the beginning of the P wave to the beginning of the Q wave, represents the time required for atrial depolarization and the delay of the impulse in the AV node prior to ventricular depolarization. The PR interval usually lasts from 0.12 to 0.20 second. The *ST segment*, from the end of the S wave to the beginning of the T wave, represents early ventricular repolarization. The *QT interval*, measured from the beginning of the Q wave to the end of the T wave, represents the total time for ventricular depolarization and repolarization.

E

THE EVIDENCE FOR PRACTICE

The U.S. Preventive Services Task Force (USPSTF) recommends against routine screening with resting electrocardiogram (ECG), exercise treadmill test (ETT), or electron beam computerized tomography (EBCT) scanning for coronary calcium, for either the presence of severe coronary artery stenosis (CAS) or the prediction of coronary heart disease (CHD) events in adults at low risk for CHD events. Because the sensitivity of these tests is limited, screening could also result in many false-negative results. *A negative test does not rule out the presence of severe CAS or a future CHD event.*

Normal Values

Normal rate, rhythm, and waveforms

Possible Meanings of Abnormal Values

Bundle branch blocks
Cardiac arrest
Conduction defects
Dysrhythmias
Electrolyte imbalances
Myocardial infarction
Myocardial ischemia
Pericarditis
Ventricular hypertrophy

Contributing Factors to Abnormal Values

- Interferences to the recording of the ECG are shown as artifacts. This may occur due to equipment failure, electrode adherence problems, electromagnetic interference, or patient movement.

Interventions/Implications

Pretest
- Explain to the patient the purpose of the test and the need for electrodes to be attached to the chest and extremities. Note that the test causes no discomfort, but that the patient will need to lie still and not speak during the procedure.
- No fasting is required prior to the test.

Procedure
- The patient is assisted to a supine position. The semi-Fowler's position may be used for patients with respiratory problems.
- The skin where electrodes are to be applied is cleansed with alcohol. Shaving of the skin may be needed to ensure proper adhesion of the electrodes.
- Electrodes are applied:
  - One monitoring electrode is applied to the left arm, right arm, and left leg.
  - A grounding electrode is placed on the right leg.
  - A total of six electrode positions are used on the chest.
- The patient is to remain still while the recording is completed.
  - Many ECG machines are now able to record all 12 leads simultaneously.

Posttest
- Remove the electrodes and cleanse the skin of any residual gel or adhesive.
- Report abnormal findings to the primary care provider.

→ **Clinical Alerts**

- Inform the patient that a normal EKG does not guarantee absence of heart disease. All risk factors of coronary artery disease should be reviewed, screening labs including lipid panel completed, and the importance of diet and exercise discussed.
- Patients should be informed of the signs and symptoms of myocardial infarction and what they should do if symptoms appear.

Electroencephalography (EEG)

Test Description
In electroencephalography (EEG), the electrical activity of the brain is recorded. This is attainable by way of electrodes attached in several locations on the scalp which pick up electrical impulses from the superficial layers of the cerebral cortex and transmit them to an electroencephalograph for recording. The resultant waveforms are then analyzed. The test is used to diagnose seizure disorders, intracranial abscesses, and tumors; to evaluate the brain's electrical activity in cases of possible cerebral damage such as that due to head injury or meningitis; and to confirm brain death, in which electrical activity of the brain is absent.

Normal Values

Normal brain waves

Possible Meanings of Abnormal Values

Brain death
Cerebral infarct
Encephalitis
Increased intracranial pressure
Intracranial abscess
Intracranial hemorrhage
Intracranial tumor
Meningitis
Seizure disorder

E

Contributing Factors to Abnormal Values

- Drugs which may alter test results: anticonvulsants, barbiturates, caffeine, sedatives, tranquilizers.
- Hypoglycemia may affect the EEG results.
- Movement of the head, body, eyes, or tongue can cause changes in the brain wave patterns.

Interventions/Implications

Pretest

- Explain to the patient the purpose of the test and the procedure to be done. Explain that there is no discomfort involved with this test. Note that no electricity enters the patient from the machine.
- No fasting is required prior to the test. However, no caffeine-containing drinks should be consumed within 8 hours of the test.
- Instruct the patient to shampoo the hair the night before the test to aid in securing the electrodes during the test.
- If a sleep-deprivation study is ordered in which the patient will need to fall asleep during the test, the patient should sleep as little as possible the night before the test.
- Medications which might influence test results should be withheld, if possible.

Procedure

- The procedure is usually conducted in an EEG laboratory. If testing for brain death, a portable EEG machine may be used at the bedside.
- The patient may either sit in a lounge chair or lie supine on a bed.
- Approximately 20 electrodes are applied to the scalp by the EEG technician in a standardized pattern using electrode paste. Grounding electrodes are applied to each ear.
- The patient is instructed to lie still with the eyes closed, while the EEG recording is made. Any movements which might affect the EEG are documented.
- The recording is interrupted periodically to allow the patient to move into a more comfortable position.
- Additional components of the EEG which might be performed include:
  - *Hyperventilation*: The patient breathes rapidly for 3 minutes. The resulting alkalosis may elicit brain wave patterns associated with seizure disorders.

- *Photostimulation*: A strobe light is flashed over the patient's face. This may elicit brain wave patterns characteristic of partial or generalized seizures.
- *Sleep EEG*: The EEG is recorded while the patient is falling asleep, during sleep, and while the patient is waking. This is used to detect brain wave abnormalities which occur during sleep, such as those associated with frontal lobe epilepsy.

Posttest

- Resume medications as taken prior to the test, with physician approval.
- Observe the patient for any seizure activity.
- Following removal of the electrodes, the electrode paste is removed. Oil, acetone, or witch hazel may help to remove the paste, then the hair should be shampooed.
- Report abnormal findings to the primary care provider.

Electromyography (EMG)

Test Description

Electromyography (EMG) is the recording of electrical activity in skeletal muscle groups. It is usually performed in conjunction with electroneurography (nerve conduction studies). Conducting both nerve conduction studies and electromyography are collectively known as *electrodiagnostic testing*. The test involves insertion of needle electrodes into the muscle. The EMG then records the state of the muscle at rest and during voluntary contraction. Muscle tissue is normally electrically silent when at rest. When muscle is voluntarily contracted, action potentials of varying rates and amplitudes appear on the EMG oscilloscope.

The information assists in determining whether the cause of muscle weakness is due to *myopathy*, a disease of the striated muscle fibers or cell membranes, or due to *neuropathy*, a disease of the lower motor neuron. EMG is most often used when people have symptoms of weakness and physical examination shows impaired muscle strength. It does not evaluate sensory fibers.

For most cases, the electrodiagnostic examination should be performed only after 21 days from the time of injury. This allows for development of fibrillation potentials (hallmark of axon degeneration). Exceptions to the suggested 21-day wait would be those cases in which it is important to locate where the lesion is along the nerve or to differentiate between axon loss and demyelinating lesions for prognostic purposes. It is likewise important to not wait too long for testing to be done. False-negative studies increase after 6-month duration.

Electromyography is best used for detection of axon loss lesions (severe compression or trauma of the nerve, ischemia of the nerve, and inflammation) and to detect muscle disorders. It is insensitive for demyelinating lesions, whereas nerve conduction studies are highly sensitive for these lesions. Thus, it is recommended in most cases to include both electroneurography (ENG) and EMG in the diagnostic plan.

Normal Values

Normal muscle electrical activity

Possible Meanings of Abnormal Values

Amyotrophic lateral sclerosis
Bell's palsy
Beriberi
Carpal tunnel syndrome
Dermatomyositis
Diabetic peripheral neuropathy
Eaton-Lambert syndrome
Guillain-Barre
Motor neuron disease
Muscular dystrophy
Myasthenia gravis
Myopathy
Myositis
Nerve dysfunction
Peripheral neuropathy
Poliomyelitis
Polymyositis
Radiculopathy

Contributing Factors to Abnormal Values

- Drugs which may interfere with test results: anticholinergics, cholinergics, skeletal muscle relaxants.

Interventions/Implications

Pretest
- Explain to the patient the purpose of the test and the procedure to be performed. Note that discomfort involved with the test is due to the insertion of the needle electrodes. Muscle aching often occurs after the procedure.
- No fasting is required prior to the test.
- Caffeine and nicotine should be avoided for 3 hours prior to the test.
- Obtain a signed informed consent.
- Trauma to the muscle from EMG may cause false results on blood tests such as creatine kinase.

Procedure
- The skin is cleansed with alcohol.
- A needle that acts as a recording electrode is inserted into the muscle being studied.
- A reference electrode is placed nearby on the skin surface.
- While the muscle is at rest, the EMG display is observed for any evidence of spontaneous electrical activity.
- The patient is then asked to slowly contract the muscle.
- Recordings are made of the muscle activity at both rest and during muscle contraction.

Posttest
- The needle is removed from the muscle and the site observed for bleeding.
- Mild analgesics may be needed to relieve muscle aching.
- Report abnormal findings to the primary care provider.

→ **Clinical Alerts**

- The EMG may alter the results of enzyme tests, such as asparate aminotransferase, creatine kinase, or lactic dehydrogenase. If ordered, such tests should be drawn prior to or 5 days after the EMG.
- Overly anxious patients may need an antianxiety medication such as lorazepam 30 minutes prior to the study.
- When ordering electrodiagnostic testing, include the suspected diagnosis. For example, use the clinical examination to narrow the diagnosis, such as "left lumbosacral radiculopathy, L5-S1" rather than "left leg pain." This will help the electrodiagnostician tailor the exam to the patient.

E

CONTRAINDICATIONS!

- Patients with bleeding disorders
- Patients receiving anticoagulants
- Patients unable to cooperate with the procedure

 Electroneurography (ENG, Nerve Conduction Studies)

Test Description

Electroneurography (ENG) is the recording of nerve conduction velocity to assist in the evaluation of peripheral nerve disease or injury. It is usually performed in conjunction with electromyography. Conducting both nerve conduction studies and electromyography are collectively known as *electrodiagnostic testing*.

Nerve conduction studies are highly sensitive in differentiating axon loss (due to severe nerve compression or trauma, ischemia of the nerve, and inflammation) from demyelination (from mild to moderate nerve compression and autoimmune disorders). The test is less uncomfortable than electromyography but nerve conduction studies are limited in terms of examination of the peripheral nervous system, unlike electromyography which allows for widespread examination of the peripheral nervous system. Nerve conduction studies are able to locate segmental demyelinating lesions, whereas electromyography is insensitive for demyelinating lesions. Thus, it is recommended in most cases to include both ENG and electromyography in the diagnostic plan.

For most cases, the electrodiagnostic examination should be performed only after 21 days from the time of injury. This allows for development of fibrillation potentials (hallmark of axon degeneration). Exceptions to the suggested 21-day wait would be those cases in which it is important to locate where the lesion is along the nerve or to differentiate between axon loss and demyelinating lesions for prognostic purposes. It is likewise important to not wait too long for testing to be done. False-negative studies increase after 6-month duration.

Normal Values

Normal nerve conduction velocity rates

Possible Meanings of Abnormal Values

Amyotrophic lateral sclerosis
Botulism
Carpal tunnel syndrome
Compressive radiculopathy (disk disease)
Guillain-Barre syndrome
Muscular dystrophy
Myasthenia gravis
Peripheral nerve disorders
Plexus disorders (brachial, lumbar)

E

Contributing Factors to Abnormal Values

- Severe pain may cause inaccurate results.
- Nerve conduction velocity slows with age.
- Poor patient cooperation during the test can limit its diagnostic usefulness.

Interventions/Implications

Pretest
- Explain to the patient the purpose of the test and the procedure to be performed. Note that discomfort involved with the test is due to minor electrical stimuli administered during the procedure.
- No fasting is required prior to the test.
- Patients who use daily analgesics can take their regular doses.
- If the exam is being done to evaluate the neuromuscular junction, such as for myasthenia gravis, medications such as pyridostigmine should be stopped at least 12 hours prior to the study.
- Obtain a signed informed consent.

Procedure
- The skin is cleansed with alcohol.
- *Sensory nerve conduction studies* are performed by placing a recording electrode on the skin directly above a sensory nerve. An electrical stimulus is applied proximally at a defined distance from the recording electrode, producing a detectable waveform called the *sensory nerve action potential.*
- *Motor nerve conduction studies* are performed by placing a recording electrode directly over the belly of the muscle and stimulating the nerve proximally. The muscle fibers depolarize, producing a waveform called a *compound motor action potential.*

Posttest
- The electrodes and paste are removed, and skin cleansed.
- Mild analgesics may be needed to relieve muscle aching.
- Report abnormal findings to the primary care provider.

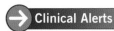

Clinical Alerts

- *It is imperative to notify the laboratory conducting the nerve conduction study if the patient has an implantable cardioverter-defibrillator or a pacemaker, as nerve conduction studies can cause a defibrillator to fire.*
    - To prevent this, arrangements need to be made for deactivating the defibrillator and for providing cardiac monitoring.
    - Regular pacemakers generally require no special precaution, but their activity will show as artifact during the nerve conduction studies.
- Overly anxious patients may need an antianxiety medication such as lorazepam 30 minutes prior to the study.
- When ordering electrodiagnostic testing, include the suspected diagnosis. For example, use the clinical examination to narrow the diagnosis, such as "left lumbosacral radiculopathy, L5-S1" rather than "left leg pain." This will help the electrodiagnostician tailor the exam to the patient.

Electronystagmography (ENG)

Test Description

Electronystagmography (ENG) is used to evaluate patients with complaints of dizziness, vertigo, or balance dysfunction. This test evaluates the oculovestibular reflex, which involves the interaction of the muscles controlling eye movement (ocular system) and the vestibular system. This reflex results in the appearance of involuntary back-and-forth eye movement, known as *nystagmus*. When the head is turned, the eyes normally deviate slowly in the opposite direction. Upon reaching the limit of their movement, they tend to quickly return to the center, and the nystagmus ceases. Abnormal nystagmus involves the same type of the movement, but it is prolonged. This can result from peripheral lesions, such as involvement of the vestibular portion of the eighth cranial nerve (acoustic nerve), or from cerebellar or brain stem involvement.

Since abnormal nystagmus is the primary sign of vestibular problems, ENG can assist in identifying the cause of dizziness, vertigo, tinnitus, or hearing loss. The ENG test consists of three parts: oculomotor evaluation, positioning/positional testing, and caloric stimulation of the vestibular system. The results of the testing are analyzed to determine whether the problem is central (brain) or peripheral. Recording of eye movement during each of the component tests is accomplished through electrodes placed near the outer canthus of each eye (for detection of lateral nystagmus), electrodes placed above and below one eye (for detection of vertical nystagmus), and a ground electrode placed above the bridge of the nose.

Normal Values

Normal waveform patterns

Possible Meanings of Abnormal Values

Brainstem lesion
Cerebellum lesion
Cerebrum lesion
Cranial nerve VIII tumor
Congenital abnormalities
Hypothyroidism
Infection
Inflammation
Labyrinthitis
Meniere's disease
Multiple sclerosis
Ototoxicity

E

Contributing Factors to Abnormal Values

- Drugs which may alter test results: antivertigo drugs, central nervous system (CNS) depressants, CNS stimulants.
- Alcohol ingestion can affect ENG test results for 72 hours post-ingestion.
- Blinking of the eyes, drowsiness, or improperly applied electrodes will alter test results.

Interventions/Implications

Pretest

- Explain to the patient the purpose of the test and the procedures to be conducted.
- No fasting is required prior to the test, however since the test may cause dizziness and/or nausea, food intake just prior to the examination should be limited.
- Alcohol, caffeine, and all medications (unless contraindicated) should be withheld for 24 to 72 hours prior to the test.
- Inspect the ear canals for intact tympanic membranes. Remove any excess wax from the canals.

Procedure

- Electrodes are placed at each of the following five points: one lateral electrode at the outer canthus of each eye, one electrode above the left eye and one below the left eye for recording of vertical nystagmus, and one electrode in the center of the forehead.
- During any of the testing, documentation is made of any complaints of dizziness by the patient.
- Testing is done with the patient seated or in a supine position.

Calibration test: This test is used to calibrate the stylus for recording of each of the subsequent tests.

- The patient looks straight ahead at a light. The light is moved 10° to the right, back to center, and then 10° to the left. The stylus is adjusted to correspond with these movements.

Gaze nystagmus test: Gaze testing is conducted to evaluate for the presence of nystagmus in the absence of vestibular stimulation.

- For gaze testing, the patient is instructed to look straight ahead and then to fixate on a target 30° to the right, left, up, and down. Fixation is maintained for approximately 30 seconds

in center gaze and 10 seconds in eccentric gaze. With some systems, the patient simply has his/her eyes closed.
- To help the patient avoid thinking of the testing, provide an arithmetic problem for the patient to calculate during the testing period.

Smooth pursuit tracking: The smooth pursuit system allows one to follow targets in the visual field. Horizontal tracking is normally smoother than vertical tracking.
- The patient looks straight ahead and follows the movement of a pendulum for 20 seconds.

Optokinetics test: For this test, the patient tracks multiple stimuli.
- The patient follows a target moving across the visual field from left to right. As one target leaves the visual field to the right, another target enters from the left.
- The procedure is repeated with the targets moving from right to left.

Positional test: The Dix-Hallpike maneuver is conducted to assess for nystagmus associated with BPPV (benign paroxysmal positional vertigo).
- The Dix-Hallpike maneuver involves turning a patient's head to the right or left and then quickly assisting him or her to a supine position with the head hanging to the right or left. The patient is left in this position for a brief period (at least 20 seconds) while eye movements are observed. Finally, the patient is returned to a sitting position. If nystagmus is observed, the test is repeated to evaluate fatigability of the response, since fatigability is one sign of BPPV.
- The examiner then places the patient in various positions for 20 to 30 seconds, assessing for nystagmus.

Caloric test: Caloric stimulation of the vestibular system assesses the lateral semicircular canal. In patients with responsive vestibular systems, cool irrigations cause nystagmus beats in the direction opposite to the stimulated ear, whereas warm irrigations cause nystagmus beats in the direction of the stimulated ear.
- The patient is positioned with the head of the bed elevated 30°.
- Protect the patient with towels and place an emesis basin under the ear being tested.
- Inform the patient that water is about to be introduced into the ear.
- With the patient's eyes closed, introduce the water so that it directly hits the tympanic membrane for 30 seconds.
- This procedure is conducted a total of four times:
    1. in the left ear, using cool water (86°F)
    2. in the right ear, using cool water (86°F)
    3. in the left ear, using warm water (111.2°F)
    4. in the right ear, using warm water (111.2°F)
- A period of rest of 3 to 5 minutes is given between steps 1 and 2 and between 3 and 4. Between steps 2 and 3, an 8 to 10 minute rest period is given.
- Note: If patient has perforated tympanic membranes, this test is modified by using water-filled finger cots.

Posttest
- Remove the electrodes and cleanse the patient's skin of any remaining paste.
- Assess the patient for weakness, dizziness, or nausea.
- Allow patient to rest as needed, and then assist with ambulation, if needed.
- Report abnormal findings to the primary care provider.

Clinical Alerts

- Normal ENG test results do not necessarily mean that a patient has typical vestibular function.
- Oculomotor stimulation with lights may cause seizures.
- Since the test may cause dizziness and/or nausea, advise patients to have someone transport them to and from the test.

E

CONTRAINDICATIONS!

- Patients with perforated eardrums
- Patients with pacemakers
- Patients unable to cooperate with the examination

 Electrophysiologic Study (EPS, Bundle of His Procedure)

Test Description

Electrophysiologic study (EPS) involves the introduction of an electrode catheter into the right atrium and the right ventricle. The catheter is usually inserted into a peripheral vein because of the greater risk for bleeding when using the arterial system for such testing. Once in place, the catheter is used to perform programmed electrical stimulation of the heart.

EPS is very useful in evaluating the conduction system of the heart. It is also used to attempt to induce any dysrhythmia which may be affecting the patient. By stimulating the occurrence of the dysrhythmia during EPS, the physician can, under controlled conditions, determine the appropriate treatment for the problem. It also provides information regarding how well antidysrhythmic drugs are working by noting how easily the arrhythmia is able to be induced.

Normal Values

Normal conduction intervals, refractory periods, and recovery times shown on EKG. No dysrhythmias induced.

Possible Meanings of Abnormal Values

Atrioventricular node defects
Cardiac arrhythmias
Electroconduction defects
Heart blocks
Sinoatrial node defects

Contributing Factors to Abnormal Values

- Drugs which may alter test results: analgesics, antidysrhythmics, sedatives, tranquilizers.

Interventions/Implications

Pretest

- Explain to the patient the purpose of the test. Provide any written teaching materials available on the subject. Note that discomfort involved with this test is due to catheter insertion, but that it will be minimized by local anesthesia to the area. The patient may also experience flushing, anxiety, dizziness, and palpitations during the procedure.
- Fasting for at least 8 hours is required prior to the test.
- For an initial study, antidysrhythmic medications may be discontinued for several days prior to the test, if possible.
- Obtain a signed informed consent.
- Perform a baseline assessment of the circulatory and neuromuscular status of the patient's legs.
- A mild sedative may be administered.

Procedure

- The patient is assisted to a supine position on the examination table in the cardiac catheterization laboratory.
- A maintenance IV line is initiated.
- Cardiac monitoring is initiated.
- Resuscitation and suctioning equipment should be readily available.
- The staff members should converse with the patient throughout the procedure to both allay patient fears, and to assess the patient's level of consciousness.
- The area of the puncture site, usually the femoral vein, is cleansed and then anesthetized.
- The needle puncture of the vein is made and the catheter is advanced to the right atrium and right ventricle. Positioning of the catheter is monitored via fluoroscopy.
- Once the catheter is in the correct position, a baseline EKG is recorded.
- Pacing is then used to induce dysrhythmias. Sustained dysrhythmias are treated with pacing, and, if unsuccessful, by cardioversion/defibrillation.
- At times, ablation of areas of the heart which are found to be causing dysrhythmias may be performed.
- When the procedure is completed, the catheter is removed and a pressure dressing is applied to the site.
- Gloves are worn throughout the procedure.

Posttest

- Monitor vital signs and neurological status every 15 minutes for 1 hour, then every 30 minutes for 2 hours, then every hour for 4 hours, and then every 4 hours.
- Assess the color, movement, temperature, and sensation (CMTS) and the pulse(s) of the affected extremity with each vital sign assessment, and compare with the other extremity.
- Check the dressing for bleeding and the area around the puncture site for swelling each time the vital signs are assessed.
- The patient is to remain on bedrest for at least 8 hours with the affected extremity immobilized.
- Resume medications as ordered.
- Report abnormal findings to the primary care provider.

→ Clinical Alerts

- Possible complications include: cardiac dysrhythmias, catheter-induced embolic stroke or myocardial infarction, hemorrhage, myocardial perforation, peripheral vascular problems, and phlebitis at catheter insertion site.

CONTRAINDICATIONS!

- Patients with acute myocardial infarction
- Patients who are unable to cooperate due to age, mental status, pain, or other factors

 # Endometrial Biopsy

Test Description

Endometrial biopsy is a procedure in which a tissue sample is obtained from the endometrium. It is used in the evaluation of abnormal or postmenopausal bleeding, and to exclude the presence of endometrial cancer or its precursors. Other uses include evaluation of uterine response to hormone therapy, evaluation of infertility, follow-up of previously diagnosed endometrial hyperplasia, and follow-up to abnormal Pap test showing cells favoring endometrial origin (especially in women over 40 years of age).

THE EVIDENCE FOR PRACTICE

Guidelines established by Brigham and Women's Hospital (2005) for management of abnormal bleeding patterns in women on hormone replacement therapy (HRT) note an endometrial biopsy is indicated for patients taking HRT in the following situations:
- Patients on cyclical HRT with unscheduled bleeding or bleeding before day 6 of progestin.
- Patients on continuous HRT with bleeding after 6 to 9 months of use.
- Patients who have bleeding after a sustained period of amenorrhea.
- Patients on the continuous regimen who have excessive bleeding (heavier than patient's past period). If the biopsy reveals only a proliferative endometrium, the dose of estrogen can be increased, or the patient can be switched to the cyclical regimen.

Normal Values

No abnormal cells

Possible Meanings of Abnormal Values

Atrophic endometrium
Atypical complex hyperplasia
Endometrial cancer
Simple hyperplasia
Uterine fibroids
Uterine polyps

Interventions/Implications

Pretest
- Explain to the patient the purpose of the test. Provide any written teaching materials available on the subject. Note that cramping may occur during the procedure.
  - Preprocedure oral nonsteroidal anti-inflammatory drug (NSAIDs), such as ibuprofen, can reduce the cramping.

- The patient must remain still during the procedure.
- No fasting is required before the test.
- Obtain a signed informed consent.

Procedure
- The procedure may be performed with or without anesthesia.
- The patient is assisted into a lithotomy position.
- A bimanual pelvic examination is performed to determine the uterine size and position.
- A speculum is inserted into the vagina.
- The cervix is visualized and anesthetized with benzocaine spray, and then is cleansed with povidone-iodine solution.
- The cervix is gently probed with the uterine sound.
    - If the cervix is too mobile, it can be stabilized by a tenaculum
    - If the sound will not pass through the internal os, the os may need to be dilated by using first a very small uterine dilator, and then successively larger dilators until the sound is able to be passed through the os.
- The endometrial biopsy catheter tip is inserted into the cervix and into the uterine fundus.
- The catheter tip is moved with an in-and-out motion at least four times to obtain adequate tissue in the catheter.
- The catheter is withdrawn, and the tenaculum is gently removed.
- Gloves are worn throughout the procedure.

Posttest
- The specimen is placed in preservative, labeled, and transported to the laboratory.
- Report abnormal findings to the primary care provider.

Clinical Alerts

- Possible complications include: bleeding, infection, perforation of the uterus, and tearing of the cervix.
- If the internal cervical os is very tight, an alternative to instrumental cervical dilation in older patients is to insert an osmotic laminaria (seaweed) dilator the morning of the procedure. This will cause slow opening of the cervix and allow the procedure to be performed in the afternoon.

CONTRAINDICATIONS!

- Pregnancy
- Patients with acute pelvic inflammatory disease
- Patients with clotting disorders
- Patients with acute cervical or vaginal infections
- Patients with cervical cancer
- Patients who are morbidly obese
- Patients with severe cervical stenosis

Endoscopic Retrograde Cholangiopancreatography (ERCP)

Test Description

Endoscopic retrograde cholangiopancreatography (ERCP) is the radiographic viewing of the pancreatic ducts and the hepatobiliary tree through an endoscope. The procedure involves injection of a contrast medium through the ampulla of Vater. ERCP and percutaneous transhepatic cholangiography are the only procedures which allow direct visualization of the biliary and pancreatic ducts. Due to the comparatively low risk of complications, ERCP is the most commonly performed of these two procedures. The procedure is especially useful in the evaluation of patients with jaundice, since visualization of the biliary ducts can occur even when the patient's bilirubin level is high. Thus the test can provide information helpful in the diagnosis of obstructive jaundice and cancer of the duodenal papilla, pancreas, and biliary ducts, and in locating calculi and stenosis in the pancreatic ducts and hepatobiliary tree. Unfortunately, pancreatitis occurs in 5% to 7% of ERCP procedures despite efforts to reduce the incidence of this complication. Newer techniques such as magnetic resonance cholangiopancreatography (MRCP) now offer a noninvasive alternative to ERCP for diagnostic purposes.

THE EVIDENCE FOR PRACTICE

ERCP is now a primarily therapeutic procedure for the management of pancreaticobiliary disorders. Diagnostic ERCP should not be undertaken in the evaluation of pancreaticobiliary pain in the absence of objective findings on other imaging studies. Routine ERCP before laparoscopic cholecystectomy should not be performed. Endoscopic therapy of postoperative biliary leaks and strictures should be undertaken as first-line therapy. (Adler, 2005).

Normal Values

Normal size and patency of the biliary and bile ducts
Absence of calculi

Possible Meanings of Abnormal Values

Biliary cirrhosis
Carcinoma of the bile ducts
Carcinoma of the duodenal papilla
Carcinoma of the head of the pancreas
Chronic pancreatitis
Pancreatic cysts
Pancreatic fibrosis
Pancreatic tumor
Papillary stenosis
Pseudocysts
Sclerosing cholangitis
Stones of the bile or pancreatic ducts
Strictures of the bile or pancreatic ducts

Contributing Factors to Abnormal Values

- Retained barium for other exams, vomiting, and diarrhea will affect test results.

Interventions/Implications

Pretest

- Explain to the patient the purpose of the test and the benefits and risks associated with the test. Provide any written teaching materials available on the subject.
- Obtain a signed informed consent from the patient.
- Inform the radiologist of any potential allergy to the contrast dye and obtain an order for an antihistamine and a steroid to be given prior to the procedure.
- Patients receiving metformin (Glucophage) for Type 2 diabetes mellitus should discontinue the drug 2 days before elective surgery or angiographic exams. This is due to the possible occurrence of lactic acidosis, a potentially fatal complication of biguanide therapy.
- Baseline labs including BUN and creatinine are obtained.
- The patient is to be NPO for 12 hours prior to the test.
- Instruct the patient to remove all objects containing metal, such as jewelry or undergarments, as these will show on the film.

Procedure

- A maintenance IV is started.
- A topical anesthetic is applied to the oropharyngeal area.
- The patient is placed in a left lateral position.
- A narcotic or sedative/hypnotic is administered.
- The endoscope is inserted through the mouth, esophagus, and stomach, and then advanced to the duodenum.
- The patient is assisted to a prone position.
- An anticholinergic drug such as atropine or glucagon is given IV to reduce duodenal spasm and to relax the ampulla of Vater.
- A catheter is inserted through the ampulla and into the common bile or pancreatic ducts.
- The contrast medium is injected and several films are taken.

Posttest

- Assess the patient's vital signs until stable.
- Withhold food and fluids until the gag reflex returns.
- Some abdominal discomfort may be present for several hours postprocedure. However, prolonged, sharp abdominal pain, especially in conjunction with nausea or vomiting, is to be reported to the physician.
- Renal function is reassessed and when appropriate, metformin may be restarted.
- Report abnormal findings to the primary care provider.

→ **Clinical Alerts**

- Possible complications include: cholangitis, hemorrhage, pancreatitis, perforation of ducts, and urinary retention.
- Observe for indications of cholangitis (hyperbilirubinemia, fever, chills) and pancreatitis (upper left quadrant pain, tenderness, elevated serum amylase levels and transient hyperbilirubinemia).

- If a barium swallow or an upper gastrointestinal and small-bowel series test is ordered, these should be completed *after* the ERCP is performed. Otherwise the barium sulfate ingested during the other exams may obscure the films made of the gallbladder.

E

CONTRAINDICATIONS!

- Pregnant women
  - Caution: A woman in her childbearing years should undergo radiography only during her menses or 12 to 14 days after its onset to avoid any exposure to a fetus.
- Patients with hypersensitivity to iodine, seafood, or contrast media
- Patients with known pancreatic and biliary problems: pancreatitis, pancreatic pseudo-cysts, stricture or obstruction of the esophagus or duodenum
- Patients with cardiac and respiratory disease
- Patients who are unable to cooperate due to age, mental status, pain, or other factors

Epstein-Barr Virus (Mononucleosis Test, EBV Antibody Test, Heterophile Antibody Titer [HAT], Monospot Test)

Test Description

Infectious mononucleosis (IM) is caused by a herpesvirus, the Epstein-Barr virus (EBV). It is characterized by fatigue, sore throat, fever, pharyngitis, lymphadenopathy, splenomegaly, and the presence of lymphocytosis. It is a self-limiting condition, with treatment aimed at symptom control.

In addition to the increased production of lymphocytes and monocytes in the lymph nodes, IM also stimulates the production of heterophile antibodies. This IgM type of antibody, which is not normally present in human beings, causes agglutination of sheep or horse red blood cells. The antibodies usually form within 4 to 7 days of the onset of the illness. The antibodies peak at weeks 2 to 5 and may persist for several months to 1 year.

A positive *heterophile antibody titer (HAT)* assists in the diagnosis of IM since it is positive in 90% of the IM cases, but it can also occur in other conditions. Typically, a positive heterophile test, done in the form of a rapid *monospot test*, along with the classic clinical picture, are sufficient for a diagnosis of infectious mononucleosis.

In the case of heterophile-negative cases and for diagnosis in atypical cases, the presence of the Epstein-Barr virus can be confirmed by EBV-specific testing. Diagnosis of IM can be established with high levels of IgM and IgG antibodies. The IgM antibodies usually disappear within 3 to 6 weeks after the onset of the illness. Previous EBV infections are identified by IgG antibodies, which usually arise from 3 weeks to several months after onset of symptoms.

Normal Values

Negative

Possible Meanings of Abnormal Values

Positive
Burkitt's lymphoma
Chronic fatigue syndrome
Cytomegalovirus
Epstein-Barr virus
Hodgkin's disease
Infectious mononucleosis
Lymphocytic leukemia
Malaria
Nasopharyngeal cancer
Pancreatic cancer
Rheumatoid arthritis
Rubella
Sarcoidosis
Systemic lupus erythematosus
Viral hepatitis

Contributing Factors to Abnormal Values

- Hemolysis of the blood sample may alter test results.

Interventions/Implications

Pretest
- Explain to the patient the purpose of the test and the need for a blood sample to be drawn.
- No fasting is required prior to the test.

Procedure
- A 7-mL blood sample is drawn in a red-top collection tube.
- Gloves are worn throughout the procedure.

Posttest
- Apply pressure at venipuncture site. Apply dressing, periodically assessing for continued bleeding.
- Label the specimen and transport it to the laboratory.
- Report abnormal findings to the primary care provider.

Clinical Alerts

- A white blood count with differential should be done concurrently to identify the lymphocytosis and the presence of atypical lymphocytes usually found in infectious mononucleosis.
- If the mono test is initially negative but mono is still suspected, a repeat mono test may be ordered in a week or so to see if heterophile antibodies have developed and/or testing for EBV antibodies may be ordered to help confirm or rule out the presence of a current EBV infection.

Erythrocyte Sedimentation Rate
(ESR, Sedimentation Rate, Sed Rate)

Test Description

The erythrocyte sedimentation rate (ESR) is a nonspecific test for inflammatory and necrotic conditions. The ESR may also be increased in situations of physiologic stress, such as pregnancy. In these types of conditions, there is a change in blood proteins which leads to a clumping of red blood cells. The ESR measures the speed with which erythrocytes settle in a tube of blood which has been mixed with an anti-coagulant. Cells which have clumped due to inflammatory and necrotic conditions settle more rapidly than single cells. Thus, the ESR, expressed in mm/h, would be increased in inflammatory and necrotic conditions. There is a direct relationship between the ESR and the course of such diseases; as the disease improves, such as due to drug therapy, the ESR decreases.

E

Normal Values

Male:	Under 50 years old: < 15 mm/hr
	Over 50 years old: < 20 mm/hr
Female:	Under 50 years old: < 20 mm/hr
	Over 50 years old: < 30 mm/hr
Child:	3–13 mm/hr
Newborn:	0–2 mm/hr

Possible Meanings of Abnormal Values

Increased	Decreased
Anemia	Congestive heart failure
Coccidioidomycosis	Factor V deficiency
Crohn's disease	Hypoalbuminemia
Hemolytic anemia	Poikilocytosis
Infection	Polycythemia vera
Inflammatory process	Sickle cell anemia
Malignancies	
Myocardial infarction	
Osteomyelitis	
Pain	
Polymyalgia rheumatica	
Rheumatoid arthritis	
Systemic lupus erythematosus	
Temporal (giant cell) arteritis	
Tissue injury	

Contributing Factors to Abnormal Values

- The ESR may be increased during menstruation, after the 12th week of pregnancy, and postpartum.
- The ESR may be decreased in the presence of elevated white blood cell count, albumin, and lipids.

- Drugs which may *increase* the ESR: dextran, heparin, oral contraceptives.
- Drugs which may *decrease* the ESR: albumin, aspirin, corticotropin, cortisone, lecithin, steroids.

Interventions/Implications

Pretest

- Explain to the patient the purpose of the test and the need for a blood sample to be drawn.
- No fasting is required before the test.

Procedure
- A 5-mL blood sample is drawn in a lavender-top collection tube containing EDTA.
- Gloves are worn throughout the procedure.

Posttest
- Invert and gently mix the sample and the anticoagulant (EDTA).
- Apply pressure at venipuncture site. Apply dressing, periodically assessing for continued bleeding.
- Label the specimen and transport it to the laboratory.
- Report abnormal findings to the primary care provider.

→ Clinical Alerts

- In polymyalgia rheumatica, the ESR is monitored frequently to guide the health-care provider in determining dosage of prednisone needed for control of symptoms.
- The ESR is usually very high (>55 mm/h) in patients with temporal arteritis. It is essential that steroids be initiated immediately to avoid complications such as blindness or stroke.

Erythropoietin (EPO)

Test Description
Erythropoietin is a glycoprotein hormone produced by the kidneys in response to tissue hypoxia. It then stimulates red blood cell (RBC) production in the bone marrow. Measuring erythropoietin assists in the diagnosis of polycythemia vera, secondary polycythemia and various anemic states, and to determine whether the amount of erythropoietin being produced is appropriate for the level of anemia present. The test may also be ordered when the hemoglobin and hematocrit indicate anemia is present, but the reticulocyte count indicates the bone marrow has not responded by increasing RBC production.

Normal Values
0–19 mU/mL

Possible Meanings of Abnormal Values

Increased	Decreased
Aplastic anemia	AIDS
Erythropoietin-producing tumors	Anemia of chronic illness
Hemolytic anemia	End-stage renal disease
Myelodysplastic syndrome	Polycythemia vera
Pregnancy	Rheumatoid arthritis
Secondary polycythemia	
Uncomplicated anemias	

Contributing Factors to Abnormal Values

- Drugs that may *increase* EPO levels: anabolic steroids, epoetin alfa, fluoxymesterone, zidovudine.
- Drugs that may *decrease* EPO levels: acetazolamide, amphotericin B, cisplatin, enalapril, epoetin alfa, furosemide.

Interventions/Implications

Pretest
- Explain to the patient the purpose of the test and the need for a blood sample to be drawn.
- No fasting is required before the test.
- Early morning blood sampling is preferred.

Procedure
- A 7-mL blood sample is drawn in a gold-top (serum separator) collection tube.
- Gloves are worn throughout the procedure.

Posttest
- Apply pressure at venipuncture site. Apply dressing, periodically assessing for continued bleeding.
- Label the specimen and transport it to the laboratory.
- Report abnormal findings to the primary care provider.

 Esophageal Manometry (Esophageal Function Studies)

Test Description

Esophageal manometry is used to assess the esophagus for normal contractile activity. The lower esophageal sphincter (LES) pressure is measured and recordings are made of the duration and sequence of peristaltic contractions. The test is conducted when the patient is experiencing difficulty in swallowing, heartburn, regurgitation, or vomiting, or has chest pain for which no explanation has been found. The test involves placement of a manometric catheter at various levels in the esophagus. A pressure transducer in the catheter is used to obtain baseline pressure measurements. The patient is then asked to swallow, after which esophageal sphincter pressures are measured and peristaltic contractions are recorded. Two other aspects of the test involve testing for acid reflux and Bernstein (acid perfusion) testing.

THE EVIDENCE FOR PRACTICE

Indications for Esophageal Manometry
- To establish the diagnosis of dysphagia in instances in which a mechanical obstruction (e.g., stricture) cannot be found.
- For placement of intraluminal devices (e.g., pH probes) when positioning is dependent on the relationship to functional landmarks, such as the lower esophageal sphincter.
- For the preoperative assessment of patients being considered for antireflux surgery if there is any question of an alternative diagnosis, especially achalasia.

Esophageal Manometry Not Indicated
- For making or confirming a suspected diagnosis of gastroesophageal reflux disease
- As the initial test for chest pain or other esophageal symptoms because of the low specificity of the findings and the low likelihood of detecting a clinically significant motility disorder. (Pandolfino & Kahrilas, 2005).

Normal Values

Pressure at the lower esophageal sphincter: 10–22 mm Hg
Normal peristaltic waves present
pH in esophagus: >5
Negative acid reflux and Bernstein tests

Possible Meanings of Abnormal Values

Achalasia
Diffuse spasm of the esophagus
Esophageal scleroderma
Gastric acid reflux
Reflux esophagitis

Interventions/Implications

Pretest
- Explain to the patient the purpose of the test. Provide any written teaching materials available on the subject. Explain to the patient that the test involves the passage of a small tube into the esophagus, which may cause the throat to be sore for a short time after the procedure.
- Fasting for 8 hours is required prior to the test.
- Tobacco and alcohol are to be avoided for 24 hours prior to the test.

Procedure
- The patient is asked to swallow the manometric catheter or the catheter is inserted into the nostril. Small holes along the sides of the catheter allow for pressure measurements to be made. The patient may gag as the catheter enters the posterior oropharynx.
- The catheter is passed into the stomach and then pulled back up into the esophagus until a large change in pressure is noted. This is location for the measurement the lower esophageal sphincter (LES) pressure.
- The patient is then asked to swallow, during which recordings of the LES pressure and peristaltic contractions are made.
- For *acid reflux* testing, a 0.1 N hydrochloric acid solution is instilled in the stomach. The pH of the esophagus is then measured. If the pH decreases, gastroesophageal (acid) reflux is present.

- For *Bernstein* testing, normal saline is first infused into the esophagus as a control. Next, 0.1 N hydrochloric acid solution is instilled for 10 minutes. This is done as an attempt to reproduce symptoms of heartburn or chest discomfort. If the patient complains of discomfort during the acid instillation, the test is considered positive.

Posttest
- Remove the catheter.
- Encourage use of throat lozenges for sore throat, if needed.
- Resume medications as taken prior to the test.
- Report abnormal findings to the primary care provider.

E

CONTRAINDICATIONS!

- Patients who are unable to cooperate due to age, mental status, pain, or other factors
- Patients with unstable vital signs

Esophagogastroduodenoscopy (EGD, Gastroscopy, Upper Gastrointestinal Endoscopy)

Test Description
Esophagogastroduodenoscopy (EGD) is the direct visualization of the esophagus, stomach, and upper duodenum through the use of a flexible fiberoptic endoscope. This endoscope is a multilumen instrument which allows viewing of the organ linings, insufflation of air, aspiration of fluid, removal of foreign objects, obtaining of tissue biopsies, and passage of a laser beam for obliteration of abnormal tissue or control of bleeding.

THE EVIDENCE FOR PRACTICE
Barrett's esophagus may be present in up to 5% of high-risk patients with gastroesophageal reflux disease (e.g., older white men) undergoing upper endoscopy. The risk of progression to dysplasia or cancer may be related to the length of Barrett's epithelium. Therefore, it is important to characterize and document the length and location of the salmon-colored mucosa during EGD.

Normal Values
Normal esophagus, stomach, and duodenum

Possible Meanings of Abnormal Values
Barrett's esophagus
Diverticula
Duodenitis
Esophageal hiatal hernia
Esophageal stenosis
Esophagitis
Gastritis

Mallory-Weiss syndrome
Pyloric stenosis
Tumors
Varices
Ulcers

Contributing Factors to Abnormal Values

- Retention of barium following an upper gastrointestinal series hinders successful completion of this test.

Interventions/Implications

Pretest

- Explain to the patient the purpose of the test. Provide any written teaching materials available on the subject. Inform the patient that a topical anesthetic will be used on the throat to minimize discomfort during scope insertion. Explain that pressure in the stomach may be experienced during movement of the endoscope and during insufflation with air or carbon dioxide.
- Obtain a signed informed consent.
- Fasting for 8 to 12 hours is required prior to the test.
- Dentures are removed.
- Resuscitation and suctioning equipment should be readily available.
- Administer preprocedure medications as ordered. An anticholinergic such as atropine may be used to decrease bronchial secretions. A medication such as midazolam may be used for sedation and relief of anxiety.

Procedure

- The patient is assisted into the left lateral decubitus position on the endoscopy table.
- Baseline vital signs are obtained. Periodic vital sign assessment is performed during the procedure.
- A maintenance IV infusion is initiated.
- A topical anesthetic is sprayed into the throat.
- The endoscope is inserted into the mouth and passed through the esophagus and stomach, and into the duodenum.
- The anatomy of the esophagus, stomach, and duodenum is inspected. Biopsy forceps may be used to remove a tissue specimen, or a cytology brush may be used to obtain cells from the surface of a lesion. Removal of foreign bodies is accomplished, if needed.
- Videotaping of the procedure is often done via a camera attached to the endoscope.
- Gloves are worn throughout the procedure.

Posttest

- Monitor vital signs every 15 minutes until stable.
- Oversedation of the patient may require administration of a narcotic antagonist, such as naloxone.
- Withhold fluids and food until the gag reflex returns (approximately 2 hours).
- Provide an emesis basis for the patient. Instruct the patient to spit out saliva rather than swallow it until the gag reflex returns.
- Inform the patient that a bloated feeling is normal.
- Report abnormal findings to the primary care provider.

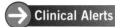

Clinical Alerts

- Possible complications: aspiration of gastric contents, bleeding, perforation, and oversedation.
- Observe the patient for indications of the following types of perforation: *esophageal perforation* (pain on swallowing and with neck movement), *thoracic perforation* (substernal or epigastric pain which increases with breathing or movement), *diaphragmatic perforation* (shoulder pain or dyspnea), and *gastric perforation* (abdominal or back pain, cyanosis, fever).

E

CONTRAINDICATIONS!

- Patients with large aortic aneurysm
- Patients with recent gastrointestinal surgery
- Patients with recent ulcer perforation
- Patients with Zenker's (esophageal) diverticulum
- Patients unable to cooperate with the exam

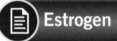

Estrogen

Test Description

Estrogen is present in the body in several forms, including estradiol, estriol, and estrone. Since estrogen is produced by the adrenal cortex, the ovaries, and testes, determination of estrogen levels can be used in evaluation of all three glands.

Estradiol is the most active of the estrogen forms, stimulating endometrial growth. It also suppresses the production of follicle-stimulating hormone (FSH) and stimulates production of luteinizing hormone (LH). Estradiol levels are used to evaluate ovarian function, and to diagnose the cause of precocious puberty in girls and gynecomastia in men. It is often used to determine whether amenorrhea is caused by menopause, pregnancy, or a medical problem. In patients with fertility problems, serial estradiol measurements are obtained prior to in vitro fertilization. Estradiol measurement can also be used to monitor effectiveness of hormone replacement therapy.

Estriol is monitored during pregnancy to assess fetal and placental function. Estriol, along with alpha-fetoprotein (AFP) and human chorionic gonadotropin (HCG), is measured as a part of the "triple marker" to assess the patient's risk of carrying a fetus with genetic abnormalities, such as Down syndrome.

Estrone is converted from androstenedione in adipose tissue. Its function is not clearly understood, but increased estrone levels, when unopposed by progesterone, have been associated with an increased risk of endometrial cancer. Estrone levels may be used to aid in the diagnosis of ovarian tumor, Turner's syndrome, hypopituitarism, gynecomastia (in men), and menopause.

Normal Values

Values variable with reference laboratory

Blood—Total Estrogen

Female: Premenopausal: 23–261 pg/mL (84–1325 pmol/L SI units)
Postmenopausal: <30 pg/mL (<110 pmol/L SI units)
Prepubertal: <20 pg/mL (<73 pmol/L SI units)

Male: <50 pg/mL (<184 pmol/L SI units)

Urine—Total Estrogen

Female: Premenopausal: 15–80 μg/24 hours (55–294 nmol/day SI units)
Postmenopausal: <20 μg/24 hours (<73 nmol/day SI units)

Male: 15–40 μg/24 hours (55–147 nmol/day SI units)

Possible Meanings of Abnormal Values

Increased	Decreased
Adrenal hyperplasia	Amenorrhea
Adrenal tumor	Anorexia nervosa
Cirrhosis	Extreme exercise
Estrogen-secreting ovarian tumor	Hypogonadism
Hepatic failure	Hypopituitarism
Klinefelter's syndrome	Menopause
Normal pregnancy	Ovarian failure
Precocious puberty	Stein-Leventhal syndrome
Renal failure	Turner's syndrome
Testicular tumor	

Contributing Factors to Abnormal Values

- Hemolysis of the blood sample may alter test results.
- Drugs which may *increase* estrogen levels: ampicillin, cascara, diethylstilbestrol, estrogens, hydrochlorothiazide, meprobamate, oral contraceptives, phenazopyridine, prochlorperazine, tetracycline.
- Drugs which may *decrease* estrogen levels: clomiphene, dexamethasone, estrogen blockers.

Interventions/Implications

Pretest
- Explain to the patient the purpose of the test and the need for a blood sample to be drawn and a 24-hour urine to be collected.
- No fasting is required before the test.
- If possible, withhold drugs which may alter test results.
- Explain 24-hour urine collection procedure to the patient.
- Stress the importance of saving *all* urine in the 24-hour period. Instruct the patient to avoid contaminating the urine with toilet paper or feces.
- Inform the patient of the presence of a preservative in the collection bottle.

Procedure
- A 7-mL blood sample is drawn in a red-top collection tube.
- Obtain the proper container containing boric acid as preservative from the laboratory.

- Begin the testing period in the morning after the patient's first voiding, which is discarded.
- Timing of the 24-hour period begins at the time the first voiding is discarded.
- *All* urine for the next 24 hours is collected in the container, which is to be kept refrigerated or on ice.
- If any urine is accidentally discarded during the 24-hour period, the test must be discontinued and a new test begun.
- The ending time of the 24-hour collection period should be posted in the patient's room.
- Gloves are worn whenever dealing with the specimen collection.

E

Posttest
- Apply pressure at venipuncture site. Apply dressing, periodically assessing for continued bleeding.
- Label the blood specimen and transport it to the laboratory.
- At the end of the 24-hour collection period, label and send the urine container on ice to the laboratory as soon as possible.
- Resume medications as taken prior to the test.
- Report abnormal findings to the primary care provider.

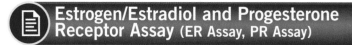

Estrogen/Estradiol and Progesterone Receptor Assay (ER Assay, PR Assay)

Test Description
Early and accurate diagnosis of breast cancer is important for optimizing treatment. Treatment of early breast cancer is less resource-intensive and generally has better outcomes. Estradiol, which is produced primarily by the ovaries, and progesterone, which is produced by the corpus luteum of the ovary, may both create a hormonal environment suitable for growth of some types of breast cancer. In this test, estrogen/estradiol receptors (ER) and progesterone receptors (PR) in the cells of a sample of breast cancer tissue are measured to decide whether the tumor is likely to respond to treatments aimed at reducing the levels of the hormone. Approximately one-half of the tumors found to be ER-positive will respond to endocrine therapy, whereas ER-negative tumors rarely respond to such therapy.

THE EVIDENCE FOR PRACTICE
In the limited-resource setting, assessment of the expression of estrogen receptors, progesterone receptors, or both is recommended only if hormonal therapy such as tamoxifen, aromatase inhibitors, or surgical or medical ovarian ablation is possible.

Normal Values
Estradiol: Negative; <3 fmol/mg of protein
Progesterone: Negative; <5 fmol/mg of protein

Possible Meanings of Abnormal Values
ER-positive and PR-positive: Cancer likely to respond to antihormone treatments

ER-negative and PR-positive: May benefit from antihormone therapy, but may have diminished response

ER-negative and PR-negative: Probably no benefit from antihormone therapy

Contributing Factors to Abnormal Values

- Antiestrogen drugs taken within the 2 months prior to the test may cause a *negative* estradiol receptor.

E

Interventions/Implications

Pretest

- Explain to the patient the purpose of the test and the sampling procedure.
- No fasting is required prior to the test.

Procedure

- The skin is cleansed with an antiseptic and draped.
- A local anesthetic is usually administered.
- At least 1 g of breast tissue is removed via excision or needle biopsy.
- Gloves are worn throughout the procedure.

Posttest

- The tissue sample is labeled and taken immediately to the laboratory to be frozen. If the sample is not frozen within 20 minutes, falsely low results will occur.
- At the conclusion of the procedure apply a dressing to the site, periodically assessing for continued bleeding.
- Administer pain medication as needed.
- Report abnormal findings to the primary care provider.

CONTRAINDICATIONS!

- Patients who have bleeding problems
- Patients who are unable to cooperate during the procedure

Ethanol (Blood Alcohol, ETOH, Ethyl Alcohol)

Test Description

Ethanol is the type of alcohol found in alcoholic beverages. It is considered a CNS depressant. This depression can result in coma and death when blood levels reach 300 mg/dL or more. Testing for blood alcohol levels is usually done as part of a legal investigation regarding impaired driving. Each state establishes its own limit for what is considered intoxication. Because of its role as legal evidence, the blood sample must be handled very carefully. The specimen is transported in a sealed plastic bag and must be signed by each person handling the specimen.

Normal Values

0 mg/dL (0 mmol/L SI units)

Possible Meanings of Abnormal Values

Increased
Alcohol ingestion

Contributing Factors to Abnormal Values
- Blood alcohol levels may be *increased* when taken concomitantly with drugs such as antihistamines, barbiturates, chlordiazepoxide, diazepam, isoniazid, meprobamate, opiates, phenytoin, and tranquilizers.

Interventions/Implications
Pretest
- Explain to the patient the purpose of the test and the need for a blood sample to be drawn.
- No fasting is required before the test.

Procedure
- If test is to be used as legal evidence, have specimen collection witnessed.
- Cleanse the venipuncture site with povidone-iodine solution instead of alcohol.
- A 5-mL blood sample is drawn in a collection containing no additives.
- *Do not* use alcohol to clean the top of the collection tube.
- Follow institutional policy regarding handling of legal evidence.
- Gloves are worn throughout the procedure.

Posttest
- Apply pressure at venipuncture site. Apply dressing, periodically assessing for continued bleeding.
- Label the specimen and transport it in a sealed plastic bag to the laboratory. The bag must be signed by each person handling the specimen.
- Report abnormal findings to the primary care provider.

  Clinical Alerts

- Other tests such as complete blood count, glucose, and electrolytes are often ordered along with ethanol since other conditions can cause symptoms similar to that of alcohol intoxication.

Euglobulin Lysis Time (Euglobulin Clot Lysis, Fibrinolysis)

Test Description
This test is used to evaluate systemic fibrinolysis, to monitor thrombolytic therapy in patients with acute myocardial infarction, and to differentiate between primary fibrinolysis and disseminated intravascular coagulation (DIC) so that correct pharmacologic therapy may be instituted.

During hemostasis, thrombin stimulates the formation of fibrin from fibrinogen. This fibrin, with the addition of fibrin stabilizing factor, forms a stable fibrin clot at the site of injury. Once the fibrin clot is no longer needed, it is dissolved by fibrinolytic agents such as plasmin, resulting in fibrin degradation products.

When the body's fibrinolytic system becomes overactive, any fibrin clot is dissolved as soon as it is formed, resulting in a bleeding disorder. This situation occurs with primary fibrinolysis caused by such things as cancer of the prostate, shock, and administration of thrombolytic agents such as urokinase.

Normal Values

No lysis of plasma clot for at least 2 hours

Possible Meanings of Abnormal Values

Increased fibrinolysis	*Decreased fibrinolysis*
(Shortened lysis time)	*(Longer lysis time)*
Acute trauma	Diabetes
Amniotic embolism	Prematurity
Antepartum hemorrhage	
Cirrhosis	
Disseminated intravascular coagulation	
Extracorporeal circulation	
Fetal death	
Hypoxia	
Incompatible blood transfusion	
Leukemia	
Pancreas cancer	
Pathologic fibrinolysis	
Postoperative period	
Prostate cancer	
Shock	
Thrombocytopenic purpura	

Contributing Factors to Abnormal Values

- *Increased* fibrinolysis may occur with exercise, hyperventilation, and increasing age.
- *Decreased* fibrinolysis may occur in newborns, obesity, postmenopausal women.
- Drugs which may *shorten* the lysis time (rapid fibrinolysis): asparaginase, clofibrate, corticotropin, dextran, steroids, thrombolytics (such as urokinase).

Interventions/Implications

Pretest
- Explain to the patient the purpose of the test and the need for a blood sample to be drawn.
- No fasting is required before the test.

Procedure
- A 7-mL blood sample is drawn in a blue-top collection tube.
- Gloves are worn throughout the procedure.

Posttest
- Apply pressure 3 to 5 minutes at venipuncture site. Apply dressing, periodically assessing for continued bleeding.
- Teach the patient to monitor the site. If the site begins to bleed, the patient should apply direct pressure and, if unable to control the bleeding, return to the lab or notify the primary care provider.
- Label the specimen, place it immediately in ice and transport it to the laboratory.
- Report abnormal findings to the primary care provider.

E

→ Clinical Alerts

- Possible complication: Hematoma at site due to prolonged bleeding time.

Evoked Potential Studies (EP Studies, Evoked Responses, Brainstem Auditory Evoked Potentials, Somatosensory Evoked Potentials, Visual Evoked Potentials)

Test Description
Evoked potentials are the electrical signals generated by the nervous system in response to sensory stimuli. Evoked potential studies measure the brain's electrical responses (evoked potentials, or responses) to stimulation of the sense organs or peripheral nerves. This aids in the diagnosis of lesions of the nervous system by evaluating the integrity of the visual, somatosensory, and auditory nerve pathways.

Somatosensory evoked potentials (SSEPs) are used to assess patients with possible spinal cord lesions, stroke, and peripheral nerve disease, as suggested by patient complaints of numbness and weakness of the extremities. *Visual evoked potentials* (VEPs) are useful in the diagnosis of lesions involving the optic nerves and optic tracts, demyelinating diseases such as multiple sclerosis, and traumatic injury. *Brainstem auditory evoked potentials* (BAEPs) are used to assess for lesions in the brain stem which involve the auditory pathway and may help uncover causes of hearing and balance problems. BAEPs can also be used to screen hearing in newborns.

Normal Values
No neural conduction delay

Possible Meanings of Abnormal Values

Abnormal SSEPs
Adrenoleukodystrophy
Cerebrovascular accident (CVA)

Cervical spondylosis
Guillain-Barre syndrome
Huntington's chorea
Intracerebral lesions
Multiple sclerosis
Parkinson's disease
Sensorimotor neuropathy
Spinal cord lesion
Spinal cord injury
Transverse myelitis

Abnormal VEPs
Amblyopia
CVA
Multiple sclerosis
Optic chiasm lesion
Optic neuritis
Optic nerve lesion
Retinopathy

Abnormal BAEPs
Acoustic neuroma
Brainstem lesion
Cochlear lesions
CVA
Hearing loss
Multiple sclerosis
Retrocochlear lesions

Contributing Factors to Abnormal Values

- Improper placement of electrodes can alter test results.
- Inability of the patient to follow directions during the test will alter test results.
- BAEPs may be affected by existing hearing loss.

Interventions/Implications

Pretest
- Explain to the patient the purpose of the test and the procedure to be done. Explain that there is no discomfort involved with this test.
- No fasting is required prior to the test. The patient should avoid caffeine use prior to the testing.
- Instruct the patient to shampoo the hair the night before the test to aid in securing the electrodes during the test.
- Have the patient remove all jewelry prior to the test.

Procedure

For somatosensory evoked potentials (SSEPs)
- The patient is placed in a comfortable position in either a lounge chair or on a bed.
- Stimulating electrodes are applied over the peripheral nerves on the wrist, knee, and ankle.
- Recording electrodes are placed on the scalp over the sensory cortex of the hemisphere opposite the limb to be stimulated.

- Other stimulating electrodes may be placed over the second cervical vertebra and the lower lumbar vertebrae.
- A painless electrical shock stimulus is delivered to the peripheral nerve through the stimulating electrode. The stimulus is enough to elicit a minor muscle response, such as a thumb twitch.
- The rate at which the electric shock stimulus is delivered to the nerve electrodes and travels to the brain is measured and documented as waveforms which can then be analyzed.

For visual evoked potentials (VEPs)

E

- The patient is placed in a comfortable position in either a lounge chair or on a bed, 1 meter from the pattern-shift stimulator.
- Electrodes are attached to the occipital, parietal, and vertex lobe areas.
- A reference electrode is attached to the ear.
- One eye is covered, and the patient is instructed to fix the gaze on a dot in the center of the screen.
- A checkerboard pattern is projected and rapidly reversed.
- The computer interprets the brain's responses to the stimuli and records them in waveforms which can then be analyzed.
- The process is repeated with the other eye covered.

For brainstem auditory evoked potentials (BAEPs)

- The patient is placed in a comfortable position in either a lounge chair or on a bed.
- Electrodes are positioned on the scalp at the vertex lobe area and on each earlobe.
- Earphones are placed in the patient's ears.
- A clicking noise stimulus is delivered into one ear while a continuous tone is delivered to the opposite ear.
- The responses to the stimuli are recorded as waveforms which can then be analyzed.

Posttest

- Following removal of the electrodes, the electrode paste is removed. Oil, acetone, or witch hazel may help remove the paste, then the hair should be shampooed.
- Report abnormal findings to the primary care provider.

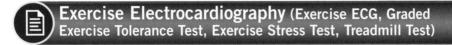

Exercise Electrocardiography (Exercise ECG, Graded Exercise Tolerance Test, Exercise Stress Test, Treadmill Test)

Test Description

Exercise electrocardiography (stress testing) measures the efficiency of the heart during physical stress. Whereas a patient may have a normal resting electrocardiogram (ECG), the same patient may have an abnormal exercise ECG. This is due to the reaction of the heart to increased demand for oxygen. To simulate patient exercise in a controlled environment, the patient walks on a treadmill or pedals a stationary bicycle while the ECG and blood pressure are monitored. The test continues until either the patient reaches the target heart rate or experiences chest pain or fatigue.

Any physical limitation that prevents a patient from exercising maximally is an indication for pharmacologic stress testing. This includes those patients with arthritis, amputation, severe peripheral vascular disease, severe chronic obstructive pulmonary disease (COPD), and debilitation. Patients taking beta blockers or other negative chronotropic agents that would not allow an adequate heart rate response to exercise, patients with left bundle branch block, and those with ventricular pacemaker are also candidates for pharmacologic stress testing.

Medications used to pharmacologically "stress" the heart include the vasodilators adenosine and dipyridamole and the catecholamine dobutamine hydrochloride. *Adenosine* is a direct coronary vasodilator. When used in this test, healthy and less-diseased coronary arteries will be able to dilate, whereas diseased coronary arteries with reduced coronary flow reserve cannot dilate further in response to the medication. *Dipyridamole* (Persantine) is an indirect coronary vasodilator that works by increasing intravascular adenosine levels. The increase in coronary blood flow induced by dipyridamole is less predictable than that of adenosine. *Dobutamine* is a synthetic catecholamine, which directly stimulates both $beta_1$ and $beta_2$ receptors, increasing heart rate, blood pressure, and myocardial contractility. Dobutamine may be used in patients who have a contraindication to vasodilator stress.

At times, an *exercise or stress echocardiogram* may be included in the stress test. This involves performance of an echocardiogram prior to the exercise stress test and again immediately following the test to view the functioning of the heart while still under the effects of exercise stress.

Exercise stress testing is often done in conjunction with myocardial perfusion imaging. See Cardiac Nuclear Scan section for discussion on this procedure.

Normal Values

Negative: No symptoms or ECG abnormalities upon attaining 85% of the maximum heart rate for the patient's age and sex

Possible Meanings of Abnormal Values

Coronary artery occlusive disease
Exercise-related hypertension
Intermittent claudication
Myocardial ischemia

Contributing Factors to Abnormal Values

- False-positive test results may occur with anemia, electrolyte imbalance, hypertension, hypoxia, left bundle branch block, left ventricular hypertrophy, valvular heart disease, Wolff-Parkinson-White syndrome.
- Drugs which may affect test results include beta blockers, calcium channel blockers, digoxin, nitroglycerin.

Interventions/Implications

Pretest
- Explain to the patient the purpose of the test and the need for electrodes to be attached to the chest. Note that the patient may become fatigued during the test and that he or she may ask for the test to be discontinued if fatigue or chest pain is experienced.
- Advise the patient to dress comfortably for the test.
- IV access is established for emergency use, if needed.
- Baseline 12-lead ECG results should be obtained if not already available.

- Obtain a signed informed consent.
- Fasting for 6 hours is required prior to the test.
- Smoking should be avoided for 6 hours prior to the test.
- Patients should refrain from ingesting caffeine for at least 24 hours prior to adenosine administration. Only caffeine-free products may be used.
- Patients should not take any medication for erectile dysfunction for 48 hours prior to the stress test due to the possibility of receiving nitroglycerin for chest pain during the test.

E

Procedure
- The skin is cleansed with alcohol and abraded with a special cream. Chest electrodes are applied and the lead wires stabilized.
- A baseline ECG tracing and blood pressure is obtained.

For the treadmill test
- The patient is assisted to step onto the treadmill.
- Ensure patient safety through use of support railings to maintain balance.
- The treadmill is turned on to slow speed at first, and increased in miles per hour and grade elevation of the treadmill.
- Absolute indications for termination of exercise testing include:
  - Drop in systolic blood pressure (SBP) of >10 mm Hg from baseline despite an increase in workload, when accompanied by other evidence of ischemia
  - Moderate-to-severe angina
  - Increasing nervous system symptoms (ataxia, dizziness, near-syncope)
  - Signs of poor perfusion (cyanosis, pallor)
  - Technical difficulties in monitoring ECG or BP
  - Patient's desire to stop
  - Sustained ventricular tachycardia
  - ST elevation (≥1mm) in leads without diagnostic Q waves
- Relative indications for terminating the test include:
  - Drop in SBP of ≥10 mm Hg from baseline without other evidence of ischemia
  - ST or QRS changes such as excessive ST depression
  - Dysrhythmias other than sustained ventricular tachycardia
  - Fatigue, shortness of breath, wheezing, leg cramps, or claudication
  - Development of bundle branch block or intraventricular conduction delay
  - Increasing chest pain
  - Hypertensive response (SBP of 250 mm Hg and/or diastolic BP of >115 mm Hg)

For the bicycle test
- The patient pedals until reaching the desired speed.
- See above for indications for terminating this test.

For pharmacologic stress test
- Patient is supine on examination table.
- IV access is established.
- Medication such as adenosine, dipyridamole, or dobutamine is administered, usually by infusion pump.
- Adenosine infusion should be terminated in the presence of severe hypotension, heart block, bronchospasm, or severe chest pain associated with ECG changes.
- Adenosine or dipyridamole-induced bronchospasm may be reversed with aminophylline.
- Reversal of dobutamine effects may be accomplished with use of beta blockers.

For all stress tests

- Throughout the testing, the ECG is monitored for changes. Blood pressure is also checked at preestablished intervals.

Posttest

- Instruct the patient to continue walking as the treadmill speed slows.
- Monitor blood pressure and ECG for at least 15 minutes after the test is completed and the patient is resting.
- Remove the electrodes and cleanse the skin of any residual gel or adhesive.
- Report abnormal findings to the primary care provider.

CONTRAINDICATIONS!

- Patients with active unstable angina
- Patients with acute myocardial infarction
- Patients with severe anemia, congestive heart failure or coronary insufficiency
- Patients with cardiac inflammation (myocarditis, pericarditis)
- Patients with uncontrolled dysrhythmias
- Patients with aortic dissection
- Patients with critical left ventricular outflow-tract obstruction
- Patients with critical aortic stenosis
- Patients with recent or active cerebral ischemia
- Patients with severe uncontrolled hypertension
- Contraindications to adenosine or dipyridamole use:
  - Patients with active bronchospasm or patients being treated for reactive airway disease
  - Patients with more than first-degree heart block (without a ventricular-demand pacemaker)
  - Patients with an SBP less than 90 mm Hg
  - Patients using dipyridamole or methylxanthines (e.g., caffeine and amino-phylline) should not undergo an adenosine stress test because these substances act as competitive inhibitors of adenosine at the receptor level, potentially decreasing or completely attenuating the vasodilatory effect of adenosine.
- Contraindications to dobutamine use:
  - Patients with recent (1 week) myocardial infarction; unstable angina; significant aortic stenosis or obstructive cardiomyopathy; atrial tachyarrhythmias with uncontrolled ventricular response; history of ventricular tachycardia, uncontrolled hypertension, or thoracic aortic aneurysm; or left bundle branch block.

Fecal Fat

Test Description

Normal absorption of fat (lipids) requires bile from the gallbladder or liver, pancreatic enzymes, and normal intestines. When a patient ingests a normal diet, the amount of fat excreted in the stool should account for no more than 20% of the total solids. A variety of fats, or lipids, are excreted in feces. They are composed of cells sloughed by the intestines, unabsorbed dietary lipids, and secretions from the gastrointestinal (GI) tract. In normal conditions, in which there are adequate biliary and pancreatic secretions, most dietary lipids are absorbed in the small intestine.

However, if malabsorption occurs, the fecal fat is excreted in the stool. This is known as **steatorrhea**, which occurs in such conditions as Crohn's disease, cystic fibrosis, and Whipple's disease.

F

Normal Values

1–7 g/day (3.5–25 mmol/day SI units)

Possible Meanings of Abnormal Values

Amyloidosis
Celiac disease/sprue
Crohn's disease
Cystic fibrosis
Diarrhea
Diverticulosis
Enteritis
Hepatobiliary disease
Lymphoma
Pancreatic disease
Post-bowel resection
Whipple's disease

Contributing Factors to Abnormal Values

- Test results may be altered by intake of barium, bismuth, castor oil, high fiber diet, mineral oil, psyllium or use of rectal suppositories.

Interventions/Implications

Pretest
- Explain to the patient the purpose of the test and the need for collection of stool.
- Instruct the patient to ingest a high-fat diet (approximately 100 g/day) for 3 days prior to the test and throughout the 3-day test period.
- Instruct the patient to collect every stool during the 3-day period so that all stools are sent to the laboratory.
- Instruct the patient to avoid contaminating the stool with urine or toilet paper. Use of a plastic collection container in the toilet will facilitate this.
- Withhold the use of castor oil or mineral oil during the entire 6-day pretest and testing period.

Procedure
- Each stool collected during the 72-hour period is either sent to the laboratory immediately, or all stools are collected in a large container kept in the freezer.
- Gloves are worn during any collection of the stool.

Posttest
- Label the specimen and transport it to the laboratory.
- Resume diet and medications as taken prior to the test.
- Report abnormal findings to the primary care provider.

 Ferritin

F

Test Description

Ferritin is the primary protein in the body which stores iron. Thus, measurement of the ferritin level provides a good indication of the size of the body's available iron stores. The ferritin level decreases before symptoms of anemia occur. For example, in Stage 1 of iron deficiency anemia, ferritin, and hemosiderin stores are depleted. In Stage 2, serum iron decreases and the total iron binding capacity increases. It is not until Stage 3, that the hemoglobin level is decreased and the iron deficiency affects heme synthesis. Assessment of the ferritin level, in conjunction with determination of the iron level and total iron-binding capacity, is used in the differential diagnosis of the various types of anemia.

THE EVIDENCE FOR PRACTICE

In the United States, race, income, education, and other socioeconomic factors are associated with iron deficiency and iron deficiency anemia. Individuals considered to be at high risk for iron deficiency include adult females, recent immigrants and, among adolescent females, fad dieters, and those who are obese. Premature and low birth weight infants are also at increased risk for iron deficiency. Measurement of ferritin can be used for screening in these individuals as it has the highest sensitivity and specificity for diagnosing iron deficiency in anemic patients.

Normal Values

Male	12–300 ng/mL (12–300 µg/L SI units)
Female	12–150 ng/mL (12–150 µg/L SI units)
Child >5 months	7–140 ng/mL (7–140 µg/L SI units)
2–5 months	50–200 ng/mL (50–200 µg/L SI units)
1 month	200–600 ng/mL (200–600 µg/L SI units)
Newborn	25–200 ng/mL (25–200 µg/L SI units)

Possible Meanings of Abnormal Values

Increased	Decreased
Acute hepatitis	Gastrointestinal surgery
Acute myocardial infarction	Hemodialysis
Anemia other than iron deficiency	Inflammatory bowel disease
Chronic inflammatory disease	Iron deficiency anemia
Chronic renal disease	Malnutrition
Cirrhosis of the liver	Menstruation
Hemochromatosis	Pregnancy
Hemosiderosis	
Hodgkin's disease	

Hyperthyroidism
Infection
Leukemia
Malignancy
Polycythemia
Rheumatoid arthritis
Thalassemia

Contributing Factors to Abnormal Values

- Falsely increased levels of ferritin may occur with:
  - intake of iron supplements and meals with a high iron content
  - after blood transfusions
  - after receipt of radiopharmaceuticals used for nuclear scans

Interventions/Implications

Pretest
- Explain to the patient the purpose of the test and the need for a blood sample to be drawn.
- No fasting is required before the test.

Procedure
- A 7-mL blood sample is drawn in a red-top collection tube.
- Gloves are worn throughout the procedure.

Posttest
- Apply pressure at venipuncture site. Apply dressing, periodically assessing for continued bleeding.
- Label the specimen and transport it to the laboratory.
- Report abnormal findings to the primary care provider.

→ Clinical Alerts

- Treatment for iron deficiency anemia with ferrous sulfate continues for 3 to 6 months beyond the point where the hemoglobin returns to normal. This allows for replenishment of the ferritin stores.
- Intake of vitamin C potentiates iron absorption.

Fetal Hemoglobin (Hemoglobin F [Hb F])

Test Description
Fetal hemoglobin, also known as Hemoglobin F (HbF), is normally found in a very small quantity in the adult. Increased Hb F in an adult may be due to sickle cell anemia, leukemia, thalassemia, or hereditary persistence of fetal hemoglobin. In the fetus, it is the primary form of hemoglobin found and is responsible for transporting oxygen

when there is little oxygen available. Usually the manufacture of Hb F decreases during the first year of life and is replaced by adult Hb A$_1$ and A$_2$.

Normal Values of Hemoglobin F

Age: 0–10 Days:	56–87%
Age: 11–20 Days:	55–83%
Age: 21–30 Days:	51–76%
Age: 31–40 Days:	46–70%
Age: 41–50 Days:	38–62%
Age: 51–60 Days:	31–54%
Age: 61–70 Days:	24–44%
Age: 71–80 Days:	17–34%
Age: 81–90 Days:	12–28%
Age: 91–100 Days:	8–24%
Age: 101–110 Days:	7–18%
Age: 111–120 Days:	5–15%
Age: 121–130 Days:	4–10%
Age: 131–140 Days:	<6.1%
Age: 141–364 Days:	<4.1%
1 year and above:	<2.1%

Possible Meanings of Abnormal Values

Increased
Hereditary persistence of fetal hemoglobin
Hyperthyroidism
Leakage of fetal blood into maternal circulation
Leukemia
Sickle cell anemia
Thalassemia major (Hb F 20–90%)
Thalassemia minor (Hb F 2–8%)

Interventions/Implications

Pretest
- Explain to the patient the purpose of the test and the need for a blood sample to be drawn.
- No fasting is required before the test.

Procedure
- A 7-mL blood sample is drawn in a lavender-top (EDTA) collection tube.
- Gloves are worn throughout the procedure.

Posttest
- Apply pressure at venipuncture site. Apply dressing, periodically assessing for continued bleeding.
- Invert and gently mix the sample and the anticoagulant.
- Label the specimen and transport it to the laboratory.
- Report abnormal findings to the primary care provider.

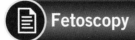
Fetoscopy

Test Description
Fetoscopy is an endoscopic procedure which allows direct visualization of the fetus. The procedure can be done for diagnostic and/or therapeutic reasons. Fetoscopy is done to evaluate the fetus for birth defects and to collect fetal blood and tissue (skin) samples. Fetoscopy can also be done for therapeutic purposes such as laser occlusion of abnormal vessels. Because the procedure involves inserting the fetoscope through the abdominal wall into the amniotic cavity, there are serious risks, including miscarriage, bleeding, and preterm labor. Because of these risks, fetoscopy is done only if there is a high probability that the fetus is not normal or there is a strong family history of birth defects. Typically other testing such as fetal ultrasound, amniocentesis, or chorionic villus sampling are the preferred testing methods whenever possible.

F

Normal Values
No birth defects or other problems detected

Possible Meanings of Abnormal Values
Birth defects such as spina bifida
Blood dyscrasias such as hemophilia, sickle cell anemia
Hereditary skin diseases

Interventions/Implications
Pretest
- Explain to the patient the purpose of the procedure. Provide any written teaching materials available on the subject. Note that discomfort involved with this procedure is due to numbing of the skin before the incision is made, and pain/pressure when the fetoscope is in the uterus.
- The patient must remain still during the procedure.
- Fasting for 8 hours is required before the procedure.
- Obtain a signed informed consent.
- Prophylactic antibiotics may be given to prevent infection.
- The fetal heart rate will be monitored.
- Often a medication such as meperidine is given to calm the fetus and decrease the woman's discomfort during the procedure.

Procedure
- The patient is assisted to a supine position on the examination table. The head of the table may be raised slightly.
- Fetal ultrasound is done to identify fetal and placental location.
- The abdominal area is cleansed and local anesthesia is administered to the area where the incision will be made.
- A small incision is made and the fetoscope is advanced into the uterus.
- Careful viewing of the fetus is done to note any physical defects. Blood and tissue sampling is done.

- The fetoscope is removed, the incision is sutured, and a dressing is applied.
- Sterile technique is maintained throughout the procedure.

Posttest

- Fetal ultrasound may be done to assess the status of the fetus and amniotic fluid level.
- The patient's vital signs are monitored and the patient is assessed for vaginal and incisional drainage.
- The patient is to avoid strenuous activity for 2 weeks after the procedure.

F

→ Clinical Alerts

- Possible complications include: hemorrhage, infection, leakage of amniotic fluid, miscarriage, preterm labor, and Rh sensitization.
- Instruct the patient to notify the obstetrician immediately for vaginal bleeding, fluid leaking from the vagina or abdominal incision, abdominal pain or cramping, fever or chills, or dizziness.
- Rh-negative women are given RhoGAM to prevent Rh sensitization (unless the fetus is known to be Rh-negative).

CONTRAINDICATIONS!

- Patients who are obese
- Very active fetus
- Patients who are unable to cooperate because of age, mental status, pain, or other factors

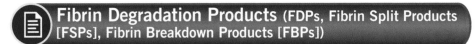

Fibrin Degradation Products (FDPs, Fibrin Split Products [FSPs], Fibrin Breakdown Products [FBPs])

Test Description

During hemostasis, fibrin, with the addition of fibrin stabilizing factor, forms a stable fibrin clot at the site of injury. Once the fibrin clot is no longer needed, it is dissolved by fibrinolytic agents such as plasmin, resulting in fibrin degradation products (FDPs). Their presence in the blood is indicative of recent clotting activity. FDPs have an anticoagulant effect and inhibit clotting.

Measurement of FDPs provides information regarding the activity of the clot-dissolving system. When high levels of FDPs are present, they indicate increased fibrinolysis, as seen in disseminated intravascular coagulation (DIC). This test is used in the diagnosis of DIC and acute occlusive vascular disease.

Normal Values

<10 µg/mL (<100 mg/L SI units)
(Note: FDP levels >40 µg/mL are highly suggestive of DIC)

Possible Meanings of Abnormal Values

Increased

Abruptio placentae
Acute leukemia
Autologous transfusions
Burns
Congenital heart disease
Disseminated intravascular coagulation
Heat stroke
Hypoxia
Infection
Intrauterine fetal death
Late pregnancy
Liver disease
Malignancy
Myocardial infarction
Portacaval shunt
Preeclampsia
Pulmonary embolism
Renal disease
Septicemia
Shock
Status post-cardiopulmonary surgery
Transfusion reaction
Transplant rejection
Venous thrombosis

Contributing Factors to Abnormal Values

- Hemolysis of the blood sample may alter test results.
- Drugs which may *increase* FDP levels: barbiturates, heparin, streptokinase, urokinase.

Interventions/Implications

Pretest
- Explain to the patient the purpose of the test and the need for a blood sample to be drawn.
- No fasting is required before the test.
- The blood sample is to be drawn prior to the initiation of heparin therapy.

Procedure
- A 7-mL blood sample is drawn into a light blue-top collection tube.
- Gloves are worn throughout the procedure.

Posttest
- Apply pressure 3 to 5 minutes at venipuncture site. Apply dressing, periodically assessing for continued bleeding.
- Teach the patient to monitor the site. If the site begins to bleed, the patient should apply direct pressure and, if unable to control the bleeding, return to the laboratory or notify the primary care provider.
- Label the specimen, place it on ice and transport it to the laboratory immediately.
- Report abnormal findings to the primary care provider.

→ **Clinical Alerts**

- Possible complication: Hematoma at site due to prolonged bleeding time

F

 Fibrinogen (Factor I)

Test Description
Fibrinogen is a polypeptide which is synthesized in the liver. During hemostasis, thrombin stimulates the formation of fibrin from fibrinogen. This fibrin, with the addition of fibrin stabilizing factor (Factor XIII), forms a stable fibrin clot at the site of injury.

Measurement of fibrinogen levels is used when investigating suspected bleeding disorders, especially when other tests of coagulation, such as prothrombin time (PT), activated partial thromboplastin time (APTT), fibrin degradation products, and D-dimer are abnormal. It can also be used to help monitor the status of progressive liver disease.

THE EVIDENCE FOR PRACTICE
Current research is investigating the significance of elevated fibrinogen levels. They may slightly to moderately increase a person's risk of developing a blood clot and over time could contribute to an increased risk for developing cardiovascular disease. Although unable to be treated, elevated fibrinogen levels may suggest the need to aggressively treat modifiable cardiac risk factors.

Normal Values
200–400 mg/dL (2.0–4.0 g/L SI units)

Possible Meanings of Abnormal Values

Increased	Decreased
Acute infection	Abortion
Burns	Abruptio placenta
Cancer (breast, kidney, stomach)	Advanced cancer
CVA	Amniotic fluid embolism
Glomerulonephritis	Anemia
Heart disease	Cirrhosis
Hepatitis	Disseminated intravascular coagulation
Inflammation	Dysfibrinogenemia
Late pregnancy	Eclampsia
Menstruation	Fat embolism
Multiple myeloma	Fibrinolysis
Myocardial infarction	Hemophilia A and B
Nephrosis	Hereditary afibrinogenemia
Pneumonia	Leukemia

Postoperative period	Liver disease
Rheumatic fever	Malnutrition
Rheumatoid arthritis	Meconium embolism
Tissue damage/injury	Septicemia
Tuberculosis	Shock
Uremia	Transfusion reaction

Contributing Factors to Abnormal Values

- Fibrinogen test results may be altered due to hemolysis of the blood sample or if the patient has received a blood transfusion within one month prior to the test.
- Drugs which may *increase* fibrinogen levels: estrogens, oral contraceptives.
- Drugs which may *decrease* fibrinogen levels: atenolol, cholesterol lowering agents, corticosteroids, estrogens, fluorouracil, progestins, thrombolytics, ticlodipine, valproic acid.

Interventions/Implications

Pretest
- Explain to the patient the purpose of the test and the need for a blood sample to be drawn.
- No fasting is required before the test.

Procedure
- A 7-mL blood sample is drawn in a light blue-top collection tube.
- Gloves are worn throughout the procedure.

Posttest
- Apply pressure 3 to 5 minutes at venipuncture site. Apply dressing, periodically assessing for continued bleeding.
- Teach the patient to monitor the site. If the site begins to bleed, the patient should apply direct pressure and, if unable to control the bleeding, return to the laboratory or notify the primary care provider.
- Label the specimen and transport it to the laboratory immediately.
- Report abnormal findings to the primary care provider.

Clinical Alerts

- Possible complication: Hematoma at site due to prolonged bleeding time.

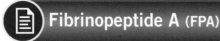

Fibrinopeptide A (FPA)

Test Description
During the process of hemostasis, intrinsic and extrinsic pathways lead to the activation of coagulation factor X. This leads to the conversion of prothrombin to thrombin. Thrombin then stimulates the formation of fibrin from fibrinogen. This fibrin, with the addition of fibrin stabilizing factor, forms a stable fibrin clot at the site of injury.

Fibrinopeptide A is a substance released as part of the clotting process. This test is used as a marker to determine the rate of conversion of fibrinogen to fibrin by thrombin. Abnormal clotting processes, such as DIC, lead to increased FPA levels.

Normal Values

0.6–1.9 ng/mL

F

Possible Meanings of Abnormal Values

Increased	Decreased
Cellulitis	Anticoagulation therapy
Disseminated intravascular coagulation	
Infection	
Leukemia	
Malignancies	
Myocardial infarction	
Pulmonary embolism	
Systemic lupus erythematosus	
Thrombosis	

Contributing Factors to Abnormal Values

- Drugs that cause *decreased* FPA levels: anticoagulants.

Interventions/Implications

Pretest
- Explain to the patient the purpose of the test and the need for a blood sample to be drawn.
- No fasting is required before the test.

Procedure
- A 7-mL blood sample is drawn in a blue-top collection tube.
- Gloves are worn throughout the procedure.

Posttest
- Apply pressure at venipuncture site. Apply dressing, periodically assessing for continued bleeding.
- Gently invert the blood collection tube.
- Label the specimen and transport it to the laboratory.
- Report abnormal findings to the primary care provider.

→ Clinical Alerts

- Possible complication: Hematoma at site due to prolonged bleeding time.
- Teach patient to monitor the site. If the site begins to bleed, the patient should apply direct pressure and, if unable to control the bleeding, return to the laboratory or notify the primary care provider.

FISH Test (Fluorescent In Situ Hybridization)

Test Description
Fluorescent in situ hybridization (FISH) is a laboratory technique that can be used to view changes in chromosomes. It can demonstrate several types of changes. If there is a gene segment which has *mutated*, the area can be made to fluoresce when it is bound by a special probe. If there is *microdeletion*, as occurs with the elastin gene on one of the two chromosomes of the seventh pair in individuals with Williams Syndrome, the area of deletion will not fluoresce. The test can also find *translocations* in which pieces of chromosomes break off and reattach to another chromosome. Malignancies such as chronic myelogenous leukemia (CML) and Burkitt's lymphoma are caused by translocations. FISH testing does not replace chromosome analysis, primarily due to its higher cost and limited availability. FISH testing is often done in addition to a standard chromosome study, depending on the condition suspected in the individual.

F

THE EVIDENCE FOR PRACTICE
When the standard karyotype is normal, a FISH study for subtelomere rearrangements is an important diagnostic component in the evaluation of the child with developmental delay/mental retardation (DD/MR).

Normal Values
Normal chromosomal composition and number

Possible Meanings of Abnormal Values

Examples of conditions tested for with FISH

Leukemias:
- Pediatric acute lymphoblastic leukemia (ALL) (12:21 translocation)
- Acute myeloid leukemia (8:21 translocation)
- Acute promyelocytic leukemia (APL) (15:17 translocation)
- B-cell chronic lymphocytic leukemia (B-CLL)
- Chronic myelogenous leukemia (9:22 translocation)

Microdeletion syndromes:
- Williams syndrome
- George syndrome
- Prader-Willi/Angelman syndrome
- Smith-Magenis syndrome
- Cri-Du-Chat syndrome
- Miller-Dieker syndrome

Interventions/Implications

Pretest
- Explain to the patient the purpose of the test. The type of condition to be tested for determines type of sample needed (blood, amniotic fluid, product of conception, bone marrow, chorionic villus sample, solid tissue, or tumor tissue).
- No fasting is required before the test.

Procedure
- For blood testing, a 7-mL blood sample is drawn in a green-top heparinized collection tube.
- Other test samples are obtained and processed per reference laboratory guidelines.
- Gloves are worn throughout the procedure.

Posttest
- Apply pressure at venipuncture site. Apply dressing, periodically assessing for continued bleeding.
- Label the specimen and transport it to the laboratory.
- Report abnormal findings to the primary care provider.

 Clinical Alerts

- Pre- and posttest counseling is recommended for discussion regarding test results and interpretation.

Folic Acid (Folate)

Test Description
Folic acid is a water-soluble vitamin formed by bacteria in the intestines and stored in the liver. It can also be found in such food sources as eggs, fruits, green leafy vegetables, liver, milk, orange juice, and yeast. This vitamin is necessary for normal functioning of red blood cells and white blood cells. It also plays a role in the metabolism of amino acids and nucleotides. An adequate folic acid level is essential for the pregnant woman to prevent neural tube defects in the developing fetus. Testing for folic acid is done in conjunction with testing for vitamin B_{12} in the diagnosis of macrocytic anemia. The body stores very little folic acid, so folic acid levels fall below normal 21 to 28 days after the beginning of the deficiency state.

THE EVIDENCE FOR PRACTICE
Periconceptional folic acid supplementation is recommended because it has been shown to reduce the occurrence and recurrence of neural tube defects (NTDs). For low-risk women, folic acid supplementation of 400 μg/day currently is recommended because nutritional sources alone are insufficient. Higher levels of supplementation should not be achieved by taking excess multivitamins because of the risk of vitamin A toxicity. For women at high risk of NTDs or who have had a previous pregnancy with an NTD, folic acid supplementation of 4 mg/day is recommended.

Normal Values
Normal: 2.7–17 ng/mL (6.1–38.5 nmol/L SI units)

Possible Meanings of Abnormal Values

Increased	Decreased
Blood transfusion	Alcoholism
Folic acid supplementation	Anorexia nervosa
Pernicious anemia	Cirrhosis
Vegetarianism	Diet (inadequate intake)
	Hemodialysis
	Hemolytic anemia
	Hyperthyroidism
	Inflammatory bowel disease
	Leukemia
	Macrocytic anemia due to pregnancy
	Malabsorption
	Megaloblastic anemia
	Neoplasia
	Pregnancy
	Sickle cell anemia
	Vitamin B_{12} deficiency

F

Contributing Factors to Abnormal Values

- Falsely increased results may occur due to hemolysis of sample.
- Falsely increased results may occur in patients with severe iron deficiency.
- Drugs which may *decrease* folic acid levels: alcohol, ampicillin, chloramphenicol, erythromycin, estrogens, methotrexate, oral contraceptives, penicillin, phenobarbital, phenytoin, tetracyclines, trimethoprim.
- Drugs which *increase* folic acid levels: folic acid.

Interventions/Implications

Pretest

- Explain to the patient the purpose of the test and the need for a blood sample to be drawn.
- Fasting is usually required for 8 hours prior to the test. Water intake is allowed. No alcohol is allowed prior to the test.

Procedure

- A 7-mL blood sample is drawn in a red-top collection tube.
- Gloves are worn throughout the procedure.

Posttest

- Apply pressure at venipuncture site. Apply dressing, periodically assessing for continued bleeding.
- Label the specimen and then protect it from light by inserting the tube into a paper bag.
- Transport the specimen to the laboratory as soon as possible.
- Report abnormal findings to the primary care provider.

→ Clinical Alerts

- Low folic acid levels can be the result of a primary vitamin B_{12} deficiency that decreases the ability of cells to take up folic acid.

Follicle-Stimulating Hormone (FSH)

Test Description

This test is used in the diagnosis of hypogonadism, infertility, menstrual disorders, precocious puberty, and menopause. Follicle-stimulating hormone (FSH) is secreted by the anterior pituitary gland. During the follicular phase of the menstrual cycle, FSH initiates the production of estradiol by the follicle, with the two hormones working together to further develop the ovarian (egg) follicle. A midcycle surge of FSH and luteinizing hormone (LH) is followed by ovulation. During the luteal phase, FSH stimulates the production of progesterone which, along with estradiol, facilitates ovarian response to LH. When menopause occurs, the ovaries stop functioning, resulting in increased FSH levels. In men, FSH stimulates the testes to produce mature sperm and also promotes the production of androgen binding proteins.

THE EVIDENCE FOR PRACTICE

In terms of infertility testing and management, elevated FSH levels on day 3 of the menstrual cycle have been correlated to poor performance with assisted reproductive technology.

- Day 3 FSH values >15 µIU/L probably reflect poor future reproductive potential.
- Day 3 FSH values <10 µIU/L represent normal follicular potential
- Values of 10–15 µIU/L probably represent an effect of aging on fertility.

Normal Values

Female:

Follicular phase	1.68–15 IU/L
Mid-cycle	21.9–56.6 IU/L
Luteal phase	0.61–16.3 IU/L
Postmenopausal	14.2–52.3 IU/L
Male	1.24–7.8 IU/L
Prepuberty	1.0–4.2 IU/L

Possible Meanings of Abnormal Values

Increased	Decreased
Acromegaly	Adrenal hyperplasia
Amenorrhea (primary)	Amenorrhea (secondary)
Anorchism	Anorexia nervosa
Castration	Delayed puberty
Gonadal failure	Hypogonadotropinism
Hyperpituitarism	Hypophysectomy
Hypogonadism	Hypothalamic dysfunction
Hypothalamic tumor	Neoplasm (adrenal, ovarian, testicular)
Hysterectomy	Prepubertal child
Klinefelter's syndrome	
Menopause	
Menstruation	
Orchiectomy	

Ovarian failure
Pituitary tumor
Precocious puberty
Stein-Leventhal syndrome
Testicular failure
Turner's syndrome

Contributing Factors to Abnormal Values

- Hemolysis of the blood sample or having a radioactive scan within 1 week of the test may alter test results.

- Drugs which may *decrease* FSH levels: chlorpromazine, estrogens, oral contraceptives, progesterone, testosterone.

Interventions/Implications

Pretest
- Explain to the patient the purpose of the test and the need for a blood sample to be drawn.
- No fasting is required before the test.
- If possible, withhold drugs which may alter test results for 48 hours prior to the test.

Procedure
- A 7-mL blood sample is drawn in a red-top collection tube.
- Gloves are worn throughout the procedure.

Posttest
- Apply pressure at venipuncture site. Apply dressing, periodically assessing for continued bleeding.
- Label the specimen and transport it to the laboratory.
- For female patients: on the laboratory slip, include the date on which the patient began her last menstrual period.
- Resume medications as taken prior to the test.
- Report abnormal findings to the primary care provider.

 Clinical Alerts

- FSH and LH are usually measured at the same time.

Free Erythrocyte Protoporphyrin (FEP)

Test Description
In the pathway of heme synthesis, erythrocyte protoporphyrin is used in the final step of heme synthesis. A vital component needed to continue the synthesis is iron. If iron is not present, the protoporphyrin cannot be synthesized into hemoglobin. This substance is then known as free erythrocyte protoporphyrin. This test measures free erythrocyte protoporphyrin (FEP) as a method of detecting iron deficiency anemia and to monitor chronic exposure to lead in adults.

Normal Values

<35 mcg/dL

Possible Meanings of Abnormal Values

Increased	Decreased
Anemia of chronic disease	Megaloblastic anemia
Hemolytic anemia	
Iron deficiency anemia	
Lead poisoning	
Thalassemia	

Contributing Factors to Abnormal Values

- Hemolysis of the blood sample may alter test results.

Interventions/Implications

Pretest
- Explain to the patient the purpose of the test and the need for a blood sample to be drawn.
- No fasting is required before the test.

Procedure
- A 5-mL blood sample is drawn in a lavender-top (EDTA) or green-top (heparinized) collection tube.
- Gloves are worn throughout the procedure.

Posttest
- Apply pressure at venipuncture site. Apply dressing, periodically assessing for continued bleeding.
- Invert and gently mix the sample and the anticoagulant.
- Label the specimen, protect it from light by wrapping it in foil, and transport it to the laboratory.
- Report abnormal findings to the primary care provider.

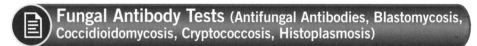

Fungal Antibody Tests (Antifungal Antibodies, Blastomycosis, Coccidioidomycosis, Cryptococcosis, Histoplasmosis)

Test Description

Of the thousands of species of fungi known, very few are considered pathogenic to humans. Susceptibility to fungal infections is most frequently seen among those individuals with debilitating or chronic diseases, those who are immunodeficient, and those undergoing drug therapy that may alter the immune system, such as steroids and antineoplastic agents.

One fungus considered pathogenic is the organism *Blastomyces dermatitidis*, which is similar in structure to tuberculosis. It causes granulomatous skin lesions and may affect visceral organs.

Coccidioidomycosis is a rare disease that carries a high mortality rate. It is caused by the organism *Coccidioides immitis*, which is endemic in the Southwestern United States, California, Mexico, Central America, and South America. Primary infections due to *Coccidioides* species most frequently manifest as community-acquired pneumonia 1 to 3 weeks after exposure, with the person usually presenting with respiratory symptoms, fever, weight loss, and fatigue.

Cryptococcosis is caused by the organism *Cryptococcus neoformans*. It is one of the most frequent fungal infections (mycoses) of the central nervous system (CNS). Susceptibility to this infection is higher in those with chronic or debilitating diseases, such as acquired immune deficiency sydrome (AIDS), and by certain types of drug therapy which may alter the immune system, such as steroids and antineoplastic agents. The disease usually begins as a respiratory infection, which then disseminates to the CNS. The organism is carried by pigeons, with the probable mode of transmission being inhalation. Symptoms range from headache and subtle changes in mental status to fever, seizures, and coma. If untreated, the disease can be fatal within a few weeks.

Histoplasmosis is the most common systemic fungal infection. This disease is caused by *Histoplasma capsulatum*, an organism that lives in moist soil, the floors of chicken houses, and bird droppings, especially those of blackbirds and starlings. The fungus is endemic to the central and eastern portions of North America. It is most often found in the states of Ohio and Missouri and the valleys of the Mississippi River. The disease is usually localized as a pulmonary disorder, often resembling tuberculosis.

THE EVIDENCE FOR PRACTICE

Being alert to common infectious respiratory diseases in one's local region and in region(s) where the patient has been can help determine the probable fungal infections involved (e.g., histoplasmosis in the Midwest, coccidioidomycosis in the Southwest and California). It is important for the primary care provider to realize that homeless people may travel from region to region and may have recently come from an area where one of these diseases is endemic.

Normal Values

No antibodies detected
Immunodiffusion: Negative
Complement fixation titer: <1:8

Possible Meanings of Abnormal Values

Positive

Blastomycosis
Coccidioidomycosis
Cryptococcosis
Histoplasmosis

Contributing Factors to Abnormal Values

- Skin tests can cause a serologic test to become positive. Thus, skin tests should be withheld until after the blood sample is drawn.

- Many mycoses cause immunosuppression, leading to low titers, or false-negative test results.
- There may be a cross-reaction between blastomycosis and histoplasmosis, resulting in falsely high titers.
- Contamination of the blood sample will alter test results.
- Hemolysis of the sample due to excessive agitation may alter results.
- Antibodies may appear early in the disease and then disappear.

Interventions/Implications

Pretest

- Obtain a travel and work history from the patient.
- Explain to the patient the purpose of the test and the need for a blood sample to be drawn.
- No fasting is required prior to the test.

Procedure

- The test should be conducted 2 to 4 weeks after exposure to the organism.
- A 7-mL blood sample is collected in a red-top tube.
- The venipuncture must not be performed on or near any fungal skin lesions.
- Gloves are worn throughout the procedure.

Posttest

- Apply pressure at venipuncture site. Apply dressing, periodically assessing for continued bleeding.
- The sample is labeled and transported to the laboratory immediately, taking care to avoid excessive agitation of the sample.
- Note on the label the specific antibody/antibodies to be tested.
- Advise the patient that other procedures to test for the suspected fungus may need to be done, including smear and culture of materials from lesions, biopsy, and skin testing.
- Report positive finding to the primary care provider.

➔ Clinical Alerts

- Confirmed cases of diseases such as coccidioidomycosis and histoplasmosis are reportable as communicable diseases to the local health department or state department of public health.

Galactose-1-Phosphate Uridyltransferase
(Gal-1-PUT, Galactosemia Screening)

Test Description
This test is used to detect the presence of galactosemia, an inherited disorder transmitted as an autosomal recessive gene. In this disorder, galactose cannot be converted to glucose. Galactose is normally converted to glucose in the liver. In order for this conversion to occur, the enzyme galactose-1-phosphate uridyltransferase is

required for conversion of galactose-1-phosphate into glucose-1-phosphate. When this enzyme is deficient, galactose-1-phosphate accumulates in the body, resulting in such problems as cataracts, liver disease, renal disease, and mental retardation.

Normal Values

18.5–28.5 U/g of hemoglobin

Possible Meanings of Abnormal Values

Decreased

Galactosemia

G

Interventions/Implications

Pretest
- Explain to the patient the purpose of the test and the need for a blood sample to be drawn.
- No fasting is required before the test.

Procedure
- In an adult, a 5-mL blood sample is drawn in a collection tube containing heparin. For infants, a heel stick or umbilical blood may be used.
- Gloves are worn throughout the procedure.

Posttest
- Apply pressure at venipuncture site. Apply dressing, periodically assessing for continued bleeding.
- Label the specimen and transport it to the laboratory.
- Report abnormal findings to the primary care provider.

Clinical Alerts

- If test results indicate the presence of galactosemia, instruct the patient (or parents) regarding the need to remove galactose-containing foods, especially milk, from the diet.

Gallbladder Scan (Hepatobiliary Imaging, Hepatobiliary Scan with Cholecystokinin [CCK], HIDA Scan)

Test Description

For a gallbladder scan, the patient is given a radionuclide compound, hydroxyl iminodiacetic acid (HIDA) labeled with technetium-99m via an IV injection. A scintillation camera is used to take a radioactivity reading from the body. These readings are fed into a computer, which translates these readings into a two-dimensional gray scale picture. These pictures are obtained at 15 to 30 minute intervals. If the biliary system has not visualized within 2 hours, the scan is repeated 2 to 4 hours later. This test is used in the diagnosis of cholecystitis. Delayed filling of the gallbladder is indicative of chronic or acalculous cholecystitis, whereas failure to visualize the gallbladder is diagnostic of an obstruction of the cystic duct, as in acute or calculus cholecystitis. If the HIDA enters the bile ducts but does not enter the small intestine, then an obstruction of the bile duct from stones or cancer is suspected.

The scan can also be done with an additional component. This involves administration of cholecystokinin (CCK). This substance causes the gallbladder to contract. This allows for estimation of the ejection fraction of the gallbladder, which is a measure of how much bile leaves the gallbladder during contraction.

G

Normal Values

Negative (visualization of gallbladder within one hour after radionuclide injection)
Normal ejection fraction (35–75%)

Possible Meanings of Abnormal Values

Acalculous cholecystitis
Acute cholecystitis
Calculous cholecystitis
Cancer of the gallbladder
Chronic cholecystitis
Obstruction of common bile duct

Contributing Factors to Abnormal Values

- Any movement by the patient may alter quality of films taken.
- Retained barium from previous exams may interfere with the test.

Interventions/Implications

Pretest
- Explain to the patient the purpose of the test. Provide any written teaching materials available on the subject. Note that discomfort involved with this test is primarily due to lying on a hard table for an extended period of time and the needle puncture. Reassure the patient that only trace amounts of the radionuclide are involved in the test.
- The patient must remain still while the scan is being performed.
- Fasting for at least 4 hours is preferred prior to the test.
- Obtain a signed informed consent.

Procedure
- The technetium-99m-labeled HIDA is administered by IV injection in a peripheral vein.
- The patient is assisted to a supine position on the examination table.
- A scintillation camera is positioned over the right upper quadrant of the patient's abdomen. This camera takes a radioactivity reading from the body. This information is transformed into a two-dimensional picture of the area.
- Scans are obtained at 15, 30, 60, and 90 minutes postinjection.
- If the gallbladder does not visualize by 2 hours postinjection, additional scans are conducted in 2 to 4 hours.
- Gloves are worn during the radionuclide injection.

Posttest
- Check the injection site for redness or swelling.
- If a woman who is lactating *must* have a nuclear scan, she should not breast-feed the infant until the radionuclide has been eliminated, possibly for 3 days.
- Although the amount of diagnostic radionuclide excreted in the urine is low, the urine should not be used for any laboratory tests for the time period indicated by the nuclear medicine department.
- Gloves are worn whenever dealing with the urine.
- Encourage fluid intake by the patient to enhance excretion of the radionuclide.
- Report abnormal findings to the primary care provider.

G

→ Clinical Alerts

- Whenever possible, schedule gallbladder scanning prior to any diagnostic tests involving barium.
- For patients with right upper quadrant pain who have a gallbladder ultrasound which shows no gallstones (acalculous biliary pain), the hepatobiliary scan with CCK is used to determine whether a hypofunctioning gallbladder may be the cause of the pain.

CONTRAINDICATIONS!

- Pregnant women
    - Caution: A woman in her childbearing years should undergo radiography only during her menses or 12 to 14 days after its onset to avoid any exposure to a fetus.
- Patients who are lactating
- Patients who are unable to cooperate due to age, mental status, pain, or other factors

Gallium Scan (Gallium [Ga] Imaging)

Test Description
The gallium scan is considered a total body scan. Although gallium can be used for scanning of individual organs, such as the liver or spleen, in this particular test, the entire body is scanned. The test is usually performed when the site of the disease, which may be malignancy, infection, or inflammation, has not been delineated. Although the liver, spleen, bones, and large bowel normally take up gallium, inflammatory and malignant processes also draw in gallium. Thus, the test is used to detect primary neoplasms, metastatic lesions, and inflammatory processes. The scan is performed 24 to 48 hours after radioactive gallium citrate has been injected. If needed, it can be performed only 4 to 6 hours after the injection, if the camera is moved slowly over the body.

THE EVIDENCE FOR PRACTICE

Several studies have suggested that PET imaging is superior to gallium imaging in staging of Hodgkin's disease.

Normal Values

Normal uptake of gallium in the liver, spleen, bones, and large bowel
No other areas of increased gallium uptake

Possible Meanings of Abnormal Values

Abscess
Hodgkin's disease
Infection
Inflammation
Malignancy
Non-Hodgkin's lymphoma

Contributing Factors to Abnormal Values

- Any movement by the patient may alter quality of films taken.
- Retained barium from previous exams may interfere with the test.

Interventions/Implications

Pretest
- Explain to the patient the purpose of the test. Provide any written teaching materials available on the subject. Note that discomfort involved with this test is primarily due to lying on a hard table for an extended period of time and the needle puncture. Reassure the patient that only trace amounts of the radionuclide are involved in the test.
- The patient must remain still while the scan is being performed.
- No fasting is required prior to the test.
- Obtain a signed informed consent.
- A laxative and/or cleansing enema may be ordered.

Procedure
- The radioactive gallium (^{67}Ga) citrate is administered by IV injection in a peripheral vein.
- At the designated time (4 to 6 hours or 24 hours post-injection), the patient is taken to the nuclear medicine department.
- The patient is assisted to a supine position on the examination table.
- A scintillation camera is used to scan the entire body. This camera takes a radioactivity reading from the body. This information is transformed into a two-dimensional picture of the area.
- Scans are also made in the prone and lateral positions.
- Additional scans may be obtained at 48 and 72 hours postinjection.
- Gloves are worn during the radionuclide injection.

Posttest
- Check the injection site for redness or swelling.
- If a woman who is lactating *must* have a nuclear scan, she should not breast-feed the infant until the radionuclide has been eliminated, possibly for 3 days.

- Although the amount of diagnostic radionuclide excreted in the urine is low, the urine should not be used for any laboratory tests for the time period indicated by the Nuclear Medicine Department.
- Gloves are worn whenever dealing with the urine.
- Encourage fluid intake by the patient to enhance excretion of the radionuclide.
- Report abnormal findings to the primary care provider.

CONTRAINDICATIONS!

- Pregnant women
  - Caution: A woman in her childbearing years should undergo radiography only during her menses or 12 to 14 days after its onset to avoid any exposure to a fetus.
- Patients who are lactating
- Patients who are unable to cooperate due to age, mental status, pain, or other factors

G

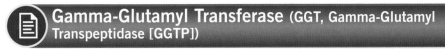

Gamma-Glutamyl Transferase (GGT, Gamma-Glutamyl Transpeptidase [GGTP])

Test Description

Measurement of gamma-glutamyl transferase (GGT) assists in the diagnosis of liver problems, especially alcoholic cirrhosis and liver tumors. GGT is an enzyme found primarily in the liver and biliary tract, and to a lesser degree in the heart, kidneys, pancreas, prostate gland, and spleen. Its function is to assist in amino acid transport across cell membranes. GGT is often measured in conjunction with alkaline phosphatase (ALP) to determine whether the ALP is increased due to liver disease. Whereas ALP may be increased with either hepatobiliary or bone disorders, the GGT is more specific for hepatobiliary problems. GGT is more sensitive than ALP, the transaminases (ALT, AST), and leucine aminopeptidase in detecting obstructive jaundice, cholangitis, and cholecystitits.

Normal Values

Female:	5–29 U/L (5–29 IU/L SI units)
Male:	5–38 U/L (5–38 IU/L SI units)
Child:	3–30 U/L (3–30 IU/L SI units)
Newborn:	5 times the child norms

Possible Meanings of Abnormal Values

Increased

Acute pancreatitis
Alcoholism
Biliary obstruction
Cholangitis
Cholecystitis
Cholelithiasis
Cirrhosis
Congestive heart failure

Hepatitis
Liver disease
Liver metastases
Myocardial infarction
Pancreatic cancer
Renal cancer
Systemic lupus erythematosus

Contributing Factors to Abnormal Values

- Hemolysis of the blood sample will alter test results.
- Drugs which may *increase* GGT levels: alcohol, aminoglycosides, barbiturates, histamine-2 blockers, NSAIDs, phenobarbital, phenytoin.
- Drugs which may *decrease* GGT levels: clofibrate, oral contraceptives.

Interventions/Implications

Pretest
- Explain to the patient the purpose of the test and the need for a blood sample to be drawn.
- Fasting for 8 hours is required prior to the test.
- No alcohol is allowed for 24 hours prior to the test.

Procedure
- A 7-mL blood sample is drawn in a red-top collection tube.
- Gloves are worn throughout the procedure.

Posttest
- Apply pressure 3 to 5 minutes at venipuncture site. Apply dressing, periodically assessing for continued bleeding.
- Label the specimen and transport it to the laboratory.
- Report abnormal findings to the primary care provider.

Clinical Alerts

- Potential complication: with liver dysfunction, patient may have prolonged clotting time.
- Teach the patient to monitor the site. If the site begins to bleed, the patient should apply direct pressure and, if unable to control the bleeding, return to the laboratory or notify the nurse.

Gastric Emptying Scan

Test Description
Delayed gastric emptying can occur for a number of reasons. There can be obstruction in the abdomen due to a tumor or ulcer. In the case of patients with diabetes, gastroparesis may be present. Patients who have gastric surgery may have obstruction

and/or gastroparesis. Regardless of the cause, delayed gastric emptying can be quite uncomfortable for the patient, leading to nausea, vomiting, abdominal pain, and diarrhea. The gastric emptying scan provides data on clearance rates of both solids and foods from the stomach.

Normal Values

No evidence of delayed gastric emptying:
 Solids cleared in <120 minutes
 Liquids cleared in <75 minutes

Possible Meanings of Abnormal Values

Increased	Decreased
Malabsorption	Gastric obstruction
Postgastric surgery	Gastroparesis
	Postradiation therapy
	Ulcer

Interventions/Implications

Pretest
- Explain to the patient the purpose of the test. Provide any written teaching materials available on the subject. Reassure the patient that only trace amounts of the radionuclide are involved in the test.
- The patient must remain still while the scan is being performed.
- Overnight fasting is required before the test.
- Obtain a signed informed consent.

Procedure
- Just prior to the test, the patient is given a radionuclide in food such as scrambled eggs for the *solid phase* of the study, followed by another type of radionuclide in water for the *liquid phase*.
  - Infants can receive the radionuclide in formula, followed by plain formula.
- The patient is assisted to a supine position on the examination table.
- Images are taken immediately to ensure the radioisotope is in the stomach.
- Imaging is repeated intermittently during the next 2 hours.
- Calculations of emptying times are provided by the computer in association with the results of the timed images.

Posttest
- If a woman who is lactating *must* have this scan, she should not breast-feed the infant until the radionuclide has been eliminated, possibly for 3 days.
- Although the amount of diagnostic radionuclide excreted in the urine is low, the urine should not be used for any laboratory tests for the time period indicated by the nuclear medicine department.
- Gloves are worn when dealing with the urine.
- Encourage fluid intake by the patient to enhance excretion of the radionuclide.
- Report abnormal findings to the primary care provider.

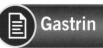

Gastrin

Test Description

Measurement of gastrin levels assists in the diagnosis of various gastric disorders. Gastrin is a polypeptide hormone produced and stored by the G-cells of the antrum of the stomach and by the islets of Langerhans of the pancreas. Gastrin facilitates digestion by triggering gastric acid secretion in the following situations: presence of proteins, calcium, or alcohol in the stomach, vagal stimulation through chewing, tasting, or smelling of food, distension of the stomach antrum, or decreased stomach acidity. When the stomach's environment becomes acidic, the secretion of gastrin is inhibited. Gastrin also stimulates release of pancreatic enzymes, the gastric enzyme pepsin, the intrinsic factor, and bile from the liver, and increases gastrointestinal motility. Abnormal gastrin secretion can occur when pathologic conditions exist. Such conditions include gastrinoma, the gastrin-secreting tumor in Zollinger-Ellison syndrome, gastric ulcers, duodenal ulcers, and pernicious anemia. Testing for gastrin provides information helpful in the diagnosis of these conditions. Provocative testing, such as through IV infusion of calcium gluconate, is used to distinguish ulcer disease from Zollinger-Ellison syndrome.

Normal Values

<100 pg/mL (<48 pmol/L SI units)

Possible Meanings of Abnormal Values

Increased

Achlorhydria
Atrophic gastritis
Duodenal ulcer
Elderly
End-stage renal disease
Gastric ulcer
G-cell hyperplasia
Hyperparathyroidism
Peptic ulcer disease
Pernicious anemia
Postvagotomy
Pyloric obstruction

Stomach cancer
Uremia
Use of acid suppressive medications (antacids, histamine-2 blockers, or proton
    pump inhibitors)
Zollinger-Ellison syndrome

Contributing Factors to Abnormal Values

- Hemolysis of the sample may alter test results.
- Falsely-increased results may occur with lipemic blood samples and intake of high-protein foods.
- Drugs which may *increase* gastrin levels: acetylcholine chloride, antacids, beta-blocking agents, calcium carbonate, calcium chloride, cholinergics, cimetidine, famotidine, insulin, nizatidine, proton pump inhibitors, ranitidine.
- Drugs which may *decrease* gastrin levels: adrenergic blockers, anticholinergics, caffeine, calcium salts, corticosteroids, ethanol, rauwolfia serpentia, reserpine, tricyclic antidepressants.

Interventions/Implications

Pretest
- Explain to the patient the purpose of the test and the need for a blood sample to be drawn.
- Fasting for 12 hours is required prior to the test. Water is permitted.
- Alcohol is to be avoided for 24 hours prior to the test.

Procedure
- A 7-mL blood sample is drawn in a red-top collection tube.
- Gloves are worn throughout the procedure.

Posttest
- Apply pressure at venipuncture site. Apply dressing, periodically assessing for continued bleeding.
- Label the specimen and transport it on ice to the laboratory.
- Report abnormal findings to the primary care provider.

Gastroesophageal Reflux Scan

Test Description

Gastroesophageal reflux occurs when the lower esophageal sphincter (LES) does not close properly and stomach contents leak back, or reflux, into the esophagus. This can lead to a variety of patient complaints, including heartburn, nausea, vomiting, dysphagia, and nocturnal cough or dyspnea. The gastroesophageal (GE) reflux scan is done to evaluate whether reflux is occurring and, if so, the degree of reflux.

Normal Values

No evidence of GE reflux

Possible Meanings of Abnormal Values

GE reflux

Interventions/Implications

Pretest

- Explain to the patient the purpose of the test. Provide any written teaching materials available on the subject. Reassure the patient that only trace amounts of the radionuclide are involved in the test.
- The patient must remain still while the scan is being performed.
- Overnight fasting is required before the test.
- Obtain a signed informed consent.

Procedure

- The patient is assisted to a supine position on the exam table.
- Just prior to the test, the patient is given a radionuclide in orange juice or food such as scrambled eggs.
    - Infants can receive the radionuclide in formula, followed by plain formula.
    - Patients with swallowing difficulties may require a nasogastric tube for ingestion of the radionuclide. The tube must be removed prior to scanning.
- Images are taken immediately to ensure the radioisotope is in the stomach.
- Imaging is repeated in 2 hours.

Posttest

- If a woman who is lactating *must* have this scan, she should not breast-feed the infant until the radionuclide has been eliminated, possibly for 3 days.
- Although the amount of diagnostic radionuclide excreted in the urine is low, the urine should not be used for any laboratory tests for the time period indicated by the nuclear medicine department.
- Gloves are worn when dealing with the urine.
- Encourage fluid intake by the patient to enhance excretion of the radionuclide.
- Report abnormal findings to the primary care provider.

Clinical Alerts

- Patients with positive GE reflux scans should be counseled on ways to minimize reflux symptoms, including dietary changes and pharmacologic treatment.

CONTRAINDICATIONS!

- Pregnant women
    - Caution: A woman in her childbearing years should undergo scanning only during her menses or 12 to 14 days after its onset to avoid any exposure to a fetus.
- Patients who are lactating
- Patients who are unable to cooperate because of age, mental status, pain, or other factors

Gastrointestinal Bleeding Scan

Test Description

The gastrointestinal (GI) bleeding scan is used to determine the site of GI bleeding. This is especially helpful for bleeding occurring in the small intestine which for the most part cannot be directly visualized with endoscopy. The GI bleeding scan involves tagging some of the patient's red blood cells (RBCs) with a radionuclide and then scanning the person's abdomen to note where bleeding might be occurring. Intermittent imaging over a period of several hours may be needed. Thus, the test can only be done on hemodynamically stable patients.

G

Normal Values

No active bleeding noted

Possible Meanings of Abnormal Values

Active gastrointestinal bleeding from:
Diverticula
Inflammatory bowel disease
Polyps
Tumors
Ulcers

Contributing Factors to Abnormal Values

- Barium studies within 24 to 48 hours will affect test results.

Interventions/Implications

Pretest
- Explain to the patient the purpose of the test. Provide any written teaching materials available on the subject. Reassure the patient that only trace amounts of the radionuclide are involved in the test.
- The patient must remain still while the scan is being performed.
- No fasting is required before the test.
- Obtain a signed informed consent.

Procedure
- 5-mL of blood is collected from the patient and combined with ^{99m}Tc.
- The ^{99m}Tc-labeled RBCs are administered intravenously to the patient.
- The patient is assisted to a supine position on the examination table.
- A scintillation camera is positioned over the patient's abdomen. This camera takes a radioactivity reading from the body. This information is transformed into a two-dimensional picture of the abdomen.
- Images are obtained every 5 to 15 minutes. In the case of very slow or intermittent bleeding, scanning may need to be done periodically for up to 24 hours.
- Gloves are worn during the radionuclide injection.

Posttest
- If a woman who is lactating *must* have this scan, she should not breast feed the infant until the radionuclide has been eliminated, possibly for 3 days.
- Although the amount of diagnostic radionuclide excreted in the urine is low, the urine should not be used for any laboratory tests for the time period indicated by the nuclear medicine department.
- Encourage fluid intake by the patient to enhance excretion of the radionuclide.
- Report abnormal findings to the primary care provider.

Clinical Alerts

- Patients undergoing a GI bleeding scan should have their vital signs assessed prior to, during, and after the procedure to ensure stability.

CONTRAINDICATIONS!

- Pregnant women
  - Caution: A woman in her childbearing years should undergo scanning only during her menses or 12 to 14 days after its onset to avoid any exposure to a fetus.
- Patients who are lactating
- Patients who are unable to cooperate because of age, mental status, pain, or other factors

Giardia Antigen (*Giardia lamblia*)

Test Description
Giardiasis is an intestinal infection caused by a protozoa, *Giardia lamblia*. After an incubation period of 1 to 2 weeks, symptoms of gastrointestinal distress may develop, including nausea, vomiting, malaise, flatulence, cramping, diarrhea, steatorrhea, and weight loss. These symptoms may last 2 to 4 weeks. Because giardiasis is spread by fecal-oral contamination, the prevalence is higher in populations with poor sanitation, close contact, and oral-anal sexual practices. It occurs where water supplies become contaminated with raw sewage. It is also frequently seen among campers who drink water from lakes or streams contaminated by various animals.

Testing for *Giardia* may be done through stool specimens for ova and parasites or through antigen assay using enzyme-linked immunosorbent assay (ELISA) or immunofluorescence to detect antibodies to trophozoites or cysts. When the antigen test is used, direct microscopy of the stool is also important since multiple infectious etiologies may be present.

Normal Values

IgG	<1:16
IgA	<1:16
IgM	<1:20

Possible Meanings of Abnormal Values

Recent or current infection: Positive IgM or a fourfold increase in IgG and/or IgA antibody titers between acute and convalescent sera

Past infection: Positive IgG and/or IgA titers without detectable IgM

Interventions/Implications

Pretest
- Explain to the patient the purpose of the test and the need for a blood sample to be drawn.
- No fasting is required before the test.

Procedure
- A 7-mL blood sample is drawn in a gold-top (serum separator) collection tube.
- Gloves are worn throughout the procedure.

Posttest
- Apply pressure at venipuncture site. Apply dressing, periodically assessing for continued bleeding.
- Label the specimen and transport it to the laboratory.
- Report abnormal findings to the primary care provider.

→ Clinical Alerts

- Patients with a positive *Giardia* antigen test are typically treated with an anti-infective such as metronidazole.

Gliadin Antibodies (Antigliadin Antibodies [AGA])

Test Description

Gliadin is part of the gluten protein found in wheat. Gliadin antibodies, also known as antigliadin antibodies (AGA) form in some individuals who are exposed to gluten over a period of time. This is one of several tests used in the diagnosis of celiac disease and other gluten-sensitive conditions. AGA testing may be used to rule out celiac disease in patients with anemia or abdominal pain, or as part of allergy testing. Typically both the IgA and IgG types of antibodies are measured.

Normal Values

Gliadin IgA & IgG antibodies:

Negative:	<20 U
Weak positive:	20–30 U
Moderate to strong positive:	>30 U

Possible Meanings of Abnormal Values

Positive
Celiac disease

Contributing Factors to Abnormal Values

- The presence of other gastrointestinal disorders, such as Crohn's disease, may cause *false-positive* results.

Interventions/Implications

Pretest
- Explain to the patient the purpose of the test and the need for a blood sample to be drawn.
- No fasting is required before the test.

Procedure
- A 7-mL blood sample is drawn in a gold-top (serum separator) collection tube.
- Gloves are worn throughout the procedure.

Posttest
- Apply pressure at venipuncture site. Apply dressing, periodically assessing for continued bleeding.
- Label the specimen and transport it to the laboratory.
- Report abnormal findings to the primary care provider.

→ Clinical Alerts

- Patients found to have celiac disease will greatly benefit from nutritional counseling regarding the removal of gluten and related proteins from the diet.

Glucagon

Test Description
Glucagon is a hormone secreted by the alpha cells of the pancreas. Its function is to elevate blood glucose levels by promoting the conversion of glycogen to glucose. Its secretion is stimulated by hypoglycemia and inhibited by the other pancreatic hormones, insulin and somatostatin. This test is used to determine the presence of a *glucagonoma* (alpha islet cell neoplasm), which causes increased glucagon levels, or hypoglycemia due to glucagon deficiency or pancreatic dysfunction, which results in decreased glucagon levels. Glucagon deficiency can be confirmed through the use of an arginine infusion in that glucagon levels will not rise as expected during the infusion.

Normal Values
50–100 pg/mL (50–100 ng/L SI units)

Possible Meanings of Abnormal Values

Increased	Decreased
Acute pancreatitis	Chronic pancreatitis
Cirrhosis	Cystic fibrosis
Diabetes mellitus	Hypoglycemia
Glucagonoma	Idiopathic glucagon deficiency
Infection	Pancreatic neoplasm
Pheochromocytoma	Postpancreatectomy
Postoperative period	
Stress	
Trauma	
Uremia	

G

Contributing Factors to Abnormal Values

- Hemolysis of the blood sample and having a radioactive scan within 48 hours prior to the test will alter test results.
- Strenuous exercise and stress may *increase* glucagon levels.
- Receipt of radionuclide within 1 week may affect test results.
- Drugs which may *increase* glucagon levels: arginine hydrochloride, danazol, glucocorticoids, gastrin, insulin, nifedipine.
- Drugs which may *decrease* glucagon levels: atenolol, propranolol, secretin.

Interventions/Implications

Pretest
- Explain to the patient the purpose of the test and the need for a blood sample to be drawn.
- Fasting for 10 to 12 hours is required prior to the test. Water is permitted.

Procedure
- A 7-mL blood sample is drawn in a collection tube containing EDTA (lavender-top).
- Gloves are worn throughout the procedure.

Posttest
- Apply pressure at venipuncture site. Apply dressing, periodically assessing for continued bleeding.
- Label the specimen and transport it on ice to the laboratory immediately.
- Report abnormal findings to the primary care provider.

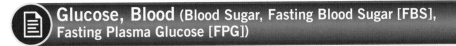

Glucose, Blood (Blood Sugar, Fasting Blood Sugar [FBS], Fasting Plasma Glucose [FPG])

Test Description

Glucose is normally formed in two ways: from the metabolism of ingested carbohydrates and from the conversion of glycogen to glucose in the liver. The maintenance of normal blood glucose is dependent upon proper functioning of two hormones. *Glucagon* causes the blood sugar to rise by speeding the breakdown of glycogen in the liver. *Insulin* allows glucose to pass into cells for use as energy, leading to a decrease in the blood glucose.

Assessment of the blood glucose allows detection of problems with glucose metabolism.

Although stressful conditions such as burns or trauma can increase the blood sugar, the most common cause of abnormal glucose metabolism is diabetes mellitus. The fasting blood sugar is an excellent screening tool for diabetes.

Criteria for the diagnosis of diabetes mellitus, as developed by the American Diabetes Association (http://care.diabetesjournals.org/cgi/content/full/27/suppl_1/s5#T2) are:

1. Symptoms of diabetes plus casual plasma glucose concentration ≥200 mg/dL (11.1 mmol/L). Casual is defined as any time of day without regard to time since last meal. The classic symptoms of diabetes include polyuria, polydipsia, and unexplained weight loss.
2. FPG ≥126 mg/dL (7.0 mmol/L). Fasting is defined as no caloric intake for at least 8 hours.
3. 2-hour postload glucose ≥200 mg/dL (11.1 mmol/L) during an oral glucose tolerance test (OGTT). The test should be performed as described by WHO, using a glucose load containing the equivalent of 75 g anhydrous glucose dissolved in water.

In the absence of unequivocal hyperglycemia, these criteria should be confirmed by repeat testing on a different day. The third measure (OGTT) is not recommended for routine clinical use.

In addition to fasting plasma glucose, a 2-hour postprandial blood glucose is sometimes assessed. In nondiabetic patients, 2-hour postprandial blood glucose levels are usually <120 to 140 mg/dL. After a meal, glucose levels peak at approximately 1 hour and then return to premeal levels within 2 to 3 hours. This variance in plasma glucose is controlled by the insulin response to food intake. In patients with type 2 diabetes, the insulin response is decreased or absent, resulting in elevated postprandial glucose. It is unknown what part the postprandial glucose levels play in overall glycemic control. Recent studies have shown premeal glucose levels to be better predictors of glycemic control.

THE EVIDENCE FOR PRACTICE

According to the American Diabetes Association (http://care.diabetesjournals.org/cgi/content/full/29/suppl_1/s4#SEC3):

- Screening to detect prediabetes (impaired fasting glucose [IFG] or impaired glucose tolerance [IGT]) and diabetes should be considered in individuals ≥45 years of age, particularly in those with a body mass index (BMI) ≥25 kg/m². Screening should also be considered for people who are <45 years of age and are overweight if they have another risk factor for diabetes. Repeat testing should be carried out at 3-year intervals.
- Screen for prediabetes and diabetes in high-risk, asymptomatic, undiagnosed adults and children within the health care setting.
- To screen for diabetes/prediabetes, either a fasting plasma glucose (FPG) test or 2-hour oral glucose tolerance test (OGTT) (75-g glucose load) or both are appropriate.
- An oral glucose tolerance test may be considered in patients with impaired fasting glucose to better define the risk of diabetes.

According to the U.S. Preventive Services Task Force (USPSTF) (http://www.ahrq.gov/ clinic/3rduspstf/ diabscr/diabetrr.htm):
- Screening for diabetes in patients with hypertension or hyperlipidemia should be part of an integrated approach to reduce cardiovascular risk. Lower targets for blood pressure (i.e., diastolic blood pressure ≤80 mm Hg) are beneficial for patients with diabetes and high blood pressure. The report of the Adult Treatment Panel III of the National Cholesterol Education Program recommends lower targets for low-density lipoprotein cholesterol for patients with diabetes.

Normal Values

Normal fasting glucose: FPG<100 mg/dL (<5.6 mmol/L SI units)

Impaired fasting glucose: FPG 100–125 mg/dL (5.6–6.9 mmol/L SI units)

Provisional diagnosis of diabetes: FPG ≥126 mg/dL (≥ 7.0 mmol/L SI units) (diagnosis must be confirmed)

Possible Meanings of Abnormal Values

Increased	Decreased
Acromegaly	Addison's disease
Adenoma of pancreas	Anxiety
Brain trauma	Bacterial sepsis
Burns	Excessive exercise
Cushing's syndrome	Glycogen storage disease
Diabetes mellitus	Hepatic necrosis
Eclampsia	Hypothyroidism
Hyperlipoproteinemia	Insulinoma
Hyperthyroidism	Islet cell carcinoma of the pancreas
Liver disease	Malabsorption
Malnutrition	Pituitary hypofunction
Myocardial infarction	Post-gastrectomy
Obesity	Reactive hypoglycemia due to
Pancreatic cancer	high carbohydrate intake
Pancreatitis	Stress
Pheochromocytoma	
Pituitary tumors	
Prolonged inactivity	
Renal failure (chronic)	
Shock	
Thyrotoxicosis	
Trauma	

Contributing Factors to Abnormal Values

- Drugs which may *increase* fasting blood glucose levels: atypical antipsychotics, azathioprine, basiliximab, beta blockers, bicalutamide, corticosteroids, diazoxide, epinephrine, estrogens, furosemide, gemfibrozil, isoniazid, levothyroxine, lithium, niacin, protease inhibitors, thiazides.
- Drugs which may *decrease* fasting blood glucose levels: acetaminophen, basiliximab, carvedilol, desipramine, ethanol, gemfibrozil, hypoglycemic agents, insulin, MAO inhibitors, phenothiazines, risperidone, theophylline.

Interventions/Implications

Pretest

- Explain to the patient the purpose of the test and the need for a blood sample to be drawn.
- Fasting of at least 8 hours is required prior to the test. Water is permitted.
- Insulin or oral hypoglycemic agents are to be withheld until after the blood sample is drawn.

Procedure

- A 7-mL blood sample is drawn in a collection tube containing a glycolytic inhibitor such as sodium fluoride.
- Gloves are worn throughout the procedure.

Posttest

- Apply pressure at venipuncture site. Apply dressing, periodically assessing for continued bleeding.
- Label the specimen and transport it to the laboratory immediately. Blood glucose levels decrease when blood is left at room temperature.
- Report abnormal findings to the primary care provider.

Clinical Alerts

- Patients with elevated fasting plasma glucose need to have the diagnosis confirmed with additional laboratory testing.
- If the patient is found to have diabetes mellitus, extensive education is needed on the condition and how to control it.

Glucose-6-Phosphate Dehydrogenase (G-6-PD)

Test Description

This test measures glucose-6-phosphate dehydrogenase (G-6-PD), one of the many enzymes normally found in the RBCs. This enzyme protects the cells from damage from oxidant chemicals. When a deficiency of G-6-PD occurs, hemolysis of the RBCs occurs, resulting in anemia.

G-6-PD deficiency is a sex-linked recessive trait carried on the X-chromosome, so males are almost exclusively affected. Females can be carriers of the trait, and in rare cases, can be affected if the trait is carried on both X chromosomes. In the United States, this genetic problem affects 10% to14% of African-Americans. The disease also tends to affect people of Middle Eastern decent, particularly those of Sephardic Jewish descent and Kurdish males.

People with the disorder are not normally anemic and display no evidence of the disease until the RBCs are exposed to an oxidant or stress. Newborns with the deficiency may experience prolonged and more pronounced neonatal jaundice than other newborns. Conditions which may precipitate hemolytic episodes in individuals affected with G-6-PD deficiency include bacterial infection, diabetic acidosis, fava bean ingestion, septicemia, and viral infection. A variety of drugs may also cause hemolytic episodes in these patients. These drugs include analgesics, antimalarials, antipyretics, antipyrines, ascorbic acid, aspirin, chloramphenicol, ciprofloxacin, dap-sone, doxorubicin, methylene blue, nalidixic acid, naphthalene, nitrofurantoin, phenazopyridine, primaquine, probenecid, quinidine, quinine, sulfacetamide, sul-famethoxazole, sulfonamides, tolbutamide, and large doses of vitamin K.

Normal Values

Screening: Negative for G-6-PD deficiency
Quantitative: 5–8.6 U/g of hemoglobin

Possible Meanings of Abnormal Values

Increased	Decreased
Chronic blood loss	Acidotic state
Hepatic coma	Congenital G-6-PD deficiency
Hyperthyroidism	Hemolytic anemia
Idiopathic thrombocytopenic purpura	Infection
Megaloblastic anemia	
Myocardial infarction	
Pernicious anemia	

Contributing Factors to Abnormal Values

- False-negative results may occur with hemolyzed samples and in patients who have had recent blood transfusions.

Interventions/Implications

Pretest
- Explain to the patient the purpose of the test and the need for a blood sample to be drawn.
- No fasting is required before the test.

Procedure
- A 5-mL sample is drawn in a collection tube containing EDTA (lavender-top) or heparin (green-top).
- Gloves are worn throughout the procedure.

Posttest
- Apply pressure at venipuncture site. Apply dressing, periodically assessing for continued bleeding.
- Label the specimen and transport it to the laboratory.
- Report abnormal findings to the primary care provider.

→ Clinical Alerts

- If a deficiency of G-6-PD is found, education of the patient is needed regard-ing the drugs and other conditions which may precipitate hemolysis. Caution must be exercised in the use of over-the-counter medications which might contain aspirin.

- If a male patient has normal G-6-PD activity levels, it is likely that they do not have a deficiency. However, if the test was performed during an episode of hemolytic anemia, it should be repeated a few weeks later when the RBC population has had time to replenish and mature.

Glucose Tolerance Test
(GTT, Oral Glucose Tolerance Test [OGTT])

G

Test Description

The oral glucose tolerance test (OGTT) is performed to rule out diabetes by evaluating the rate at which glucose is removed from the blood stream. Following administration of an oral glucose load, blood samples are drawn in 1/2, 1, 2, and 3 hours. For nondiabetic patients, the rise in blood glucose is relatively minor. For diabetic patients, however, the glucose level shows a dramatic increase and remains greatly elevated for several hours. This test is also used in screening for gestational diabetes during pregnancy.

According to the American Diabetes Association (http://care.diabetesjournals.org/cgi/content/full/27/supplµ1/s5#T2), the corresponding categories when the OGTT is used are the following:

- 2-hour postload glucose <140 mg/dL = normal glucose tolerance;
- 2-hour postload glucose 140–199 mg/dL = impaired glucose tolerance (IGT);
- 2-hour postload glucose ≥200 mg/dL = provisional diagnosis of diabetes (the diagnosis must be confirmed).

THE EVIDENCE FOR PRACTICE

To screen for diabetes/prediabetes, either a fasting plasma glucose (FPG) test or 2-hour oral glucose tolerance test (OGTT) (75-g glucose load) or both are appropriate.

Normal Values

For 75-gram OGTT used to check for Type 2 diabetes mellitus
Fasting: 60–100 mg/dL (3.3–5.6 mmol/L SI units)
1 hour: <200 mg/dL (11.1 mmol/L SI units)
2 hours: <140 mg/dL (7.8 mmol/L SI units)

For 50-gram OGTT used to screen for gestational diabetes
1 hour: <140 mg/dL (7.8 mmol/L SI units)

For 100-gram OGTT used to screen for gestational diabetes
Fasting: <95 mg/dL (<5.3 mmol/L SI units)
1 hour: <180 mg/dL (<10 mmol/L SI units)
2 hours: <155 mg/dL (<8.6 mmol/L SI units)
3 hours: <140 mg/dL (7.8 mmol/L SI units)

Possible Meanings of Abnormal Values

Increased Tolerance	Decreased Tolerance
Addison's disease	Central nervous system lesions
Hypoparathyroidism	Cushing's syndrome
Hypothyroidism	Diabetes mellitus
Liver disease	Gastrectomy
Pancreatic islet cell hyperplasia	Gestational diabetes
Pancreatic islet cell tumor	Hemochromatosis
Reactive hypoglycemia	Hyperlipidemia
	Hyperthyroidism
	Impaired glucose tolerance
	Pheochromocytoma
	Severe liver damage

G

Contributing Factors to Abnormal Values

- Bedrest, infections, smoking, and stress may alter test results.
- Intake of low carbohydrate diet may falsely suggest diabetes mellitus or IGT.
- Drugs which may *increase* glucose tolerance: hypoglycemic agents, insulin.
- Drugs which may *decrease* glucose tolerance: corticosteroids, estrogens, niacin, thiazide diuretics.

Interventions/Implications

Pretest
- Explain to the patient the purpose of the test and the need for multiple blood samples.
- Fasting for 8 hours is required prior to the test. Water is permitted.
- No alcohol or coffee intake or excessive physical activity is allowed for 8 hours prior to the test.
- No smoking is allowed during the testing period.
- If possible, drugs which may influence test results are withheld for 3 days before the test.

Procedure
- A 7-mL blood sample is drawn in a collection tube containing a glycolytic inhibitor such as sodium fluoride (gray-top tube).
- The patient is given an oral glucose load: 75–100 g of glucose dissolved in water or lemon juice (to improve taste of very sweet substance).
- Additional blood samples are drawn at 30 minutes, 1 hour, 2 hours, and 3 hours.
- Water is permitted and encouraged during the testing period.
- The patient should rest quietly throughout the testing period.
- Gloves are worn throughout the procedure.

Posttest
- The patient should be observed for weakness, tremors, anxiety, sweating, or fainting. If symptoms occur, a blood sample is drawn and tested for glucose level. For hypoglycemia (low blood sugar), administer orange juice with sugar added or IV glucose. For hyperglycemia, insulin will be administered. In either case, the test is discontinued.
- Apply pressure at venipuncture site. Apply dressing, periodically assessing for continued bleeding.

- Label each specimen and transport to the laboratory immediately. Blood glucose levels decrease when blood is left at room temperature.
- The patient should eat and resume medications as before the test.
- Report abnormal findings to the primary care provider.

Clinical Alerts

- Possible complication: hypoglycemia, hyperglycemia
- The OGTT is not typically used in children

G

CONTRAINDICATIONS!

- Any conditions in which there is altered carbohydrate tolerance: endocrine disorders, myocardial infarction, postpartum, recent surgery, serious infections

Glycosylated Hemoglobin (G-Hb, Glycated Hgb, Glycohemoglobin, Hemoglobin A$_{1c}$, [HbA$_{1c}$])

Test Description

There are several forms of hemoglobin (Hb), with HbA comprising 90% of the total. A portion of HbA, denoted as HbA$_1$, is glycolated, meaning it absorbs glucose. When blood glucose levels are above normal for an extended period of time, the hemoglobin of the red blood cells becomes saturated with glucose in the form of *glycohemoglobin*. This saturation is present for the 120-day lifespan of the red blood cell. By testing for glycosylated hemoglobin, the primary care provider discovers what the average blood glucose level has been for the previous 2 to 3 months. This is especially valuable when monitoring diabetics whose blood sugars change dramatically from day-to-day and to monitor long-term diabetic control. Whereas a fasting blood sugar may be influenced by the patient's recent adherence to the prescribed treatment regimen, the glycosylated hemoglobin is irreversible; it shows what type of diabetic control has occurred over several months. Because of this, the glycosylated hemoglobin test has become a valued component of diabetic care.

In reviewing test results, it is important to know what is being measured. Some laboratories report glycosylated Hb as a whole, which includes A$_{1a}$, A$_{1b}$, and A$_{1c}$, while others report only HbA$_{1c}$, which can be 2% to 4% less than the value for glycosylated Hb.

The correlation between the HbA$_{1c}$ level and the average plasma glucose level is that a 1% rise in HbA$_{1c}$ is equivalent to an increase of 35 mg/dL in the average plasma glucose. Thus:

$$4\% \text{ HbA}_{1c} = 65 \text{ mg/dL average plasma glucose}$$
$$5\% \text{ HbA}_{1c} = 100 \text{ mg/dL average plasma glucose}$$
$$6\% \text{ HbA}_{1c} = 135 \text{ mg/dL average plasma glucose}$$

7% HbA_{1c} = 170 mg/dL average plasma glucose
8% HbA_{1c} = 205 mg/dL average plasma glucose
9% HbA_{1c} = 240 mg/dL average plasma glucose
10% HbA_{1c} = 275 mg/dL average plasma glucose
11% HbA_{1c} = 310 mg/dL average plasma glucose
12% HbA_{1c} = 345 mg/dL average plasma glucose

Glycemic control is based on research findings that lowering the HbA_{1c} is associated with a reduction in the complications of diabetes. According to the American Diabetes Association (ADA) (http://care.diabetesjournals.org/cgi/content/full/29/suppl_1/s4#SEC6), the goal for patients in general is an HbA_{1c} <7%, with goals *for the individual patient* being as close to normal (<6%) as possible without significant hypoglycemia. This goal may not be appropriate for patients with a history of severe hypoglycemia, patients with limited life expectancies, very young children or older adults, and individuals with comorbid conditions.

G

THE EVIDENCE FOR PRACTICE
The use of glycated hemoglobin test (A_{1c}) for the diagnosis of diabetes is not recommended at this time.

Normal Values of HbA_{1c}
 (Values vary with reference laboratory)
  Nondiabetic adult: 2.2–5 %
  Diabetic adult: <7% (ADA guideline)

Possible Meanings of Abnormal Values

Increased	Decreased
Alcohol	Chronic loss of blood
Hyperglycemia	Chronic renal failure
Lead poisoning	Hemolytic anemia
Newly diagnosed diabetic	Pregnancy
Poor diabetic control	Sickle cell anemia
	Splenectomy
	Thalassemia

Interventions/Implications

Pretest
- Explain to the patient the purpose of the test and the need for a blood sample to be drawn.
- No fasting is required before the test.

Procedure
- A 7-mL blood sample is drawn in a lavender-top collection tube.
- Gloves are worn throughout the procedure.

Posttest
- Apply pressure at venipuncture site. Apply dressing, periodically assessing for continued bleeding.

- Label the specimen and transport it to the laboratory.
- Report abnormal findings to the primary care provider.

Clinical Alerts

- This test is not affected by the time the blood sample is drawn, by food intake, by exercise, by stress, or by the prior administration of diabetic medications.
- The HbA$_{1c}$ test should be performed:
  - At least two times a year in patients who are meeting treatment goals and who have stable glycemic control.
  - Quarterly in patients whose therapy has changed or who are not meeting glycemic goals.
  - As needed to assist with decision-making on therapy changes.
- Glycemic goals should be individualized. More stringent goals (<6%) reduce complications of diabetes, but have increased risk of hypoglycemia. Children, pregnant women, elderly, and anyone with severe or frequent hypoglycemia require special considerations.
- If goals are not met despite reaching premeal glucose goals, more emphasis may be needed on evaluating postprandial glucose levels.
- Patients need to be instructed on home glucose monitoring, with the results being reviewed by the primary care provider on a regular basis.

Gonorrhea Culture

Test Description

Gonorrhea, a common venereal disease, results from sexual transmission of *Neisseria gonorrhoeae*. This infection is responsible for approximately 50% of all cases of pelvic inflammatory disease in women. Cultures may be taken from the urethra in males and the endocervical canal in women. Other culture sites are the throat and rectum, if the person has had oral or anal intercourse.

Treatment is usually begun after a culture is found to be positive. However, if the patient is exhibiting symptoms or has had intercourse with an infected individual, treatment is begun once the specimen is obtained.

THE EVIDENCE FOR PRACTICE

The U.S. Preventive Services Task Force (USPSTF) recommends that clinicians screen all sexually active women, including those who are pregnant, for gonorrhea infection if they are at increased risk for infection, that is, if they are young or have other individual or population risk factors. The USPSTF guidelines (http://www.ahrq.gov/clinic/uspstf/uspsgono.htm) state:

- Women and men under the age of 25—including sexually active adolescents—are at highest risk for genital gonorrhea infection. Risk factors for gonorrhea include a history of previous gonorrhea infection, other sexually transmitted infections, new or multiple sexual partners, inconsistent condom use, sex work, and drug use. Risk factors for pregnant women are the same as for nonpregnant women. Prevalence of gonorrhea infection varies widely among communities and patient populations. African Americans and men who have sex with men have a higher prevalence of infection than the general population in many communities and settings.

Normal Values
Negative

Possible Meanings of Abnormal Values

G

Positive
Gonorrhea

Contributing Factors to Abnormal Values
- Voiding by males within 1 hour of a urethral culture may make fewer organisms available for culture.
- Douching by females within 24 hours of a cervical culture may make fewer organisms available for culture.
- Use of lubricant can alter test results.

Interventions/Implications
Pretest
- Explain to the patient the purpose of the test and the type of specimen to be collected.
- No fasting is required prior to the test.
- Females should avoid douching or tub baths prior to the test if an endocervical swab is to be obtained.

Procedure
- Cultures may be obtained using a dry, sterile cotton swab which is then applied to a Thayer-Martin medium, or a special gel transport medium swab.
- Gloves are worn throughout any of the following procedures.

For an endocervical culture
- The female patient is assisted into the lithotomy position, draped, and encouraged to relax through deep breathing techniques.
- A vaginal speculum lubricated with only warm water is inserted.
- Cervical mucus is removed using a large cotton swab.
- A dry, sterile cotton swab is then inserted into the endocervical canal and rotated from side to side, remaining there for 10 to 30 seconds to allow absorption of organisms onto the swab.

For a urethral culture
- The male patient is assisted into a supine position. This position is recommended to avoid falling if vasovagal syncope occurs during the procedure. Such a reaction would be characterized by profound hypotension, bradycardia, pallor, and diaphoresis.
- The urethral meatus is cleansed with sterile gauze.
- A calcium alginate swab or a sterile bacteriologic wire loop is inserted 2 to 3 cm into the urethra and rotated from side to side.

For a rectal culture

- Following the collection of an endocervical or urethral specimen, another sterile cotton swab is inserted approximately 1 in. into the anal canal, and moved from side to side to obtain the specimen. If the swab becomes contaminated with stool, it is discarded and the specimen collection is repeated with a clean swab.

For a throat culture

- The patient's head is tilted back. The posterior pharynx and tonsillar crypts are swabbed with the sterile swab, while avoiding any contact with the tongue or lips.

Posttest

- After obtaining the specimen, roll the swab in a Z pattern in a Thayer-Martin medium or insert into a commercially available gel transport container.
- Label and transport the specimen to the laboratory as soon as possible.
- Advise the patient to avoid all sexual contact until test results are available.
- Report abnormal findings to the primary care provider.

G

→ **Clinical Alerts**

- Patients with positive test results should have their sexual partners examined.
- DNA testing using polymerase chain reaction (PCR) methodology is the newest method of testing for gonorrhea. This can be done on a urine specimen. If used, instruct the patient not to urinate for 1 hour prior to collection. The patient should collect the first 15–50 mL of voided urine (the first part of the stream) in a plastic, preservative-free, sterile urine collection cup.

Growth Hormone: Growth Hormone Stimulation/Suppression Test
(GH, Human Growth Hormone [hGH], Somatotropin)

Test Description

Growth hormone (GH) is a polypeptide produced by the anterior pituitary gland. Its primary function is to stimulate growth of the body. It also plays important roles in protein synthesis, fatty acid utilization, insulin mobilization, and RNA production. The synthesis and release of GH is regulated by the hypothalamus via growth hormone-releasing factor (GHRF) and growth hormone release-inhibiting factor (GHRIH, or somatostatin).

Hyposecretion of GH in children results in dwarfism, whereas hypersecretion of GH in children leads to gigantism and in adults, acromegaly. This test is used to determine hypo- and hyperfunctioning of the pituitary gland, so that appropriate intervention can be initiated.

A random test for GH level may be insufficient to diagnose a deficiency. To provide additional information, GH stimulation and/or suppression tests may be done. The *growth hormone stimulation test* is performed to diagnose growth hormone deficiency. A variety of methods are used to stimulate growth hormone secretion for this test. These include insulin-induced hypoglycemia, vigorous exercise, and drugs such as arginine hydrochloride, glucagon, levodopa, and clonidine hydrochloride. The *growth hormone suppression test* is used to diagnose hypersecretion of GH. Suppression of GH release in a person with normal levels of GH is induced through use of the oral glucose tolerance test (GTT), whereas with hypersecretion of GH, the GTT will cause little or no decrease in GH.

Normal Values

GH levels (random specimen)
Males: <5 ng/mL (<5 μg/L SI units)
Females: <10 ng/mL (<10 μg/L SI units)

GH stimulation test
>10 ng/ml (>10 μg/L SI units)

GH suppression test
<2 ng/ml (<2 μg/L SI units)

Possible Meanings of Abnormal Values

Random specimen

Increased	Decreased
Acromegaly	Dwarfism
Anorexia nervosa	Failure to thrive
Gigantism	Growth hormone deficiency
Hypoglycemia	Hyperglycemia
Hypothalamic tumor	Hypopituitarism
Hyperpituitarism	
Pituitary tumor	
Sleep (2 hours after)	
Starvation	
Surgery	

Stimulation test

Lack of GH increase
Growth hormone deficiency

Suppression test

Slight or no decrease in GH
Acromegaly

Contributing Factors to Abnormal Values
- Levels of growth hormone may vary with exercise, nutritional status, sleep, and stress.
- Any testing for growth hormone should be scheduled no sooner than 48 hours after any diagnostic tests using radioactive materials.
- Drugs which may *increase* levels of growth hormone: amphetamines, arginine, clonidine, dopamine, estrogens, glucagon, indomethacin, insulin, interferon, levodopa, niacin, oral contraceptives, phenytoin.

- Drugs which may *decrease* levels of growth hormone: antipsychotics, bromocriptine, corticosteroids, dexamethasone, octreotide, progestins, valproic acid.

Interventions/Implications

Pretest

Random specimen
- Explain to the patient the purpose of the test and the need for a blood sample to be drawn.
- Fasting for 8 hours is required prior to the test. Water is permitted.
- The patient should be at rest in a stress free environment for 30 minutes prior to the test.

Stimulation/suppression test
- All steroid medications should be withheld prior to the test, if possible. If they must be given, record the drug name on the laboratory slip.
- Explain to the patient the purpose of the test and that the test will usually involve the intravenous infusion of a drug (stimulation test) or administration of an oral glucose load (suppression test). Note that several blood samples will need to be drawn.
- Fasting for 8 to 10 hours is required prior to the test. Water is permitted.
- The patient should be at rest in a stress free environment for 90 minutes prior to the test.

Procedure

Random specimen
- A 7-mL blood sample is drawn in a red-top collection tube.
- Gloves are worn throughout the procedure.

Stimulation test
- A baseline blood sample of 5 to 7 mL is drawn in a red-top collection tube.
- Procedures will vary depending on the type of stimulator used. Check with reference laboratory for specific procedures.
  - For example, use of arginine, an amino acid, involves IV infusion of the drug over 30 minutes. Blood samples are then drawn 30, 60, and 90 minutes after the infusion is complete.
- Gloves are worn throughout the procedure.

Suppression test
- A baseline blood sample of 5 to 7 mL is drawn in a red-top collection tube.
- An oral glucose load is administered. Check with reference laboratory for specific procedures.
- Blood samples are then drawn 30, 60, and 90 minutes after the infusion is complete.
- Gloves are worn throughout the procedure.

Posttest
- Apply pressure at venipuncture site. Apply dressing, periodically assessing for continued bleeding.
- Carefully label any blood samples as to the time drawn. Samples must be taken to the laboratory immediately, since growth hormone has a half-life of only 20 to 25 minutes.
- Resume diet and medications as prior to the test.
- Report abnormal findings to the primary care provider.

Clinical Alerts

- For stimulation/suppression tests, use of an intermittent infusion device, such as a saline lock, will allow drug administration and blood sampling without the need for numerous venipunctures.

CONTRAINDICATIONS!

- Patients with cerebrovascular disease
- Patients with seizure disorders
- Patients with low basal plasma cortisol levels
- Patients who have had a myocardial infarction

H

Ham's Test (Acidified Serum Lysis Test, Paroxysmal Nocturnal Hemoglobinuria [PNH] Test)

Test Description

Ham's test is named after Dr. Thomas Hale Ham, an American physician known for his work in hematology, especially in the area of hemolysis. Ham's test evaluates whether RBCs become more fragile when they are placed in mild acid. The test is conducted to identify paroxysmal nocturnal hemoglobinuria (PNH), a rare condition in which hemoglobin is found in the urine during and after sleep. This condition is thought to be related to the hypersensitivity of RBCs to higher levels of carbon dioxide (acidic) and the resulting decrease in blood pH (acidic environment). To perform the test, the patient's blood sample is mixed with ABO-compatible normal serum and dilute acid, maintained at 37°C, and then examined for hemolysis. Normally, RBCs do not undergo hemolysis. However, RBCs from patients with PNH are especially susceptible to lysis under these conditions.

Normal Values

Negative

Possible Meanings of Abnormal Values

Increased

Aplastic anemia
Dyserythropoietic anemia
Leukemia
Paroxysmal nocturnal hemoglobinuria (PNH)
Spherocytosis

Contributing Factors to Abnormal Values

- Hemolysis of the blood sample may alter test results.
- Transfusion of whole blood or packed cells within 3 weeks of this test may cause false-negative results.

Interventions/Implications

Pretest
- Explain to the patient the purpose of the test and the need for a blood sample to be drawn.
- No fasting is required before the test.

Procedure
- A 7-mL blood sample is drawn in a collection tube containing EDTA (lavender-top)
- Gloves are worn throughout the procedure.

Posttest
- Apply pressure at venipuncture site. Apply dressing, periodically assessing for continued bleeding.
- Label the specimen and transport it to the laboratory.
- Report abnormal findings to the primary care provider.

CONTRAINDICATIONS!

- Patients who have received a blood transfusion within 3 weeks prior to the test

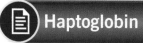

Haptoglobin

Test Description

Haptoglobin is an alpha$_2$ globulin protein produced in the liver. Its function is to bind with free hemoglobin in the blood. Normally there is very little free hemoglobin in the circulation. However, when RBCs are destroyed, their hemoglobin is released. After haptoglobin attaches to this free hemoglobin, the resulting complex is transported back to the liver where its components, such as iron and heme, are recycled.

This action conserves the body's iron stores by preventing their excretion in the urine. This recycling process destroys the haptoglobin.

When large numbers of RBCs are destroyed, the rate of haptoglobin destruction by the liver is higher than the rate at which new haptoglobin is created. Thus, the levels of haptoglobin in the blood will decrease. Any condition which destroys RBCs can thus deplete haptoglobin levels very rapidly, because it cannot be replaced quickly enough. Examples of such conditions are hemolytic anemia, mechanical disruption as from prosthetic heart valves, and antibodies, as seen in transfusion reactions.

Haptoglobin levels are also affected by the presence of liver disease. Liver damage may result in decreased haptoglobin production and decreased clearing of the haptoglobin-free hemoglobin complexes.

Normal Values

27–139 mg/dL (0.27–1.39 g/L SI units)

Possible Meanings of Abnormal Values

Increased	Decreased
Acute infection	Autoimmune hemolytic anemia
Acute rheumatic disease	Congenital ahaptoglobinemia
Arterial disease	Erythroblastosis fetalis
Biliary obstruction	G-6-PD deficiency
Chronic infection	Hemolysis
Granulomatous disease	Hepatocellular disease
Inflammation	Hereditary spherocytosis
Malignant neoplasms	Hypertension
Peptic ulcer	Infectious mononucleosis
Pneumonia	Liver disease
Post-myocardial infarction	Malarial infestation
Pregnancy	Paroxysmal nocturnal hemoglobinuria
Tissue necrosis	Prosthetic heart valves
Tuberculosis	Sickle cell disease
Ulcerative colitis	Systemic lupus erythematosus
	Thalassemia
	Thrombotic thrombocytopenic purpura
	Transfusion reaction
	Uremia

H

Contributing Factors to Abnormal Values

- Hemolysis of the blood sample will alter test results.
- Drugs which may *increase* haptoglobin levels: androgens, corticosteroids.
- Drugs which may *decrease* haptoglobin levels: chlorpromazine, diphenhydramine, estrogens, indomethacin, isoniazid, nitrofurantoin, oral contraceptives, quinidine, streptomycin.

Interventions/Implications

Pretest
- Explain to the patient the purpose of the test and the need for a blood sample to be drawn.
- No fasting is required before the test.

Procedure
- A 7-mL blood sample is drawn in a red-top collection tube.
- Gloves are worn throughout the procedure.

Posttest
- Apply pressure at venipuncture site. Apply dressing, periodically assessing for continued bleeding.
- Label the specimen and transport it to the laboratory immediately, taking care not to shake it, as this will cause unwanted hemolysis.
- Report abnormal findings to the primary care provider.

→ Clinical Alerts

- In evaluation of anemia, haptoglobin levels may be evaluated in conjunction with measurement of the reticulocyte count and complete blood count.

- Hemolytic anemia will usually result in decreased haptoglobin levels, increased reticulocyte count, and decreased RBC count, hemoglobin, and hematocrit.
- If the haptoglobin level is normal in the presence of an increased reticulocyte count, the RBC destruction is not likely to be intravascular. It is more likely to be occurring in the spleen and liver. In this situation, there is no free hemoglobin released into the circulation, so there is no binding with haptoglobin.
- If both the haptoglobin level and the reticulocyte count are normal, the anemia is most likely not due to RBC hemolysis.

H

Helicobacter Pylori Testing (*H. Pylori*)

Test Description

Helicobacter pylori is a very common bacterium which primarily resides in the stomach. The prevalence in the United States was 30% to 40% in the 1990s, but has decreased somewhat since that time. Segments of the U.S. population with increased, probability of *H. pylori* infection include African Americans, Hispanics/Latinos, immigrants from developing counties, persons of low socioeconomic status, Native Americans from Alaska, and people older than 50 years of age. Most people infected with the bacterium are asymptomatic, with the primary effect of the infection being a chronic gastritis. *H. pylori* has been found to be associated with development of peptic ulcer disease, gastric cancer, mucosa-associated lymphoid tissue lymphoma, and dyspepsia uninvestigated by endoscopy or imaging.

Testing for *H. pylori* includes invasive techniques such as endoscopy and biopsy, and several noninvasive tests, including serologic tests, the stool antigen test, and the urea breath test. These tests vary not only in methodology, but also in their sensitivity for documenting *active* infection. Serologic testing typically involves testing for specific IgG antibodies to *H. pylori* in the patient's serum. A positive IgG antibody test indicates either a past infection which might have been eradicated or an ongoing infection. Thus, sensitivity for active infection is only 85%. Thus a positive serologic test does not assist the primary care provider in knowing whether or not to treat, since it is unknown whether it is active or perhaps gone. Also testing for IgM and IgA helps improve the sensitivity.

Two tests *do* test for active infection. The *stool antigen test* is an enzymatic immunoassay (ELISA) that identifies *H. pylori* antigen in a stool specimen. This test is considered a sensitive measure of active infection with 93.1% sensitivity. Similar sensitivity for active infection is found with the *urea breath test* (94.7%). In this test, the patient takes urea orally which is labeled with an isotope. If *H. pylori* is present in the stomach, labeled carbon dioxide is produced as a result of the interaction. This carbon dioxide can be detected in the patient's breath within minutes of the urea ingestion. The patient breathes into a collection bag or onto a flat breath card.

Normal Values

Negative

Possible Meanings of Abnormal Values

Positive IgG

Active *H. pylori* infection
Past *H. pylori* infection

Positive Stool or Breath Test

Active *H. pylori* infection

Contributing Factors to Abnormal Values

H

- Intake of antibiotics, proton-pump inhibitors or bismuth preparations within 2 weeks of the urea breath test can cause *false-negative* test.

Interventions/Implications

Pretest

- Explain to the patient the purpose of the test and the need for a blood, stool, or breath sample to be collected.
- No fasting is required before the test for blood or stool testing.
- Fasting for 1 hour is required before the urea breath test.
- For the urea breath test, the patient must not take antibiotics, proton-pump inhibitors, or bismuth preparations for 2 weeks prior to the test.

Procedure

- Gloves are worn when handling any specimen.

For serologic tests

- A 7-mL blood sample is drawn in a red-top collection tube.

For stool antigen test

- Collect 0.5 mL of semisolid stool (not diarrheal) in a sterile cup.

For urea breath test

- The patient ingests a capsule containing isotope labeled urea.
  - A radioactive or nonradioactive isotope may be used. For pregnant women and children, the nonradioactive isotope is used.
- The capsule is taken with a test meal to delay gastric emptying and allow sufficient time for the urea to be in contact with the abdominal mucosa.
- Breath samples are collected for up to 20 minutes in a special collection bag or the patient may be instructed to breathe onto a special card.

Posttest

For serologic testing

- Apply pressure at venipuncture site. Apply dressing, periodically assessing for continued bleeding.

For all testing

- Label the specimen and transport it to the laboratory.
- Report abnormal findings to the primary care provider.

Hematocrit (Hct, Packed Cell Volume [PCV])

Test Description

Hematocrit is defined as the proportion of red blood cells to plasma within a sample of blood. Following collection of the sample, the specimen is centrifuged. Due to their weight, the red blood cells are forced to the bottom of the test tube. A determination of the percentage of these packed cells in comparison to the plasma is then made.

Hematocrit can be used to assess the extent of a patient's blood loss. A drop of 3% in hematocrit equals approximately one unit of blood loss. It is important to note, however, that the drop in hematocrit does not occur immediately. As a result of a large blood loss, there is a loss of equal proportions of red blood cells and plasma. Thus the hematocrit remains normal for a period of time. In an attempt to compensate for the blood loss and return the plasma volume to normal, the body shifts fluid from the intracellular and interstitial compartments to the intravascular compartment. Red blood cells, however, are not able to be replaced in such a short time. Thus, the relative percentage of red blood cells, as denoted by the hematocrit, will decrease.

Hematocrit is a useful measure only if the patient's hydration level is normal. When normal hydration is present and the total red blood cell count and hemoglobin are both normal, the hematocrit is approximately three times the hemoglobin result.

Normal Values

Female:	37–48% (0.37–0.48 SI units)
Male:	42–52% (0.42–0.52 SI units)
Pregnancy:	Decreased (dilutional)
Elderly:	Slightly decreased
Newborn:	Increased

Possible Meanings of Abnormal Values

Increased	Decreased
Burns	Addison's disease
Cardiovascular disease	Anemia
Chronic lung disease	Bone marrow suppression
Congenital heart defect	Chronic infection
Cushing's disease	Cirrhosis
Dehydration (hemoconcentration)	Hemorrhage
Erythrocytosis	Hodgkin's disease
Hepatic cancer	Hypothyroidism
Polycythemia vera	Leukemia
Renal cyst	Lymphoma
Secondary polycythemia	Malnutrition
Shock	Multiple myeloma
	Overhydration (hemodilution)
	Pregnancy
	Prosthetic heart values
	Renal disease
	Rheumatic fever

Subacute bacterial endocarditis
Systemic lupus erythematosus
Vitamin deficiency (B_6, B_{12}, folic acid)

Contributing Factors to Abnormal Values

- Tests results may be affected by problems with procedure technique:
  - Taking the sample from the arm in which an IV is infusing results in hemodilution and a decreased hematocrit.
  - Leaving the tourniquet in place for more than 1 minute during the procedure will result in hemoconcentration. This can increase the hematocrit by 2.5% to 5%.
- False increases may occur when the blood glucose is greater than 400 mg/dL, when the patient is dehydrated, or in the presence of leukocytosis.
- Pregnancy causes slight decreases in hematocrit due to higher total blood volume (dilutional effect).
- Individuals living in high altitudes have increased hematocrit results.
- Hemolysis of the sample can alter test results.

Interventions/Implications

Pretest
- Explain to the patient the purpose of the test and the need for a blood sample to be drawn.
- No fasting is required before the test.

Procedure
- Obtain the sample before the patient's bath, shower, or massage, as these activities can temporarily increase the hematocrit.
- The blood sample can be obtained in one of two ways:
  - Hematocrit can be performed on capillary blood, so a finger stick (or heel stick for infants) may be used.
    - After the puncture is made, discard the first drop of blood.
    - Use a capillary tube for collection of a 0.5-mL sample.
    - Do *not* squeeze the tissue to increase the bleeding, as this adds tissue fluids and causes dilution of the sample.
  - Venipuncture may also be used. A 5-mL sample is drawn in a collection tube containing EDTA (lavender-top)
- Gloves are worn throughout the procedure.

Posttest
- If venipuncture is used, invert the tube and gently mix the sample with the anticoagulant.
- Apply pressure at venipuncture or stick site. Apply dressing, periodically assessing for continued bleeding.
- Label the specimen and transport it to the laboratory. Note on the laboratory order slip if the stick method is used.

→ Clinical Alerts

- Hematocrit results may be 5% to 10% higher when capillary blood is used rather than venous blood.
- Hematocrit is usually performed in conjunction with hemoglobin measurement.

- Hematocrit and hemoglobin may be assessed serially to evaluate for blood loss or to evaluate response to treatment for anemia.
- When analyzing data, take into consideration that a shift in fluid from the vascular system to surrounding tissue will yield an increase in hematocrit, because the fluid shift increases the concentration of RBCs.
- A physical condition (such as lung disease) that decreases a person's ability to oxygenate their blood will yield an increase in hemoglobin and hematocrit. The body is trying to compensate for the decrease in oxygen by providing more oxygen carriers.
- After a large loss of blood, as with trauma or a gastrointestinal bleed, the hematocrit will remain normal because equal proportion of RBCs and plasma will be lost. Compensation by the body to increase its vascular capacity will then pull fluid from surrounding tissues and cause a decrease in hematocrit. Hemoglobin will decrease immediately after blood loss.

H

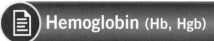

Hemoglobin (Hb, Hgb)

Test Description

Hemoglobin is composed of the *heme* portion, which contains iron and the red pigment porphyrin, and the *globin* portion, which is a protein. By measuring the hemoglobin concentration of the blood, one is determining the oxygen-carrying capacity of the blood. Both high and low hemoglobin counts indicate defects in the balance of red blood cells in the blood, and may indicate disease. This test is usually used to assess for the presence of anemia and polycythemia and to monitor response to treatment for each. When the patient's hydration status is normal, the hemoglobin is approximately one-third of the hematocrit value.

THE EVIDENCE FOR PRACTICE

Practice guidelines for perioperative blood transfusion developed by the American Society of Anesthesiologists (2006) state:

> *Monitoring for transfusion indications.* Measure hemoglobin or hematocrit when substantial blood loss or any indication of organ ischemia occurs. Red blood cells should usually be administered when the hemoglobin concentration is low (e.g., less than 6 g/dL in a young, healthy patient), especially when the anemia is acute. Red blood cells are usually unnecessary when the hemoglobin concentration is more than 10 g/dL. These conclusions may be altered in the presence of anticipated blood loss. The determination of whether intermediate hemoglobin concentrations (i.e., 6 to 10 g/dL) justify or require red blood cell transfusion should be based on any ongoing indication of organ ischemia, potential or actual ongoing bleeding (rate and magnitude), the patient's intravascular volume status, and the patient's risk factors for complications of inadequate oxygenation. These risk factors include a low cardiopulmonary reserve and high oxygen consumption.

Normal Values

Female:	12–16 g/dL (7.4–9.9 mmol/L SI units)
Male:	13–18 g/dL (8.1–11.2 mmol/L SI units)
Pregnancy:	Decreased (dilutional)
Elderly:	Slightly decreased
Newborn:	Increased

Possible Meanings of Abnormal Values

Increased	Decreased
Burns	Addison's disease
Cardiovascular disease	Anemia
Chronic lung disease	Bone marrow suppression
Congenital heart defect	Chronic infection
Cushing's disease	Cirrhosis
Dehydration (hemoconcentration)	Hemorrhage
Erythrocytosis	Hodgkin's disease
Hepatic cancer	Hypothyroidism
Polycythemia vera	Leukemia
Renal cyst	Lymphoma
Secondary polycythemia	Malnutrition
Shock	Multiple myeloma
	Overhydration (hemodilution)
	Pregnancy
	Prosthetic heart values
	Renal disease
	Rheumatic fever
	Subacute bacterial endocarditis
	Systemic lupus erythematosus
	Vitamin deficiency (B_6, B_{12}, folic acid)

Contributing Factors to Abnormal Values

- Leaving the tourniquet in place for more than 1 minute during the procedure will result in hemoconcentration.
- False increases may occur with lipemic samples and when leukocytosis is present.
- Individuals living in high altitudes have increased hemoglobin results.
- Smokers have increased hemoglobin levels.
- Hemolysis of the sample can alter test results.
- Drugs which may *increase* hemoglobin level: gentamicin, methyldopa.
- Drugs which may *decrease* hemoglobin level: antibiotics, antineoplastic agents, apresoline, aspirin, indomethacin, MAO inhibitors, primaquine, rifampin, sulfonamides.

Interventions/Implications

Pretest
- Explain to the patient the purpose of the test and the need for a blood sample to be drawn.
- No fasting is required before the test.

Procedure
- The blood sample can be obtained in one of two ways:
  - Hemoglobin can be performed on capillary blood, so a finger stick (or heel stick for infants) may be used.
    - After the puncture is made, discard the first drop of blood.
    - Use a capillary tube for collection of a 0.5-mL sample.
    - Do *not* squeeze the tissue to increase the bleeding, as this adds tissue fluids and causes dilution of the sample.
  - Venipuncture may also be used. A 5-mL sample is drawn in a collection tube containing EDTA (lavender-top).
- Gloves are worn throughout the procedure.

Posttest
- If venipuncture is used, invert the tube and gently mix the sample with the anticoagulant.
- Apply pressure at venipuncture site. Apply dressing, periodically assessing for continued bleeding.
- Label the specimen and transport it to the laboratory.
- Report abnormal findings to the primary care provider.

→ Clinical Alerts

- Hemoglobin is usually performed in conjunction with hematocrit measurement.
- Hemoglobin and hematocrit may be assessed serially to evaluate for blood loss or to evaluate response to treatment for anemia.
- A physical condition (such as lung disease) that decreases a person's ability to oxygenate their blood will yield an increase in hemoglobin and hematocrit. The body is trying to compensate for the decrease in oxygen by providing more oxygen carriers.
- After a large loss of blood, as with trauma or a gastrointestinal bleed, hemoglobin will decrease immediately and the hematocrit will remain normal because equal proportion of RBCs and plasma will be lost.

Hemoglobin Electrophoresis (Hgb Electrophoresis)

Test Description
Hemoglobin electrophoresis is used to identify abnormal types or amounts of hemoglobin, the oxygen-carrying component of the blood. The hemoglobin molecules are placed in a solution through which an electrical current is sent. The various types of hemoglobin migrate through the solution at different rates, depending on the strength or weakness of their electrical charges. This movement allows a mapping of the types and relative percentages of hemoglobin present in the sample.

The types of hemoglobin which may be included in the electrophoresis are the following:

Hemoglobins normally found in the body

Hemoglobin A$_1$:   This is the major adult hemoglobin normally found in the body.

Hemoglobin A$_2$:   This is a minor hemoglobin normally found in the body.

Hemoglobin F: This hemoglobin, known as fetal hemoglobin, is normally found in the body in a very small quantity in the adult. Increased Hgb F in an adult may be due to sickle cell anemia, leukemia, thalassemia, or hereditary persistence of fetal hemoglobin. In the fetus, it is the primary form of hemoglobin found and is responsible for transporting oxygen when there is little oxygen available.

Hemoglobins usually absent from the body

Hemoglobin C: This hemoglobin causes the RBCs to lyse more easily than normal. These RBCs have a decreased lifespan.

Hemoglobins D/E: When these hemoglobins are present in a patient with sickle cell anemia or thalassemia, the disease tends to be of a more serious nature.

Hemoglobin H: This hemoglobin disrupts normal transport of oxygen to the tissues of the body. Hgb H binds with the oxygen, which prevents it from being available to the tissues.

Hemoglobin S: This hemoglobin causes the RBCs to distort into a sickle shape in response to decreased oxygen levels. Its presence is the basis for the diagnosis of *sickle cell trait*, which occurs in approximately 10% of American blacks, and *sickle cell anemia*, which affects 1 in every 625 American blacks.

H

Normal Values

Adult:	Hgb A$_1$ 95–98%
	Hgb A$_2$ 2–3%
	Hgb F <0.8–2%
	Hgb C, D, E, and H: 0%
Newborn:	Hgb F 50–80%
6 months:	Hgb F 8%
>6 months:	Hgb F 1–2%

Possible Meanings of Abnormal Values

Hemoglobin C trait:	Hgb C >45%
Hemoglobin C disease:	Hgb C >90%
Hemolytic anemia:	Hgb D and Hgb E present
Sickle cell trait:	Hgb S 20–40%
	Hgb A$_1$ 60–80%
	Hgb F <2%
Sickle cell disease:	Hgb S 80–100%
	Hgb F <2%
	HgbA$_1$ is absent
Thalassemia minor:	Hgb F 2–8%
	Hgb A$_2$ <1%

Thalassemia major: Hgb F 20–90%

HgbA₁ is decreased

HgbA₂ may be normal, low, or high

Contributing Factors to Abnormal Values

- Blood transfusions received in the past 3–4 months may alter test results.
- Hemolysis of the sample may alter test results.

Interventions/Implications

Pretest

- Explain to the patient the purpose of the test and the need for a blood sample to be drawn.
- No fasting is required before the test.

Procedure

- A 7-mL blood sample is drawn in a collection tube containing EDTA (lavender-top)
- Gloves are worn throughout the procedure.

Posttest

- Invert and gently mix the sample and the anticoagulant.
- Apply pressure at venipuncture site. Apply dressing, periodically assessing for continued bleeding.
- Label the specimen and transport it to the laboratory.
- Report abnormal findings to the primary care provider.

→ Clinical Alerts

- If hemoglobin abnormalities such as sickle cell trait or sickle cell disease are found, genetic counseling should be offered.

Hepatitis Virus (Hepatitis A, Hepatitis B, Hepatitis C, Hepatitis D, Hepatitis E)

Test Description

Hepatitis is inflammation of the liver which may be caused by a virus, bacteria, or a toxic substance. There are five major types of viral hepatitis which have been identified. Each is caused by a different virus and differs in its incubation period, mode of transmission, and severity.

Hepatitis A virus (HAV), formerly called infectious hepatitis, has an incubation period of 2 to 7 weeks (average of 4 weeks) and is primarily transmitted by the oral-fecal route. This type of hepatitis does not lead to chronic disease. Vaccination is available against HAV. Testing for HAV involves checking IgM and IgG antibodies.

Hepatitis B (HBV), previously known as serum hepatitis, has an incubation period of 6 to 23 weeks (average of 17 weeks). It is spread primarily by blood and body secretions. Hepatitis B is also spread through use of contaminated needles, including those used for tattooing and body piercing. This form of hepatitis is more serious than hepatitis A. It causes liver cell damage, leading to cirrhosis and cancer, and may be fatal. Treatment involves use of interferon and antiviral medication to attempt to control replication of the virus. HBV vaccination provides protection for 20 plus years.

The Hepatitis B virus is composed of an outer capsule surrounding an inner core. The outer capsule contains a protein called the Hepatitis B surface antigen (HBsAg). The inner core contains the Hepatitis B core antigen (HBcAg). The inner core also contains yet another protein called HBeAg. The body responds to the presence of these antigens by producing antibodies against them. Thus, testing includes checking for the presence of the antigens as well as the antibodies (HBsAb, HBcAb, and HBeAb).

Hepatitis C (HCV), was at one time called "non-A, non-B hepatitis". It has an incubation period of 2 to 25 weeks (average 7 to 9 weeks). It is spread primarily by contact with blood and body fluids. It can also be spread through contaminated IV needles and those used for tattooing and body piercing. Clinically, this form of hepatitis is similar to hepatitis B, but of less severity. It is also associated with development of liver cancer and frequently progresses to chronic hepatitis and cirrhosis of the liver. Testing for HCV involves checking for the presence of HCV antibodies.

Hepatitis D (HDV), previously known as delta hepatitis, is caused by the delta virus, an RNA virus. This type of hepatitis only infects people who already have hepatitis B. Its incubation period is 2 to 8 weeks. Vaccination to HBV also prevents HDV infection. Testing for anti-HDV antibodies is usually not done unless the person is found to have HBV.

Hepatitis E (HEV) is rare in the United States. Outbreaks of this virus are associated with use of contaminated water supply. Its incubation period is 2 to 9 weeks (average 40 days). There is no chronic state which develops with this virus, so treatment is not needed. Currently there is no testing for HEV.

Testing for hepatitis

Hepatitis A antibody, IgM and IgG (HAV-Ab)
This test measures antibodies to the hepatitis A virus. If the antibodies are found to be of the IgM type, this is indicative of a current infection with hepatitis A. IgM antibodies appear 2 to 4 weeks after exposure to hepatitis and are detectable for only approximately 4 to 8 weeks. If the antibodies are of the IgG type, this indicates a past infection with hepatitis A and probable immunity to the disease. IgG antibodies are the second type of immunoglobulins which appear in an immune response. These immunoglobulins are present for life, which provides immunity from reinfection with this type of hepatitis.

Hepatitis B surface antigen (HBsAg)
This test measures the surface antigen of the hepatitis B virus. It is used to screen potential blood donors and to diagnose hepatitis B virus. HBsAg is the earliest indicator of hepatitis B, often rising before clinical symptoms appear. This antigen usually appears 4 to 12 weeks after infection, and is indicative of active hepatitis B. If the level of HBsAg continues above normal, the person is considered to be a carrier of hepatitis B. A negative result indicates that the person has never been exposed to the virus or has recovered from acute hepatitis and has rid themselves of the

H

virus. A positive result indicates an active infection but does not indicate whether the virus can be passed to others.

Hepatitis B surface antibody (HBsAb, anti-HBs)

This test measures antibodies to the hepatitis B surface antigen. This antibody appears 2 to 16 weeks after the hepatitis B surface antigen has disappeared. The presence of this antibody demonstrates immunity to the hepatitis B virus, except for a few rare subtypes. This test is used to determine if a vaccine is needed for persons at risk for hepatitis B. A positive result indicates immunity to hepatitis B from vaccination or recovery from an infection.

Hepatitis B core antigen (HBcAg)

This test measures a core antigen of the hepatitis B virus in liver cells. It is used only for research purposes.

Hepatitis B core antibody (HBcAb, anti-HBc)

This test measures antibodies to the core antigen of hepatitis B. This antibody appears in the serum 1 to 4 weeks after contraction of the hepatitis B virus, rises during the chronic phase of the illness, and remains present for the patient's lifetime. The HBcAb is elevated during the time between the disappearance of the surface antigen (HBsAg) and the appearance of the surface antibody (HBsAb). This time period is the "core window" phase. Thus, it is the most reliable test to determine the presence of hepatitis B infection when both the surface antibody and surface antigen are absent.

Hepatitis B e antigen (HBeAg)

This test measures the e antigen of the hepatitis B virus. This antigen usually appears within 4 to 12 weeks of the infection, and is present for only 3 to 6 weeks. Unlike the surface antigen, the e-antigen is found in the blood only when there are viruses also present. The HBeAg level correlates with titers of the virus, so the test is used primarily to evaluate the degree of infectivity. Thus, the presence of HBeAg indicates the virus can be passed to others. If this antigen persists in the blood for more than 3 months, chronic liver disease is probable. Measurement of HBeAg may also be used to monitor the effectiveness of HBV treatment, since successful treatment should lead to no HBeAg remaining in the blood and to the presence of anti-HBe.

Hepatitis B e antibody (HBeAb, anti-HBe)

This test measures antibodies to the e antigen of the hepatitis B virus. This antibody appears 8 to 16 weeks after the infection and usually indicates the acute infection is over. The presence of this antibody along with a positive result in testing for the hepatitis B surface antigen (HBsAg) usually indicates a carrier state.

Hepatitis C antibody (anti-HCV)

This test measures antibodies to the hepatitis C virus. Most cases of posttransfusion hepatitis are hepatitis C in nature. The presence of anti-HCV antibodies indicate exposure to HCV, but do not indicate whether there is acute, chronic, or resolved disease.

Hepatitis D antibody (anti-HDV)

This test measures antibodies to the delta hepatitis virus. A positive test result suggests recent infection or carrier state for the virus, which only occurs in conjunction with the hepatitis B virus.

THE EVIDENCE FOR PRACTICE

Currently the U.S. Preventive Services Task Force (USPSTF):

- Recommends against routine screening for hepatitis C virus (HCV) infection in asymptomatic adults who are not at increased risk (general population) for infection.
- Found insufficient evidence to recommend for or against routine screening for HCV infection in adults at high risk for infection (noting no evidence was found showing such screening leads to improved long-term health outcomes).

Normal Values

Negative

Possible Meanings of Abnormal Values

H

Positive

Hepatitis A Antibody (HAV-Ab)
Positive, IgM: Acute hepatitis A infection
Positive, IgG: Past exposure to hepatitis A, probable immunity

Hepatitis B surface antigen (HBsAg)
Either active/chronic hepatitis B or a carrier state

Hepatitis B surface antibody (HBsAb, anti-HBs)
Immunity to hepatitis B (due to natural infection or Hepatitis B vaccination)

Hepatitis B core antibody (HBcAb, anti-HBc)
Hepatitis B infection

Hepatitis B e antigen (HBeAg)
Hepatitis B infection

Hepatitis B e antibody (HBeAb, anti-HBe)
Hepatitis B infection or carrier state

Hepatitis C antibody (anti-HCV)
Hepatitis C (acute, chronic, or resolved)

Hepatitis D antibody (anti-HDV)
Hepatitis D infection or carrier state

Contributing Factors to Abnormal Values

- Diagnostic testing in which radionuclides were used within 1 week prior to this test may falsely elevate test results.

Interventions/Implications

Pretest
- Explain to the patient the purpose of the test and the need for a blood sample to be drawn.
- No fasting is required before the test.

Procedure
- A 7-mL blood sample is drawn in a red-top collection tube.
- Gloves are worn throughout the procedure.

Posttest
- Apply pressure at venipuncture site. Apply dressing, periodically assessing for continued bleeding.
- Label the specimen and transport it to the laboratory.
- Report abnormal findings to the primary care provider.

Clinical Alerts

- A helpful table for interpreting Hepatitis B tests can be found at the website for the Centers for Disease Control and Prevention, National Center for Infectious Diseases at: http://www.cdc.gov/ncidod/diseases/hepatitis/b/Bserology.htm.
- Close monitoring of patients with hepatitis is needed regarding liver function and continuation of treatment regimens, when appropriate.

Herpes Simplex Antibody (Herpes Simplex Virus [HSV], HSV-1, HSV-2, Herpesvirus)

Test Description
This test measures antibodies to the herpes simplex virus. Herpes simplex is a common viral infection transmitted through contact with mucous membrane secretions. Herpes simplex 1 (HSV-1) is caused by the *human herpesvirus 1* and is usually found in the respiratory tract, eyes, or mouth (cold sores). Herpes simplex 2 (HSV-2) is caused by the *human herpesvirus 2* and is generally found in the genitourinary tract. HSV-2 is also known as genital herpes (herpes genitalis). At least 50 million persons in the United States have genital HSV infection.

The common pattern of infection with the herpes virus is primary infection, latency, and reactivation (secondary infection). Both type-specific and nontype-specific antibodies to HSV develop during the first several weeks after infection and persist indefinitely.

A newborn may become infected (neonatal herpes) during vaginal delivery if the mother is infected with genital herpes at the time of delivery. Should a woman acquire the herpes virus during pregnancy, the fetus may have congenital herpes, resulting in disorders of the central nervous system and brain damage.

Both IgG and IgM titers may be performed. HSV Antibody IgG titers typically rise approximately 1 to 2 weeks after a primary infection, peak 6 to 8 weeks after infection, and then decline. An increase in the HSV Antibody IgM titer occurs several days after initial HSV infection.

THE EVIDENCE FOR PRACTICE
Cesarean delivery should be performed on women with first-episode HSV who have active genital lesions at delivery.

Normal Values
Negative

Possible Meanings of Abnormal Values

Positive
HSV infection

Contributing Factors to Abnormal Values
- Hemolysis of the sample will alter test results.

Interventions/Implications

Pretest
- Explain to the patient the purpose of the test and the need for a blood sample to be drawn.
- No fasting is required before the test.

Procedure
- A 7-mL blood sample is drawn in a red-top collection tube.
- A culture of any lesions may also be obtained to isolate the type of HSV.
- Gloves are worn throughout the procedure.

Posttest
- Apply pressure at venipuncture site. Apply dressing, periodically assessing for continued bleeding.
- Label the specimen and transport it to the laboratory.
- Report abnormal findings to the primary care provider.

→ Clinical Alerts

- Explain to the pregnant patient that, should genital herpes be present at the time of delivery, cesarean section may be necessary.
- Sexual partners of patients testing positive for HSV-2 should also be tested. Education is needed regarding prevention of transmission, treatment during active infection, and suppression therapy.

Hexosaminidase (HEX A, HEX B)

Test Description
Hexosaminidase is an enzyme involved in the hydrolysis of molecules containing hexose. There are hexosaminidase A, B, and S. With a deficiency of hexosaminidase, certain lipids accumulate in lysosomes. The primary example of resulting disease is Tay-Sachs disease, in which lysosomes fill with GM2 gangliosides due to a deficiency of hexosaminidase A. In the acute infantile form of Tay-Sachs disease, symptoms begin between 3 and 6 months of age. Progressive neurodegeneration leads to total incapacitation and death, usually by age 4 years. Juvenile (subacute) and adult-onset variants of the deficiency have later onsets and slower progression of symptoms.

The diagnosis of hexosaminidase A deficiency relies upon the demonstration of absent to near-absent beta-hexosaminidase A (HEX A) enzymatic activity in the serum or white blood cells of a symptomatic individual in the presence of normal or elevated activity of the beta-hexosaminidase B (HEX B) isoenzyme. Hexosaminidase A deficiency is inherited in an autosomal recessive manner. Serum testing can be done in males and nonpregnant females. Leukocyte testing is the only testing which can be done on a pregnant female. Serum testing is contraindicated in the pregnant female because pregnancy normally causes lower levels of HEX A, thus testing during pregnancy would give a false appearance of being a carrier of Tay-Sachs disease.

Normal Values

See reference laboratory for values

Possible Meanings of Abnormal Values

Decreased

Hexosaminidase A: Tay-Sachs disease
Hexosaminidase A and B: Sandhoff disease

Contributing Factors to Abnormal Values

- Pregnancy and oral contraceptives cause *falsely-decreased* levels of hexosaminidase A. Serum testing is *not* to be done during pregnancy or if taking OCPs.

Interventions/Implications

Pretest
- Explain to the patient the purpose of the test and the need for a blood sample to be drawn.
- Overnight fasting is required before the test.

Procedure
- A 7-mL blood sample is drawn in a red-top collection tube.
- Gloves are worn throughout the procedure.

Posttest
- Apply pressure at venipuncture site. Apply dressing, periodically assessing for continued bleeding.
- Label the specimen and transport it to the laboratory.
- Report abnormal findings to the primary care provider.

→ Clinical Alerts

- Genetic counseling is recommended prior to pregnancy.

CONTRAINDICATIONS!

- Pregnancy
- Use of oral contraceptives

High-Density Lipoprotein (HDL)

Test Description
Cholesterol is synthesized in the liver from dietary fats. It is transported in the blood by the low density lipoproteins (LDLs, or "bad" cholesterol) and high-density lipoproteins (HDLs, or "good" cholesterol). HDLs carry excess cholesterol back to the liver, where it is broken down and removed from the body in bile. Thus, higher levels of HDL are desired as they seem to be associated with a decreased risk for coronary heart disease.

The high-density lipoprotein (HDL) level is measured as part of the lipid profile. A low HDL level (<40 mg/dL) is considered a major risk factor for cardiovascular disease, and thus has an impact on the patient's LDL goal. A high HDL (≥60 mg/dL) is considered a "negative" risk factor. That is, its presence removes one risk factor from the person's total. Low HDL (<40 mg/dL for men, <50 mg/dL for women) is also one of the risk factors for metabolic syndrome.

THE EVIDENCE FOR PRACTICE
According to the Third Report of the National Cholesterol Education Program (NCEP) Expert Panel on Detection, Evaluation, and Treatment of High Blood Cholesterol in Adults (http://www.nhlbi.nih.gov/guidelines/cholesterol/atp3_rpt.htm):
* In all adults aged 20 years or older, a fasting lipoprotein profile (total cholesterol, LDL cholesterol, HDL cholesterol, and triglycerides) should be obtained once every 5 years. If the testing opportunity is nonfasting, only the values for total cholesterol and HDL cholesterol will be usable. In such a case, if total cholesterol is ≥200 mg/dL or high density lipoprotein is <40 mg/dL, a follow-up lipoprotein profile is needed for appropriate management based on LDL.

Normal Values
40–60 mg/dL (1.04–1.55 mmol/L SI units)
Values >60 mg/dL: Considered a *negative* risk factor for heart disease
Values <40 mg/dL: Considered a major risk factor for heart disease

Possible Meanings of Abnormal Values

Increased	Decreased
Alcoholism	Chronic inactivity
Chronic liver disease	Diabetes mellitus
Decreased risk for CHD	End-stage liver disease
Long-term aerobic exercises	Hyperthyroidism
	Hypertriglyceridemia
	Increased risk of CHD
	Metabolic syndrome
	Obesity
	Renal failure
	Smoking
	Stress

Contributing Factors to Abnormal Values

- Radiologic contrast agents and recent weight changes may alter test results.
- HDL levels may be affected by acute illness, stress, and pregnancy. HDL assessment should be postponed until 6 weeks after resolution.
- Drugs which may *increase* HDL levels: alpha blockers, carbamazepine, cholesterol lowering agents, estrogens, hydroxychloroquine, indapamide, insulin, oral hypoglycemic agents, phenobarbital, phenytoin.
- Drugs which may *decrease* HDL levels: anabolic steroids, beta blockers, methimazole, methyldopa, neomycin, oral contraceptives, progestins, raloxifene, tamoxifen, thiazide diuretics, verapamil.

Interventions/Implications

Pretest
- Explain to the patient the purpose of the test and the need for a blood sample to be drawn.
- Fasting for 12 hours is required prior to the test. Water is permitted.

Procedure
- A 7-mL blood sample is drawn in a lavender-top collection tube.
- Gloves are worn throughout the procedure.

Posttest
- Apply pressure at venipuncture site. Apply dressing, periodically assessing for continued bleeding.
- Label the specimen and transport it to the laboratory.
- Report abnormal findings to the primary care provider.

Clinical Alerts

- If the test result is <40 mg/dL, NCEP guidelines suggest first reaching the LDL goal, then intensifying weight management and increasing physical activity.
- Depending on levels of other lipoproteins and the degree of hypercholesterolemia present, cholesterol-lowering medication may be initiated, along with lifestyle modifications.

HIV Antibody Tests (Human Immunodeficiency Virus [HIV] Antibody Test, Acquired Immunodeficiency Syndrome [AIDS] Serology, ELISA for HIV, Western Blot for HIV)

Test Description

Human immunodeficiency virus (HIV) is the virus which causes acquired immunodeficiency syndrome (AIDS). HIV attacks the body's helper T cells which are important components of cell-mediated immunity. This results in immunosuppression and susceptibility to opportunistic infections such as *Pneumocystis carinii* and *Candida albicans*. Modes of transmission of the virus include direct contact between the blood of the infected person with that of an uninfected person and through sexual and body fluid transmission. Thus, individuals at high risk for AIDS include sexually active homosexuals, individuals with multiple sexual partners, intravenous drug users who have shared needles, persons who have received numerous transfusions of blood products (such as hemophiliacs), and newborn infants of infected women.

Multiple tests are available for HIV testing. The most common is the enzyme-linked immunosorbent assay, or *ELISA*. This test is used to screen for HIV, but is not considered to be a confirmatory test. This is due to false-negative and false-positive test results which are possible with this testing method. ELISA detects antibodies to HIV, not the HIV antigens. Therefore, a positive ELISA will not occur until antibodies have had time to form. If the ELISA is positive, the test is repeated using the same blood sample. If the test is again positive, the *Western blot* is performed. The Western blot test uses electrophoresis techniques to separate out component proteins of HIV, thus allowing detection of HIV antibodies. Should the Western blot test also be positive, the person is considered to have serologic evidence of HIV infection. It is important to note, and inform the patient, that this means there has been exposure to the virus and the virus is present in the body, but this does not necessarily indicate the occurrence of clinical AIDS. If the ELISA testing is positive, but this is not confirmed by the Western blot test, repeat testing is required in 3 to 6 months.

H

THE EVIDENCE FOR PRACTICE

According to the Centers for Disease Control and Prevention (CDC) (http://www.cdc.gov/mmwr/PDF/rr/rr5514.pdf):

- In all health-care settings, screening for HIV infection should be performed routinely for all patients aged 13 to 64 years. Health-care providers should initiate screening unless prevalence of undiagnosed HIV infection in their patients has been documented to be <0.1%. In the absence of existing data for HIV prevalence, health-care providers should initiate voluntary HIV screening until they establish that the diagnostic yield is <1 per 1000 patients screened, at which point such screening is no longer warranted.
- All patients initiating treatment for TB should be screened routinely for HIV infection.
- All patients seeking treatment for STDs, including all patients attending STD clinics, should be screened routinely for HIV during each visit for a new complaint, regardless of whether the patient is known or suspected to have specific behavior risks for HIV infection.
- Screening should be voluntary and undertaken only with the patient's knowledge and understanding that HIV testing is planned.

Normal Values

Negative for antibodies to HIV

Possible Meanings of Abnormal Values

Increased
AIDS
HIV exposure

Contributing Factors to Abnormal Values

- Antibody results may be negative for up to 3 to 6 months after infection with HIV. This is due to the latency period of the virus. During this period of time, known as the "window phase", the patient shows no symptoms of the infection. However, the patient may pass on the infection to others during this phase.

Interventions/Implications

Pretest

- Explain to the patient the purpose of the test and the need for a blood sample to be drawn.
- No fasting is required before the test.

Procedure

- A 7-mL blood sample is drawn in a red-top collection tube.
- An informed written consent is usually required.
- Gloves are worn throughout the procedure.

Posttest

- Apply pressure at venipuncture site. Apply dressing, periodically assessing for continued bleeding.
- Label the specimen, following institutional policy regarding maintaining confidentiality of patient's identity and test results. Transport the specimen to the laboratory.
- Report abnormal findings to the primary care provider.

→ Clinical Alerts

- Possible complication: risk of infection at venipuncture site due to immunocompromised state. Teach patient to notify health-care provider if drainage, redness, warmth, edema, or pain at the site or fever occur.
- Provide to the patient emotional support, counseling, and education prior to and following HIV testing.
- When HIV infection is diagnosed, health-care providers should strongly encourage patients to disclose their HIV status to their spouses, current sex partners, and previous sex partners and recommend that these partners be tested for HIV infection.
- Notifying a patient that routine HIV testing will be performed might result in acknowledgement of risk behaviors and offers an opportunity to discuss HIV infection and how it can be prevented.

Homocysteine (HCY)

Test Description

Homocysteine is a sulfur-containing amino acid formed in the conversion of methionine to cysteine. Methionine is one of the essential amino acids the body receives from dietary intake. In healthy cells, homocysteine is quickly converted to other products.

Since the 1990s, it has been known that a high plasma homocysteine level is associated with increased risk of cardiovascular disease. What is not known is whether the elevated homocysteine level causes cardiovascular disease or is a consequence of having cardiovascular disease.

Folate, Vitamin B_6, and Vitamin B_{12} are needed to metabolize homocysteine. In deficiency of these vitamins, homocysteine levels rise, sometimes before the vitamin deficiency is found. Adding folic acid and other B vitamins to the diet is effective in lowering homocysteine levels, but whether this reduction improves the clinical outlook for the patient is unknown.

Another cause of increased homocysteine levels is a rare inherited disorder called *homocystinuria*. In this condition, the person has a dysfunctional enzyme that does not allow the usual breakdown of methionine. Methionine and homocysteine build up in the body, resulting in very high levels of homocysteine in the blood and urine. Individuals with homocystinuria experience skeletal deformities, ocular abnormalities, mental retardation, hepatic steatosis, and premature death. They also have a very high risk of thromboembolism and atherosclerosis, leading to premature cardiovascular disease.

H

THE EVIDENCE FOR PRACTICE

The American Heart Association (AHA) has not yet called hyperhomocysteinemia a major risk factor for cardiovascular disease. While recognizing that homocysteine may promote atherosclerosis by damaging the inner lining of arteries and promoting blood clots, the AHA notes that a causal link has not yet been established, and no controlled treatment study has shown that folic acid supplements reduce the risk of atherosclerosis or that taking these vitamins affects the development or recurrence of cardiovascular disease. The AHA does recommend a healthy, balanced diet containing the recommended daily value of folic acid of 400 µg.

Normal Values

Male: 1–2.12 mg/L (7.4–15.7 µmol/L SI units)
Female: 0.53–2 mg/L (3.9–14.8 µmol/L SI units)

Possible Meanings of Abnormal Values

Increased (Hyperhomocysteinemia)
CVD risk factor
Homocystinuria
Smoking
Vitamin deficiencies (folate, B_6, B_{12})

Contributing Factors to Abnormal Values

- Homocysteine levels can increase with age and with smoking.
- Drugs that *increase* homocysteine levels: carbamazepine, cycloserine, isoniazid, methotrexate, penicillamine, phenytoin, procarbazine.

Interventions/Implications

Pretest
- Explain to the patient the purpose of the test and the need for a blood sample to be drawn.
- No fasting is required before the test.

Procedure
- A 7-mL blood sample is drawn in a gold-top (serum separator) collection tube.
- Gloves are worn throughout the procedure.

Posttest
- Apply pressure at venipuncture site. Apply dressing, periodically assessing for continued bleeding.
- Label the specimen and transport it to the laboratory.
- Report abnormal findings to the primary care provider.

Human Leukocyte Antigen Test (HLA Test, HLA Typing, Histocompatibility Antigen Test, Tissue Typing)

Test Description

Human leukocyte antigens (HLAs) are glycoproteins found on almost all nucleated cells in the body, but have their highest concentrations on the surface of leukocytes. HLAs are the primary components used by the body's immune system for determining whether a substance is self or nonself (foreign). Many HLAs have been identified and research continues to discover more. Some specific antigens have been found to be associated with certain diseases. The most common example of this is HLA-B27, which has been found in patients with ankylosing spondylitis, Reiter's syndrome, and rheumatoid arthritis. Others have been found to be associated with celiac disease and diabetes mellitus Type 1.

The HLA test is done to determine what leukocyte antigens are present on the surface of the cells. This information is crucial when organ transplantation is being considered, since histocompatibility (tissue compatibility) *must* be present in order to minimize the chance for organ rejection. For bone marrow transplantation, HLA A, B, C, plus HLA-DR, DQ phenotype antigen identity is usually recommended.

Another use of HLA typing is paternity testing. In this situation, the HLAs of a child are compared with those of the potential father. If the HLA typing does not match, it disqualifies the man from being the father. However, if the HLA typing does match, it indicates that man *might* be the father.

Normal Values

Requires interpretation of HLA antigen combination

Examples of Possible Meanings of Abnormal Values

Positive for HLA-B27:	Ankylosing spondylitis, Reiter's syndrome, Rheumatoid arthritis, Graves' disease
Positive for DR2/DQ1:	Idiopathic narcolepsy

Positive for B8:	Celiac disease, Chronic active hepatitis, Sarcoidosis
Positive for A3:	Hemochromatosis
Positive for Bw15 plus B8:	Diabetes mellitus Type 1

Contributing Factors to Abnormal Values

- Hemolysis of the blood sample may alter test results.
- Receipt of a blood transfusion within 72 hours prior to the test will alter test results.

Interventions/Implications

Pretest
- Explain to the patient the purpose of the test and the need for a blood sample to be drawn.
- No fasting is required before the test.

Procedure
- A 7-mL blood sample is drawn in a collection tube containing heparin (green-top).
- Gloves are worn throughout the procedure.

Posttest
- Apply pressure at venipuncture site. Apply dressing, periodically assessing for continued bleeding.
- Label the specimen and transport it to the laboratory.
- Report abnormal findings to the primary care provider.

H

➔ Clinical Alerts

- The presence of a specific HLA is not necessarily indicative of disease. For example, HLA-B27 antigen is found in 80% to 90% of people with ankylosing spondylitis, but HLA-B27 is also present in 5% to 7% of people without autoimmune disease. Thus, the HLA finding must be considered in association with any symptoms the patient is experiencing.

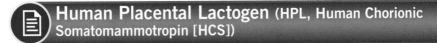

Human Placental Lactogen (HPL, Human Chorionic Somatomammotropin [HCS])

Test Description
This test is used to evaluate placental functioning. Human placental lactogen (HPL) is a protein hormone produced by the placenta. In pregnancy, HPL promotes increased blood glucose levels. The level of HPL slowly increases throughout pregnancy, reaching a level of 7 mcg/mL at term, and dropping abruptly to zero after delivery. Low HPL values during pregnancy may indicate fetal distress and warrant further assessment of fetal viability with nonstress testing and amniocentesis.

Normal Values
Value rises during pregnancy:

5th–27th week:	<4.6 µg/mL
28th–31st week:	2.4–6.1 µg/mL

32nd–35th week: 3.7–7.7 µg/mL
36th week to term: 5–8.6 µg/mL

Possible Meanings of Abnormal Values

Increased	Decreased
Maternal diabetes mellitus	Choriocarcinoma
Maternal liver disease	Fetal distress
Maternal sickle cell disease	Hydatidiform mole
Multiple pregnancies	Intrauterine growth retardation (IUGR)
Rh isoimmunization	Placental insufficiency
	Postmaturity syndrome
	Threatened abortion
	Toxemia of pregnancy

Contributing Factors to Abnormal Values

- Hemolysis of the blood sample and recent radioactive scans may alter test results

Interventions/Implications

Pretest
- Explain to the patient the purpose of the test and the need for a blood sample to be drawn.
- No fasting is required before the test.

Procedure
- A 7-mL blood sample is drawn in a red-top collection tube.
- Gloves are worn throughout the procedure.

Posttest
- Apply pressure at venipuncture site. Apply dressing, periodically assessing for continued bleeding.
- Label the specimen and transport it to the laboratory.
- Report abnormal findings to the primary care provider.

Human T-Cell Lymphotrophic I/II Antibody (HTLV-I, HTLV-II)

Test Description
Human T-cell lymphotrophic virus (HTLV) is the name for several different retroviruses. HTLV-III is the former name of the human immunodeficiency virus (HIV) known to cause acquired immunodeficiency syndrome (AIDS). HTLV-I and HTLV-II do not cause AIDS. They are, however, associated with other types of diseases. HTLV-I is linked with adult T-cell leukemia. HTLV-II is associated with adult hairy-cell leukemia. However, presence of the antibody to these viruses in the blood does not necessarily mean the person will develop the disease.

Normal Values
Negative

Possible Meanings of Abnormal Values

Positive

Acute HTLV infection
Adult T-cell leukemia
Adult hairy-cell leukemia
Demyelinating neurological disorders
Tropical spastic paraparesis

Interventions/Implications

Pretest
- Explain to the patient the purpose of the test and the need for a blood sample to be drawn.
- No fasting is required before the test.

Procedure
- A 7-mL blood sample is drawn in a red-top collection tube.
- Gloves are worn throughout the procedure.

Posttest
- Apply pressure at venipuncture site. Apply dressing, periodically assessing for continued bleeding.
- Label the specimen and transport it on ice to the laboratory.
- Report abnormal findings to the primary care provider.

17-Hydroxycorticosteroids (17-OHCS, Porter-Silber Test)

Test Description

The adrenal cortex secretes three types of hormones: the glucocorticoids (primarily cortisol), the mineralocorticoids (aldosterone), and the sex hormones (androgens, estrogen, progesterone). The test for 17-hydroxycorticosteroids (17-OHCS) measures the metabolites, or products, of the breakdown of the glucocorticoids known as cortisone and hydrocortisone. It is thus a test of adrenal cortical function. This test has been used in the differential diagnosis of Cushing's syndrome and Addison's disease. Urinary cortisol levels and plasma cortisol levels are more sensitive tests and are replacing this test.

Normal Values

Female: 2.0–6.0 mg/day (5.5–17 µmol/day SI units)
Male: 3.0–10.0 mg/day (8–28 µmol/day SI units)

Possible Meanings of Abnormal Values

Increased	Decreased
Acetonuria	Addison's disease
Acromegaly	Adrenal infarction
Acute illness	Adrenal hemorrhage
Adrenal hyperplasia	Anorexia nervosa

Adrenal tumor
Cushing's syndrome
Ectopic ACTH-producing tumor
Glucosuria
Fructosuria
Hirsutism
Hypertension (severe)
Insomnia
Obesity
Pituitary tumor
Pregnancy
Stress
Thyrotoxicosis
Virilism

Congenital adrenal hyperplasia
Hypopituitarism
Hypothyroidism

Contributing Factors to Abnormal Values

- Drugs which may *increase* 17-OHCS levels: acetazolamide, ascorbic acid, cefoxitin, chloral hydrate, chlordiazepoxide, chlorpromazine, colchicine, corticotropin, cortisone acetate, digitalis, erythromycin, gonadotropins, hydrocortisone, hydroxyzine, iodides, meprobamate, methenamine, methicillin, paraldehyde, quinidine, quinine, spironolactone.
- Drugs which may *decrease* 17-OHCS levels: apresoline, carbamazepine, corticosteroids, estrogens, medroxyprogesterone acetate, meperidine, morphine, oral contraceptives, pentazocine, phenothiazines, phenytoin, promethazine, reserpine, salicylates, thiazides.

Interventions/Implications

Pretest
- Explain 24-hour urine collection procedure to the patient.
- Stress the importance of saving *all* urine in the 24-hour period. Instruct the patient to avoid contaminating the urine with toilet paper or feces.
- Inform the patient of the presence of a preservative in the collection bottle.
- If possible, withhold any drugs which may interfere with test results.

Procedure
- Obtain the proper container containing 1 g of boric acid as preservative from the laboratory.
- Begin the testing period in the morning after the patient's first voiding, which is discarded.
- Timing of the 24-hour period begins at the time the first voiding is discarded.
- *All* urine for the next 24 hours is collected in the container, which is to be kept refrigerated or on ice.
- If any urine is accidentally discarded during the 24-hour period, the test must be discontinued and a new test begun.
- The ending time of the 24-hour collection period should be posted in the patient's room.
- Gloves are worn whenever dealing with the specimen collection.

Posttest
- At the end of the 24-hour collection period, label and send the urine container on ice to the laboratory as soon as possible.
- Report abnormal findings to the primary care provider.

5-Hydroxyindoleacetic Acid (5-HIAA)

Test Description
Serotonin is synthesized from the amino acid tryptophan by hormone-producing enterochromaffin cells in the gut and bronchi. The functions of serotonin are many and include vasodilation and regulation of smooth muscle contraction, such as that occurring during peristalsis. Serotonin is metabolized in the liver, resulting in the production of 5-hydroxyindoleacetic acid (5-HIAA), which is excreted in the urine. Early carcinoid tumors of the intestine secrete abnormal amounts of serotonin. This abnormal secretion, which can reach as high as 300 to 1000 mg/24 hours, can be found through measurement of 5-HIAA in the urine.

H

Normal Values

Qualitative random sample:	Negative
Quantitative:	2–9 mg/24 hours (10–47 µmol/day SI units)
	Lower in women than in men

Possible Meanings of Abnormal Values

Increased
Benign or malignant carcinoid tumors of the intestine
Intake of foods high in indoles (see Contributing Factors to Abnormal Values)
Mastocytosis
Tumors in other organs, including endocrine tumors

Contributing Factors to Abnormal Values
- Test results may be altered by improper 24-hour urine collection technique, severe diarrhea, or ingestion of foods containing large amounts of serotonin, such as avocados, bananas, eggplants, pineapples, red plums, tomatoes, and walnuts.
- Drugs which may interfere with testing due to physiologic response: acetaminophen, alpha blockers, beta blockers, atenolol, bromocriptine, bronchodilators, clonidine, digoxin, isoniazid, L-dopa, labetelol, methyldopa, MAO inhibitors, nitroglycerin, sympathomimetic amines, phenobarbital, phenothiazines, pentolamine, reserpine, salicylates, tricyclic antidepressants.

Interventions/Implications
Pretest
- Explain 24-hour urine collection procedure to the patient.
- Stress the importance of saving *all* urine in the 24-hour period. Instruct the patient to avoid contaminating the urine with toilet paper or feces.
- Inform the patient of the presence of a preservative in the collection bottle.
- Instruct the patient to avoid tobacco, tea, and coffee for 3 days prior to specimen collection.
- Instruct patient to maintain a diet low in indoles (see Contributing Factors to Abnormal Values) for 3 days before the test.

- Check with the laboratory regarding any questionable medications that patient may be taking to determine the need to hold any medications prior to the test.
- Notify the health-care provider of the patient's medications which may alter the test results.

Procedure
- Obtain the proper container containing 1 g of boric acid as preservative from the laboratory.
- Begin the testing period in the morning after the patient's first voiding, which is discarded.
- Timing of the 24-hour period begins at the time the first voiding is discarded.
- *All* urine for the next 24 hours is collected in the container, which is to be kept refrigerated or on ice.
- If any urine is accidentally discarded during the 24-hour period, the test must be discontinued and a new test begun.
- The ending time of the 24-hour collection period should be posted in the patient's room.
- Gloves are worn whenever dealing with the specimen collection.

Posttest
- At the end of the 24-hour collection period, label and send the urine container on ice to the laboratory as soon as possible.
- Resume the patient's usual diet and medications following test completion.
- Report abnormal findings to the primary care provider.

Hysterosalpingography (Uterosalpingography)

Test Description
Hysterosalpingography is used to detect blocked fallopian tubes. It can also confirm the presence of uterine abnormalities. The test is used primarily as a portion of an infertility workup. A cannula is inserted into the cervix through which contrast medium is injected. This allows for viewing of the uterus and the fallopian tubes by fluoroscopy. The incidence of allergic reaction to the dye is reduced, since the dye is usually not absorbed when administered in this way. Radiographic films are taken throughout the procedure.

THE EVIDENCE FOR PRACTICE
The basic workup of the infertile couple should include complete history and physical, ovulation documentation, semen analysis, and hysterosalpingography.

Normal Values
Normal size, shape, position of uterus and fallopian tubes
Patent fallopian tubes

Possible Meanings of Abnormal Values
Ectopic pregnancy
Intrauterine adhesions

Intrauterine fibroids
Intrauterine foreign body
Partial or complete blockage of fallopian tube(s)
Uterine fistula

Contributing Factors to Abnormal Values

- Retained barium, gas, or stool in the intestines may result in poor quality films.

Interventions/Implications

Pretest

- Explain to the patient the purpose of the test. Provide any written teaching materials available on the subject. Note that discomfort during this test is due to menstrual-like cramping due to injection of the dye. Shoulder pain may be experienced as the contrast medium normally leaks into the peritoneal cavity, irritating the diaphragm and stimulating the phrenic nerve.
- Check for allergies to iodine, shellfish, or contrast medium dye. Inform the radiologist of such possible allergy.
- Obtain a signed informed consent.
- No fasting is required prior to the test.
- A laxative the night prior to the test, or an enema or suppository the morning of the test may be ordered.
- The patient should empty the bladder prior to the test.
- Preprocedure sedation may be ordered.

Procedure

- The patient is placed in the lithotomy position.
- A plain abdominal x-ray is taken to check for absence of retained barium, gas, or stool in the intestine.
- A speculum is inserted into the vagina.
- The cervix is cleansed, and a cannula is inserted into the cervix.
- Contrast medium is injected through the cannula.
- The flow of the dye is followed fluoroscopically through the uterus and fallopian tubes.
- Films are taken throughout the procedure.
- Gloves are worn throughout the procedure.

Posttest

- Most allergic reactions to radiopaque dye occur within 30 minutes of administration of the contrast medium. Observe the patient closely for: respiratory distress, hypotension, edema, hives, rash, tachycardia, and/or laryngeal stridor. Emergency resuscitation equipment must be readily accessible.
- Observe for allergic reaction to the dye for 24 hours.
- A perineal pad is applied. Inform the patient that a bloody vaginal discharge may be present for 1 to 2 days after the procedure.
- Monitor vital signs at least every 4 hours for 24 hours.
- Observe for indications of infection, including elevated temperature, chills, flushing, tachycardia, and abdominal pain.
- Report abnormal findings to the primary care provider.

→ **Clinical Alerts**

- Possible complications include: allergic reaction to dye, infection of the endometrium or fallopian tubes, and uterine perforation.

CONTRAINDICATIONS!

- Patients who are allergic to iodine, shellfish, or contrast medium dye
- Patients who are pregnant or suspected of being pregnant
- Patients who are in their menses
- Patients with undiagnosed vaginal bleeding
- Patients with pelvic inflammatory disease

Immunoelectrophoresis (Gamma Globulin Electrophoresis, Immunoglobulin Electrophoresis)

Test Description
The total blood protein consists of albumin and globulin, which is further divided into the alpha, beta, and gamma globulins. The gamma globulins are called *immunoglobulins*, since, as components of antibodies, they play a vital role in the immune process. Five types of immunoglobulins are measured during electrophoresis: IgA, IgD, IgE, IgG, and IgM.

Immunoglobulin G (IgG) is the most abundant of the gamma globulins, accounting for approximately 75% of the total. IgG provides protection against viruses, bacteria, and toxins, and is the only immunoglobulin which crosses the placenta. IgG is particularly important in the secondary response of the immune system. When the immune system is confronted with an antigen for the first time, the *primary* response is made by IgM and is soon followed by an elevation of the IgG level. IgG retains memory of the antigen, so that the next time the immune system is challenged by the antigen, IgG is ready to immediately respond.

Immunoglobulin A (IgA), which makes up 10% to 15% of the total gamma globulins, is the second most abundant gamma globulin. IgA is present in several body fluids, including colostrum, saliva, and tears. This immunoglobulin is considered the first line of defense against organisms attempting to invade the respiratory, gastrointestinal, and urinary tracts.

Immunoglobulin M (IgM) accounts for 7% to 10% of the gamma globulins. It is the first immunoglobulin to respond to an antigen coming in contact with the immune system for the first time. Thus, since the IgM level is the first to increase in the primary response, the IgM level is an indicator of an acute infection. IgM is also responsible for the formation of natural antibodies, such as the ABO blood groups.

Immunoglobulin E (IgE) is present in very small amounts. It plays a role in allergic responses, such as hypersensitivity and anaphylactic reactions. Its level also increases in parasitic infestations.

Immunoglobulin D (IgD) is also present in very small amounts. Its function is unknown.

To conduct *immunoelectrophoresis*, an electrical current is passed through the blood serum, causing the various immunoglobulins to separate according to their electrical charge. Each immunoglobulin forms a band which has a characteristic appearance. This appearance is altered when an abnormality of a particular immunoglobulin is present.

Normal Values

Adult:

    IgG: 639–1349 mg/dL (6.39–13.49 g/L SI units)

    IgA: 70–312 mg/dL (0.70–3.12 g/L SI units)

    IgM: 56–352 mg/dL (0.56–3.52 g/L SI units)

    IgD: 0.5–3 mg/dL (0.005–0.03 g/L SI units)

    IgE: 0.01–0.04 mg/dL (0.0001–0.0004 g/L SI units)

Newborn:

    IgG: 640–1,250 mg/dL (6.40–12.50 g/L SI units)

    IgA: 0–11 mg/dL (0–0.11 g/L SI units)

    IgM: 5–30 mg/dL (0.05–0.30 g/L SI units)

    IgD and IgE: Negligible

Possible Meanings of Abnormal Values

IgG

Increased	Decreased
IgG myeloma	Agammaglobulinemia
Infectious disease	AIDS
Liver disease	Bacterial infections
Lymphomas	Humoral immune deficiency
Multiple sclerosis	IgA myeloma
Neurosyphilis	Leukemia
Parasitic disease	Lymphoid aplasia
Rheumatic fever	Preeclampsia
Rheumatoid arthritis	
Sarcoidosis	
Sjögren's syndrome	
Severe malnutrition	
Systemic lupus erythematosus	

IgA

Increased	Decreased
Alcoholism	Agammaglobulinemia
Carcinoma	Chronic sinopulmonary disease
Cirrhosis	Hereditary ataxia- telangiectasia
Chronic infections	Humoral immune deficiency
Dysproteinemia	Hypogammaglobulinemia
Exercise	Inflammatory bowel disease
Liver disease	Late pregnancy
Multiple myeloma	Leukemia
Obstructive jaundice	Nephrotic syndrome

Rheumatoid arthritis
Sinusitis

IgM

Increased	Decreased
Actinomycosis	Agammaglobulinemia
Bartonellosis	Amyloidosis
Fungal infections	Humoral immune deficiency
Infectious mononucleosis	Hypogammaglobulinemia
Malaria	IgG and IgA myeloma
Rheumatoid arthritis	Inflammatory bowel disease
Systemic lupus erythematosus	Leukemia
Trypanosomiasis	Lymphoid aplasia
Waldenström's macroglobulinemia	Nephrotic syndrome

IgE

Increased	Decreased
Asthma	Advanced carcinoma
Dermatitis	Agammaglobulinemia
Eczema	AIDS
Food and drug allergies	Ataxia-telangiectasia
Hay fever	IgE deficiency
IgE myeloma	Non-IgE myeloma
Pemphigoid	
Periarteritis nodosa	
Rhinitis	
Sinusitis	
Wiskott-Aldrich syndrome	

IgD

Increased	Decreased
Autoimmune disease	AIDS
Chronic infections	Non-IgD myeloma
Dysproteinemia	
IgD myeloma	

Contributing Factors to Abnormal Values

- Drugs which may *increase* immunoglobulins: carbamazepine, chlorpromazine, dextran, estrogens, gold compounds, methylprednisolone, oral contraceptives, penicillamine, phenytoin, valproic acid.
- Immunization within the previous 6 months can *increase* immunoglobulins.

Interventions/Implications

Pretest
- Explain to the patient the purpose of the test and the need for a blood sample to be drawn.
- No fasting is required before the test.

Procedure
- A 7-mL blood sample is drawn in a red-top collection tube.
- Gloves are worn throughout the procedure.

Posttest
- Apply pressure at venipuncture site. Apply dressing, periodically assessing for continued bleeding.
- Label the specimen and transport it to the laboratory.
- Report abnormal findings to the primary care provider.

 Immunoscintigraphy

Test Description
Immunoscintigraphy is based upon the use of monoclonal antibody technology. In this type of testing, radioactive antibodies travel to specific sites within the body for the detection of certain malignancies. Although in the future more types of cancer will be able to be tested for in this way, the current testing is limited to detecting recurrent metastatic colorectal or ovarian cancer. The monoclonal antibodies for this test have the radionuclide indium chloride-111 attached to them. After the antibodies are injected and located on cancer cells, the radionuclide is able to be detected through scanning.

Normal Values
No areas of increased radionuclide uptake in the body

Possible Meanings of Abnormal Values
Ovarian cancer
Recurrent colorectal cancer

Contributing Factors to Abnormal Values
- Any movement by the patient may alter quality of films taken.
- *False-positive* results can occur due to uptake of the radionuclide in degenerative joint disease, abdominal aortic aneurysm, and inflammatory gastrointestinal diseases.

Interventions/Implications
Pretest
- Explain to the patient the purpose of the test. Provide any written teaching materials available on the subject. Note that discomfort involved with this test is limited to the venipuncture. Reassure the patient that only trace amounts of the radionuclide are involved in the test.
- The patient must remain still while the scan is being performed.
- No fasting is required prior to the test.
- Obtain a signed informed consent.

Procedure
- The radiolabeled monoclonal antibody is administered by IV injection in a peripheral vein.
- At the designated time (48 to 72 hours postinjection), the patient is taken to the nuclear medicine department.
- The patient is assisted to a supine position on the examination table.

- Scans are made of the anterior and posterior chest, abdomen, and pelvis.
- Gloves are worn during the radionuclide injection.

Posttest
- Check the injection site for redness or swelling.
- If a woman who is lactating *must* have a nuclear scan, she should not breast feed the infant until the radionuclide has been eliminated, possibly for 3 days.
- Although the amount of diagnostic radionuclide excreted in the urine is low, the urine should not be used for any laboratory tests for the time period indicated by the nuclear medicine department.
- Gloves are worn whenever dealing with the urine.
- Encourage fluid intake by the patient to enhance excretion of the radionuclide.
- Report abnormal findings to the primary care provider.

CONTRAINDICATIONS!

- Pregnant women
  - Caution: A woman in her childbearing years should undergo radiography only during her menses or 12 to 14 days after its onset to avoid any exposure to a fetus.
- Patients who are lactating
- Patients who are unable to cooperate due to age, mental status, pain, or other factors

Influenza A & B

Test Description
Influenza type A and B virus cause seasonal outbreaks of the flu, resulting in significant morbidity and mortality. If diagnosed within 48 hours of onset, influenza may be treated with antiviral medications. Thus, rapid and accurate diagnosis is needed. Use of a traditional viral culture is very accurate, but can take 3 to 7 days to be completed. A rapid method is now available in which a cell culture using two different cell lines are in a single cell well. Upon inoculation, the mixed cell culture is incubated for 24 hours and then analyzed using monoclonal fluorescent antibody typing.

Normal Values
Negative

Possible Meanings of Abnormal Values
Influenza A/B

Interventions/Implications
Pretest
- Explain to the patient the purpose of the test. Provide any written teaching materials available on the subject.
- No fasting is required before the test.

Procedure
- Ask the patient to cough and then tilt the head back (coughing helps decrease the occurrence of gagging)
- Insert a sterile wire-shafted nasopharyngeal swab through the nostril into the space just beneath the inferior turbinate (nasopharynx).
- The swab is gently rotated, allowing a few seconds for the swab to absorb the secretions, and is then removed.
- Gloves are worn during the procedure.

Posttest
- Report abnormal findings to the primary care provider.

Insulin (Insulin Assay, Serum Insulin)

Test Description
This test measures the level of insulin in the serum. Insulin is a hormone secreted by the beta cells of the islets of Langerhans of the pancreas. It regulates the metabolism and transport of carbohydrates, amino acids, proteins, and lipids and facilitates glucose uptake by adipose tissue and skeletal muscle. Insulin also stimulates the synthesis and storage of triglycerides and proteins. Insulin secretion occurs when the plasma level of glucose increases. As the plasma glucose level decreases, secretion of insulin ceases.

This test can provide information about the presence of insulin resistance. If the insulin level is high with a normal or elevated blood sugar, the problem may be that the pancreas is working harder than it should to keep the blood sugar under control. This insulin resistance is one characteristic of *metabolic syndrome*, a condition which puts people at risk of coronary heart disease and Type 2 diabetes.

Measurement of the serum insulin level is also used to assist in the diagnosis of hypoglycemic states and diabetes mellitus. Assessing the insulin level is sometimes done in conjunction with performance of a glucose tolerance test (GTT). In the case of an islet cell transplant, the insulin level may be monitored to assess viability of the transplant.

Normal Values
6–29 µIU/mL (43–208 pmol/L SI units)

Possible Meanings of Abnormal Values

Increased	Decreased
Acromegaly	Hyperglycemia
Cushing's syndrome	Hypopituitarism
Fructose intolerance	Diabetes mellitus Type 1
Galactose intolerance	
Hyperinsulinism	
Hypoglycemia	

Injection of exogenous insulin
Insulinoma
Liver disease
Diabetes mellitus Type 2
Obesity
Pancreatic islet cell lesion
Sulfonylurea-induced hypoglycemia

Contributing Factors to Abnormal Values

- Radioactive scans within 7 days prior to the test will alter test results.
- Hemodialysis destroys insulin.
- Presence of anti-insulin antibodies may alter test results.
- Drug which may *increase* insulin levels: albuterol, calcium gluconate in the newborn, epinephrine, fructose, glucagon, glucose, insulin, levodopa, medroxyprogesterone acetate, oral contraceptives, prednisolone, quinidine, spironolactone, sucrose, terbutaline, thyroid hormones, tolazamide, tolbutamide.
- Drugs which may *decrease* insulin levels: asparaginase, beta-adrenergic blockers, calcitonin, cimetidine, ethacrynic acid, ethanol, ether, furosemide, metformin, nifedipine, phenobarbital, phenytoin, thiazide diuretics.

Interventions/Implications

Pretest

- Explain to the patient the purpose of the test and the need for a blood sample to be drawn.
- Fasting for 8 hours is required prior to the test. Water is permitted.
- Insulin should be withheld prior to the test.
- If done in conjunction with a GTT, the insulin level should be drawn prior to administration of the glucose load.

Procedure

- A 7-mL blood sample is drawn in a red-top collection tube.
- Gloves are worn throughout the procedure.

Posttest

- Apply pressure at venipuncture site. Apply dressing, periodically assessing for continued bleeding.
- Label the specimen, place it in ice and transport it to the laboratory immediately.
- Resume medications as taken prior to the test.
- Report abnormal findings to the primary care provider.

→ Clinical Alerts

- For hypoglycemia workups, other tests, such as glucose, proinsulin, anti-insulin antibodies, and insulin c-peptide may also be done.
- It is not unusual for individuals with newly diagnosed diabetes mellitus Type 2 to have hypertriglyceridemia as well. Normalizing of the blood glucose through treatment can have a parallel effect of lowering the triglyceride level.

Intravenous Pyelography
(IVP, Excretory Urography, Intravenous Urography)

Test Description

Intravenous pyelography (IVP) uses radiopaque contrast dye to allow visualization of the kidneys, ureters, and bladder. This test is performed in cases of suspected renal disease or urinary tract dysfunction. Following injection of the dye, serial films are made as the dye filters through the kidneys and is excreted into the ureters and bladder. At the end of the procedure, a postvoiding film is also taken. This test provides a great deal of information regarding the structure of the kidneys and their ability to excrete the dye. It also is used for assessment of the ureters and bladder for obstruction, hematuria, stones, and trauma.

THE EVIDENCE FOR PRACTICE

Noncontrast CT is the most rapid and accurate technique for the evaluation of flank pain. If there is uncertainty about whether a calcific density represents a ureteral calculus or a phlebolith, contrast medium can be injected and the scan repeated for definitive diagnosis. The IVP is the technique of choice if CT is not available.

Normal Values

Normal size, shape, position, and functioning of kidneys, ureters, and bladder

Possible Meanings of Abnormal Values

Absence of one kidney
Bladder tumor
Chronic pyelonephritis
Congenital abnormalities
Glomerulonephritis
Hydronephrosis
Polycystic kidney disease
Prostatic enlargement
Renal calculi
Renal cysts
Renal tuberculosis
Renal tumor
Renovascular hypertension
Supernumerary kidney
Trauma
Ureteral calculi

Contributing Factors to Abnormal Values

- Retained barium, gas, or stool in the intestines may result in poor quality films.
- Any movement by the patient may alter quality of films taken.

Interventions/Implications

Pretest
- Explain to the patient the purpose of the test. Provide any written teaching materials available on the subject. Note that minimal discomfort during the test is due to the venipuncture, and that during injection of the dye, transient sensations including warmth, flushing, a salty taste, and nausea may be experienced.
- Check for allergies to iodine, shellfish, or contrast medium dye. Inform the radiologist of such possible allergy so that a hypoallergenic nonionic contrast medium may be used for the test.
- Patients receiving metformin (Glucophage) for Type 2 diabetes mellitus should discontinue the drug 2 days before receipt of contrast medium. This is due to the possible occurrence of lactic acidosis, a potentially fatal complication of biguanide therapy.
- Baseline BUN and creatinine is obtained.
- Fasting for 8 hours is required prior to the test. The patient should be well hydrated prior to the beginning of the fasting period.
- A laxative the night prior to the test, or an enema or suppository the morning of the test may be ordered.
- Resuscitation and suctioning equipment should be readily available.

Procedure
- The patient is assisted to a supine position on the radiography table.
- A kidney, ureter, and bladder (KUB) film is taken to assess for gross abnormalities of the urinary tract.
- A maintenance IV line is initiated.
- The contrast dye is administered by IV injection.
- Serial films are made, usually at 1, 5, 10, 15, 20, and 30 minutes postinjection.
- The patient is then asked to void, after which a postvoiding film is taken.
- Gloves are worn during the venipuncture.

Posttest
- Most allergic reactions to radiopaque dye occur within 30 minutes of administration of the contrast medium. Observe the patient closely for respiratory distress, hypotension, edema, hives, rash, tachycardia, and/or laryngeal stridor. Emergency resuscitation equipment must be readily accessible.
- Observe for allergic reaction to the dye for 24 hours.
- Apply pressure at venipuncture site. Apply dressing, periodically assessing for continued bleeding.
- Resume the patient's diet. Encourage fluid intake of at least three glasses of liquid to speed the excretion of the dye from the body.
- BUN and creatinine should be reassessed prior to resuming metformin.
- Report abnormal findings to the primary care provider.

→ **Clinical Alerts**

- Possible complication: Allergic reaction to dye.
- If barium studies are also ordered, they are to be performed *after* this procedure has been successfully completed.

- Patients who are allergic to iodine, shellfish, or contrast medium dye
- Pregnant women
  - Caution: A woman in her childbearing years should undergo radiography only during her menses or 12 to 14 days after its onset to avoid any exposure to a fetus.
- Patients who are unable to cooperate due to age, mental status, pain, or other factors
- Patients with renal failure or those susceptible to dye-induced renal failure (dehydrated patients)

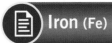

Iron (Fe)

Test Description

Iron is found primarily in the hemoglobin of the red blood cells (65%) and in storage as ferritin or hemosiderin (30%) in the liver, bone marrow, and spleen. It functions to carry oxygen to the tissues and indirectly assists in returning carbon dioxide to the lungs. Measurement of iron levels assists in the diagnosis of anemia. If the hemoglobin and hematocrit are low, iron testing can be useful in determining the cause of the anemia. It can also be tested to assess a person's response to iron supplementation as a treatment for anemia. Another use of the test is to aid in the diagnosis of hemochromatosis, an inherited disorder of iron metabolism in which the person absorbs more iron than the body needs.

Iron levels are typically assessed in conjunction with other tests, including ferritin, total iron binding capacity, and transferrin. Iron levels vary throughout the day; therefore, laboratories usually specify the time the blood sample should be drawn.

THE EVIDENCE FOR PRACTICE

The USPSTF recommends routine screening for iron deficiency anemia in asymptomatic pregnant women.

Normal Values

50–150 µg/dL (9.0–26.9 µmol/L SI units)
Elderly: Decreased

Possible Meanings of Abnormal Values

Increased	Decreased
Acute liver damage	Blood loss
Aplastic anemia	Burns

Hemochromatosis	Cancer
Hemolytic anemia	Infection
Hemosiderosis of excessive	Inflammation
iron intake	Myocardial infarction
Lead poisoning	Nephrosis
Nephritis	Pregnancy
Pernicious anemia	Rheumatoid arthritis
Polycythemia	Uremia
Thalassemia	

Contributing Factors to Abnormal Values

- Falsely increased iron levels may occur due to intake of vitamin B_{12} within 48 hours prior to testing the iron level or hemolysis of the sample
- Iron levels are highest in the morning and lowest in the evening.
- Falsely decreased iron levels may occur due to a lipemic specimen or in the presence of inflammatory states.
- Drugs which may *increase* the iron level: cefotaxime, chloramphenicol, estrogens, ferrous sulfate, methimazole, methotrexate.
- Drugs which may *decrease* the iron level: allopurinal, aspirin, cholestyramine, corticotropin, metformin, pergolide, progestins, risperidone, testosterone.

Interventions/Implications

Pretest

- Explain to the patient the purpose of the test and the need for a blood sample to be drawn.
- Fasting is required for 12 hours prior to the test. Water intake is allowed.
- No iron supplements are to be taken within 24 to 48 hours prior to the test.

Procedure

- Obtain the blood sample in the morning, usually after 10 AM.
- A 5-mL blood sample is obtained in a red-top collection tube.
- Gloves are worn throughout the procedure.

Posttest

- Apply pressure at venipuncture site. Apply dressing, periodically assessing for continued bleeding.
- Label the specimen and transport it to the laboratory.
- Report abnormal findings to the primary care provider.

→ Clinical Alerts

- Should the iron level be found to be low, provide the patient with information regarding dietary sources of iron.
- Should iron supplementation be needed, its absorption can be enhanced by taking it with orange juice.
- Ferritin, TIBC, transferrin, and percent transferrin saturation are usually measured at the same time serum iron is measured.

17-Ketosteroids (17-KS)

Test Description

This test provides an indication of adrenal function. The adrenal cortex secretes three types of hormones: the glucocorticoids (primarily cortisol), the mineralocorticoids (aldosterone), and the sex hormones (androgens, estrogen, progesterone). The test for 17-ketosteroids (17-KS) measures the adrenal hormones and metabolites of testicular androgens. All 17-KS are not androgens, but do produce androgenic effects. Testosterone, which is the most potent androgen, is not measured by this test in that testosterone is not a 17-KS. Thus this test is but an approximation of androgenic activity. To provide a more complete representation of androgenic activity, plasma testosterone levels should also be measured. With the availability of specific hormone and hormone metabolite tests, this assay is less useful than in the past.

Normal Values

Female >15 years:	5.0–15.0 mg/day (17.3–52.0 µmol/day SI units)
Male >15 years:	9.0–22.0 mg/day (31.2–76.3 µmol/day SI units)
11–14 years:	2.0–7.0 mg/day (6.9–24.2 µmol/day SI units)
0–10 years:	0.1–3.0 mg/day (0.4–10.4 µmol/day SI units)

K

Possible Meanings of Abnormal Values

Increased	Decreased
Adrenal hyperplasia	Addison's disease
Adrenocortical tumors	Castration
Adrenogenital syndrome	Chronic illness
Cushing's syndrome	Gout
Female pseudohermaphrodism	Hypogonadism
Hirsutism	Hypopituitarism
Hyperpituitarism	Klinefelter's syndrome
Infection (severe)	Myxedema
Obesity	Menopause
Ovarian luteal cell tumors	Nephrosis
Pregnancy	Thyrotoxicosis
Premature infants	
Stein-Leventhal syndrome	
Stress	
Testicular interstitial cell tumors	

Contributing Factors to Abnormal Values

- Stress and exercise may alter test results.
- Drugs which may *increase* 17-KS levels: ampicillin, ascorbic acid, cephalothin, chloramphenicol, chlordiazepoxide, chlorpromazine, cloxacillin, corticotropin, cortisone, dexamethasone, digitoxin, erythromycin, hydralazine, meprobamate, methicillin, morphine, nalidixic acid, oxacillin, penicillin, phenazopyridine, phenothiazines, piperidine, quinidine, quinine, salicylates, secobarbital, spironolactone, testosterone.

- Drugs which may *decrease* 17-KS levels: chlordiazepoxide, chlorpromazine, corticosteroids, dexamethasone, digoxin, estrogens, glucose, meprobamate, metyrapone, oral contraceptives, paraldehyde, penicillin, phenytoin, probenecid, promazine, propoxyphene, pyrazinamide, quinine, quinidine, reserpine, salicylates, secobarbital, spironolactone.

Interventions/Implications

Pretest
- Explain 24-hour urine collection procedure to the patient.
- Stress the importance of saving *all* urine in the 24-hour period. Instruct the patient to avoid contaminating the urine with toilet paper or feces.
- Inform the patient of the presence of a preservative in the collection bottle.
- Encourage the patient to avoid excessive physical activity and stress during the testing period.
- If possible, withhold medications which may alter test results.

Procedure
- Obtain the proper container containing 1 g of boric acid as preservative from the laboratory.
- Begin the testing period in the morning after the patient's first voiding, which is discarded.
- Timing of the 24-hour period begins at the time the first voiding is discarded.
- *All* urine for the next 24 hours is collected in the container, which is to be kept refrigerated or on ice.
- If any urine is accidentally discarded during the 24-hour period, the test must be discontinued and a new test begun.
- The ending time of the 24-hour collection period should be posted in the patient's room.
- Gloves are worn whenever dealing with the specimen collection.

Posttest
- At the end of the 24-hour collection period, label and send the urine container on ice to the laboratory as soon as possible.
- Resume medications as taken prior to the test.
- Report abnormal findings to the primary care provider.

Kidney Sonogram (Renal Ultrasonography)

Test Description
Ultrasonography is a noninvasive method of diagnostic testing in which ultrasound waves are sent into the body with a small transducer pressed against the skin. The transducer then receives any returning sound waves, which are deflected back as they bounce off various structures. The transducer converts the returning sound waves into electric signals that are then transformed by a computer into a visual display on a monitor.

In renal ultrasonography, the transducer is passed over the flank area. This allows visualization of the kidneys and the perirenal tissues. This test is especially valuable for use in patients who are unable to have other renal examinations because of hypersensitivity to contrast media or pregnancy. It can also be used for post-transplant evaluation and guidance for biopsy, aspiration, or nephrostomy tube insertion.

Normal Values

Normal size, shape, and location of kidneys
Absence of calculi, cysts, hydronephrosis, obstruction, or tumor

Possible Meanings of Abnormal Values

Hydronephrosis
Perirenal hematoma
Renal calculi
Renal cyst
Renal tumor
Ureteral obstruction

Contributing Factors to Abnormal Values

- The transducer must be in good contact with the skin as it is being moved. A water-based gel is used to ensure good contact with the skin.
- Retained barium from previous tests may hinder testing.
- Obesity may interfere with the clarity of the images.

Interventions/Implications

Pretest
- Explain to the patient the purpose of the test. Provide any written teaching materials available on the subject. Note that there is no discomfort involved with this test.
- No fasting is required before the test.

Procedure
- The patient is assisted to a prone position on the ultrasonography table.
- A coupling agent, such as a water-based gel, is applied to the flank area.
- A transducer is placed on the skin and moved as needed to provide good visualization of the kidneys.
- The sound waves are transformed into a visual display on the monitor. Printed copies of this display are made.

Posttest
- Cleanse the patient's skin of any lubricant.
- Report abnormal findings to the primary care provider.

Lactic Acid (Blood Lactate)

Test Description

Lactic acid is produced by anaerobic glycolysis. In other words, lactic acid is produced as a result of carbohydrate metabolism in an environment where the cells do not have enough oxygen to allow for conversion of fuel to carbon dioxide and water. An example of this type of situation is strenuous exercise. Lactic acid is used for muscle contraction when energy needs exceed the supply of oxygen. Lactic acid accumulates in situations where there is an excess production of lactate and removal of the lactic acid from the blood by the liver is decreased, as can occur in liver disease.

Normal Values

0.5–2.2 mEq/L (0.5–2.2 mmol/L SI units)

Possible Meanings of Abnormal Values

Increased	Decreased
Alcoholism	Hypothermia
Cardiac arrest	
Congestive heart failure	
Dehydration	
Diabetes mellitus	
Hemorrhage	
Hepatic coma	
Hyperthermia	
Hypoxia	
Lactic acidosis	
Liver disease	
Malignancy	
Peritonitis	
Renal failure	
Respiratory failure	
Shock	
Strenuous exercise	

Contributing Factors to Abnormal Values

- Hemolysis of the blood sample may alter test results.
- During exercise, blood lactate can increase up to ten times the normal level.
- Lactic acid levels may be falsely low in the presence of high LDH levels.
- Drugs which may *increase* lactic acid levels: alcohol, epinephrine, glucose, sodium bicarbonate.

Interventions/Implications

Pretest

- Explain to the patient the purpose of the test and the need for a blood sample to be drawn.

- No fasting is required before the test.
- No exercise for several hours prior to the test.

Procedure
- A 7-mL blood sample is drawn in a grey-top collection tube, avoiding use of a tourniquet and clenching of the patient's hand when possible.
- Collected blood should be cooled on ice immediately.
- Gloves are worn throughout the procedure.

Posttest
- Apply pressure at venipuncture site. Apply dressing, periodically assessing for continued bleeding.
- Label the specimen and transport it to the laboratory.
- Report abnormal findings to the primary care provider.

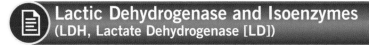

Lactic Dehydrogenase and Isoenzymes
(LDH, Lactate Dehydrogenase [LD])

Test Description

Lactic dehydrogenase (LDH) is an intracellular enzyme found primarily in the heart, liver, skeletal muscles, and the erythrocytes. It is present in smaller amounts in the brain, kidneys, lungs, pancreas, and spleen. LDH is released after damage has occurred to the tissue.

LDH can be measured as the total enzyme in the serum, or each of its five isoenzymes may be measured. Measuring the isoenzymes can help to differentiate the source of the elevated total LDH. The isoenzymes and their primary sources include:

LDH_1: Heart muscle and erythrocytes
LDH_2: Reticuloendothelial system (normally in serum)
LDH_3: Lungs
LDH_4: Kidneys, pancreas, and placenta
LDH_5: Liver and skeletal muscle

LDH, along with asparate aminotransferase (AST) and creatine kinase (CK), have traditionally been assessed in the case of suspected myocardial infarction (MI). However, the availability of testing for troponin has decreased the use of LDH for diagnosing MI. It typically appears in the bloodstream within 12 hours of the tissue injury, with peak values occurring 24 to 48 hours postinjury. The peak value may reach 300 to 800 IU/L following an MI. LDH levels are usually elevated for approximately 10 days. Thus, LDH becomes elevated after CK following an MI. In diagnosing a suspected MI, the total LDH, along with LDH_1 and LDH_2 are usually evaluated, with LDH_1 being greater than LDH_2. Isolated increases of LDH may occur in the absence of physical problems.

Normal Values

Total LDH: 110–210 IU/L (1.83–3.50 µkat/L SI units)
Isoenzymes: LDH_1: 17–27%
              LDH_2: 28–38%

LDH$_3$: 17–28%
LDH$_4$: 5–15%
LDH$_5$: 5–15%

Possible Meanings of Abnormal Values

Increased

Abruptio placenta
Acute pancreatitis
Anemia of chronic disease
Biliary obstruction
Bone metastases
Cancer of prostate
Congestive heart failure
Delirium tremens
Eclampsia
Fractures
Hemolytic anemia
Hepatitis
Hyperthermia
Hypothyroidism
Infectious mononucleosis
Leukemia
Liver cancer
Liver damage
Macrocytic anemias
Malignant tumors
Muscular dystrophy
Myocardial infarction
Pernicious anemia
Pneumonia (*Pneumocystis carinii*)
Pulmonary infarction
Seizure
Shock
Skeletal muscle disease
Trauma

Contributing Factors to Abnormal Values

- Hemolysis of the blood sample and strenuous exercise prior to the test will alter test results.
- Drugs which may *increase* LDH levels: alcohol, anabolic steroids, anesthetics, antibiotics, aspirin, beta blockers, clofibrate, diltiazem, fluorides, itraconazole, levodopa, narcotics, NSAIDs, nifedipine, paroxetine, procainamide, propylthiouracil, sulfasalazine, verapamil.
- Drugs which may *decrease* LDH levels: ascorbic acid, oxalates.

Interventions/Implications

Pretest
- Explain to the patient the purpose of the test and the need for a blood sample to be drawn.
- No fasting is required before the test.

Procedure
- A 7-mL blood sample is drawn in a red-top collection tube.
- Gloves are worn throughout the procedure.

Posttest
- Apply pressure at venipuncture site. Apply dressing, periodically assessing for continued bleeding.
- Label the specimen and transport it to the laboratory.
- Report abnormal findings to the primary care provider.

 ## Lactose Tolerance Test (Breath Hydrogen Test)

Test Description
Lactase is an enzyme which is found in the small intestine. Its function is the digestion of lactose, a sugar found in milk. In some people, there is a deficiency of lactase. When individuals who are lactase deficient ingest milk, the lactose builds up in the intestine, where it is metabolized by the bacteria normally found there. This results in abdominal cramping, bloating, and diarrhea.

L

This test, used to test for lactose intolerance, can be done two different ways, both of which occur after the patient ingests a lactose solution. The noninvasive method is the measurement of breath hydrogen content. Breath samples are collected during exhalation and analyzed for hydrogen, a byproduct of bacteria that breakdown the lactose that is not absorbed. If the breath test is not available, blood samples are drawn at several designated time intervals to monitor the blood glucose level. At the same time, the patient is observed for any of the physical symptoms associated with lactose intolerance. If the gastrointestinal symptoms appear and the blood glucose level increases by less than 20 mg/dL, lactase insufficiency is indicated.

Normal Values
A rise in plasma glucose levels of >20 mg/dL and no abdominal symptoms (abdominal pain, bloating, flatus, diarrhea)
In the breath test, a peak rise in hydrogen content of 12 parts per million over the fasting (baseline) level is considered positive.

Possible Meanings of Abnormal Values

Decreased
Enterogenous diarrhea
Lactase insufficiency

Contributing Factors to Abnormal Values
- Strenuous exercise and smoking may alter the test results.
- Drugs which may alter test results: benzodiazepines, insulin, oral contraceptives, propranolol, thiazide diuretics.

Interventions/Implications

Pretest

- Explain to the patient the purpose of the test and the need for multiple blood samples to be drawn.
- Fasting and avoidance of strenuous exercise for 8 hours are required prior to the test.
- No smoking is allowed during the test.

Procedure

- A 7-mL blood sample is drawn in a grey-top collection tube.
- The adult patient is given 50–100 g of lactose in 200 mL of water. (Note: The dose for a child is based upon body weight.)
- Additional blood samples are drawn at 30 minutes, 1 hour, and 2 hours after lactose ingestion.
- Gloves are worn throughout the procedure.
- For breath test, contact reference laboratory for collection protocol.

Posttest

- Apply pressure at venipuncture site. Apply dressing, periodically assessing for continued bleeding.
- Label the specimen and transport it to the laboratory.
- Report abnormal findings to the primary care provider.

L

→ Clinical Alerts

- Patients with abnormal test results will require additional testing for other types of sugar intolerance, such as glucose or galactose.

Laparoscopy (Gynecologic Laparoscopy, Pelvic Endoscopy, Pelviscopy, Peritoneoscopy)

Test Description

Laparoscopy is the direct visualization of the peritoneal cavity via a laparoscope inserted through the anterior abdominal wall. During the procedure, one or two small incisions are made to allow insertion of the laparoscope and other instruments. The limited incisional size is advantageous in shortening the surgical time and recovery time from this procedure.

This procedure is used to evaluate patients complaining of abdominal/pelvic pain, for detecting carcinoma, ectopic pregnancy, endometriosis, pelvic inflammatory disease, and abdominal/pelvic masses, for staging of cancer, for evaluating ascites, to view the fallopian tubes as part of an infertility workup, and with some types of abdominal trauma. Laparoscopy is also used to perform such procedures as lysis of adhesions, ovarian biopsy, and tubal ligation. Laparoscopic surgery can also be used for other types of surgery such as cholecystectomy and appendectomy.

Normal Values

Normal uterus, fallopian tubes, and ovaries
Normal abdominal organs

Possible Meanings of Abnormal Values

Abdominal organ abnormalities
Adhesions
Ascites
Cancer
Ectopic pregnancy
Endometriosis
Hydrosalpinx
Ovarian cyst
Ovarian tumor
Pelvic inflammatory disease
Salpingitis
Uterine fibroids

Interventions/Implications

Pretest

- Explain to the patient the purpose of the test and the procedure to be done. Note that some abdominal and shoulder pain will be felt for 24 to 36 hours after the procedure, but that mild analgesics will control it. Shoulder pain is due to pressure on the diaphragm by carbon dioxide used during the procedure.
- Fasting for 8 hours is required prior to the test.
- Obtain a signed written consent.
- An enema prior to the procedure is sometimes ordered.
- Ask the patient to void prior to the procedure.
- The patient's abdomen is shaved as ordered.

Procedure

- This sterile procedure is usually conducted in the operating room.
- For gynecologic procedures:
    - The patient is typically given a general anesthetic and is then placed in the lithotomy position with her legs supported in the stirrups. A Trendelenburg position may be used to move the intestines away from the pelvic organs.
    - The bladder may be catheterized and a bimanual examination of the pelvis performed to detect abnormalities.
    - A uterine manipulator is inserted through the vagina and cervix and into the uterus to permit the pelvic organs to be moved for better visualization.
- For abdominal procedures, the patient is supine.
- The abdomen is cleansed and draped.
- A small incision is made in the subumbilical area into the peritoneal cavity.
- The Veres (pneumoperitoneum) needle is inserted into the incision and used to fill the peritoneal cavity with approximately 3 L of carbon dioxide. This gas lifts the abdominal wall from the intra-abdominal viscera.
- The needle is removed and a trocar and sheath are inserted into the peritoneal cavity.
- The trocar is removed and replaced with the laparoscope.

- When visual examination and any other planned procedures, such as tubal ligation, are completed, the laparoscope is removed, the carbon dioxide is evacuated, and the sheath is removed.
- The incision is closed with sutures, clips, or Steri-strips, and a dressing is applied.
- The uterine manipulator is removed and a perineal pad is applied.
- Videotaping of the procedure is usually done via a camera attached to the laparoscope.

Posttest
- Remind the patient that abdominal and shoulder discomfort is not unusual following the procedure. Analgesics may be taken.
- Instruct the patient to report immediately any excessive pain.
- Monitor vital signs and urinary output until stable.
- Resume diet as taken prior to the procedure.
- Instruct the patient to restrict activity for 2 to 7 days.
- Report abnormal findings to the primary care provider.

→ Clinical Alerts

- Possible complications include: hemorrhage, punctured visceral organ, such as the intestine. The patient should be periodically assessed for abdominal tenderness and distention, fever, decreased bowel sounds, tachycardia, and hypotension.

CONTRAINDICATIONS!

- Patients with advanced abdominal wall malignancy
- Patients with advanced respiratory or cardiovascular disease
- Patients with intestinal obstruction, abdominal mass, or abdominal hernia
- Patients with chronic tuberculosis
- Patients with history of peritonitis
- Patients with possible adhesions due to multiple previous surgical procedures
- Patients with suspected intra-abdominal hemorrhage

Lead

Test Description
Lead is a heavy metal used in paint, leaded gasoline, insecticides, and pottery glaze. Because of its presence in paint, lead is a hazard in older homes with peeling paint easily accessible to young children. It is usually present in the body in minute amounts due to environmental exposure. Such low levels in adults do not appear to cause problems, however, in children, relatively low levels of lead can lead to toxicity that may cause deficits in intellectual or cognitive development. Lead

screening is performed on at risk children, as well as industrial workers who are exposed to lead. Lead levels are also used to monitor response to treatment for elevated lead levels.

THE EVIDENCE FOR PRACTICE

The Centers for Disease Control and Prevention and the American Academy of Pediatrics recommend that, at a minimum, screening be offered to:

- every Medicaid-eligible child and those children whose families are part of an assistance program. These children should be screened at age 1 and again at 2 years of age.
- at risk children 3 to 6 years of age who have not been previously tested.
- children who live in or regularly visit a house or apartment built before 1950, or before 1978 if the dwelling has been/or is undergoing renovation or remodeling.
- children with a playmate or sibling who has or did have *lead poisoning*.

Normal Values

Adults:	<20 µg/dL (<0.95 µmol/L SI units)
Children:	<10 µg/dL (<0.48 µmol/L SI units)

Possible Meanings of Abnormal Values

Increased

Lead poisoning

Interventions/Implications

Pretest
- Explain to the patient the purpose of the test and the need for a blood sample to be drawn.
- No fasting is required before the test.

Procedure
- A 7-mL blood sample is drawn in a lead-free tan-top or lavender-top collection tube.
- Gloves are worn throughout the procedure.

Posttest
- Apply pressure at venipuncture site. Apply dressing, periodically assessing for continued bleeding.
- Label the specimen and transport it to the laboratory.
- Report abnormal findings to the primary care provider.

→ **Clinical Alerts**

- Workers exposed to lead should have blood lead levels <40 µg/dL.
- In children with blood lead levels >10 µg/mL, the source of the lead exposure must be identified and removed. Treatment is needed for levels >25 µg/dL.
- Red blood cell studies usually show a microcytic anemia when lead poisoning is present.

Legionnaire's Disease Antibody Test

Test Description

Legionnaire's disease is a type of atypical pneumonia caused by *Legionella pneumophila*. It is characterized by flulike symptoms, including high fever, mental confusion, headache, pleuritic pain, myalgias, dyspnea, productive cough, and hemoptysis. It occurs most often among middle-aged and older men, smokers, and individuals with chronic diseases or receiving immunosuppressive therapy. The bacteria that cause Legionnaire's disease have been found in water delivery systems and can survive in the warm, moist, air conditioning systems of large buildings including hospitals. The organism has also been isolated from soil; those working with or living near soil excavations are at risk of contracting the disease.

Diagnosis of Legionnaire's disease is made through determination of the presence of *Legionella* antibodies. Antibody titers are low during the first week, rise the second and third weeks, peak at 5 weeks, and then drop slowly over several years. One antibody titer is performed within the first week of the illness (acute phase) and a second is done 3 to 6 weeks after the fever began (convalescent phase). A fourfold rise in titer >1:128 between these two antibody assessments is diagnostic of the disease. A single titer of at least 1:256 indicates a previous infection with *Legionella*, but is not confirmation of Legionnaire's disease, since 1% to 16% of healthy adults have similar titer levels.

Normal Values

Negative

Possible Meanings of Abnormal Values

Increased

Legionnaire's disease

Contributing Factors to Abnormal Values

- Hemolysis of the blood sample will alter test results.

Interventions/Implications

Pretest
- Explain to the patient the purpose of the test and the need for a blood sample to be drawn.
- No fasting is required before the test.

Procedure
- A 7-mL blood sample is drawn in a red-top collection tube.
- Gloves are worn throughout the procedure.

Posttest
- Apply pressure at venipuncture site. Apply dressing, periodically assessing for continued bleeding.

- Label the specimen and transport it to the laboratory.
- Report abnormal findings to the primary care provider.

→ **Clinical Alerts**

- For patients diagnosed with Legionnaire's disease, treatment includes administration of antibiotics such as quinolones and macrolides.

 Leucine Aminopeptidase (LAP)

Test Description
Leucine aminopeptidase (LAP) is an enzyme normally found in the hepatocytes of the liver and is present in the blood, bile, and urine. It is released into the blood after damage to liver cells from hepatotoxic drugs or infection, such as hepatitis. LAP may also be released into the blood by tumors in the liver, thus it may also serve as a tumor marker.

This test is useful in diagnosis of conditions when the alkaline phosphatase is elevated. LAP changes parallel those of alkaline phosphatase except that LAP is usually normal in bone diseases or malabsorption problems, but serves as an indicator of liver damage. LAP is generally not as sensitive as testing other liver enzymes such as ALT, AST, ALP, LDH, and GGT. Unlike other liver enzymes LAP can also be measured in the urine.

Normal Values
Female:	75–185 U/mL (18.0–44.4 U/L SI units)
Male:	80–200 U/mL (19.2–48.0 U/L SI units)

Possible Meanings of Abnormal Values

Increased
Cholelithiasis
Cirrhosis
Hepatitis
Jaundice
Liver cancer
Liver dysfunction
Pancreatic cancer
Pancreatitis
Pregnancy
Systemic lupus erythematosus

Contributing Factors to Abnormal Values
- Drugs which may *increase* LAP levels: estrogens, hepatotoxic drugs, progesterones.

Interventions/Implications

Pretest

- Explain to the patient the purpose of the test and the need for a blood sample to be drawn.
- No fasting is usually required prior to the test. Some laboratories may require an 8-hour fast.

Procedure

- A 7-mL blood sample is drawn in a red-top collection tube.
- Gloves are worn throughout the procedure.

Posttest

- Apply pressure 3 to 5 minutes at venipuncture site. Apply dressing, periodically assessing for continued bleeding.
- Label the specimen and transport it to the laboratory.
- Report abnormal findings to the primary care provider.

 Clinical Alerts

- Possible complication: Prolonged bleeding at site due to vitamin K deficiency due to liver dysfunction
- Teach the patient to monitor the site. If the site begins to bleed, the patient should apply direct pressure and, if unable to control the bleeding, return to the laboratory or notify the health-care provider.

 Leukoagglutinin Test

Test Description

Patients requiring transfusion receive blood which is compatible with their own blood based on testing for ABO blood type and Rh factor. During and after administration of blood, the patient is monitored for signs and symptoms of a transfusion reaction. One such reaction would be a hemolytic reaction due to ABO incompatibility. This type of reaction can result in hemoglobinemia, hemoglobinuria, disseminated intravascular coagulation (DIC), renal failure, and cardiovascular collapse.

Nonhemolytic febrile reactions can also occur. In this case, the patient experiences an apparent transfusion reaction despite receiving compatible blood. This type of reaction can range in severity from fever to dyspnea and hypotension. This reaction is thought to be due to the patient forming antibodies against the white blood cells (WBCs) of the donor blood, although the formation of cytokines during the storage of the blood is also a possible explanation.

If a nonhemolytic febrile reaction occurs and the blood is found to be ABO compatible, the leukoagglutinin test should be done. If the test is positive, the patient should receive leukocyte-poor blood for future transfusions.

Normal Values

Negative

Possible Meanings of Abnormal Values

Positive
Blood transfusion reaction

Contributing Factors to Abnormal Values

- Receipt of previous blood transfusions and pregnancy may cause WBC antibodies to form.

Interventions/Implications

Pretest
- Explain to the patient the purpose of the test and the need for a blood sample to be drawn.
- No fasting is required before the test.

Procedure
- A 7-mL blood sample is drawn in a red-top collection tube.
- Gloves are worn throughout the procedure.

Posttest
- Apply pressure at venipuncture site. Apply dressing, periodically assessing for continued bleeding.
- Label the specimen and transport it to the laboratory.
- Report abnormal findings to the primary care provider.

 Leukocytes in Stool (Stool for WBCs, Fecal Leukocytes)

Test Description
The presence of leukocytes in stool is an indicator of inflammation as a result of bacteria-host interaction. Leukocyte analysis is useful for the differentiation of bacillary dysentery, demonstrating a preponderance of polymorphonuclear leuko-cytes (neutrophils). The presence of fecal leukocytes warrants a stool culture to determine the actual microorganism and assist in the planning of treatment.

Normal Values

None detected

Possible Meanings of Abnormal Values

Positive
Campylobacter
Clostridium difficile

Escherichia coli
Salmonella
Shigella
Ulcerative colitis

Contributing Factors to Abnormal Values

- Stool cannot be processed if submitted in formalin, contains barium, or if unpreserved for more than 24 hours.

Interventions/Implications

Pretest

- Explain to the patient the purpose of the test. Provide any written teaching materials available on the subject.
- No fasting is required before the test.

Procedure

- A small, random stool specimen is collected in a vial containing polyvinyl alcohol.

Posttest

- Report abnormal findings to the primary care provider.

L

→ Clinical Alerts

- If stool is positive for leukocytes, a follow-up culture is needed. Appropriate treatment is instituted based on organism identified.

Lipase

Test Description

Lipase is an enzyme produced by the pancreas which converts fats and triglycerides into fatty acids and glycerol. Measurement of this enzyme is done to distinguish abdominal pain due to acute pancreatitis from that due to other causes which might benefit from surgical intervention. Lipase is usually evaluated in conjunction with serum amylase. Lipase increases in the blood within 24 to 36 hours after the onset of acute pancreatitis, which is after amylase increases. Lipase remains elevated up to 14 days longer than amylase.

THE EVIDENCE FOR PRACTICE

Acute pancreatitis is suspected in patients presenting with epigastric upper abdominal pain that is acute in onset, rapidly increasing in severity, and persistent without relief. Serum amylase and/or lipase levels can be considered diagnostic when the reported value(s) is ≥3 times normal.

Normal Values

0–160 U/L (0–160 U/L SI units)

Possible Meanings of Abnormal Values

Increased

Acute pancreatitis
Acute cholecystitis
Biliary obstruction
Chronic relapsing pancreatitis
Diabetic ketoacidosis
Intestinal obstruction
Liver disease
Pancreatic cancer
Pancreatic pseudocyst
Peritonitis
Renal failure

Contributing Factors to Abnormal Values

- Hemolysis of the blood sample may alter test results.
- Drugs which may *increase* lipase levels: ACE-inhibitors, acetaminophen, aminosalicylic acid, antivirals, azathioprine, bethanecol, cholinergics, codeine, corticosteroids, corticotropin, dexamethasone, ethacrynic acid, ethanol, furosemide, heparin, indomethacin, meperidine, mercaptopurine, methacholine, morphine, oral contraceptives, phenformin, statins, triamcinolone.
- Drugs which may *decrease* lipase levels: calcium ions.

Interventions/Implications

Pretest
- Explain to the patient the purpose of the test and the need for a blood sample to be drawn.
- Fasting for 8 to 12 hours is required prior to the test. Water is permitted.

Procedure
- A 7-mL blood sample is drawn in a red-top collection tube.
- Gloves are worn throughout the procedure.

Posttest
- Apply pressure at venipuncture site. Apply dressing, periodically assessing for continued bleeding.
- Label the specimen and transport it to the laboratory.
- Report abnormal findings to the primary care provider.

Clinical Alerts

- Serum amylase and lipase are typically both evaluated in suspected pancreatitis.
- In some patients, acute pancreatitis may be present in the absence of enzyme abnormalities.

Liver and Pancreatobiliary System Sonogram
(Gallbladder and Biliary System Sonogram, Liver Sonogram, Pancreas Sonogram)

Test Description

Ultrasonography is a noninvasive method of diagnostic testing in which ultrasound waves are sent into the body with a small transducer pressed against the skin. The transducer then receives any returning sound waves, which are deflected back as they bounce off various structures. The transducer converts the returning sound waves into electric signals that are then transformed by a computer into a visual display on a monitor.

In this particular type of ultrasonography, the areas evaluated include the gallbladder, biliary system, liver, and pancreas. This procedure is now used much more frequently than oral cholescystography, since ultrasonography involves no radiation exposure for the patient. This test is used for evaluating jaundice, hepatomegaly, and abdominal trauma, and in the diagnosis of acute cholecystitis, suspected metastatic tumors of the liver, and suspected pancreatic carcinoma. It can also be used to guide the insertion of a biopsy needle.

L

Normal Values

Normal gallbladder, bile ducts, liver, and pancreas

Possible Meanings of Abnormal Values

- Acute cholecystitis
- Biliary obstruction
- Cholelithiasis
- Dilation of the bile ducts
- Gallbladder carcinoma
- Gallbladder polyps
- Hematoma
- Hepatic abscess
- Hepatocellular disease
- Liver cyst
- Liver metastases
- Pancreatic carcinoma
- Pancreatitis
- Primary hepatic tumor
- Pseudocyst of the pancreas
- Subphrenic abscess

Contributing Factors to Abnormal Values

- The transducer must be in good contact with the skin as it is being moved. A water-based gel is used to ensure good contact with the skin.
- Test results are hindered by the presence of bowel gas, retained barium, or obesity.

Interventions/Implications

Pretest
- Explain to the patient the purpose of the test. Provide any written teaching materials available on the subject. Note that there is no discomfort involved with this test.
- The patient is to eat a fat-free meal in the evening and then fast for 8 to 12 hours before the test. This promotes accumulation of bile in the gallbladder, resulting in better visualization during ultrasonography.

Procedure
- The patient is assisted to a supine position on the ultrasonography table.
- A coupling agent, such as a water-based gel, is applied to the area to be evaluated.
- A transducer is placed on the skin and moved as needed to provide good visualization of the structures.
- The sound waves are transformed into a visual display on the monitor. Printed copies of this display are made.

Posttest
- Cleanse the patient's skin of any lubricant.
- Report abnormal findings to the primary care provider.

Liver Biopsy (Percutaneous Needle Biopsy of the Liver)

Test Description

Although the liver can be evaluated in a number of ways, including measurement of liver enzymes, ultrasonography, and CT scanning, only liver biopsy can provide actual tissue samples for histopathologic evaluation. Indications for performing liver biopsy include: persistently elevated liver enzymes, jaundice of unknown etiology, hepatomegaly of unknown etiology, infiltrative diseases such as sarcoidosis or amyloidosis, and suspected disease of the liver, such as tumors, cysts, or cirrhosis.

A percutaneous needle biopsy of the liver is considered a closed procedure and can be performed at the bedside. A 14 to 18 gauge tissue core needle is inserted directly through the skin into the liver, either blindly or guided through the concurrent use of ultrasonography or CT scan, and a sample of liver tissue is aspirated. An open procedure, where the biopsy is performed through a surgical incision, is an alternate method. Regardless of the type of biopsy procedure used, the biopsied tissue is placed in a collection container and covered with an appropriate solution (e.g., 10% formalin, Ringer's solution). The laboratory will appropriately fix, prepare, and stain the tissue for microscopic examination by a pathologist.

THE EVIDENCE FOR PRACTICE

According to the American Gastroenterological Association, patients (with chronic hepatitis C) in whom antiviral therapy is being considered are candidates for liver biopsy, the gold standard for determining histologic grade and stage, unless the potential for complications is unacceptably high.

Normal Values

Absence of abnormal cells and tissue

Possible Meanings of Abnormal Values

Alcoholic liver disease
Amyloidosis
Benign tumor
Biliary atresia
Cirrhosis
Cyst
Coccidioidomycosis (disseminated)
Hemochromatosis
Hemosiderosis
Hepatitis
Hepatocellular carcinoma
Hodgkin's lymphoma
Liver abscess
Malignant tumor (primary or metastatic)
Metabolic disorders
Nonalcoholic steatohepatitis (NASH)
Non-Hodgkin's lymphoma
Primary biliary cirrhosis
Sarcoidosis
Schistosomiasis
Sclerosing cholangitis
Tuberculosis
Weil's disease
Wilson's disease

Interventions/Implications

Pretest

- Explain the procedure to the patient. Have the patient practice holding breath after exhalation. Explain that the patient may feel discomfort in right shoulder and/or the biopsy site during the procedure.
- Instruct the patient to remain NPO for at least 6 hours prior to the test.
- Obtain signed informed consent.
- Assess for coagulation deficiencies. Monitor prothrombin time (PT), partial thromboplastin time (PTT), and platelet count. Treatment regimen to reverse coagulopathies may include administration of vitamin K, fresh frozen plasma transfusion, or platelet transfusion.
- Obtain baseline hematocrit.
- Administer sedation, if ordered.

Procedure

- The procedure is usually performed at the bedside by the physician.
- Baseline vital signs are taken and recorded. Vital signs are also taken periodically during the procedure.
- The patient is placed in the supine or left lateral position. The patient's right hand should be under the head, and the head turned to the left.

- A local anesthetic is administered.
- Conscious sedation, typically using midazolam with fentanyl or meperidine, may be used.
- The patient is instructed to inhale and exhale deeply several times and then to hold the breath following a full expiration. This maintains the diaphragm in its highest position to minimize chance of puncture during the procedure.
- The needle is inserted in the right midaxillary line at the sixth to seventh or eighth to ninth intercostal space, depending on the level of maximal liver dullness. This position may vary if a specific area is the target for the biopsy and the biopsy is being guided by ultrasound or CT scan.
- The tissue sample is aspirated, and the needle is quickly removed.
- Once the needle is removed, the patient is allowed to breathe normally.
- The tissue sample is placed in a specimen bottle containing a 10% formalin solution and sent to pathology.
- A pressure dressing is applied to the site.
- The entire procedure usually takes approximately 10 to 15 minutes.
- Gloves are worn throughout the procedure.

Posttest

- Monitor vital signs frequently, following the institution's policy for postoperative care. Assess for signs of hemorrhage (elevated pulse, decreasing blood pressure) and peritonitis (elevated temperature).
- Assess rate, rhythm, and depth of respirations. Assess breath sounds. Assess for dyspnea, pleuritic chest pain, cyanosis, hypotension, and restlessness.
- Assess for hemorrhage by observing dressing for bleeding. Do **not** remove pressure dressing to look for bleeding. Obtain hematocrit 6 to 8 hours after the test. Report any drop from pretest level immediately.
- Observe for pain.
- Right upper quadrant pain may be due to subscapular accumulation of blood or bile.
- Right shoulder pain may be due to blood on the undersurface of the diaphragm.
- Maintain pressure on the biopsy site by turning patient on right side for 1 to 4 hours, placing a rolled towel or small towel under the costal margin, and maintaining bedrest for at least 6 hours.
- Instruct the patient to avoid coughing or straining, which increases intra-abdominal pressure. Strenuous activities or heavy lifting are to be avoided for 1 to 2 weeks.
- Report abnormal findings to the primary care provider.

L

→ Clinical Alerts

- Possible complications include: bile peritonitis, hemorrhage, perforation of an abdominal organ (diaphragm, gallbladder, or kidney), pneumothorax, and shock. Frequent checks needed of vital signs, pulmonary assessment, abdominal assessment, pain assessment, mental status, and observation of pressure dressing.

CONTRAINDICATIONS!

- Patients with bleeding disorders
- Patients with prothrombin times in the anticoagulant range (2–3 times the control value)

- Patients with decreased platelet count (<50,000/mm³)
- Patients with platelet dysfunction due to aspirin use or renal failure
- Patients in which there is difficulty in determining liver location, as in presence of ascites or morbid obesity (in these cases use of transjugular biopsy may be an alternative)
- Patients with extrahepatic obstruction
- Patients with infection (subdiaphragmatic, right hemithoracic, or biliary tract)
- Patients with suspected vascular tumor (hemangioma) of the liver
- Patients who are unable to cooperate during the procedures (anyone unable to remain still and/or unable to hold their breath following exhalation)

Liver/Spleen Scan

Test Description

For a liver/spleen scan, the patient is given a radionuclide compound, usually a technetium-99m radiopharmaceutical via an IV injection. A scintillation camera is used to take a radioactivity reading from the body. These readings are fed into a computer, which translates these readings into a two-dimensional gray scale picture. These pictures are obtained 30 minutes following the injection. This test is used in the diagnosis of abscesses, hematomas, tumors, and infiltrative processes of the liver and/or spleen, and to evaluate jaundice.

Normal Values

Normal size, shape, and position of liver and spleen

Possible Meanings of Abnormal Values

Abscesses of the liver/spleen
Amyloidosis of the liver/spleen
Budd-Chiari syndrome
Cirrhosis
Granulomas of the liver/spleen
Hepatitis
Hematomas of the liver/spleen
Hepatic cysts
Infection
Injury
Portal hypertension
Primary or metastatic tumors of the liver/spleen
Sarcoidosis of the liver/spleen

Contributing Factors to Abnormal Values

- Any movement by the patient may alter quality of films taken.
- Retained barium from previous exams may interfere with the test.

Interventions/Implications

Pretest
- Explain to the patient the purpose of the test. Provide any written teaching materials available on the subject. Note that discomfort involved with this test is primarily due to lying on a hard table for an extended period of time and the needle puncture. Reassure the patient that only trace amounts of the radionuclide are involved in the test.
- The patient must remain still while the scan is being performed.
- No fasting is required prior to the test.
- Obtain a signed informed consent.

Procedure
- The radiopharmaceutical is administered by IV injection in a peripheral vein.
- The patient is assisted to a supine position on the examination table.
- A scintillation camera is positioned over the right upper quadrant of the patient's abdomen. This camera takes a radioactivity reading from the body. This information is transformed into a two-dimensional picture of the area.
- Scans are obtained 30 minutes postinjection. Scans with the patient in the lateral and prone positions are also performed.
- Gloves are worn during the radionuclide injection.

Posttest
- Check the injection site for redness or swelling.
- If a woman who is lactating *must* have a nuclear scan, she should not breast-feed the infant until the radionuclide has been eliminated, possibly for 3 days.
- Although the amount of diagnostic radionuclide excreted in the urine is low, the urine should not be used for any laboratory tests for the time period indicated by the nuclear medicine department.
- Gloves are worn whenever dealing with the urine.
- Encourage fluid intake by the patient to enhance excretion of the radionuclide.
- Report abnormal findings to the primary care provider.

Clinical Alerts

- Whenever possible, schedule the liver/spleen scan prior to any testing involving barium.

CONTRAINDICATIONS!

- Pregnant women
  - Caution: A woman in her childbearing years should undergo radiography only during her menses or 12 to 14 days after its onset to avoid any exposure to a fetus.
- Patients who are lactating
- Patients who are unable to cooperate due to age, mental status, pain, or other factors

Low-Density Lipoprotein (LDL)

Test Description

Cholesterol is synthesized in the liver from dietary fats. It is transported in the blood by the low density lipoproteins (LDLs, or "bad" cholesterol) and high density lipoproteins (HDLs, or "good" cholesterol). LDLs carry cholesterol from the liver to other parts of the body where it can cause atherosclerotic disease. High levels of LDL are associated with an increased risk for coronary artery disease (CAD).

To determine a target goal for LDL, risk factors must be determined. These include:

- Cigarette smoking
- Hypertension
- HDL <40 mg/dL
- Family history of premature CHD (male <age 55, female <age 65)
- Age (male ≥45, female ≥55)

If the HDL is ≥60 mg/dL, this is considered a "negative" risk factor, which removes one risk factor from the total count. The presence of diabetes mellitus is regarded as a CHD risk equivalent.

Target LDL levels, according to Adult Treatment Panel III (ATP III) guidelines, are:

With 0–1 cardiac risk factors:	<160 mg/dL (<4.14 mmol/L SI units)
With ≥2 cardiac risk factors:	<130 mg/dL (<3.36 mmol/L SI units)
With CAD or diabetes:	<100 mg/dL (<2.6 mmol/L SI units)

It is now suggested by some research studies that individuals at very high risk of heart disease should have an LDL of <70 mg/dL.

As a part of evaluating this risk, the low-density lipoprotein (LDL) level is measured as part of the lipid profile. In addition to actual measurement of the LDL, it can be calculated with the following formula:

$$LDL = Total Cholesterol - HDL - (Triglycerides/5)$$

THE EVIDENCE FOR PRACTICE

According to the Third Report of the National Cholesterol Education Program (NCEP) Expert Panel on Detection, Evaluation, and Treatment of High Blood Cholesterol in Adults (http://www.nhlbi.nih.gov/guidelines/cholesterol/atp3_rpt.htm):

- In all adults aged 20 years or older, a fasting lipoprotein profile (total cholesterol, low density lipoprotein cholesterol, high density lipoprotein [HDL] cholesterol, and triglycerides) should be obtained once every 5 years. If the testing opportunity is nonfasting, only the values for total cholesterol and HDL cholesterol will be usable. In such a case, if total cholesterol is ≥200 mg/dL or high density lipoprotein is <40 mg/dL, a follow-up lipoprotein profile is needed for appropriate management based on low density lipoprotein.

Normal Values

Optimal:	<100 mg/dL (<2.6 mmol/L SI units)
Near Optimal:	100–129 mg/dL (2.6–3.35 mmol/L SI units)

Abnormal Values

Borderline high risk: 130–159 mg/dL (3.36–4.11 mmol/L SI units)
High risk: >159 mg/dL (>4.11 mmol/L SI units)

Possible Meanings of Abnormal Values

Increased	Decreased
Cholestasis	Cancer
Chronic renal failure	Malabsorption
Diabetes mellitus	Malnutrition
Hepatic disease	Myeloproliferative disease
High cholesterol diet	
Hyperlipidemia	
Hypothyroidism	
Multiple myeloma	
Nephrotic syndrome	
Porphyria	
Pregnancy	

Contributing Factors to Abnormal Values

- Drugs which may *increase* LDL levels: anabolic steroids, aspirin, carbamazepine, corticosteroids, oral contraceptives, phenothiazines, progestins, sulfonamides.
- Drugs which may *decrease* LDL levels: cholestyramine, clofibrate, estrogens, neomycin sulfate, nicotinic acid, statin drugs, thyroxine.

Interventions/Implications

Pretest
- Explain to the patient the purpose of the test and the need for a blood sample to be drawn.
- Fasting for 12 hours is required prior to the test. Water is permitted.

Procedure
- A 7-mL blood sample is drawn in a lavender-top collection tube.
- Gloves are worn throughout the procedure.

Posttest
- Apply pressure at venipuncture site. Apply dressing, periodically assessing for continued bleeding.
- Label the specimen and transport it to the laboratory.
- Report abnormal findings to the primary care provider.

Clinical Alerts

- For individuals with elevated LDL levels, counseling is needed regarding dietary changes, weight loss, and exercise. Drug therapy may also be instituted.

Lumbar Puncture with Cerebrospinal Fluid (CSF) Analysis (LP, Spinal Tap)

Test Description

Cerebrospinal fluid (CSF) is a clear protein substance which circulates in the sub-arachnoid space. Its functions include protection of the brain and spinal cord from injury and transportation of substances through the central nervous system (CNS). Samples of CSF are most commonly obtained via a lumbar puncture; however they may also be obtained during myelography, cisternal puncture, or ventricular puncture. In a *lumbar puncture*, the spinal needle is inserted between two of the lumbar verte-brae. The *cisternal puncture* involves the insertion of the needle between the first cer-vical vertebra and the rim of the foramen magnum. The cisternal puncture is rarely used due to the needle's proximity to the brainstem. The *ventricular puncture*, also rarely used, involves drilling a hole in the skull and inserting a needle into a lateral ventricle. This procedure is used when the other methods might cause such compli-cations as brainstem herniation. The analysis of the CSF provides information to assist in the diagnosis of a wide variety of CNS diseases, including infectious diseases.

THE EVIDENCE FOR PRACTICE

Adult patients with headache exhibiting signs of increased intracranial pressure including papilledema, absent venous pulsations on funduscopic examination, altered mental status, or focal neurologic deficits should undergo a neuroimaging study before having an LP. In the absence of findings suggestive of increased intracranial pressure, an LP can be per-formed without obtaining a neuroimaging study. (Note: An LP does not assess for all causes of a sudden severe headache.) (ACEP, 2002)

Normal Values

Cell count

White blood cells:	0–5 mononuclear cells/μL ($0–5 \times 10^6$ cells/L SI units)
Red blood cells:	None
Chloride:	110–125 mEq/L (110–125 mmol/L SI units)
Color:	Clear, colorless
Glucose:	50–75 mg/dL (2.8–4.2 mmol/L SI units)
Pressure:	50–180 mm H_2O
Protein:	15–45 mg/dL (0.15–0.45 g/L SI units)
Gamma globulin:	3–12% of total protein

Possible Meanings of Abnormal Values

Cell count

Increased WBCs	Increased RBCs
Abscess	Hemorrhage
Acute infection	Traumatic tap
Brain infarction	
Demyelinating disease	
Meningitis	

Onset of chronic illness
Tumor

Chloride

| **Decreased** |
| Meningitis |
| Tuberculosis |

Color

Bloody:	Subarachnoid, intracerebral, or intraventricular hemorrhage
	Spinal cord obstruction
	Traumatic tap
Cloudy:	Infection
	Protein in CSF
Orange, yellow, or brown:	Erythrocyte breakdown (old blood), elevated protein

Glucose

Increased	**Decreased**
Systemic hyperglycemia	Bacterial infection
	Fungal infection
	Meningitis
	Mumps
	Postsubarachnoid hemorrhage
	Systemic hypoglycemia
	Tuberculosis

Pressure

Increased	**Decreased**
Hemorrhage	Diabetic coma
Infection	Shock
Trauma	Spinal subarachnoid obstruction
Tumor	(spinal cord tumor)
	Syncope

Protein

Increased	**Decreased**
Blood in CSF	Rapid CSF production
Diabetes mellitus	
Hemorrhage	
Infection	
Inflammatory process	
Polyneuritis	
Syphilis	
Trauma	
Tumors	

Gamma globulin

| **Increased** |
| Demyelinating disease (e.g., multiple sclerosis) |
| Guillain-Barre syndrome |
| Neurosyphilis |

Contributing Factors to Abnormal Values

- Coughing, crying, or straining during the procedure may increase the CSF pressure.

Interventions/Implications

Pretest

- Explain to the patient the purpose of the test. Provide any written teaching materials available on the subject. Note that discomfort during the test is due to the injection of the local anesthetic and penetration of the dura mater with the needle
- The patient must remain still while the procedure is performed.
- No fasting is required before the procedure.
- Obtain a signed informed consent.

Procedure

- The patient is assisted into a side-lying position with the knees drawn up to the abdomen and the chin on the chest. This flexion of the spine provides easy access to the lumbar subarachnoid space.
- Assist the patient in maintaining the proper position by placing one arm around the patient's knees and the other arm around his or her neck.
- The skin is cleansed and draped. A local anesthetic is administered to the area.
- Ask the patient to report any pain or tingling sensations throughout the procedure which may indicate irritation or puncture of a nerve root.
- The spinal needle is inserted in the midline, usually between the third and fourth lumbar vertebrae.
- The stylet is removed from the needle and a stopcock and manometer are attached to the needle to measure initial CSF pressure.
- A sample of the CSF is collected in a sterile container.
- A final pressure reading is taken, and the needle is removed.
- A sterile dressing is applied to the puncture site.
- Gloves are worn throughout the procedure.

Posttest

- Instruct the patient to maintain bedrest for 8 hours with no more than a 30° elevation of the head of the bed. This will help to minimize the occurrence of postlumbar puncture headache.
- Encourage the patient to take in fluids.
- Observe the puncture site for swelling and drainage and assess the movement and sensation to the lower extremities frequently for the first 4 hours after the procedure.
- Report abnormal findings to the primary care provider.

→ Clinical Alerts

- Possible complications include: bleeding into the spinal canal, CSF leakage causing severe headache, meningitis, spinal cord damage, transient back or leg pain or paresthesias
- Life-threatening complications include: brainstem herniation resulting in brain damage or death, retroperitoneal hemorrhage due to puncture of the aorta or vena cava

- Patients with increased intracranial pressure (CSF removal can lead to brainstem herniation)
- Patients with infection at the puncture site
- Patients who are unable to cooperate because of age, mental status, pain, or other factors

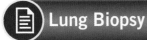

Lung Biopsy

Test Description

Lesions of the lung may be studied through such tests as chest x-ray, computed tomography (CT) scan, and bronchoscopy. However, determination of the nature of a lesion, that is, whether a mass is benign or malignant, can only be made by obtaining a biopsy of the tissue. In a lung biopsy, a sample of lung tissue is removed for histologic study. The tissue sample may be obtained by needle biopsy through the chest wall, by tissue sampling during fiberoptic bronchoscopy, or by open biopsy during a thoracotomy. This discussion will be limited to that of needle biopsy of the lung.

L

Normal Values

No abnormal cells or tissue present

Possible Meanings of Abnormal Values

Adenocarcinoma
Granuloma
Pulmonary infection
Oat cell carcinoma
Sarcoidosis
Squamous cell carcinoma

Interventions/Implications

Pretest
- Explain to the patient the purpose of the test and the procedure to be done. Explain to the patient that a local anesthetic will be used, but that transient sharp pain may be experienced when the biopsy needle touches the lung. Remind the patient that no movement, such as coughing, can occur during the biopsy.
- Obtain baseline chest x-ray and coagulation tests (partial thromboplastin time, platelet count, prothrombin time).
- Fasting after midnight prior to the test is usually required.
- Obtain a signed informed consent.
- Obtain baseline vital signs.

Procedure
- The patient is assisted to a sitting position with the arms supported on a pillow on an overbed table.

- The skin is cleansed with an antiseptic and draped.
- A local anesthetic is administered.
- A small incision is made in the posterior chest wall at the selected intercostal space.
- The biopsy needle is introduced through the incision, chest wall, and pleura, and into the tissue or mass to be biopsied.
- The specimen is obtained and the needle removed.
- A portion of the tissue to be studied for histology is placed in a container with a formaldehyde solution. The remaining tissue sample is placed in a sterile container for microbiological study.
- Pressure is exerted on the biopsy site, followed by application of a sterile dressing.
- Gloves are worn throughout the procedure.

Posttest
- Assist the patient into a semi-Fowler's position.
- Monitor the patient's vital signs, breath sounds, and comfort level, and check the dressing for drainage every 15 to 30 minutes until stable.
- Observe for indications of hemothorax or pneumothorax: rapid, shallow respirations, dyspnea, air hunger, chest pain, cough, hemoptysis, and absence of breath sounds over area.
- Observe for signs of infection: elevated temperature, chest pain, yellow sputum, and abnormal breath sounds.
- Administer analgesics as needed.
- Provide emotional support as the patient awaits test results.
- Report abnormal findings to the primary care provider.

→ **Clinical Alerts**

- Possible complications include: bleeding, hemothorax, infection, and pneumothorax.
- A postprocedure chest x-ray is obtained to assess for complications.

CONTRAINDICATIONS!

- Patients with bleeding disorders
- Patients with hypoxia, pulmonary hypertension, or cardiac disease with cor pulmonale
- Patients with hyperinflation of the lung
- Patients unable to cooperate with the examination

Lung Scan (Ventilation/Perfusion Scan, V/Q Scan)

Test Description
The *lung perfusion scan* is performed to detect pulmonary emboli (PE), and to assess arterial perfusion of the lungs. The scan involves injection of a radiopharmaceutical, followed by scanning. The radiolabeled particles filter out of the capillary membrane and become trapped in the lung tissue, allowing the camera to detect

areas of obstructed blood flow. The lung perfusion scan is performed prior to, but in association with, the lung ventilation scan. The *lung ventilation scan* is used to delineate areas of the lung ventilated during respiration. For this scan, the patient inhales a radioactive gas. The results of both scans are reviewed to help in diagnosis.

A decreased uptake of the radioisotope during a perfusion scan indicates a blood flow problem. If generalized, there could be an occlusion of the pulmonary arteries. A localized decrease in perfusion with normal ventilation may indicate pulmonary embolism.

A decreased uptake of the radioactive gas during a ventilation scan may indicate airway obstruction, pneumonia, or chronic obstructive pulmonary disease (COPD). With these conditions, perfusion will usually be normal.

THE EVIDENCE FOR PRACTICE

The American College of Emergency Physicians' clinical policy on pulmonary embolism states:

- In patients with a low-to-moderate pretest probability of PE, a normal perfusion scan reliably excludes clinically significant PE.
- In patients with a low-to-moderate pretest probability of PE and a nondiagnostic V/Q scan, use one of the following tests instead of pulmonary arteriogram to exclude clinically significant PE:
    1. A negative quantitative D-dimer assay (turbidimetric or ELISA).
    2. A negative whole blood cell qualitative D-dimer assay in conjunction with a Wells' score of 4 or less.
    3. A negative single bilateral venous ultrasonographic scan for low-probability patients.
    4. A negative serial* bilateral venous ultrasonographic scan for moderate-probability patients.

The group also notes that thin collimation spiral CT scan of the thorax with 1- to 2-mm image reconstruction may be used as an alternative to V/Q scan during the diagnostic evaluation of patients with suspected PE.

Normal Values

Uniform uptake pattern during both perfusion and ventilation portions of the test

Possible Meanings of Abnormal Values

Airway obstruction
Asthma
Atelectasis
Bronchitis
COPD
Emphysema
Pneumonia
Pneumonitis

---

*serial venous ultrasonography refers to scheduling a patient for follow-up examination in the emergency department within 3 to 7 days or referring to a primary care physician for follow-up.

Pulmonary embolism

Tumors

Tuberculosis

Contributing Factors to Abnormal Values

- Any movement by the patient may alter quality of films taken.
- Pulmonary parenchymal problems such as pneumonia may mimic a perfusion defect.

Interventions/Implications

Pretest

- Explain to the patient the purpose of the test. Provide any written teaching materials available on the subject. Note that discomfort involved with this test is primarily due to lying on a hard table for an extended period of time and the needle puncture. Reassure the patient that only trace amounts of the radionuclide are involved in the test.
- The patient must remain still while the scan is being performed.
- No fasting is required prior to the test, unless sedation is going to be used during the test. If so, fasting for 4 hours is required prior to the test.
- Obtain a signed informed consent.

Procedure

For the perfusion scan

- The radiopharmaceutical is administered by IV injection in a peripheral vein.
- The patient is assisted to a supine position on the examination table.
- A scintillation camera is positioned over the patient's chest. This camera takes a radioactivity reading from the body. This information is transformed into a two-dimensional picture of the area.
- Scans with the patient in the prone and several lateral positions are also performed.
- Gloves are worn during the radionuclide injection.

For the ventilation scan

- The patient breathes the radioactive gas (krypton 85 or xenon 133) through a face mask.
- Scanning of the chest to show gas distribution is completed.

Posttest

- Check the injection site for redness or swelling.
- If a woman who is lactating *must* have a nuclear scan, she should not breast-feed the infant until the radionuclide has been eliminated, possibly for 3 days.
- Although the amount of diagnostic radionuclide excreted in the urine is low, the urine should not be used for any laboratory tests for the time period indicated by the nuclear medicine department.
- Gloves are worn whenever dealing with the urine.
- Encourage fluid intake by the patient to enhance excretion of the radionuclide.
- Report abnormal findings to the primary care provider.

→ **Clinical Alerts**

- A chest x-ray should be performed either prior to or immediately following a V/Q scan. This assists with evaluation of the scan.

CONTRAINDICATIONS!

- Pregnant women
  - Caution: A woman in her childbearing years should undergo radiography only during her menses or 12 to 14 days after its onset to avoid any exposure to a fetus.
- Patients who are lactating
- Patients who are unable to cooperate due to age, mental status, pain, or other factors

 Luteinizing Hormone (LH)

Test Description

Luteinizing hormone (LH), like follicle-stimulating hormone (FSH), is secreted by the anterior pituitary gland. FSH promotes maturation of the ovarian follicle, which is needed for production of estrogen. As estrogen levels rise, luteinizing hormone (LH) is produced. High levels of FSH and LH are both needed in order for ovulation to occur in women and for the transformation of the ovarian follicle into the corpus luteum, a process known as *luteinization*. After ovulation occurs, LH maintains the corpus luteum, which synthesizes progesterone. If pregnancy does not occur, the corpus luteum disintegrates after about 10 days. LH also stimulates the ovaries to produce steroids, primarily estradiol. These steroids help the pituitary to regulate the production of LH. At menopause, the ovaries stop functioning and LH levels rise. In males, LH and FSH stimulate the testes to release testosterone, which is needed for spermatogenesis to occur. This test is used to determine whether ovulation has occurred, and to evaluate amenorrhea and infertility.

L

Normal Values

Females:
Follicular phase:	5–30 mIU/mL (5–30 IU/L SI units)
Midcycle:	75–150 mIU/mL (75–150 IU/L SI units)
Luteal phase:	3–40 mIU/mL (3–40 IU/L SI units)
Postmenopausal:	30–200 mIU/mL (30–200 IU/L SI units)
Males:	6–23 mIU/mL (6–23 IU/L SI units)

Possible Meanings of Abnormal Values

Increased	Decreased
Acromegaly (early)	Anorexia nervosa
Alcohol abuse	Hypogonadotropism
Amenorrhea	Hypopituitarism
Congenital absence of ovaries	Hypothalamic dysfunction
Hyperpituitarism	Malnutrition
Klinefelter's syndrome	Prolactinoma
Menopause	Sheehan's syndrome
Menstruation	
Ovarian failure	

Polycystic ovarian disease
Precocious puberty
Primary gonadal dysfunction
Stein-Leventhal syndrome
Turner's syndrome

Contributing Factors to Abnormal Values

- Hemolysis of the blood sample or having a radioactive scan within 1 week of the test may alter test results.
- Drugs which may *increase* LH levels: bromocriptine, clomiphene, finasteride, hydrocortisone, ketoconazole, lupron, spironolactone, tamoxifen, valproic acid.
- Drugs which may *decrease* LH levels: anabolic steroids, anticonvulsants, digoxin, estrogens, ketoconazole, metformin, octreotide, phenothiazines, progestins, tamoxifen.

Interventions/Implications

Pretest

- Explain to the patient the purpose of the test and the need for a blood sample to be drawn.
- No fasting is required before the test.
- If possible, withhold drugs which may alter test results for 48 hours prior to the test.

Procedure

- A 7-mL blood sample is drawn in a red-top collection tube.
- Gloves are worn throughout the procedure.

Posttest

- Apply pressure at venipuncture site. Apply dressing, periodically assessing for continued bleeding.
- Label the specimen and transport it to the laboratory.
- For female patients: on the laboratory slip, include the date on which the patient began her last menstrual period.
- Resume medications as taken prior to the test.
- Report abnormal findings to the primary care provider.

Clinical Alerts

- FSH and LH are usually measured at the same time.
- Pooled blood specimens are sometimes used to provide a more accurate assessment of LH.

Lyme Disease Antibody Test

Test Description

Lyme disease is caused by the tick-transmitted spirochete *Borrelia burgdorferi*. The incubation period for the infection is 14 to 23 days. Lyme disease has three stages. The first stage involves a lesion and erythema around the bite, followed by regional lymphadenopathy, malaise, fever, headache, myalgias, arthralgias, and possibly conjunctivitis. The second stage, which occurs weeks to months later, may be associated with a rash and neurologic abnormalities, including meningitis, encephalitis, and Bell's palsy. The third stage, the chronic form of the disease, is characterized by arthritis, skin lesions, and additional neurologic problems.

Diagnosis of Lyme disease is made through determination of the presence of *Borrelia* antibodies. Antibody titers are usually low during the first several weeks of the illness, reach peak levels months later, and remain elevated for several years. ELISA (enzyme-linked immunosorbent assay) testing is done and if positive, a Western blot test is done to confirm the diagnosis. A DNA-based test using polymerase chain reaction (PCR) methodology can also be done. This test is highly specific for identification of the organism.

THE EVIDENCE FOR PRACTICE

According to the International Lyme and Associated Diseases Society, treatment decisions should not be based routinely or exclusively on laboratory findings. The two-tier diagnostic criteria, requiring both a positive enzyme-linked immunosorbent assay (ELISA) and western blot, lacks sensitivity and leaves a significant number of individuals with Lyme disease undiagnosed and untreated. Thus, laboratory results should not be used to exclude an individual from treatment.

Normal Values

Negative

Possible Meanings of Abnormal Values

Positive/Increased

Lyme disease

Contributing Factors to Abnormal Values

- False-positive results may occur in persons with high rheumatoid factor (RF) levels, spirochete infections, or previous Lyme disease infections.

Interventions/Implications

Pretest
- Explain to the patient the purpose of the test and the need for a blood sample to be drawn.
- No fasting is required before the test.

Procedure
- A 7-mL blood sample is drawn in a red-top collection tube.
- Gloves are worn throughout the procedure.

Posttest
- Apply pressure at venipuncture site. Apply dressing, periodically assessing for continued bleeding.
- Label the specimen and transport it to the laboratory.
- Report abnormal findings to the primary care provider.

→ **Clinical Alerts**

- If the patient is diagnosed with Lyme disease, treatment with antibiotics such as doxycycline should begin as soon as possible to avoid recurrent or refractory Lyme disease.

 Lymphangiography (Lymphography)

Test Description
Lymphangiography is the term used to indicate visualization of the lymphatic system. A contrast medium is injected into each foot. Visualization is then possible of the lymphatic system from the feet up to the thoracic duct. The test is used to detect and stage lymphomas and to assist in the differential diagnosis of lymphedema. When used with lymph node biopsy, the lymphangiogram can be used to determine the possible spread of cancer and effectiveness of cancer therapy. The contrast medium remains in the body for 1 to 2 years, thus allowing subsequent films to be made in order to monitor disease progression and assess any response of the patient to therapy.

Normal Values
Normal lymphatic vessels and nodes

Possible Meanings of Abnormal Values
Hodgkin's lymphoma
Lymphadenopathy
Non-Hodgkin's lymphoma
Metastatic involvement of the lymph nodes
Primary lymphedema
Secondary lymphedema

Contributing Factors to Abnormal Values
- Any movement by the patient may alter quality of films taken

Interventions/Implications
Pretest
- Explain to the patient the purpose of the test. Provide any written teaching materials available on the subject. Note that discomfort involved with this test is primarily due to lying on a hard table for an extended period of time and the needle punctures. Explain that some discomfort may be felt in the popliteal or inguinal areas when the dye is first injected.
- Check for allergies to iodine, shellfish, or contrast medium dye. Inform the radiologist of such possible allergy and obtain order for an antihistamine and steroid to be administered prior to the test.
- Patients receiving metformin (Glucophage) for Type 2 diabetes mellitus should discontinue the drug 2 days before elective surgery or angiographic exams. This is due to the possible occurrence of lactic acidosis, a potentially fatal complication of biguanide therapy.

- Baseline BUN and creatinine levels should be obtained.
- No fasting is required prior to the test.
- Obtain a signed informed consent.

Procedure
- The patient is assisted to a supine position on the examination table.
- The skin over the dorsum of each foot is cleansed. Blue contrast dye is injected intradermally between each of the first three toes of each foot. In 15 to 30 minutes the lymphatic vessels will appear as small blue lines.
- In the dorsum of each foot, a local anesthetic is injected and a 1-inch incision is made.
- Due to the extremely small diameter of the lymphatic vessels, a 30-gauge needle is inserted into the vessel. The contrast dye is then infused over a 60- to 90-minute period of time.
- Fluoroscopy is used to visualize the movement of the contrast dye. When the dye reaches the level of the third and fourth lumbar vertebrae, the infusion is discontinued.
- The needles are removed, the incisions sutured, and sterile dressings are applied.
- Radiographic films are taken at this time and again in 24 hours.
- Gloves are worn throughout the procedure.

Posttest
- Most allergic reactions to radiopaque dye occur within 30 minutes of administration of the contrast medium. Observe the patient closely for: respiratory distress, hypotension, edema, hives, rash, tachycardia, and/or laryngeal stridor. Emergency resuscitation equipment must be readily accessible.
- Continue to observe the patient for allergic reaction for 24 hours.
- Check the incisional sites for bleeding and signs of infection at frequent intervals. Sutures are removed in 7 to 10 days.
- The patient should maintain bedrest with the feet elevated for 24 hours. Ice bags may be applied to the feet to help reduce swelling.
- Observe for signs of pulmonary complications: shortness of breath, pleuritic pain, hypotension, low-grade fever, and cyanosis.
- Recheck the BUN and creatinine to verify adequate renal functioning prior to restarting metformin.
- Report abnormal findings to the primary care provider.

➡ Clinical Alerts

- Possible complications include: allergic reaction to dye, bleeding at the puncture site, infection at the puncture site, lipid pneumonia from embolization of the contrast medium, and renal failure
- Inform the patient that the dye will turn the urine and stool blue for 48 hours. The patient's skin and vision may have a blue tint for 48 hours.

CONTRAINDICATIONS!

- Patients who are allergic to iodine, shellfish, or contrast medium dye
- Pregnant women
  - Caution: A woman in her childbearing years should undergo radiography only during her menses or 12 to 14 days after its onset to avoid any exposure to a fetus.

- Patients who are unable to cooperate due to age, mental status, pain, or other factors
- Patients with renal failure or those susceptible to dye-induced renal failure (dehydrated patients)
- Patients with compromised functioning of the cardiac, pulmonary, hepatic, or renal systems

Lymphocyte Immunophenotyping
(T- and B-Cell Lymphocyte Counts)

Test Description

The immune system is composed of two subsystems: the humoral immune system and the cellular immune system. The primary cell of the humoral immune system is the *B-lymphocyte*, which matures in the bone marrow. B cells circulate in the blood in an inactive state. When the B cell is exposed to a specific protein or microorganism (antigen) for the first time, it produces antibodies (immunoglobulins) that bind with the antigen. This antibody production can take weeks to years, but antibodies are usually detectable in the blood within 6 months. In subsequent exposures to the same antigen, the antibodies formed against it are already present in the blood, so the response occurs almost immediately.

T-lymphocytes, which mature in the thymus gland, comprise the cellular immune system. When a T cell encounters a specific protein or microorganism to which it has been programmed to respond, it can directly attack and destroy the substance. Several types of T cells are produced. *Cytotoxic T cells* release toxic chemicals that directly destroy the antigen. *Helper T cells*, which carry the CD4 marker, stimulate the response of all other T cells. They also stimulate the humoral immune response. The *suppressor T cells*, which carry the CD8 marker, are responsible for stopping both humoral and cell-mediated immune responses, when appropriate. *Memory cells* are able to remember antigens that they have previously encountered. These cells thus provide for immediate response to the antigen when it is next encountered.

Testing of T- and B-lymphocyte counts is conducted to evaluate the status of the immune system. It is typical for the measurement of T- and B-lymphocyte counts to be included within testing for immunologic status in patients infected with the human immunodeficiency virus (HIV). Lymphocyte counts decrease as immune function decreases. The number of suppressor T cells remains normal or may increase. As helper T cells (CD4) become infected by HIV, their numbers decrease. Thus, as the CD4 cell count decreases, the predominant cell becomes the suppressor T cells, keeping the immune system suppressed and unable to fight infection.

Normal Values

Lymphocytes:	0.66–4.60 thousand/µL
B cells:	3–21% (92–392 cells/µL)
T cells:	60–88% (644–2201 cells/µL)
Helper T cells (CD4):	34–67% (493–1191 cells/µL)
Suppressor T cells (CD8):	10–42% (182–785 cells/µL)

Lymphocyte ratio:
Helper T cell to suppressor T cell ratio: >1.0

Possible Meanings of Abnormal Values

T cells

Increased	Decreased
Graves' disease	Acute viral infection
	DeGeorge's syndrome
	HIV infection
	Hodgkin's disease
	Increased risk for clinical AIDS
	Increased risk for opportunistic infections
	Malignancies
	Nezelof's syndrome
	Wiskott-Aldrich syndrome

B cells

Increased	Decreased
Chronic lymphocytic leukemia	Deficiency of IgG, IgA, IgM
Systemic lupus erythematosus	Hypogammaglobulinemia
	Lymphomas
	Multiple myeloma
	Nephrotic syndrome

L

Contributing Factors to Abnormal Values

- There is a diurnal variation in test values.

Interventions/Implications

Pretest
- Explain to the patient the purpose of the test and the need for a blood sample to be drawn.
- No fasting is required before the test.

Procedure
- A 7-mL blood sample is drawn in a green-top heparinized collection tube.
- Gloves are worn throughout the procedure.

Posttest
- Apply pressure at venipuncture site. Apply dressing, periodically assessing for continued bleeding.
- Label the specimen and transport it to the laboratory.
- Report abnormal findings to the primary care provider.

→ Clinical Alerts

- Potential complication: Infection at venipuncture site due to immunocompromised state.

- Teach the patient to monitor the site and to notify the primary care provider if signs or symptoms of infection occur, such as drainage, redness, warmth, edema, pain at the site, or fever.
- Periodic determinations of CD4 counts can be extremely stressful for the individual. Provide counseling and other referral sources as appropriate.

 Magnesium

Test Description

Magnesium (Mg^{++}) is primarily an ion of the intracellular fluid. Magnesium is essential for proper neuromuscular functioning, for energy production, for blood clotting, and for the activation of some enzymes. Only a very small amount of magnesium is found in the blood. The majority of magnesium is found in the bones, combined with calcium and phosphorus. Because of this close relationship among these electrolytes, changes in serum magnesium also affect serum levels of calcium and phosphorus. The body maintains magnesium levels by controlling its absorption from the intestines and its excretion or absorption by the kidneys. Thus, many of the causes of abnormal magnesium levels involve the gastrointestinal and renal systems.

Patients experiencing increased serum magnesium levels (*hypermagnesemia*) will have lethargy, flushing, hypotension, respiratory depression, bradycardia, and weak or absent deep tendon reflexes. Patients with *hypomagnesemia*, or decreased serum magnesium levels, will have muscle twitching and tremors, tetany, cardiac arrhythmias, and hyperactive deep tendon reflexes.

Normal Values

1.5–2.0 mEq/L (0.8–1.0 mmol/L SI units)

Possible Meanings of Abnormal Values

Increased (Hypermagnesemia)	Decreased (Hypomagnesemia)
Addison's disease	Alcoholism
Adrenalectomy	Chronic malnutrition
Dehydration	Chronic pancreatitis
Diabetic acidosis	Chronic renal disease
Hyperparathyroidism	Diarrhea (prolonged)
Hypothyroidism	Draining GI fistulas
IV administration of	Hemodialysis
magnesium sulfate	Hepatic cirrhosis
Multiple myeloma	Hyperaldosteronism
Renal failure	Hypercalcemia

M

| Use of magnesium-containing antacids or laxatives | Hyperthyroidism
Hypoalbuminemia
Hypoparathyroidism
Low dietary intake
Malabsorption
Pancreatitis
Toxemia of pregnancy
Ulcerative colitis
Uncontrolled diabetes |

Contributing Factors to Abnormal Values

- Use of a tourniquet during acquisition of the blood sample may alter test results.
- Hemolysis of the blood sample may alter test results.
- Drugs which may *increase* serum magnesium levels: amiloride, aminoglycosides, antacids, aspirin, calcitrol, cathartics, Epsom salts, felodipine, IV magnesium sulfate, lithium, medroxyprogesterone, salicylates, tacrolimus, triamterene.
- Drugs which may *decrease* serum magnesium levels: amphotericin, azathioprine, calcium gluconate, cisplatin, cyclosporine, digoxin, diuretics, haloperidol, insulin, neomycin, oral contraceptives, theophylline, trastuzumab.

Interventions/Implications

M

Pretest

- Explain to the patient the purpose of the test and the need for a blood sample to be drawn.
- No fasting is required prior to the test.
- Drugs containing magnesium salts, such as milk of magnesia, should be withheld for 3 days prior to the test.

Procedure

- A 7-mL blood sample is drawn in a red-top collection tube, avoiding use of a tourniquet, if possible.
- Gloves are worn throughout the procedure.

Posttest

- Apply pressure at venipuncture site. Apply dressing, periodically assessing for continued bleeding.
- Label the specimen and transport it to the laboratory.
- Report abnormal findings to the primary care provider.

➔ Clinical Alerts

- Frequent monitoring of magnesium levels may be done to monitor response to treatment with magnesium supplements.
- Magnesium may be monitored along with calcium and phosphorus levels to monitor response to calcium supplementation.

Magnetic Resonance Imaging (MRI)

Test Description

Magnetic resonance imaging (MRI) is based upon the knowledge that a magnetic field causes atoms, especially the nuclei of hydrogen ions, to line up in a parallel configuration. Radio-frequency energy is then directed at the atoms, knocking them out of their alignment and causing them to spin. When the radio-frequency energy is discontinued, the atoms realign themselves within the magnetic field. During their realignment, the atoms emit radio-frequency energy as a tissue-specific signal based on the relative density of their nuclei and their realignment time. These signals are interpreted by the MRI computer, which then produces a very high-resolution image.

The MRI holds several advantages over computed tomography (CT). The image provided by the procedure is of excellent quality. The MRI uses no contrast medium and no radiation, thus it presents no hazards of allergic reaction or radiation exposure to the patient. Bone artifacts which can obscure the viewing in a CT scan do not occur with an MRI. Blood vessels appear dark on the MRI, so that they can be easily viewed. MRI is quickly replacing other diagnostic tests as the standard of care for various conditions. MRI can evaluate cerebral infarction within hours of the event. It is used for diagnosis of most abnormalities of the brain and spine, has almost entirely replaced arthrography for diagnosis of knee injuries, and has virtually eliminated the need for myelography. A disadvantage is that the MRI is more expensive to perform than the CT; however, its diagnostic value is well worth the additional cost. CT is more effective than MRI in studying the chest.

The MRI machine is enclosed in a special room designed to protect it from interference by outside radio signals. The magnetic field in the room is always present and will cause watches to stop and will erase the magnetic strips found on the back of credit cards. The magnetic field also affects the functioning of computer-based equipment such as electronic infusion devices and ventilators. The magnet may move metal objects which may be present in the body, thus the test is contraindicated for any patient with a pacemaker, intracranial aneurysm clips, inner ear implants, metal fragments in the eyes, or gunshot wounds to the head. The patient is put on a moving pallet that is pushed into a large cylinder which houses the magnet.

Examples of MRI use include:

MRI of the abdomen/pelvis

MRI can be used to evaluate organs within the abdomen and pelvis. MRI is especially useful for imaging of the liver, male and female pelvis, pancreas, kidneys, and adrenals. It is also good for staging of cancers that involve retroperitoneal structures (lymph nodes) and peritoneal metastases.

MRI of the brain

When choosing between CT and MRI, it is best to use unenhanced CT to evaluate patients with an acute neurologic event (such as acute head injury, stroke, and subarachnoid hemorrhage). The MRI is used for all other suspected neurologic processes, including venous occlusion, neoplasm, demyelination, cerebral or cerebellar abscess, neurodegenerative disease, cysts, hydrocephalus, congenital or developmental defects. Evaluation of suspected tumors requires gadolinium-enhanced MRI.

MRI of the breast
Breast MRI has been shown to have high sensitivity for cancer detection. It is increasingly used following mammography to evaluate suspicious breast lesions.

MRI of the heart
Use of cardiac MRI is expanding, Due to its superior resolution, cardiac MRI provides detailed information about cardiac function, chamber volumes, and valvular function. It is also useful for assessing the direction and velocity of blood flow, evaluating congenital defects, and diagnosing cardiomyopathy. Gadolinium enhanced imaging done soon after myocardial infarction can distinguish between reversible and irreversible myocardial dysfunction.

MRI of the spine
MRI of the spine can demonstrate spinal cord lesions, causes of cord compression, disk herniation, and spinal stenosis. Only if MRI is contraindicated or unavailable, should a CT plus myelography be used to evaluate these conditions.

Magnetic resonance angiography (MRA)
MRA works well in the evaluation of major arteries of the body, especially the carotid, vertebrobasilar, and intracranial vessels. However, it is unable to detect subtle changes in smaller, distal vessels.

Magnetic resonance venography (MRV)
MRV images the venous side of the intracerebral circulation. It can be done along with MRI and MRA studies. Uses include pseudotumor cerebri, coagulopathies, or follow-up assessment of infectious processes.

M

THE EVIDENCE FOR PRACTICE
In women at high genetic or familial risk of breast cancer, MRI has high sensitivity (up to 94%) for the detection of breast cancer when used as an adjunct to mammography. This increase in sensitivity may lead to an earlier diagnosis of malignant breast lesions. However, MRI and mammography combined may lead to an increase in false positives, resulting in higher rate of benign biopsies. (ICSI, 2005).

Normal Values
No evidence of pathology

Possible Meanings of Abnormal Values
Abscesses
Acute tubular necrosis
Aortic aneurysm
Arteriovenous malformation
Atherosclerotic plaques
Avascular necrosis
Cerebral infarction
Cerebral lesions
Congenital heart disease

Degenerative vertebral disks
Dementia
Edema
Gaucher's disease
Glomerulonephritis
Hemorrhage
Hydronephrosis
Hyperparathyroidism
Joint disorders
Marfan's syndrome
Multiple sclerosis
Myocardial infarction
Osteomyelitis
Renal vein thrombosis
Seizures
Spinal cord injuries
Subarachnoid hemorrhage
Tumor detection and staging

Contributing Factors to Abnormal Values

M

- Excessive movement by the patient can blur images.

Interventions/Implications

Pretest

- Explain to the patient the purpose of the test and the procedure to be performed. Note that no radiation exposure is involved in this test. Explain that the patient will be moved into a large cylinder for the test and will need to remain completely still during the test. A variety of noises will be heard during the test.
- No fasting is required prior to the test.
- Obtain a signed informed consent.
- Preprocedure medication with antianxiety drugs for those patients with claustrophobia may be needed.
- Remove all metal objects from the body, including medication patches, prior to the test.
- Instruct the patient to void prior to the test.
- Sedation may be ordered for patients who are very young, who are uncooperative, or who are claustrophobic.

Procedure

- The patient is assisted to a supine position on the padded table and moved into the MRI cylinder.
- The patient and MRI staff may communicate via microphone during the procedure.
- As the radio signals are switched on and off and images produced, the patient hears a variety of noises.

Posttest

- If sedation was given prior to the exam, ensure the patient is fully awake prior to ambulation.
- Report abnormal findings to the primary care provider.

Clinical Alerts

- Use of an "open" MRI is an option for claustrophobic patients, however, the "closed" MRI provides a higher quality result.
- Medication patches, such as nitroglycerin, contraception, or nicotine patches, must be removed prior to scanning. Many of these have a small metal wire inside and can cause thermal injury.
- Some eye makeup has a metallic base and may cause fluttering of the eyelids. It is best to remove all eye makeup before having an MRI of the brain/head.
- Patients with embedded wires, stimulators, or batteries cannot be scanned.

CONTRAINDICATIONS!

- Patients who are morbidly obese
- Patients who are pregnant, although there is no evidence of teratogenic or development abnormalities associated with MRI
- Patients who are unable to cooperate during the procedure
- Patients who are claustrophobic
- Patients who require continuous life-support equipment which cannot be used inside the MRI room
- Patients with implantable metal objects such as pacemakers, intracranial aneurysm clips, infusion pumps, inner ear implants, or heart valves manufactured prior to 1964, or those with metal fragments in the eye(s) or gunshot wounds of the head. *(Note: Most stainless steel orthopedic implants and prosthetic devices are not ferromagnetic and are not affected by MRI.)*

M

Mammography

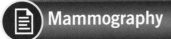

Test Description

Mammography is a radiographic technique in which x-ray films are made of the breast. The mammogram is considered a routine screening procedure to detect the presence of tumors too small to be discovered by palpation. It is also used to further investigate questionable areas found on breast palpation. The test can also be used to evaluate symptomatic breast disease such as nipple discharge, breast pain, nipple retraction, or dimpling of the skin on the breast. Suspicious areas found by mammography are then biopsied in order to confirm the presence of malignancy. The test has a high rate of false-positive results, meaning the percentage of women recalled for further testing. Other imaging techniques being studied for breast cancer screening include computer-aided mammography and magnetic resonance imaging (MRI).

Although age 40 is the suggested age to begin mammography screening, women considered high risk due to fibrocystic breast disease, family history of breast cancer, or personal history of any type of cancer, should begin screening at an earlier age and may be tested on a more frequent basis.

THE EVIDENCE FOR PRACTICE

The U.S. Preventive Services Task Force (USPSTF) recommends screening mammography, with or without clinical breast examination, every 1 to 2 years for women aged 40 and older. The American Cancer Society recommends screening mammography begin at age 40. Screening decisions in older women should be individualized by considering the potential benefits and risks of mammography in the context of current health status and estimated life expectancy. As long as a woman is in reasonably good health and would be a candidate for treatment, she should continue to be screened with mammography.

Normal Values

Negative

Possible Meanings of Abnormal Values

Benign cyst
Breast abscess
Fibrocystic changes
Malignant tumor
Suppurative mastitis

Contributing Factors to Abnormal Values

M

- Very glandular breast tissue, previous breast surgery, and breast implants hinder accurate analysis of the mammogram.
- Powders and salves on the breast or use of deodorant may appear as calcifications on the mammograms, thus causing false-positive results.

Interventions/Implications

Pretest

- Explain to the patient the purpose of the test and the procedure to be performed. Note that some discomfort will be felt during compression of the breast.
- No fasting is required prior to the test.
- All jewelry and clothing is to be removed from above the waist. An x-ray gown which opens in the front is worn for the test.
- No deodorants, powders, or other substances should be used on the breasts or underarms prior to the test.

Procedure

- The patient is either seated on a chair or standing in front of the mammogram machine.
- One breast is placed on a platform above the x-ray plate.
- The breast is compressed from above as the craniocaudal film is taken.
- The machine is then rotated, the breast is compressed from the side, and the lateral, or axillary, film is taken.
- The procedure is repeated for the other breast.

Posttest

- The patient is asked to remain in the x-ray department until the films are developed and found to be readable.
- Instruct the patient in breast self-examination, as appropriate.
- Report abnormal findings to the primary care provider.

Clinical Alerts

- Mammography does not eliminate the need for a clinical breast exam by the health-care provider.
- Diagnostic mammography using spot compression views are used if a palpable abnormality is noted during a clinical breast exam.
- When discussing need for mammograms, it is important to note that a woman of 70 is almost twice as likely to develop breast cancer in the next year as a woman aged 50, and that >80% of breast cancers are diagnosed in women who have no family history of breast cancer.
- It is important to remember that, although rare, breast cancer can also occur in men.

CONTRAINDICATIONS!

- Pregnant women
  - Caution: A woman in her childbearing years should undergo radiography only during her menses or 12 to 14 days after its onset to avoid any exposure to a fetus.

Measles (Rubeola) Antibody Test

M

Test Description

Measles (rubeola) is a viral infection which is spread by droplets from the nose, mouth, or throat. The incubation period is typically 8 to 12 days from exposure to the virus until symptoms appear. Symptoms of measles include fever, cough, runny nose, sore throat, myalgias, conjunctivitis, photophobia, Koplik's spots in the mouth, and a rash. The rash usually appears 3 to 5 days after generalized symptoms begin and lasts 4 to 7 days. It usually starts on the head and moves down the body. Treatment for measles is usually symptomatic. Serum immune globulin given 6 days after exposure to the virus can reduce the risk of developing measles or decrease the severity of the disease.

Immunization against measles is recommended using two doses of the measles, mumps, and rubella (MMR) vaccine. The first dose is given at 12 to 15 months and the second is given at 4 to 6 years of age. The rubeola antibody test measures IgG and IgM antibody formation against the rubeola virus. It can be used to diagnose rubeola and to determine whether the person is immune to the virus either from having had the measles infection or from having been vaccinated. A diagnosis of rubeola is made when a fourfold increase between the acute titer and the convalescent titer occurs (a period of 10 to 14 days). Demonstration of specific IgG on a serum sample is evidence of immunity to rubeola.

Normal Values

Negative for IgM and IgG:	Susceptible to rubeola
Positive for IgM:	Current or recent rubeola infection
Positive for IgG:	Immunity to rubeola

Possible Meanings of Abnormal Values

Positive	Negative
Immunity to rubeola (IgG)	Susceptible to rubeola
Rubeola infection (IgM)	

Contributing Factors to Abnormal Values

- Hemolysis due to excessive agitation of the blood sample may alter test results.

Interventions/Implications

Pretest
- Explain to the patient the purpose of the test and the need for a blood sample to be drawn.
- No fasting is required before the test.

Procedure
- A 7-mL blood sample is drawn in a red-top collection tube.
- Gloves are worn throughout the procedure.

Posttest
- Apply pressure at venipuncture site. Apply dressing, periodically assessing for continued bleeding.
- Label the specimen and transport it to the laboratory.
- Report abnormal findings to the primary care provider.

Meckel's Diverticulum Nuclear Scan (Meckel Scan)

Test Description
The causes of abdominal pain or occult gastrointestinal bleeding are many, but one, Meckel's diverticulum, is a common congenital abnormality of the intestinal tract. Meckel's diverticulum is a remnant of structures within the fetal digestive tract that were not fully reabsorbed before birth. Although located in the intestinal tract, Meckel's diverticulum is lined with *gastric* mucosa. This type of mucosa secretes acid, which causes ulceration of intestinal tissue. This results in the abdominal pain and occult blood in stools which causes the patient to seek health care.

In the Meckel's diverticulum nuclear scan, technetium-99m pertechnetate is administered by IV injection. This particular radionuclide concentrates in gastric mucosal tissue, whether it is located in the stomach or in Meckel's diverticulum. Scanning then detects this concentration. The scan will not detect Meckel's diverticulum which does not contain gastric mucosa.

Normal Values
Negative (normal radionuclide distribution)

Possible Meanings of Abnormal Values
Meckel's diverticulum

Contributing Factors to Abnormal Values

- Any movement by the patient may alter quality of films taken.
- Retained barium from previous exams may interfere with the test.

Interventions/Implications

Pretest

- Explain to the patient the purpose of the test. Provide any written teaching materials available on the subject. Note that discomfort involved with this test is primarily due to lying on a hard table for an extended period of time and the needle puncture. Reassure the patient that only trace amounts of the radionuclide are involved in the test.
- The patient must remain still while the scan is being performed.
- Fasting for 6 to 12 hours is required prior to the test.
- Obtain a signed informed consent.
- Administer a histamine H_2-receptor antagonist 1 to 2 days prior to the test, as ordered to prevent the radionuclide from being forced from Meckel's diverticulum by gastric acid.

Procedure

- The patient should empty the bladder prior to the exam.
- The radiopharmaceutical is administered by IV injection in a peripheral vein.
- The patient is assisted to a supine position on the exam table.
- A scintillation camera is positioned over the right lower quadrant of the patient's abdomen. This camera takes a radioactivity reading from the body. This information is transformed into a two-dimensional picture of the area.
- Scans are obtained every 5 minutes for up to 1 hour.
- Gloves are worn during the radionuclide injection.

Posttest

- Check the injection site for redness or swelling.
- If a woman who is lactating *must* have a nuclear scan, she should not breast-feed the infant until the radionuclide has been eliminated, possibly for 3 days.
- Although the amount of diagnostic radionuclide excreted in the urine is low, the urine should not be used for any laboratory tests for the time period indicated by the nuclear medicine department.
- Gloves are worn whenever dealing with the urine.
- Encourage fluid intake by the patient to enhance excretion of the radionuclide.
- Report abnormal findings to the primary care provider.

M

→ Clinical Alerts

- If possible, schedule the Meckel scan prior to any tests involving barium.

CONTRAINDICATIONS!

- Pregnant women
  - Caution: A woman in her childbearing years should undergo radiography only during her menses or 12 to14 days after its onset to avoid any exposure to a fetus.
- Patients who are lactating
- Patients who are unable to cooperate due to age, mental status, pain, or other factors

Mediastinoscopy

Test Description

Mediastinoscopy is the direct visualization of the contents of the mediastinum, including the heart and its vessels, the trachea, esophagus, thymus, and lymph nodes. This is accomplished via a mediastinoscope inserted at the suprasternal notch. Biopsy of the lymph nodes can be performed, allowing detection of lymphoma, sarcoidosis, and staging of lung cancer. Diagnosis of bronchogenic carcinoma can be made at an early stage using this procedure. This procedure is useful for diagnosing diseases when other tests such as sputum cytology, lung scans, and biopsies via bronchoscopy do not provide a diagnosis.

THE EVIDENCE FOR PRACTICE

In patients suspected of having nonsmall cell lung cancer (NSCLC), who have no evidence of distant metastases, and who have enlarged, discrete mediastinal nodes by computed tomography (CT) (because of a high false-positive rate of CT), mediastinoscopy is the invasive procedure of choice to rule in mediastinal node involvement. (Detterbeck, 2005).

Normal Values

Normal mediastinal lymph nodes

Possible Meanings of Abnormal Values

Coccidioidomycosis
Esophageal cancer
Histoplasmosis
Hodgkin's disease
Lung cancer
Lymphoma
Metastasis
Pneumocystis carinii
Sarcoidosis
Tuberculosis

Interventions/Implications

Pretest

- Explain to the patient the purpose of the test and the procedure to be done. Note that the patient will receive a general anesthetic and may experience a sore throat after the procedure due to having had an endotracheal tube in place. Note that temporary chest and incisional pain is also common.
- Fasting for 8 hours is required prior to the test.
- Obtain a signed written consent.
- Administer preprocedure medication as ordered.

Procedure

- This sterile procedure is conducted in the operating room.

- The patient is given a general anesthetic, and an endotracheal tube is inserted.
- A small incision is made in the suprasternal notch.
- The mediastinoscope is inserted, and tissue samples of the mediastinal lymph nodes are collected.
- Videotaping of the procedure may be done via a camera attached to the mediastinoscope.
- The mediastinoscope is removed, the incision is closed with sutures, and a sterile dressing is applied.

Posttest
- Monitor vital signs every 15 minutes for 1 hour, every 30 minutes for 2 hours, every hour for 4 hours, and then every 4 hours.
- Check the dressing for drainage, and the wound for hematoma formation.
- Assess the patient for fever, crepitus, dyspnea, cyanosis, diminished breath sounds, tachycardia, and hypotension.
- Send tissue specimen to the laboratory immediately.
- When fully awake, resume diet as taken prior to the procedure.
- Report abnormal findings to the primary care provider.

Clinical Alerts

- Possible complications include: hemorrhage, laryngeal nerve damage, pneumothorax, and puncture of the esophagus, trachea, or blood vessels
- Careful observation is needed of the vital signs, pulmonary assessment, and palpation of the neck for subcutaneous emphysema.

M

CONTRAINDICATIONS!

- Patients with scarring of the mediastinal area from previous mediastinoscopy
- Patients with superior vena cava syndrome due to extensive collateral neovascularization
- Patients who have had previous mediastinal radiation treatments
- Patients with median sternotomy or tracheostomy
- Patients with an aneurysm of the aortic arch

Methemoglobin (Hemoglobin M)

Test Description

Normally, hemoglobin is the carrier of oxygen in the blood. In certain conditions or exposure to certain substances, the hemoglobin is altered so that it can no longer carry oxygen. This leads to the appearance of cyanosis. This altered form of hemoglobin is known as *methemoglobin* or *hemoglobin M*.

Methemoglobinemia (elevated levels of hemoglobin M in the blood) can be acquired through introduction of certain substances into the blood, including aniline, chlorates, dapsone, nitrates, nitrites, phenacetin, and sulfonamides. It can also be due to an autosomal dominant genetic condition in which hemoglobin M is pro-duced (Hb M disease), or there can be an autosomal recessive congenital deficiency of the enzyme (NADH cytochrome b5 reductase) needed to reduce hemoglobin M to normal hemoglobin. Treatment for these diseases involves ascorbic acid or meth-ylene blue. The greatest risk of nitrate poisoning occurs in infants fed well water contaminated with nitrates. The nitrate nitrogen concentration of the water should be <10 ppm.

THE EVIDENCE FOR PRACTICE

Health-care professionals who suspect that an infant has methemoglobinemia are advised to consult with the local poison control center or a toxicologist to help guide management. An asymptomatic infant with cyanosis who has a methemoglobin concentration of <20% usually requires no treatment other than identifying and eliminating the source of exposure (assuming a normal hematocrit). Anemic children will display toxicity at lower methemo-globin concentrations. (Greer & Shannon, 2005).

Normal Values

0.4–1.5% of total hemoglobin

M

Possible Meanings of Abnormal Values

Increased

Hb M disease
NADH cytochrome b5 reductase deficiency
Nitrate poisoning
Toxic effects of drugs

Interventions/Implications

Pretest
- Explain to the patient the purpose of the test and the need for a blood sample to be drawn.
- No fasting is required before the test.

Procedure
- A 7-mL blood sample is drawn in a green-top collection tube.
- Gloves are worn throughout the procedure.

Posttest
- Apply pressure at venipuncture site. Apply dressing, periodically assessing for continued bleeding.
- Label the specimen and transport it to the laboratory.
- Report abnormal findings to the primary care provider.

➔ Clinical Alerts

- Water with high nitrate concentrations should not be ingested by the infant or used for preparation of infant formulas or infant foods.

Metyrapone Test

Test Description

Metyrapone is an inhibitor of 11-beta hydroxylase, an enzyme which converts 11-deoxycortisol to cortisol. With administration of metyrapone, less cortisol is produced, which normally stimulates the pituitary to produce adrenocorticotropic hormone (ACTH) through a negative feedback mechanism. Although cortisol itself will not be able to be synthesized, the cortisol precursors such as 11-deoxycortisol will be present in the blood or the urine. Thus, this test measures the ability of the pituitary gland to secrete ACTH in response to decreased serum cortisol.

This test is used in the differential diagnosis of adrenal hyperplasia from a primary adrenal tumor. If adrenal hyperplasia is present, the amount of cortisol precursors will be significantly increased. If, however, the problem is due to an adrenal tumor, there will be no response to metyrapone administration.

There are two different types of metyrapone tests. The first is an overnight test. A single dose of metyrapone is given at 11 p.m. and blood is drawn at 8 a.m. for measurement of serum cortisol, ACTH, and 11-deoxycortisol. In the second type of test, metyrapone is given 6 times a day for 24 hours and then a 24-hour urine sample is collected for measurement of 17-OHCS (a metabolic product of cortisol). Blood samples for serum cortisol, ACTH, and 11-deoxycortisol may also be drawn.

M

Normal Values

Blood:

11-Deoxycortisol:	>7 µg/dL (> 202 nmol/L SI units)
Cortisol:	<3 µg/dL (< 83 nmol/L SI units)

24-hour urine:

17-Ketosteroids:	>2 times base level
17-OHCS:	3–5 times base level

Possible Meanings of Abnormal Values

Increased	Decreased
Cushing's syndrome	Addison's disease
Hypopituitarism	

Contributing Factors to Abnormal Values

- Radioactive scans within 7 days prior to the test will alter test results.
- Drugs which may *decrease* plasma metyrapone levels: amitriptyline, chlordiazepoxide, chlorpromazine, corticosteroids, estrogens, glucocorticoids, oral contraceptives, phenobarbital, phenothiazines, phenytoin, progestins, rifampin.
- Abnormal thyroid function can affect this test.

Interventions/Implications

Pretest

- Explain to the patient the purpose of the test and the need for two blood samples to be drawn. Also explain the need for multiple 24-hour urine collections.
- Stress the importance of saving *all* urine in the 24-hour period. Instruct the patient to avoid contaminating the urine with toilet paper or feces.
- Inform the patient of the presence of a preservative in the collection bottle.
- No fasting is required prior to the test.
- Drugs that may affect the test should be discontinued if possible prior to the test.

Procedure

Blood

- A 7-mL blood sample is drawn in a red-top collection tube. This is the baseline cortisol level.
- Administer metyrapone (30 mg/kg) orally at 11 PM.
- Another 7-mL blood sample is drawn the next morning at 8 AM.
- Gloves are worn throughout the procedure.

24-hour urine

- A baseline 24-hour urine specimen is collected.
- Obtain the proper container containing the appropriate preservative from the laboratory.
- Begin the testing period in the morning following the patient's first voiding, which is discarded.
- Timing of the 24-hour period begins at the time the first voiding is discarded.
- *All* urine for the next 24-hours is collected in the container, which is to be kept refrigerated or on ice.
- If any urine is accidentally discarded during the 24-hour period, the test must be discontinued and a new test begun.
- The ending time of the 24-hour collection period should be posted in the patient's room.
- Administer adult patients metyrapone 500 to750 mg orally every 4 hours for 6 doses (dosage for children is reduced; refer to reference laboratory) beginning at 11 PM.
- Begin additional 24-hour urine collection at 8 AM the next morning, following the same collection procedure as above.
- Gloves are to be worn whenever dealing with the specimen collection.

Posttest

- Monitor for symptoms of Addisonian crisis: muscle weakness, mental and emotional changes, anorexia, nausea, vomiting, hypotension, hyperkalemia, severe abdominal, back, and leg pain, hyperpyrexia followed by hypothermia, vascular collapse.
- Resume pretest medications.

Blood

- Apply pressure at venipuncture site. Apply dressing, periodically assessing for continued bleeding.
- Label specimen and transport it to the laboratory.

24-hour urine

- Label the container and transport it on ice to the laboratory as soon as possible following the end of each of the 24-hour collection periods.
- Report abnormal findings to the primary care provider.

> **→ Clinical Alerts**
>
> - Potential complications: addisonian crisis (adrenal insufficiency).
> - If Addisonian crisis occurs, treatment goals include: reverse shock, restore blood circulation, replenish body with essential steroids (hydrocortisone).

CONTRAINDICATIONS!

- Do *not* perform this test if primary adrenal insufficiency is likely. Metyrapone inhibits cortisol production.

Microalbumin (MA, Microalbumin/Creatinine Ratio)

M

Test Description
Albumin is one of the proteins present in the body. Protein molecules are usually not found in the urine, since their size prevents them from filtering through the glomerular basement membrane (GBM). Albumin molecules are comparatively small, so if there is a problem with the GBM and it becomes "leaky," albumin molecules are going to be the first proteins able to pass through the membrane and into the urine. This type of problem, known as albuminuria, can be seen in diabetic nephropathy and in patients with hypertension.

What is important in the care of the patient with diabetes is that kidney problems be found early so that intervention can be done. Early onset of kidney problems is indicated by the presence of *microalbuminuria (MA)*, in which minute amounts of albumin appear in the urine. MA can be present for several years before significant kidney damage is apparent. When significant damage occurs, there is *macroalbuminuria*.

MA can be measured in several ways: random urine sample, timed urine sample, and 24-hour urine. Albumin levels vary throughout a 24-hour period, so collection of a 24-hour urine provides the most accurate measurement of microalbumin. However it obviously is time consuming and its accuracy is based on *all* urine being collected. *Timed urine samples* can also be used. These are usually urine collections of 4 hours or overnight. Results of timed urine samples are not as accurate as 24-hour urines, but they can be corrected using creatinine measurement since creatinine is excreted on a consistent basis. Most commonly used for MA assessment is the *random urine*, since it requires only one urine sample and no preparation. The random urine can also be corrected using the creatinine value, a result known as the *microalbumin/creatinine ratio*. This ratio is calculated thus:

$$(\text{Urine albumin in mg}/\text{Urine creatinine in mg}) \times 1000$$

THE EVIDENCE FOR PRACTICE
The American Diabetes Association notes the following regarding nephropathy screening:
- Perform an annual test for the presence of microalbuminuria in Type 1 diabetic patients with diabetes duration of ≥ 5 years and in all Type 2 diabetic patients, starting at diagnosis and during pregnancy.

- Serum creatinine should be measured at least annually for the estimation of glomerular filtration rate (GFR) in all adults with diabetes regardless of the degree of urine albumin excretion. The serum creatinine alone should not be used as a measure of kidney function but instead used to estimate GFR and stage the level of chronic kidney disease.

Normal Values

0–23 mg/L

Possible Meanings of Abnormal Values

Increased
Atherosclerosis
Diabetic nephropathy
Hypertensive nephropathy
Nephropathy
Nephrotoxic drugs
Preeclampsia
Pregnancy
Protein loading (supplements)
Urinary tract infection
Vigorous exercise

Contributing Factors to Abnormal Values

- Exercise, smoking, menstruation, and dehydration can affect the results of microalbumin testing.

Interventions/Implications

Pretest
- Explain urine collection procedure to the patient, noting whether it is a random urine, a timed urine, or a 24-hour urine.
- For 24-hour urines, stress the importance of saving *all* urine in the 24-hour period. Instruct the patient to avoid contaminating the urine with toilet paper or feces.

Procedure
- Random urine is simply one urine specimen collected at the provider's office.
- A timed urine sample is to be collected for a specific length of time (4 hour, overnight).

For 24-hour urine collection
- Obtain the proper container containing no preservative from the laboratory.
- Begin the testing period in the morning after the patient's first voiding, which is discarded.
- Timing of the 24-hour period begins at the time the first voiding is discarded.
- *All* urine for the next 24 hours is collected in the container, which is to be kept refrigerated or on ice.
- If any urine is accidentally discarded during the 24-hour period, the test must be discontinued and a new test begun.

- The ending time of the 24-hour collection period should be posted in the patient's room.
- Gloves are worn whenever dealing with the specimen collection.

Posttest
- Label the urine container and transport it to the laboratory as soon as possible.
- Report abnormal findings to the primary care provider.

Clinical Alerts

- Because exercise, smoking, and menstruation can affect the results and albumin excretion can vary from day to day, an abnormal value should be repeated.
  - The diagnosis of persistent abnormal microalbumin excretion requires documentation of two of three consecutive abnormal values obtained on different days.
- Confirmed, persistently elevated microalbumin levels should be treated with an angiotensin-converting enzyme (ACE) inhibitor titrated to normalization of microalbumin excretion. ARBs can also be used. The goal is to delay the progression of microalbuminuria to macroalbuminuria.

M

 ## Mumps Antibody Test

Test Description

Mumps is a viral infection which is spread by respiratory droplets and by contact with items contaminated by saliva of the infected person. Symptoms include facial pain, swelling of the parotid glands, fever, headache, and sore throat. The infection is usually self-limiting, but in some cases can infect the testes, causing testicular pain and scrotal swelling. The incubation period between exposure to the virus and appearance of symptoms is 12 to 24 days. It is most common in children aged 2 to 12 who have not been vaccinated against mumps.

Immunization against mumps is recommended using two doses of the measles, mumps, and rubella (MMR) vaccine. The first dose is given at 12 to 18 months and the second is given at 4 to 6 years of age. The mumps antibody test measures IgG and IgM antibody formation against the mumps virus. It can be used to diagnose mumps and to determine whether the person is immune to the virus either from having had the mumps infection or from having been vaccinated. A diagnosis of mumps is made when a fourfold increase between the acute titer and the convalescent titer occurs (a period of 10 to 14 days). Demonstration of specific IgG on a serum sample is evidence of immunity to mumps.

Normal Values

Negative for IgM and IgG:	Susceptible to mumps
Positive for IgM:	Current or recent mumps infection
Positive for IgG:	Immunity to mumps

Possible Meanings of Abnormal Values

Positive	Negative
Immunity to mumps (IgG)	Susceptible to mumps
Mumps infection (IgM)	

Contributing Factors to Abnormal Values

- Hemolysis due to excessive agitation of the blood sample may alter test results.

Interventions/Implications

Pretest

- Explain to the patient the purpose of the test and the need for a blood sample to be drawn.
- No fasting is required before the test.

Procedure

- A 7-mL blood sample is drawn in a red-top collection tube.
- Gloves are worn throughout the procedure.

Posttest

- Apply pressure at venipuncture site. Apply dressing, periodically assessing for continued bleeding.
- Label the specimen and transport it to the laboratory.
- Report abnormal findings to the primary care provider.

 Myelography

Test Description

Myelography is the radiographic study of the subarachnoid space of the spinal column. This is accomplished through injection of a water-soluble contrast dye into the spinal subarachnoid space via a lumbar puncture. Oil-based dye or air can also be used. The filling of the space with the dye can be viewed via fluoroscopy. Disorders which can be visualized through use of myelography include tumors, changes in bone structure, and herniations or protrusions of intervertebral disks.

Before the advent of CT and MRI scans, myelography was the best method to determine the cause of spinal problems. Today, myelography is more likely to be performed when other tests such as CT or MRI have not provided adequate information regarding the cause of the patient's pain or other spinal symptoms. It is also useful for patients who are unable to have an MRI, such as with patients who have metal plates and screws in their spine.

Myelography is usually combined with CT scanning to obtain a much more detailed view of the spine and the spinal nerves. The myelogram itself usually takes 30 to 60 minutes, with another 30 to 60 minutes required for the CT scan to be completed.

Normal Values

Normal spinal canal with no obstruction or structural abnormalities

Possible Meanings of Abnormal Values

Arachnoiditis
Arthritic bone spurs
Congenital abnormalities
Herniated intervertebral disks
Infection
Inflammation
Meningiomas
Metastatic tumors
Neurofibromas
Primary tumors
Spinal nerve root injury
Spinal stenosis
Traumatic injury

Interventions/Implications

Pretest

- Explain to the patient the purpose of the test. Provide any written teaching materials available on the subject. Note that discomfort during the test is due to insertion of the needle, and that during injection of the dye, transient sensations including warmth, flushing, a salty taste, and nausea may be experienced. Explain that movement will not be allowed during the test.
- Check for allergies to iodine, shellfish, or contrast medium dye. Inform the radiologist of such possible allergy and obtain order for an antihistamine and steroid to be administered prior to the test. A hypoallergenic nonionic contrast medium may be used for the test in allergic patients.
- Patients receiving metformin (Glucophage) for Type 2 diabetes mellitus should discontinue the drug 2 days before the procedure. This is due to the possible occurrence of lactic acidosis, a potentially fatal complication of biguanide therapy.
- Fasting for 8 hours is required prior to the test. The patient should be well hydrated prior to the beginning of the fasting period, and may continue liquids during the fasting period.
- Instruct the patient to void prior to the procedure.
- If a water-soluble contrast medium such as metrizamide (Amipaque) is to be used during the procedure, drugs which decrease the seizure threshold should be withheld for 48 hours prior to the test. These drugs include phenothiazines, tricyclic antidepressants, CNS stimulants, and amphetamines.
- Some institutions require discontinuing warfarin in preparation for the test.
- Patients who smoke should refrain from smoking beginning the day before the test to lessen the chance of postprocedure nausea and headache.

Procedure

- The patient is assisted to a side-lying position on the radiography table, with the knees drawn up to the abdomen and the chin on the chest.
- A lumbar puncture is performed. Fifteen milliliters of cerebrospinal fluid is removed and an equal amount of contrast dye is injected.
- With the needle in place, the patient is turned to the prone position and the table is tilted to assist with the flow of the dye. The chin is hyperextended to prevent the dye from entering the cranium.

- Radiographic films are taken.
- At the end of the procedure, the needle is removed and a sterile dressing is applied to the site.
- Gloves are worn during the venipuncture.

Posttest

- Most allergic reactions to radiopaque dye occur within 30 minutes of administration of the contrast medium. Observe the patient closely for: respiratory distress, hypotension, edema, hives, rash, tachycardia, and/or laryngeal stridor. Emergency resuscitation equipment must be readily accessible.
- Observe for allergic reaction to the dye for at least 6 hours post-procedure.
- The patient is to remain on bedrest for 8 hours with the head of the bed elevated no more than 45°. Specific positioning instructions may vary due to type of dye used.
- Observe the patient for indications of meningeal irritation, as characterized by headache, irritability, neck stiffness, fever, and photophobia. If present, keep the room quiet and dark, and provide analgesic medication.
- Monitor vital signs at least every 30 minutes for 4 hours, then every 4 hours for 24 hours.
- Check the dressing for drainage with each vital sign assessment.
- Assess the patient's ability to void.
- Encourage fluid intake to enhance excretion of the dye.
- The patient may resume preprocedure diet and activities the day following the test. A clear liquid diet is usually preferred following the test.
- Renal function should be assessed before metformin is restarted.
- Report abnormal findings to the primary care provider.

→ Clinical Alerts

- Possible Complications include: allergic reaction to dye, bleeding around the spinal sac, herniation of the brain, meningitis, seizures, and spinal headache.
- Headache following a myelogram may not occur for several days after the procedure. Typically rest and increased fluid intake will resolve a mild headache; medication may be needed for moderate to severe headache.
  - For unresolved spinal headache, an additional procedure may be required to stop leakage of cerebrospinal fluid from the puncture site.
- The patient should be instructed to notify the primary care provider if fever, excessive nausea or vomiting, severe unresolved headache, stiff neck, paresthesias of the legs, or dysfunction of the bladder or bowel occurs.

CONTRAINDICATIONS!

- Patients who are allergic to iodine, shellfish, or contrast medium dye
- Pregnant women
  - Caution: A woman in her childbearing years should undergo radiography only during her menses or 12 to 14 days after its onset to avoid any exposure to a fetus.
- Patients with increased intracranial pressure
- Patients with infection at the puncture site
- Patients with multiple sclerosis
- Patients who are unable to cooperate due to age, mental status, pain, or other factors

Myoglobin

Test Description

Myoglobin is a heme-containing, oxygen-binding protein which is present in the cytoplasm of cardiac and skeletal muscle cells. It serves as a reservoir of oxygen to meet very short-term needs. When muscle cell injury occurs through disease, as in myocardial infarction, or through trauma, myoglobin is released into the blood. This usually begins within 2 to 6 hours following muscle tissue damage, peaks in 8 to 12 hours, and returns to a normal level in about 1 day. Myoglobin is excreted by the kidneys (myoglobinuria) and is detected in the urine up to 1 week following muscle tissue injury.

Normal Values

<85 ng/mL (<85 µg/L SI units)

Possible Meanings of Abnormal Values

Increased

Malignant hyperthermia
Muscular dystrophy
Myocardial infarction
Muscle enzyme deficiencies
Muscle injury
Polymyositis
Renal failure
Rhabdomyolysis
Seizures
Severe burns
Shock
Surgical procedure
Trauma
Vigorous exercise

Contributing Factors to Abnormal Values

- Hemolysis of the blood sample and recent radioactive scans will alter test results.
- IM injections may *increase* myoglobin levels.
- Drugs that may *increase* myoglobin levels: statins, theophylline.

Interventions/Implications

Pretest
- Explain to the patient the purpose of the test and the need for a blood sample to be drawn.
- No fasting is required before the test.

Procedure
- A 7-mL blood sample is drawn in a collection tube.
- Gloves are worn throughout the procedure.

Posttest
- Apply pressure at venipuncture site. Apply dressing, periodically assessing for continued bleeding.
- Label the specimen and transport it to the laboratory.
- Report abnormal findings to the primary care provider.

Clinical Alerts

- Since myoglobin is found in skeletal as well as cardiac muscle, other tests such as CK-MB or troponin are usually required to determine whether elevated myoglobin levels are due to cardiac damage.

Nasopharyngeal Culture

Test Description
Nasopharyngeal culture involves obtaining a sample of secretions from the nasopharynx. The sample is then grown in a culture medium. The type of organism is identified, and if appropriate, the culture can be used to then determine which antibiotic therapy will be effective against the organism (sensitivity testing).

Normal Values
Normal flora

Possible Meanings of Abnormal Values
Bacterial infection (including *S. aureus, B. pertussis, N. meningitides*)
Fungal infection
Viral infection

Interventions/Implications
Pretest
- Explain to the patient the purpose of the test. Provide any written teaching materials available on the subject.
- No fasting is required before the test.

Procedure
- Ask the patient to cough and then tilt the head back (coughing helps decrease the occurrence of gagging).
- A sterile swab is inserted through the nostril into the space just beneath the inferior turbinate.
- The swab is gently rotated, allowing a few seconds for the swab to absorb the secretions, and is then removed.
- Gloves are worn during the procedure.

Posttest
• Report abnormal findings to the primary care provider.

 Clinical Alerts

• If testing for *C. diphtheriae*, a throat swab is also taken.

 Natriuretic Peptides (Atrial Natriuretic Peptide [ANP], A-Type Natriuretic Peptide, Brain Natriuretic Peptide [BNP], B-Type Natriuretic Peptide, N-Terminal ProBNP [NT-ProBNP])

Test Description

Natriuretic peptides are structurally similar peptides produced by cells throughout the body. Two of these, A-type natriuretic peptide (also known as *atrial natriuretic peptide, or ANP*) and B-type natriuretic peptide (also known as *brain natriuretic peptide, or BNP*) are produced by the myocardial cells. ANP is made exclusively by atrial myocytes, while BNP is produced by both atrial and ventricular myocytes. ANP and BNP maintain homeostasis by promoting diuresis and natriuresis. BNP is released from the ventricles, especially the left ventricle, during pressure or volume overload. It causes dilation of arteries and veins and also decreases levels of vaso-constricting and sodium-retaining neurohormones. It is now known that ventricular overload results in release of both BNP and N-terminal proBNP (NT-proBNP).

Although ANP was the first natriuretic peptide, it is the BNP that is widely used clinically. This is due in part to its longer half-life (20 minutes for BNP versus 3 minutes for ANP). Also, BNP levels are not affected by exertion or exercise, whereas ANP levels can be affected by routine activity. NT-proBNP has a half-life of 120 minutes, making it somewhat less useful for monitoring acute changes. However, it is used in diagnosing heart failure and studies are suggesting it as a strong predictor of mortality.

The use of BNP in helping to diagnose heart failure is well-documented. Levels of BNP are elevated in individuals with symptomatic heart failure in a noncompensated state. However, patients who have left ventricular dysfunction that is compensated due to medical therapy may have normal BNP levels. BNP testing is especially useful in helping health-care providers distinguish between dyspnea due to heart failure and dyspnea due to other causes.

N

THE EVIDENCE FOR PRACTICE

According to the Heart Failure Society of America (2006):

> The diagnosis of decompensated heart failure (HF) should be based primarily on signs and symptoms. When the diagnosis is uncertain, determination of plasma B-type natriuretic pep-tide (BNP) or N-terminal pro-B-type natriuretic peptide (NT-proBNP) concentration should be considered in patients being evaluated for dyspnea who have signs and symptoms com-patible with HF. The natriuretic peptide concentration should not be interpreted in isolation, but in the context of all available clinical data bearing on the diagnosis of HF.

Normal Values

BNP:	<100 pg/mL (<100 ng/L SI units)
NT-proBNP:	<400 pg/mL (<400 ng/L SI units)

Possible Meanings of Abnormal Values

Increased	Decreased
Acute lung injury	Therapeutic response to antihypertensive
Acute myocardial infarction	therapy
Chronic renal failure	Therapeutic response to diuretic therapy
Cirrhosis	
Congestive heart failure	
Coronary angioplasty	
Hypertension	
Hypervolemic states	
Left ventricular hypertrophy	
Nesiritide infusion	
Pulmonary hypertension	

Contributing Factors to Abnormal Values

- BNP levels are increased with age, female gender.
- Obesity may cause *falsely decreased* BNP levels.
- Patients in renal failure or on dialysis may have elevated BNP levels whether or not heart failure is present.
- Patients with right-sided heart failure (due to cor pulmonale, pulmonary emboli, pulmonary hypertension) have elevated levels (300–400 pg/mL).
- Nesiritide infusion causes BNP levels of 3000 pg/mL.

Interventions/Implications

Pretest
- Explain to the patient the purpose of the test and the need for a blood sample to be drawn.
- No fasting is required before the test.

Procedure
- A 7-mL blood sample is drawn in a white-top EDTA (nonglass) collection tube.
- Plasma must be separated from cells by centrifuge within 2 hours and frozen.
- Gloves are worn throughout the procedure.

Posttest
- Apply pressure at venipuncture site. Apply dressing, periodically assessing for continued bleeding.
- Label the specimen and transport it to the laboratory.
- Report abnormal findings to the primary care provider.

→ Clinical Alerts

- Patients in chronic heart failure have elevated BNP levels, but may be stable.
- Patients with newly elevated BNP require further evaluation, including echocardiogram.

- Although BNP and NT-proBNP are secreted in a 1:1 ratio, the NT-proBNP level may be much higher in the same patient because of its longer half-life.

 ## Nonstress Test (NST, Fetal Activity Study)

Test Description

The nonstress test (NST) is a noninvasive technique used to evaluate the status of the fetus. Common reasons for an NST include: the patient having diabetes or hypertension, the fetus being small or not growing properly, and pregnancies extending past the due date.

Unlike the contraction stress test, the NST does not include stimulation with oxytocin. The fetal activity monitored in this test may be spontaneous or induced by uterine contraction or external manipulation. Normally, the fetal heart rate (FHR) should accelerate in response to fetal movement. The fetus is reported as being "reactive" when two or more FHR accelerations are detected within a 20-minute period. Each of the accelerations must be at least 15 beats per minute and last for at least 15 seconds. The NST is highly reliable for determining fetal viability. Only with a "nonreactive" result, is a contraction stress test (CST) indicated.

N

Normal Values

Reactive

Possible Meanings of Abnormal Values

Nonreactive fetus

Contributing Factors to Abnormal Values

- Fetal immaturity, especially fetuses <28 weeks gestation, can cause a nonreactive NST.
- Fetal sleep.

Interventions/Implications

Pretest

- Explain to the patient the purpose of the test and the procedure to be done. Note that there is no discomfort associated with the NST.
- No fasting is required prior to the test. Instruct the patient to eat prior to the test to ensure a high maternal serum glucose level, which enhances fetal activity.

Procedure

- The patient is instructed to void.
- The patient is assisted into a Sims' position.
- An external fetal monitor is applied to the patient's abdomen, which will provide a graph of FHR and uterine contractions.

- The patient is instructed to push a button on the fetal monitor whenever she feels fetal movement. This is then indicated on the graph, allowing correlation to be made with the FHR at that time.
- If there is no fetal movement for 20 minutes, the fetus is externally stimulated by rubbing or compressing the patient's abdomen or by producing a loud noise near the abdomen.
- If there is no fetal movement for 40 minutes, the test is considered nonreactive.

Posttest
- Report abnormal findings to the primary care provider.

Clinical Alerts

- If the test finds the fetus to be nonreactive (no change in the fetal heart rate when the fetus moves), the patient is scheduled for a CST.
- Explain to the patient that a nonreactive NST does not always mean there is a problem with the fetus. Conducting the test during the fetus' sleep cycle may cause it to be nonreactive.

5'-Nucleotidase (5'-N)

Test Description
Testing for 5'-nucleotidase (5'-N) is used in conjunction with alkaline phosphatase (ALP) to differentiate between hepatobiliary diseases and bone diseases. 5'-N is an enzyme found in the plasma membranes of liver cells and cells of the bile duct. Its limited location makes this test relatively specific in nature. When both 5'-N and ALP are elevated, the presence of liver metastases is probable.

Normal Values
1–11 U/L (0.02–0.18 µkat/L SI units)

Possible Meanings of Abnormal Values

Increased
Biliary obstruction
Cholestasis
Cirrhosis
Hepatitis
Late pregnancy
Liver disease
Liver metastases

Contributing Factors to Abnormal Values

- Drugs which may *increase* 5'-N levels: anabolic steroids, antibiotics, aspirin, codeine, hepatotoxic drugs, imipramine, indomethacin, meperidine, morphine, phenothiazines, phenytoin, thiazide diuretics.

Interventions/Implications

Pretest

- Explain to the patient the purpose of the test and the need for a blood sample to be drawn.
- No fasting is required before the test.

Procedure

- A 7-mL blood sample is drawn in a red-top collection tube.
- Gloves are worn throughout the procedure.

Posttest

- Apply pressure 3 to 5 minutes at venipuncture site. Apply dressing, periodically assessing for continued bleeding.
- Teach the patient to monitor the site. If the site begins to bleed, the patient should apply direct pressure and, if unable to control the bleeding, return to the laboratory or notify the primary care provider.
- Label the specimen and transport it to the laboratory.
- Report abnormal findings to the primary care provider.

 Clinical Alerts

- With liver dysfunction, the patient may have prolonged clotting time.

O

 Osmolality, Blood (Serum Osmolality)

Test Description

The osmolality of the blood measures the number of osmotically active particles in the serum. The test is useful in assessing fluid and electrolyte imbalances and in determining fluid requirements. It provides valuable information regarding a patient's hydration status, the concentration of the urine, and the status of ADH (antidiuretic hormone) secretion, and is used in toxicology workups. Serum osmolality is primarily ordered to investigate hyponatremia. Hyponatremia may be due to sodium loss through the urine or due to increased fluid in the bloodstream.

Normal Values

280–296 mOsm/kg of H_2O (280–296 mmol/kg SI units)

Possible Meanings of Abnormal Values

Increased	Decreased
Acidosis	Addison's disease
Advanced liver disease	Congestive heart failure
Alcohol overdose	Edema

Azotemia
Burns
Convulsions
Dehydration
Diabetes insipidus
Diabetes mellitus
Edema
Ethylene glycol overdose
High protein diet
Hyperaldosteronism
Hyperbilirubinemia
Hypercalcemia
Hyperglycemia
Hypernatremia
Hypokalemia
Ketoacidosis
Methanol overdose
Shock
Trauma
Uremia

Hepatic cirrhosis
Hepatic failure with ascites
Lung cancer
Overhydration
Postoperative
Syndrome of inappropriate
   ADH secretion (SIADH)

Contributing Factors to Abnormal Values

- Test results may be altered due to hemolysis of the blood sample.
- Drugs which may alter test results: mineralocorticoids, osmotic diuretics.

Interventions/Implications

Pretest
- Explain to the patient the purpose of the test and the need for a blood sample to be drawn.
- No fasting is required before the test.

Procedure
- A 7-mL blood sample is drawn in a red-top collection tube.
- Gloves are worn throughout the procedure.

Posttest
- Apply pressure at venipuncture site. Apply dressing, periodically assessing for continued bleeding.
- Label the specimen and transport it to the laboratory.
- Report abnormal findings to the primary care provider.

→ Clinical Alerts

- Elevated serum osmolality levels result in worsening clinical condition:
  - >385 mOsm/kg H_2O → stupor in hyperglycemia
  - >400 mOsm/kg H_2O → grand mal seizures
  - >420 mOsm/kg H_2O → death

Osmolality, Urine (Urine Osmolality)

Test Description

The urine osmolality measures the number of osmotically active particles in the urine, or the concentration of the urine. This, in turn, reflects the ability of the kidneys to concentrate urine. The test is useful in assessing fluid and electrolyte imbalances and in determining fluid requirements. It is especially useful in the evaluation of hyponatremia and hypernatremia, and to distinguish prerenal azotemia from ischemic acute tubular necrosis. Following an overnight fast, the urine osmolality should be at least three times the osmolality of the blood.

Normal Values

Random specimen: 50–1200 mOsm/kg H_2O (50–1200 mmol/kg SI units)
After 12–14 hour fast: >850 mOsm/kg H_2O (>850 mmol/kg SI units)

Possible Meanings of Abnormal Values

Increased	Decreased
Addison's disease	Acute renal failure
Azotemia	Aldosteronism
Congestive heart failure	Diabetes insipidus
Dehydration	Edema
Diabetes mellitus	Fever
Diarrhea	Glomerulonephritis
Edema	High protein diet
Glycosuria	Hypercalcemia
Hepatic cirrhosis	Hypokalemia
High protein diet	Hyponatremia
Hyperglycemia	Multiple myeloma
Hypernatremia	Overhydration
Ketoacidosis	Sickle cell anemia
Postoperative	Urinary tract obstruction
Prerenal azotemia	Water intoxication
Sodium overload	
Syndrome of inappropriate ADH secretion (SIADH)	
Uremia	

0

Contributing Factors to Abnormal Values

- Abnormal results may occur with intake of antibiotics, antidepressants, antipsychotics, bromocriptine, chemotherapy, dextran, diuretics, glucose, mannitol, and radiographic contrast agents.

Interventions/Implications

Pretest

- Explain to the patient the purpose of the test and the need for a urine specimen.

- No fasting is required for random testing.
- Overnight fasting is required prior to the test, if ordered as a fasting urine specimen.

Procedure
- 10-mL of urine is collected in a plastic specimen container.
- Gloves are worn throughout the procedure.

Posttest
- Label the specimen and transport it to the laboratory immediately.
- Report abnormal findings to the primary care provider.

 ## Osteocalcin (Bone G1a Protein)

Test Description
Osteocalcin (bone G1a protein) is a protein synthesized in bone by osteoblasts. After production, some of it is incorporated into the bone matrix and some enters the circulation. The bone matrix then mineralizes to create new bone. Research has found that the circulating level of osteocalcin reflects the rate of bone formation. Thus, measurement of osteocalcin is useful for identifying individuals at risk for developing osteoporosis, for monitoring bone metabolism during and after menopause, and for monitoring response to antiresorptive therapy. The effect of antiresorptive therapy on osteocalcin levels can be assessed much sooner (in 3 to 6 months) than can be seen on bone density testing (1 to 2 years).

Normal Values
Male:	8–37 ng/mL (1.37–6.33 nmol/L SI units)
Female:	7–38 ng/mL (1.20–6.50 nmol/L SI units)
Osteoporosis:	17–49 ng/mL (2.91–8.38 nmol/L SI units)

Possible Meanings of Abnormal Values

Increased	Decreased
Acromegaly	Antiresorptive therapy
Fracture	Hypoparathyroidism
Hyperparathyroidism	
Osteoporosis	

Contributing Factors to Abnormal Values
- There is a diurnal variation in osteocalcin levels.

Interventions/Implications
Pretest
- Explain to the patient the purpose of the test and the need for a blood sample to be drawn.
- No fasting is required before the test.

Procedure
- A 7-mL blood sample is drawn in a red-top collection tube at 7 AM.
- Gloves are worn throughout the procedure.

Posttest
- Apply pressure at venipuncture site. Apply dressing, periodically assessing for continued bleeding.
- Label the specimen and transport it to the laboratory.
- Report abnormal findings to the primary care provider.

Oximetry (Ear Oximetry, Pulse Oximetry, Oxygen Saturation, SaO_2)

Test Description
Oximetry is a noninvasive procedure used to monitor the oxygen saturation of arterial blood. Due to the simplicity and convenience of the procedure, oximetry is used in a variety of settings where monitoring of oxygenation status is needed. Examples of oximetry use include during surgical procedures, during mechanical ventilation, and during diagnostic testing such as stress testing.

Oximetry measures the percentage of oxygen being carried by the hemoglobin. To perform this measurement, a light-emitting sensor is attached to a site such as a finger. The sensor emits beams of light through the skin tissue. A light-detecting sensor then records the amount of light absorbed by the oxygenated hemoglobin. This absorption rate is converted to the percentage of oxygen saturation present in the blood, which is shown on the monitor.

THE EVIDENCE FOR PRACTICE
Screening for nocturnal hypoxia can be done easily and inexpensively with overnight pulse oximetry in the home. The oximeter is returned to the clinic, where the overnight oximetry and heart rate data are downloaded. If a significant portion of the night's data indicates oxygen saturations below 88%, supplemental oxygen can be provided empirically at 1 to 2 L/min. Home oximetry can be repeated at that level to verify correction of hypoxia. (ICSI, 2007)

Normal Values
≥95%

Possible Meanings of Abnormal Values

Increased	Decreased
Adequate oxygen therapy	Excessive blood loss
	Carbon monoxide poisoning
	Chronic obstructive lung disease
	Hypoventilation
	Hypoxia
	Inadequate available oxygen
	Pulmonary embolism
	Smoking

Contributing Factors to Abnormal Values

- False alarms may occur due to movement of the site to which the sensor is attached, equipment problems, or inadequate blood flow to the site.
- Inaccurate readings may occur if the patient is anemic or has received contrast media, or if there are bright lights in the room.

Interventions/Implications

Pretest
- Explain to the patient the purpose of the test, noting that no discomfort is associated with this procedure.
- Inform the patient of the presence of alarms. Explain that the alarm will sound should the sensor become displaced. Also inform the patient of steps which will be taken should the oxygen saturation be found to be low.
- No fasting is required prior to the test.

Procedure
- The site must have good circulation. Examples of possible sites include fingers, earlobes, and toes.
- Ensure that the skin is clean and dry. Rub the area to increase its blood flow.
- Apply the sensor to the chosen site.

Posttest
- Report abnormal findings to the primary care provider.

 Clinical Alerts

- Medicare currently provides coverage for home oxygen for beneficiaries with partial pressure measurements at or below 55 mm Hg or oxygen saturation at or below 88 percent. If certain other diseases/conditions are present, coverage is provided for patients with an oxygen partial pressure of 56 to 60 mm Hg or an oxygen saturation of 89%.
  - Claims must be supported by valid qualifying test results, including oximetry testing.

http://www.cms.hhs.gov/apps/media/press/release.asp?Counter=1815
http://www.cms.hhs.gov/transmittals/downloads/R166OTN.pdf

 Papanicolaou Test (Exfoliative Cytologic Study, Pap Smear, Pap Test, Thin Prep)

Test Description
The Papanicolaou (Pap) smear can be performed on many body secretions, including gastric secretions, prostatic secretions, sputum, and urine. However, the term is most commonly associated with the test for detection of cervical cancer. A vaginal examination is performed and cells are obtained from the cervix. In the case of

a woman who has had a total hysterectomy (removal of the uterus and cervix), cells may be obtained from the vaginal wall. The cells are then classified according to a grading system such as the Bethesda System. The system was reviewed and updated by representatives of 45 professional societies at the 2001 conference, with the following components now included in Pap test results (Available at: http://www.bethesda2001.cancer.gov/terminology.html).

The "Specimen Type" notes whether the specimen is of the conventional smear type or the newer liquid-based preparation. With liquid-based Pap tests, DNA testing can be performed to check for the presence of high-risk types of human papilloma virus (HPV) which have been associated with the development of cervical cancer.

The "Specimen Adequacy" is noted as being either satisfactory (with presence or absence of endocervical/transformation zone component noted) or unsatisfactory for evaluation. A reason is noted for an unsatisfactory specimen, such as an inadequate number of cells or lubricant interfering with the evaluation. Even with a satisfactory specimen, there can be situations in which the quality of the specimen is somewhat compromised, such as partially obscuring blood or inflammation.

The "Interpretation/Result" section states "Negative for Intraepithelial Lesion or Malignancy" when there is no cellular evidence of neoplasia. If present, *Trichomonas*, fungal organisms (*Candida*), bacteria consistent with *Actinomyces*, cellular changes consistent with herpes simplex virus, or a shift in flora suggestive of bacterial vaginosis will be identified, as will reactive cellular changes (associated with inflammation, radiation, or presence of intrauterine device), glandular cells (after hysterectomy), or atrophy (postmenopausal). If endometrial cells are seen in a woman age 40 and older, this is considered an abnormality and is noted in the report. Epithelial cell abnormalities may include any of the following:

- Squamous cell
  - ASC-US (atypical squamous cells of undetermined significance)
  - LSIL (low grade squamous intraepithelial lesion)
  - HSIL (high grade squamous intraepithelial lesion)
  - Features suspicious for invasion
  - Squamous cell carcinoma
- Glandular cell
  - Atypical endocervical/endometrial/glandular cells
  - Atypia, favoring neoplasia
  - Endocervical adenocarcinoma in situ
  - Adenocarcinoma (endocervical, endometrial, extrauterine)

THE EVIDENCE FOR PRACTICE

According to American Cancer Society and American College of Obstetricians and Gynecologists (ACOG) guidelines:

- All women should begin cervical cancer screening about 3 years after they begin having vaginal intercourse, but no later than when they are 21 years old. Screening should be done every year with the regular Pap test or every 2 years using the newer liquid-based Pap test.
- Beginning at age 30, women who have had 3 normal Pap test results in a row may get screened every 2 to 3 years. Women who have certain risk factors such as diethylstilbestrol (DES) exposure before birth, HIV infection, or a weakened immune system due to

organ transplant, chemotherapy, or chronic steroid use should continue to be screened annually.

- Women 70 years of age or older who have had 3 or more normal Pap tests in a row and no abnormal Pap test results in the last 10 years may choose to stop having cervical cancer screening. Women with a history of cervical cancer, DES exposure before birth, HIV infection, or a weakened immune system should continue to have screening as long as they are in good health.
- Women who have had a total hysterectomy (removal of the uterus and cervix) may also choose to stop having cervical cancer screening, unless the surgery was done as a treatment for cervical cancer or precancer. Women who have had a hysterectomy without removal of the cervix should continue to follow the guidelines above.
- Women need to be educated that an annual pelvic exam is still needed, even when a Pap test is not done.

Normal Values

Satisfactory for evaluation
Negative for intraepithelial lesion or malignancy
No organisms or other findings

Possible Meanings of Abnormal Values

Atrophy
Bacterial vaginosis
Cervical cancer
Fungal infection
Inflammation
Sexually transmitted infection (*Trichomonas,* herpes simplex virus)

Contributing Factors to Abnormal Values

- Pap test results may be altered by allowing the cells of the specimen to dry if using smear technique, using lubricating jelly on the vaginal speculum, douching, tub bathing, menstrual flow, and infections.
- Drugs that may alter test results include digitalis and tetracycline.
- Insufficient number of cells collected will not allow interpretation of the specimen.

Interventions/Implications

Pretest
- Explain to the patient the purpose of the test and the need for a vaginal examination to be done. Note that minimal discomfort is felt during the insertion of the vaginal speculum.
- Instruct the patient to not use douches, tampons, vaginal medications, sprays, or powders for at least 24 hours before having a Pap test.
- Instruct the patient to void before the examination
- The health-care provider should allow discussion of concerns or fears, especially for women who have had problems with pelvic exams in the past, survivors of rape or sexual abuse, and for those who have never had a pelvic exam.

Procedure
- The patient is asked to remove clothing from the waist down and is provided with a drape for privacy.
- The patient is assisted into the lithotomy position with her legs supported in stirrups.
- A vaginal speculum lubricated only with warm water is inserted into the vagina. Asking the patient to breathe deeply will help her pelvic muscles relax, allowing easier insertion of the speculum.
- Once the cervix is visualized, several samples of cells are obtained from the cervix (using a spatula) and the cervical os (using a cytobrush). A broomlike collection device is available for use with liquid-based Pap testing which samples both areas at one time.
- In women who do not have a cervix, cells from the vagina are collected if a Pap test is needed.
- For a Pap smear, the specimen is smeared onto a glass slide. A fixative must be applied before the cells air-dry.
- For a liquid-based Pap test, the collection device is vigorously swirled in the solution to ensure release of the collected cells. If a broom device is used, it should be pushed against the bottom of the solution vial 10 times, then swirled in the solution
- The specimen is labeled with patient identification information and sent to the laboratory. A requisition form typically must accompany the specimen, which includes identification information, date of birth, date of last menstrual period, and relevant clinical history.
- Gloves are worn throughout the procedure.

Posttest
- Assist the patient to a sitting position.
- Explain to the patient that a very small amount of bleeding from the cervix may occur after the procedure and may require use of a small pad.
- Report results to the patient.

Clinical Alerts

- Should results be abnormal, management should follow established guidelines of the American Society for Colposcopy and Cervical Pathology (ASCCP) available at http://www.asccp.org/pdfs/consensus/algorithms.pdf.
- In cases of a satisfactory specimen, but lacking transformation zone components, it is recommended that repeat testing in 6 months be done for women at higher risk for neoplasia (immunocompromised, HIV positive, previous smear with ASC-US, history of HPV). Women at low risk can be screened with a repeat test in 12 months.
- Women age 40 and older whose Pap report notes presence of endometrial cells should be referred to gynecology for follow-up. This may involve a repeat Pap, endometrial biopsy, or possibly D&C.

CONTRAINDICATIONS!

- If currently having menses
- If douched or used vaginal products within 24 hours of examination

Paracentesis (Abdominal Paracentesis, Abdominal Tap, Peritoneal Fluid Analysis, Peritoneal Tap)

Test Description

Paracentesis refers to the removal of fluid from the peritoneal cavity. This cavity is the space between the visceral peritoneum, which covers the abdominal organs, and the parietal peritoneum, which lines the abdominal cavity. In some conditions, such as cardiac disease, infection, neoplasia, sodium retention, and cirrhosis of the liver, serous fluid accumulates in the peritoneal cavity, an assessment finding known as *ascites*.

Paracentesis may be done for diagnostic purposes to determine the cause of the ascites, or for therapeutic purposes to remove tense ascites causing respiratory difficulties or pain. The test is also performed in cases of abdominal trauma to check for bleeding into the peritoneal cavity.

Based on laboratory analysis, the fluid is categorized as either "exudative" or "transudative."

Normal Values

Gross appearance:	Clear to pale yellow in color, odorless
Amount:	<50 mL
Bacteria:	None
Cell counts:	Red blood cells: Negative
	White blood cells: <300/μL
Cytology:	No malignant cells present
Fungi:	None
Protein:	0.3 to 4.1 g/dL

Possible Meanings of Abnormal Values

Based on laboratory analysis, the fluid is categorized as either "exudative" or "transudative."

Transudative ascites

Laboratory findings
- Protein <3g/dL
- Protein ascites/serum ratio <0.5
- LD ascites/serum ratio <0.6
- Albumin gradient[a] >1.1, LD <200 U/L

Causes: hepatic cirrhosis, congestive heart failure, constrictive pericarditis, Budd-Chiari syndrome, inferior venal caval obstruction, nephrotic syndrome

Exudative ascites

Laboratory findings
- Protein >3 g/dL
- Protein ascites/serum ratio >0.5

---

[a]Albumin gradient = serum albumin − ascites albumin

- LD ascites/serum ratio >0.6
- Albumin gradient <1.1
- WBC >500/mm³ with >250 mm³ polymorphonuclear cells (if infection)
- Ascites CEA >10 ng/mL (with malignancy)

Causes: peritoneal membrane permeability defects including malignancy, spontaneous bacterial peritonitis, tuberculosis, vasculitis, pancreatitis, myxedema

Contributing Factors to Abnormal Values

- Injury to underlying organs may contaminate the sample with bile, blood, urine, or feces.
- Contamination of the specimen will alter white blood cell count.

Interventions/Implications

Pretest

- Explain to the patient the purpose of the test and the procedure to be done. Explain that a local anesthetic will be used, but that a pressure-like pain will occur as the needle pierces the peritoneum.
- No fasting is required prior to the test.
- CBC, platelet count, and coagulation studies are obtained.
- Obtain a signed informed consent.
- The patient needs to empty the bladder prior to the procedure to avoid accidental puncture of the bladder.
- Obtain baseline assessment information, including vital signs, weight, and abdominal girth.

Procedure

- Assist the patient to a sitting position with the feet on the floor and the back well supported. If the patient cannot tolerate this position, a high Fowler's position may be used.
- Monitor vital signs every 15 minutes during the procedure.
- Sterile technique is used throughout the procedure.
- The usual site to be used for the puncture is located midway between the umbilicus and the symphysis pubis. Alternate sites are the flank, the iliac fossa, the border of the rectus, or, when assessing for abdominal bleeding, at each quadrant of the abdomen.
    - For smaller ascitic volume, abdominal ultrasound may be needed to locate fluid accumulation.
- The area is shaved, cleansed, and draped.
- A local anesthetic is administered.
- A small incision is made at the site if a trocar and cannula are to be inserted. Otherwise, a needle is inserted through the peritoneum.
    - If for diagnostic purposes, 18 g needle is sufficient.
    - For drainage of large volumes of fluid, a 14 g needle is usually required.
- A sample of the fluid is obtained.
- If additional fluid is to be drained, connect a tubing between the cannula and the collection receptacle.
- A maximum of 1000 mL is allowed to drain slowly from the site. Rapid drainage, and thus hypovolemia, can be avoided by either raising the collection receptacle to slow the draining or by clamping the tubing.
- When the procedure is complete, the trocar or needle is removed. A pressure dressing is applied.

Posttest
- Monitor vital signs until stable.
- Check the dressing frequently for drainage. Assess for hemorrhage, for increasing pain, and for abdominal tenderness.
- If a large amount of fluid is drained from the peritoneal cavity, a fluid shift may occur from the vascular space to the peritoneal cavity. Assess for elevated pulse and respirations, decreased blood pressure, mental status changes, and dizziness. Intravenous fluids or albumin may be ordered.
- Observe for hepatic coma in patients with severe hepatic disease, as evidenced by mental status changes, drowsiness, and stupor.
- Weigh the patient and measure the abdominal girth for comparison with pretest values, as indications of fluid loss.
- Monitor urinary output for 24 hours. Observe for hematuria.
- Label the specimen and transport it to the laboratory immediately.
- Report abnormal findings to the primary care provider.

→ Clinical Alerts

- Possible complications include: hemorrhage, hepatic coma, perforation of abdominal organs, peritonitis, shock and hypovolemia.

CONTRAINDICATIONS!

- Patients with bleeding disorders
- Patients with intestinal obstruction
- Patients with an infected abdominal wall
- Patients who are unable to cooperate during the procedure
- Patients with severe portal hypertension with abdominal collateral circulation

Parathyroid Hormone (PTH, Parathormone)

Test Description
Parathyroid hormone (PTH) is produced by the parathyroid glands, four glands located within the fascial capsule of the thyroid gland. PTH plays a major role in maintaining calcium and phosphorus levels in the body. This balance is accomplished through promotion of intestinal absorption of calcium, mobilization of calcium and phosphorus from the bone, and renal tubular reabsorption of calcium and excretion of phosphorus. PTH breaks down into three molecular fragments including N-terminal, C-terminal, and mid-region fragment. However, intact PTH, as the major biologically active form, is the form more frequently measured. PTH levels are typically assessed when the patient has an abnormal calcium level and to monitor conditions which may affect calcium levels, such as chronic renal failure.

THE EVIDENCE FOR PRACTICE

PTH levels are usually not evaluated in isolation. Because PTH can affect both calcium and phosphorus levels, these levels are also typically assessed. Kidney function can affect PTH levels, so serum creatinine levels may also be monitored. Likewise, serum levels of calcium, phosphorus, and intact plasma PTH should be measured in all patients with chronic kidney disease (CKD) and glomerular filtration rate (GFR) <60 mL/min/1.73 m².

Normal Values

10–60 pg/mL (10–60 ng/L SI units)

Possible Meanings of Abnormal Values

Increased	Decreased
Calcium malabsorption	Autoimmune disease
Chronic renal failure	Graves' disease
Ectopic PTH production	Hypercalcemia
Hypocalcemia	Hypoparathyroidism
Lactation	Milk-alkali syndrome
Pregnancy	Parathyroidectomy
Primary hyperparathyroidism	Sarcoidosis
Renal hypercalciuria	Vitamin A and D toxicity
Rickets	
Secondary hyperparathyroidism	
Squamous cell carcinoma	
Vitamin D deficiency	

Contributing Factors to Abnormal Values

- Drugs that can *increase* PTH levels include anticonvulsants, furosemide, isoniazid, lithium, rifampin, steroids, thiazide diuretics, and medications that contain phosphate.
- Drugs that can slightly *decrease* PTH levels include cimetidine and propranolol.
- Falsely low values may occur following ingestion of milk.
- Other factors which may impact PTH levels: pregnancy, breast-feeding, hyperlipidemia, and radioactive scan within previous week.

Interventions/Implications

Pretest
- Explain to the patient the purpose of the test and the need for a blood sample to be drawn.
- Fasting for 8 to 10 hours is required before the test.
- PTH levels will vary during the day, peaking at about 2 a.m. Specimens are usually drawn about 8 a.m.

Procedure
- A 5-mL blood sample is collected in a red-top tube.
- Gloves are worn throughout the procedure.

Posttest
- Apply pressure at venipuncture site. Apply dressing, periodically assessing for continued bleeding.

- The sample is labeled and transported to the laboratory where it is centrifuged. The serum is frozen until ready for processing.
- Report results to the primary care provider.

 Clinical Alerts

- With elevated serum PTH and serum calcium levels, the patient may be at risk for a variety of clinical conditions, including kidney stones due to hypercalciuria, osteoporosis from calcium loss from bones, kidney failure, and hypertension.

 # Parotid Gland Imaging (Salivary Gland Imaging)

Test Description
There are three pairs of salivary glands. The largest of these are the parotid, which are located over the jaw in the preauricular area bilaterally. The parotid glands produce saliva to aid in chewing and swallowing and which contains enzymes to begin food digestion. The parotid glands may become infected or inflamed or become obstructed due to tumor, cyst, or stone. Nuclear imaging is used to determine the cause of facial swelling or pain, abnormal tastes, or dry mouth.

Normal Values

Normal parotid gland structure and function

Possible Meanings of Abnormal Values
Abscess
Acute parotitis
Benign tumor
Cyst
Malignant tumor
Sialadinitis
Sjögren's syndrome

Interventions/Implications
Pretest
- Explain to the patient the purpose of the test. Provide any written teaching materials available on the subject. Reassure the patient that only trace amounts of the radionuclide are involved in the test.
- The patient must remain still while the scan is being performed.
- No fasting is required before the test.
- Obtain a signed informed consent.

Procedure
- Radionuclide is injected intravenously.

- Images of the parotid glands are taken every 1 to 3 minutes for 30 minutes.
- To assess patency of salivary ducts, the patient may be asked to use a lemon slice or swish lemon juice in the mouth. This causes emptying of the parotid gland if the ducts are patent.
- Gloves are worn during the radionuclide injection.

Posttest
- Although the amount of diagnostic radionuclide excreted in the urine is low, the urine should not be used for any laboratory tests for the time period indicated by the nuclear medicine department.
- Encourage fluid intake by the patient to enhance excretion of the radionuclide.
- Report abnormal findings to the primary care provider.

CONTRAINDICATIONS!

- Pregnant women
  - Caution: A woman in her childbearing years should undergo scanning only during her menses or 12 to 14 days after its onset to avoid any exposure to a fetus.
- Patients who are lactating
- Patients who are unable to cooperate because of age, mental status, pain, or other factors

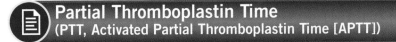

Partial Thromboplastin Time
(PTT, Activated Partial Thromboplastin Time [APTT])

P

Test Description

The process of hemostasis involves numerous steps and the proper functioning of a variety of coagulating factors and other substances. The *partial thromboplastin time (PTT)* or *activated partial thromboplastin time (APTT)* is used to evaluate how well the coagulation process is functioning. This test is useful for detecting bleeding disorders caused by either deficient or defective coagulation factors that compose the intrinsic system. These factors include I, II, V, VIII, IX, X, XI, and XII. Normal APTTs may reflect normal clotting function but moderate single factor deficiencies may still exist. They will not be reflected in the APTT until they have decreased to 30% to 40% of normal.

The PTT is also used to monitor heparin therapy. Heparin inactivates prothrombin and prevents the formation of thromboplastin. Thus, in conditions in which prevention of thrombus formation is essential, heparin is given, usually in the form of a continuous intravenous infusion. It is important that the patient's response to this anticoagulant therapy be appropriate; that is, enough for prevention of clot formation, but not so much as to cause spontaneous bleeding. This delicate balance can be monitored through use of the PTT.

The PTT involves measuring the amount of time it takes for a clot to form in a plasma sample to which calcium and partial thromboplastin have been added. If additional chemicals are added to standardize and accelerate the test, the result is reported as an *activated partial thromboplastin time, or APTT*. A normal range for

PTT is 60 to 90 seconds, whereas for APTT the normal range is 25 to 35 seconds. Laboratories report the actual PTT or APTT values along with the control value for reference. The therapeutic level for a patient receiving heparin is 1.5 to 2.5 times the control value. If the value falls below the therapeutic level for a patient on heparin, an increase in anticoagulation, and thus, dosage is needed. If the APTT is greater than 100 seconds, the patient is at high risk for spontaneous bleeding. In the case of heparin overdose with resultant hemorrhage, the antidote is protamine sulfate, with each 1 mg reversing 100 units of heparin.

Normal Values

APTT: 25–35 seconds
PTT: 60–90 seconds
Therapeutic level for anticoagulant therapy: 1.5–2.5 times the control value

Possible Meanings of Abnormal Values

Increased	Decreased
Abruptio placentae	Acute hemorrhage
Afibrinogenemia	Advanced cancer
Autologous blood transfusion	Hypercoagulability
Bleeding disorders	Very early DIC
Cardiac surgery	
Cirrhosis	
Disseminated intravascular coagulation	
Dysfibrinogenemia	
Factor XII deficiency	
Hemodialysis	
Hemophilia A (factor VIII deficiency)	
Hemophilia B (factor IX deficiency)	
Heparin therapy	
Hypoprothrombinemia	
Liver disease	
Malabsorption	
Vitamin K deficiency	
von Willebrand's disease	

Contributing Factors to Abnormal Values

- Hemolysis of the blood sample may alter test results.
- Presence of lupus anticoagulant can *increase* PTT results.
- High or low hematocrit levels may interfere with test results due to effect on citrate concentration.
- Drugs which may *increase* PTT: antibiotics, asparaginase, aspirin, cholestyramine, cyclophosphamide, enoxaparin, quinine, thrombolytics, warfarin

Interventions/Implications

Pretest
- Explain to the patient the purpose of the test and the need for a blood sample to be drawn.

- If the patient is receiving a continuous heparin infusion, inform the patient that a blood sample will be drawn daily for monitoring response to the medication.
- No fasting is required prior to the test.
- If the patient is receiving heparin intermittently, draw the PTT 30 to 60 minutes before the next dose. If receiving heparin by continuous infusion, the PTT can be drawn at any time.
- Do *not* draw the sample from the arm in which heparin is infusing.
- If the blood sample is to be drawn from an arterial line with a heparin-flush pressure bag, withdraw at least 10 mL of blood before drawing the sample for the PTT.

Procedure
- A 7-mL blood sample is drawn in a light blue-top collection tube containing sodium citrate.
- Gloves are worn throughout the procedure.

Posttest
- Apply pressure 3 to 5 minutes at venipuncture site. Apply dressing, periodically assessing for continued bleeding.
- Teach the patient to monitor the site. If the site begins to bleed, the patient should apply direct pressure and, if unable to control the bleeding, return to the laboratory or notify the primary care provider.
- Report abnormal findings to the primary care provider.

Clinical Alerts

- Possible complications include: Hematoma at site due to prolonged bleeding time
- Spontaneous bleeding can occur with APTT >100 seconds.
    - Assess patient for spontaneous bleeding: epistaxis, bleeding gums, low back pain from possible retroperitoneal bleeding, joint pain, bruising, petechiae, hematuria, or melena.

P

Parvovirus B-19 Antibody Test

Test Description
Parvovirus B-19, known as "fifth disease," primarily affects children in the form of a rash. A bright red rash on both cheeks with a "slapped face" pattern first appears, followed by a rash on the arms, legs, and trunk. The rash typically fades from the center outwards, giving it a lacy appearance. Although it usually lasts for 5 to 14 days, the rash may appear intermittently for several weeks. Sunlight, heat, exercise, fever, or emotional stress can cause the rash to reappear.

Parvovirus B-19 can also affect adults. Joint pain and swelling are more common symptoms in adults. The majority of adults have antibodies to the parvovirus, meaning they have been exposed to the virus and likely had no or very minor symptoms.

However, the disease can be serious for some people. Patients with sickle cell anemia or similar types of chronic anemia can suffer from acute anemia during this illness. If a pregnant woman becomes infected with parvovirus B-19 during the first half of pregnancy, there is a <5% risk that the fetus will have severe anemia and miscarriage may occur.

THE EVIDENCE FOR PRACTICE

Pregnant women exposed to parvovirus B-19 should have serologic screening performed to determine if they are at risk for seroconversion.

Normal Values

Negative

Possible Meanings of Abnormal Values

Increased

IgM—active infection with parvovirus B-19
IgG—previous exposure to parvovirus B-19; lifetime immunity

Interventions/Implications

Pretest

- Explain to the patient the purpose of the test and the need for a blood sample to be drawn.
- No fasting is required before the test.

Procedure

- A 7-mL blood sample is drawn in a red-top collection tube.
- Gloves are worn throughout the procedure.

Posttest

- Apply pressure at venipuncture site. Apply dressing, periodically assessing for continued bleeding.
- Label the specimen and transport it to the laboratory.
- Report abnormal findings to the primary care provider.

Pelvic Sonogram (Gynecologic Sonogram, Obstetric Sonogram, Pelvic Echogram, Pelvic Ultrasound, Transvaginal Ultrasound)

Test Description

Ultrasonography is a noninvasive method of diagnostic testing in which ultrasound waves are sent into the body with a small transducer pressed against the skin. The transducer then receives any returning sound waves, which are deflected back as they bounce off various structures. The transducer converts the returning sound waves into electric signals that are then transformed by a computer into a visual display on a monitor.

The purpose of the pelvic ultrasound is to provide images of the structures in the pelvic region. There are three types of pelvic ultrasound:

- *Transabdominal—*
  - Used for women and men to help identify kidney stones, tumors, and other disorders in the urinary bladder
  - Used for women to evaluate the bladder, ovaries, uterus, cervix, and fallopian tubes
  - Used for women to assess, if present, the fetus and fetal sac. It is helpful in the diagnosis of fetal death, placenta previa, and abruptio placentae. It also provides guidance for amniocentesis, fetoscopy, or intrauterine procedures
  - Used for men to evaluate the bladder and seminal vesicles
- *Transvaginal—*used for women to evaluate the endometrium and muscle walls of the uterus
- *Transrectal—*used for men to study the prostate gland (see "Prostate Sonogram" for discussion of this approach)

THE EVIDENCE FOR PRACTICE

A common problem among menstruating women is a painful ovarian cyst (often a hemorrhagic luteal cyst) which can cause unilateral pelvic pain. Diagnosis can be confirmed by pelvic ultrasound. Repeating the ultrasound after the next cycle (preferably 3 to 7 days after last menstrual period) should show resolution of the cyst.

P

Normal Values

Normal fetal and placental size and position
No pelvic organ abnormalities

Possible Meanings of Abnormal Values

Abnormal fetal structure
Abruptio placentae
Abscesses
Ectopic pregnancy
Fetal death
Fetal malpresentation (breech, transverse)
Fibroid
Foreign body (e.g., intrauterine device)
Hydatidiform mole
Inappropriate fetal size
Multiple pregnancy
Pelvic tumor
Placenta previa
Uterine anomalies
Uterine cancer

Contributing Factors to Abnormal Values

- The transducer must be in good contact with the skin as it is being moved. A water-based gel is used to ensure good contact with the skin.
- Retained barium from previous exams or bowel gas may alter test results.

Interventions/Implications

Pretest

- Explain to the patient the purpose of the test. Provide any written teaching materials available on the subject. Note that there is no pain involved with this test, although a pressure feeling may occur.
- No fasting is required before the test.
- A full bladder is needed during the examination. Instruct the patient to drink 1 L of water 1 hour before the procedure and remind her not to void until the test is completed.
- For a transvaginal ultrasound, explain that the transducer is smaller than a vaginal speculum.

Procedure

Transabdominal

- The patient is assisted to a supine position on the ultrasonography table.
- A coupling agent, such as a water-based gel, is applied to the abdominal and pelvic area.
- A transducer is placed on the skin and moved as needed to provide good visualization of the pelvic structures and the fetus.
- The sound waves are transformed into a visual display on the monitor. Printed copies of the display are made.

Transvaginal

- The patient first empties her bladder, and is then assisted to a supine position, possibly with her feet in stirrups.
- A protective cover is placed over the transducer, lubricated with a small amount of gel, and inserted 2 to 3 in into the vagina.
- The transducer is moved in different orientations to provide views of the uterus and ovaries.
- The sound waves are transformed into a visual display on the monitor. Printed copies of the display are made.
- Gloves are worn throughout the procedure.

Posttest

- Cleanse the patient's skin of any lubricant.
- Allow the patient to void immediately after the transabdominal test is completed.
- Report abnormal findings to the primary care provider.

→ **Clinical Alerts**

- In the case of pregnancy, pelvic ultrasound often allows determination of the gender of the fetus. It should be confirmed that the patient desires to know the gender before informing her of the results.

Pericardiocentesis (Pericardial Fluid Analysis)

Test Description

Pericardiocentesis refers to the removal of fluid from the pericardial cavity. This cavity is the space between the visceral pericardium, which is the serous inner layer of the pericardium, and the parietal pericardium, which is the outer fibrous layer of the pericardium. In some conditions, such as inflammatory diseases of the heart, myocardial rupture, and penetrating trauma to the heart, a large amount of fluid may accumulate in the pericardial cavity, an assessment finding known as *pericardial effusion*.

Pericardiocentesis may be done as a diagnostic procedure to determine the cause of the fluid production, or for emergency therapeutic purposes. In the case of penetrating trauma, the rapidly forming effusion causes increased intrapericardial pressure which reduces cardiac output, a situation known as *cardiac tamponade*. In this type of emergency, the pericardiocentesis must be done immediately, without waiting for signed informed consent.

Normal Values

<50 mL of clear, straw-colored fluid
Absence of bacteria, red blood cells, white blood cells
No abnormal cells present

Possible Meanings of Abnormal Values

Acute myocardial infarction
Bacterial pericarditis
Cardiac trauma
Congestive heart failure
Fungal pericarditis
Myocardial rupture
Neoplasm
Pericarditis
Rheumatoid disease
Rupture of ventricular aneurysm
Systemic lupus erythematosus
Traumatic tap
Tuberculous pericarditis

Contributing Factors to Abnormal Values

- Antimicrobial therapy, if started prior to the test, may decrease the bacterial count.
- Contamination of the specimen through break in sterile technique will alter white blood cell count.

Interventions/Implications

Pretest
- Explain to the patient the purpose of the test and the procedure to be done. Explain that a local anesthetic will be used, but that a pressure-like pain will occur as the needle pierces the pericardial sac. Explain that no movement, including deep breathing or coughing, can occur during the test.
- Fasting is required for 6 hours prior to the test.
- Obtain a signed informed consent.
  - Note: If emergency situation, inform the patient's family of the immediate need for the procedure.
- Echocardiography should be performed prior to the test to locate the fluid and to avoid accidental puncture of the heart.
- Obtain baseline vital signs.
- Resuscitation and suctioning equipment must be readily available.
- Pulse oximetry may be ordered for use throughout the procedure.

Procedure
- Assist the patient to the supine position with the head of the bed elevated 60°.
- Initiate a maintenance IV, and administer premedication as ordered.
- Monitor vital signs every 15 minutes during the procedure.
- Sterile technique is used throughout the procedure.
- The skin from the left costal margin to the xiphoid process is cleansed and draped.
- A local anesthetic is administered.
- A 16- to 18-gauge cardiac needle attached to a 50-mL syringe and a three-way stopcock is inserted through the chest wall between the left costal margin and the xiphoid process (in the subxyphoid space) into the pericardial sac. An ECG lead is attached to the needle with a clip. The ECG must be monitored throughout the procedure for the following changes:
  - *Elevation of the PR segment* indicates the needle is touching the atrial surface.
  - An *ST-segment elevation* indicates the needle is touching the epicardial surface and needs to be pulled back slightly.
  - An *abnormally shaped QRS complex* may indicate myocardial perforation.
  - *Premature ventricular contractions* usually indicate the needle is touching the ventricular wall.
- When the pocket of fluid is reached, a Kelly clamp is applied to the needle at the skin surface to prevent it from entering further. A 50-mL sample of the fluid is then obtained.
- When the procedure is complete, the needle is removed. Pressure is immediately applied and maintained for 3 to 5 minutes. A dressing is then applied.

Posttest
- Monitor vital signs every 15 minutes for 1 hour, every 30 minutes for 2 hours, every hour for 4 hours, and then every 4 hours.
- Check the dressing frequently for drainage.
- Continue to observe the patient for any respiratory or cardiac distress: muffled and distant heart sounds, distended neck veins, paradoxical pulse, and shock.
- Label the specimen and transport it to the laboratory immediately.
- Report abnormal findings to the primary care provider.

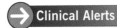

Clinical Alerts

- Possible complications include: cardiac tamponade syndrome from laceration of coronary artery or rapid reaccumulation of fluid; myocardial laceration, pleural effusion, puncture of lung, liver, or stomach, vasovagal arrest, and ventricular fibrillation.

CONTRAINDICATIONS!

- Patients with bleeding disorders
- Patients who are unable to cooperate during the procedure

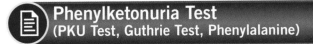

Phenylketonuria Test
(PKU Test, Guthrie Test, Phenylalanine)

Test Description
Phenylalanine hydroxylase is an enzyme which converts phenylalanine to tyrosine. A deficiency of this enzyme leads to a buildup of phenylalanine which results in severe mental retardation. This condition, known as *phenylketonuria (PKU)*, is an autosomal recessive inborn error of metabolism. Screening of all newborns for PKU is required in all states. Testing is done either on the serum (Guthrie test) or on the urine. Testing is not valid until the newborn has ingested an ample amount of the amino acid phenylalanine, which is found in human and cow's milk. Two or three days of intake are usually sufficient for the Guthrie test. Urine PKU testing is usually done after the infant is 4 to 6 weeks old.

P

THE EVIDENCE FOR PRACTICE
The American Academy of Family Physicians *strongly recommends* ordering screening test for phenylketonuria in neonates.

Normal Values
    Blood: Negative
    Urine: No green discoloration

Possible Meanings of Abnormal Values

Increased
Delayed enzyme system development
Galactosemia
Hepatic disease
Hyperphenylalaninemia
Low birth weight
Phenylketonuria

Contributing Factors to Abnormal Values

- Testing for PKU too early may lead to *false-negative* results. Blood sample should be collected from infants older than 24 hours and younger than 7 days.
- Drugs which may alter test results: antibiotics, aspirin, salicylates.

Interventions/Implications

Pretest

- Explain the purpose of the test to the mother and the need for a blood sample to be obtained.
- No fasting is required prior to the test.

Procedure

For Guthrie (serum) test

- After the newborn has been taking in ample amounts of milk for 2 to 3 days, the test may be performed.
- Cleanse the newborn's heel with alcohol and allow to air dry.
- Puncture the heel with a lancet, allowing several drops of blood to collect on the filter paper for the Guthrie test.

For urine test

- Urine testing for PKU may be performed after 4 to 6 weeks of age.
- This is accomplished by either dropping 10% ferric chloride on a diaper containing fresh urine, or by pressing a Phenistix test stick against the urine on the diaper.
- With either method, a green discoloration is indicative of PKU.
- Gloves are worn throughout the above procedures.

Posttest

- Apply pressure on the newborn's heel for 5 to 10 minutes and then leave the site open to the air for healing.
- Report abnormal findings to the primary care provider.

→ Clinical Alerts

- Treatment for PKU is a low phenylalanine diet. This should be implemented as soon as possible in the neonatal period. Adherence to a low-phenylalanine diet should be life-long.
- Food must be chosen only from special lists and weighed or measured accurately so that the daily intake of phenylalanine is the amount prescribed.
  - High protein foods (such as fish, chicken, eggs, milk, cheese, dried beans, nuts, and tofu) cannot be eaten.
  - Any product containing the artificial sweetener aspartame must be avoided
  - A special infant formula called Lofenalac is made for infants with PKU. It can be used throughout life as a protein source that is extremely low in phenylalanine and balanced for the remaining essential amino acids. Adjustments are made in the formula content based on frequent monitoring of phenylalanine in the blood.

Phosphorus (P, Phosphate, PO_4)

Test Description

Most of the body's phosphorus is combined with calcium in the bones. About 15%, however, exists in the blood, making phosphorus the main anion in the intracellular fluid. It has several functions, including a role in glucose and lipid metabolism, storage and transfer of energy within the body, generation of bony tissue, and maintenance of acid-base balance. Like calcium, phosphorus is controlled by the parathyroid hormone (PTH). It holds an inverse relationship with calcium; an excess in the serum of one results in the kidneys excreting the other. PTH increases calcium and phosphate release from bone and decreases loss of calcium and increases loss of phosphate in the urine. An elevated serum phosphorus level is known as *hyperphosphatemia*; decreased level, *hypophosphatemia*.

THE EVIDENCE FOR PRACTICE

Serum levels of calcium, phosphorus, alkaline phosphatase, total carbon dioxide (CO_2), and parathyroid hormone (PTH) should be measured in all patients with chronic kidney disease (CKD) Stages 2 through 5. The frequency of these measurements should be based on the stage of CKD.

Normal Values

2.4–4.1 mg/dL (0.78–1.34 mmol/L SI units)

Possible Meanings of Abnormal Values

Increased (Hyperphosphatemia)	Decreased (Hypophosphatemia)
Acromegaly	Antacid abuse
Addison's disease	Carbohydrate loading
Bone tumors	Chronic alcoholism
Diabetic ketoacidosis (early)	Diabetic ketoacidosis (after treatment)
Healing fracture	Diuresis
Hypocalcemia	Hypercalcemia
Hypoparathyroidism	Hyperinsulinism
Massive blood transfusions	Hypokalemia
Milk-alkali syndrome	Hyperparathyroidism
Nephritis	Hypothyroidism
Phosphate supplementation	Malabsorption
Prepuberty	Malnutrition
Renal failure	Osteomalacia
Sarcoidosis	Renal disease
Sickle cell anemia	Rickets
Thyrotoxicosis	Salicylate intoxication
Tissue damage	Severe burns
Uremia	Vitamin D deficiency
Vitamin D intoxication	

P

Contributing Factors to Abnormal Values

- Use of a tourniquet during acquisition of the blood sample may alter test results.
- Hemolysis of the blood sample may alter test results.
- Due to increased carbohydrate metabolism causing decreased phosphorus levels, glucose solutions should not be infused prior to the test.
- Drugs which may *increase* serum phosphorus levels: antibiotics, epoetin, etidronate, furosemide, hydrochlorothiazide, naproxen, nifedipine, phosphate enemas, risedronate, risperidone, testosterone, venlafaxine, vitamin D.
- Drugs which may *decrease* serum phosphorus levels: amlodipine, anabolic steroids, anticonvulsants, azathioprine, calcitonin, calcitrol, cisplatin, diuretics, doxorubicin, insulin, IV dextrose, lithium, niacin, nicardipine, phenothiazines, phosphate binding antacids, raloxifene, theophylline overdose, venlafaxine.

Interventions/Implications

Pretest
- Explain to the patient the purpose of the test and the need for a blood sample to be drawn.
- No fasting is required before the test.

Procedure
- A 7-mL blood sample is drawn in a red-top collection tube, avoiding use of a tourniquet, if possible.
- Gloves are worn throughout the procedure.

Posttest
- Apply pressure at venipuncture site. Apply dressing, periodically assessing for continued bleeding.
- Label the specimen and transport it to the laboratory.
- Report abnormal findings to the primary care provider.

→ Clinical Alerts

- Serum phosphorus results should be correlated with serum calcium levels to determine possible causes.
    - Increased phosphorus with decreased calcium: hypoparathyroidism, renal disease
    - Increased phosphorus with normal or increased calcium: milk-alkali syndrome, hypervitaminosis D
    - Decreased phosphorus with increased calcium: hyperparathyroidism, sarcoidosis
    - Decreased phosphorus and calcium: malabsorption, vitamin D deficiency, renal tubular acidosis

📄 Plasminogen (Fibrinolysin)

Test Description

When injury to a blood vessel or tissue occurs, the process of hemostasis is initiated and results in the formation of a fibrin clot. Plasminogen is a beta-globulin protein normally found in fibrin clots in an inactive form. Once healing has occurred and the fibrin clots are no longer needed, enzymes within the endothelial cells trigger the conversion of plasminogen to plasmin. The production of plasmin, which is a fibrinolytic enzyme, results in lysis of the fibrin clot.

Plasmin cannot be directly measured since it is not present in the circulation in its active form. Thus, measurement of its inactive form, plasminogen, is used to evaluate this fibrinolytic system. The test is performed by adding a plasminogen activator to the patient's blood sample. This causes plasminogen to convert to active plasmin, which in turn causes a chemical substance in the solution to change color. This colored substance, which can be measured, is proportional to the functional plasminogen level.

Normal Values

3.36 ± 0.44 CTA (Council on Thrombolytic Agents) U/mL

Possible Meanings of Abnormal Values

Increased	Decreased
Anxiety	Cirrhosis
Infection	Disseminated intravascular coagulation
Inflammation	Eclampsia
Pregnancy	Hyaline membrane disease
Stress	Liver disease
	Nephrosis
	Preeclampsia
	Thrombosis
	Tumors

Contributing Factors to Abnormal Values

- Hemolysis of the blood sample may alter test results.
- Falsely decreased values may occur if the tourniquet remains in place a prolonged time prior to the venipuncture.
- Vigorous exercise increases plasminogen levels.
- Drugs which may *increase* plasminogen levels: anabolic steroids, oral contraceptives.
- Drugs which may *decrease* plasminogen levels: thrombolytic agents.

Interventions/Implications

Pretest
- Explain to the patient the purpose of the test and the need for a blood sample to be drawn.
- No fasting is required before the test.

Procedure
- A 7-mL blood sample is drawn in a light blue-top collection tube.
- Gloves are worn throughout the procedure.

Posttest
- Apply pressure 3 to 5 minutes at venipuncture site. Apply dressing, periodically assessing for continued bleeding.

- Teach the patient to monitor the site. If the site begins to bleed, the patient should apply direct pressure and, if unable to control the bleeding, return to the laboratory or notify the primary care provider.
- Label the specimen and transport it to the laboratory.
- Report abnormal findings to the primary care provider.

 Clinical Alerts

- Decreased plasminogen levels indicate an increased risk of thrombosis.

 Platelet Aggregation Test

Test Description

The *platelet aggregation test* evaluates the ability of the platelets to adhere to each other. When there is an injury to the wall of a blood vessel, any bleeding through the vessel wall is brought under control through the formation of a platelet plug. Several substances and processes are required for this plug to form. There must be an adequate number of platelets in the circulation. There must also be platelet agonists, such as thrombin, which assist the platelets to aggregate or clump, and proteins such as fibrinogen which are able to bind to the surface of the platelets.

In this test, the patient's platelets are mixed with platelet agonists such as adenosine diphosphate (ADP), arachidonic acid, collagen, epinephrine, ristocetin, and thrombin. After clumping of the platelets has occurred, a measurement is made of the amount of light passing through the solution. The transmission of light through the plasma solution should be increased after platelet aggregation.

Normal Values

Norm varies with reagent used.

Possible Meanings of Abnormal Values

Increased	Decreased
Atheromatosis	Afibrinogenemia
Hypercoagulability	Autoimmune disorders
Hyperlipemia	Bernard-Soulier syndrome
Polycythemia vera	Beta-thalassemia major
	Cirrhosis
	Glanzmann's thrombasthenia
	Idiopathic thrombocytopenic purpura
	Macroglobulinemia
	Myeloproliferative disorders
	Recent cardiopulmonary bypass
	Recent dialysis
	Scurvy

Systemic lupus erythematosus
Thrombocythemia
Uremia
Vasculitis
von Willlebrand's disease
Wiskott-Aldrich syndrome

Contributing Factors to Abnormal Values

- Hemolysis of the blood sample, lipemia, hemoglobinemia, or bilirubinemia may alter the test results.
- Drugs which may *decrease* platelet aggregation: aspirin, carbenicillin, cephalothin, chlordiazepoxide, chloroquine, clofibrate, cocaine, corticosteroids, cyproheptadine, diazepam, diphenhydramine, dipyridamole, furosemide, gentamicin, guaifenesin, heparin, ibuprofen, imipramine, indomethacin, marijuana, mefenamic acid, naproxen, nitrofurantoin, nortriptyline, penicillin G, phenothiazines, phenylbutazone, promethazine, propranolol, pyrimidine compounds, warfarin, sulfinpyrazone, theophylline, vitamin E.

Interventions/Implications

Pretest
- Explain to the patient the purpose of the test and the need for a blood sample to be drawn.
- No fasting is required before the test.

Procedure
- A 7-mL blood sample is drawn in a light blue-top collection tube.
- Gloves are worn throughout the procedure.

Posttest
- Apply pressure 3 to 5 minutes at venipuncture site. Apply dressing, periodically assessing for continued bleeding.
- Teach the patient to monitor the site. If the site begins to bleed, the patient should apply direct pressure and, if unable to control the bleeding, return to the laboratory or notify the primary care provider.
- Label the specimen and transport it to the laboratory.
- Report abnormal findings to the primary care provider.

P

Clinical Alerts

- Possible complication: Hematoma at site due to prolonged bleeding time

Platelet Antibody Test (Antiplatelet Antibody Detection, Platelet Antibody Detection Test)

Test Description

The platelet antibody test may be ordered when the person has a low platelet count (thrombocytopenia) which is unresponsive to platelet transfusion. Platelet autoantibodies are IgG immunoglobulins which develop in individuals when they become sensitized to platelet antigens of transfused blood. When platelet autoantibodies are present, both donor and recipient platelets are destroyed. At times, antiplatelet antibodies may appear in the blood for unknown reasons, a condition known as idiopathic thrombo-cytopenic purpura (ITP), or as an adverse effect of certain drugs. Drug-induced immunologic thrombocytopenia may be caused by such drugs as chlordiazepoxide, gold, heparin, phenytoin, quinidine, quinine sulfate, and sulfa drugs.

Normal Values

Negative

Possible Meanings of Abnormal Values

Increased

Drug-induced immunologic thrombocytopenia
Idiopathic thrombocytopenic purpura
Neonatal thrombocytopenia
Paroxysmal hemoglobinuria
Posttransfusion purpura

Contributing Factors to Abnormal Values

- Hemolysis of the blood sample will alter test results.
- Blood transfusions may result in the development of isoantibodies.

Interventions/Implications

Pretest
- Explain to the patient the purpose of the test and the need for a blood sample to be drawn.
- If possible, the blood sample should be drawn prior to any blood transfusion.
- No fasting is required before the test.

Procedure
- A 10- to 30-mL blood sample is drawn in red-top collection tubes.
- Gloves are worn throughout the procedure.

Posttest
- Apply pressure 3 to 5 minutes at venipuncture site. Apply dressing, periodically assess-ing for continued bleeding.
- Teach the patient to monitor the site. If the site begins to bleed, the patient should apply direct pressure and, if unable to control the bleeding, return to the laboratory or notify the primary care provider.
- Label the specimen and transport it to the laboratory.
- Report abnormal findings to the primary care provider.

→ Clinical Alerts

- Possible complication: Prolonged bleeding due to thrombocytopenia

Platelet Count (Thrombocyte Count)

Test Description

Platelets, or thrombocytes, are fragments of megakaryocytes which are formed in the bone marrow. They circulate in the bloodstream for a life span of 8 to 12 days, at which time they are removed from the circulation by the spleen. Platelets are essential to hemostasis and blood clotting. When a blood vessel wall is injured, the platelets adhere to its wall and aggregate, forming a platelet plug. They also release phospholipids which are required by the intrinsic coagulation pathway.

Patients with platelet counts between 50,000 and 150,000/mm³ usually show few, if any, signs of bleeding. Spontaneous bleeding of a minor nature and prolonged bleeding following surgery or trauma are seen in patients with platelet counts ranging between 20,000 and 50,000/mm³. The most serious risk lies with patients whose platelet counts are fewer than 20,000/mm³. In these patients, spontaneous bleeding of a more serious nature occurs.

The platelet count may be done by machine or by microscopic examination. Obtaining the platelet count is helpful in the diagnosis of *thrombocytopenia* (decreased platelet count) and *thrombocytosis* (increased number of platelets), provides information about platelet production, and allows monitoring of the effect of antineoplastic drug therapy and radiation therapy on platelet production.

THE EVIDENCE FOR PRACTICE

Normal Values

150,000–400,000/mm³ (150–400 X 10⁹/L SI units)

Possible Meanings of Abnormal Values

Increased (Thrombocytosis)	Decreased (Thrombocytopenia)
Acute infection	Acute leukemia
Asphyxiation	AIDS
Chronic leukemia	Allergic conditions
Chronic pancreatitis	Aplastic anemia
Cirrhosis	Autotransfusion
Collagen disease	Clostridial infection
Heart disease	Disseminated intravascular coagulation
Inflammation	Exposure to DDT
Iron deficiency anemia	Extracorporeal bypass
Malignant tumors	Hemolytic anemia
Multiple myeloma	Hypersplenism
Myeloproliferative disease	Idiopathic thrombocytopenic purpura
Polycythemia vera	Lymphoproliferative diseases
Posthemorrhagic anemia	Menstruation
Postpartum	Multiple myeloma
Post-splenectomy	Pernicious anemia
Pregnancy	Prosthetic heart valve
Rheumatoid arthritis	Radiation
Sickle cell anemia	Splenomegaly

P

Trauma
Tuberculosis
Viral infections

Systemic lupus erythematosus

Contributing Factors to Abnormal Values

- Conditions in which platelet count is *increased*: high altitudes, persistent cold temperatures, strenuous exercise, excitement.
- Condition in which platelet count is *decreased*: prior to menstruation.
- Drugs which may *increase* the platelet count: cephalosporins, clindamycin, clozapine, corticosteroids, danazol, dipyridamole, donepezil, epoetin, gemfibrozil, lithium, oral contraceptives, zidovudine.
- Drugs which may *decrease* the platelet count: ACE-inhibitors, acetaminophen, allopurinol, antiarrhythmics, antibiotics, barbiturates, chemotherapeutic agents, diuretics, donepezil, infliximab, NSAIDs, phenothiazines.

Interventions/Implications

Pretest

- Explain to the patient the purpose of the test and the need for a blood sample to be drawn.
- No fasting is required before the test.

Procedure

- A 7-mL blood sample is drawn in a lavender-top collection tube.
- Gloves are worn throughout the procedure.

Posttest

- Apply pressure 3 to 5 minutes at venipuncture site. Apply dressing, periodically assessing for continued bleeding.
- Teach the patient to monitor the site. If the site begins to bleed, the patient should apply direct pressure and, if unable to control the bleeding, return to the laboratory or notify the nurse.
- Label the specimen and transport it to the laboratory.
- Report abnormal findings to the primary care provider.

→ Clinical Alerts

- Possible complications include:
    - Hematoma at site due to prolonged bleeding time.
    - Spontaneous bleeding with platelet count <20,000/mm³.
- Assess patient for spontaneous bleeding: epistaxis, bleeding gums, low back pain from possible retroperitoneal bleeding, joint pain, bruising, petechiae, hematuria, or melena.

Platelet, Mean Volume (Mean Platelet Volume, [MPV])

Test Description
Platelets, or thrombocytes, are fragments of megakaryocytes which are formed in the bone marrow. They are essential to hemostasis and blood clotting. When a blood

vessel wall is injured, the platelets adhere to its wall and aggregate, or clump, forming a platelet plug. It is advantageous to this process for the platelets to be large. When bone marrow function declines, the megakaryocytes are small, resulting in small platelets. If a condition other than bone marrow dysfunction is the cause of a low platelet count, the bone marrow tries to compensate by releasing larger platelets. Thus, measurement of the mean platelet volume assists in the diagnosis of thrombocytopenic disorders, those conditions in which there is a decreased platelet count.

Normal Values

25 μm in diameter (8–10 fL SI units)

Possible Meanings of Abnormal Values

Increased	Decreased
Bernard-Soulier syndrome	Aplastic anemia
Diabetes mellitus	Hypersplenism
Disseminated intravascular coagulation	Inflammatory bowel disease (active)
Hyperthyroidism	Megaloblastic anemia
Leukemia	Wiskott-Aldrich syndrome
May-Hegglin anomaly	
Myeloproliferative disorders	
Rheumatic heart disease	
Systemic lupus erythematosus	
Valvular heart disease	

Interventions/Implications

Pretest
- Explain to the patient the purpose of the test and the need for a blood sample to be drawn.
- No fasting is required before the test.

Procedure
- A 7-mL blood sample is drawn in a lavender-top collection tube.
- Gloves are worn throughout the procedure.

Posttest
- Apply pressure 3 to 5 minutes at venipuncture site. Apply dressing, periodically assessing for continued bleeding.
- Teach the patient to monitor the site. If the site begins to bleed, the patient should apply direct pressure and, if unable to control the bleeding, return to the laboratory or notify the primary care provider.
- Label the specimen and transport it to the laboratory.
- Report abnormal findings to the primary care provider.

→ Clinical Alerts

- Possible complication: Hematoma at site due to prolonged bleeding time

Plethysmography, Arterial (Pneumoplethysmography)

Test Description
Arterial plethysmography is a manometric test which evaluates the arterial blood flow in the lower extremities. This test involves the placement of pressure cuffs at various levels on the legs. Arterial waveforms are then recorded. A normal waveform is characterized by a sharp rise to a peak, a dicrotic notch, and then a downslope to the baseline. In the case of arterial occlusive disease, the waveforms are abnormal, with a lower height, a rounding of the peaks, and a loss of the dicrotic notch. With the availability of ultrasound and computed tomographic scanning, the use of plethysmography is becoming much less frequent.

Normal Values
Normal arterial waveforms

Possible Meanings of Abnormal Values
Arterial embolism
Arterial insufficiency
Arterial trauma
Arteriosclerosis
Diabetic ischemia
Raynaud's disease

Contributing Factors to Abnormal Values
- Since nicotine constricts the blood vessels, smoking within 2 hours prior to the exam will affect the test results.
- The temperature of the testing area may alter the peripheral circulation, thus affecting the test results.
- Arterial occlusion proximal to the extremity can prevent blood flow to the limb and affect the test results.

Interventions/Implications
Pretest
- Explain to the patient the purpose of the test and the procedure to be done.
- Inform the patient that the procedure is painless, but that no movement of the extremities can occur during the test.
- No fasting is required prior to the test.
- All clothing must be removed from the extremities.
- Obtain signed informed consent if required by the institution.

Procedure
- The patient is assisted into a semi-Fowler's position.
- Pressure cuffs are applied to the upper thigh, above the knee, below the knee, and above the ankle of each leg.

- The first cuff is inflated to 75 mm Hg for 2 seconds and then lowered to 65 mm Hg. The waveforms are recorded.
- The procedure is repeated for each cuff on each leg.

Posttest
- The cuffs are removed and the patient is allowed to dress.
- Ensure that each set of waveforms are labeled with the correct cuff site.
- Report abnormal findings to the primary care provider.

CONTRAINDICATIONS!

- The test should not be performed on an extremity which is cold and pale or cyanotic, since blood flow is obviously compromised to the limb.

 # Plethysmography, Venous (Impedance Plethysmography)

Test Description

Venous plethysmography is a manometric test which evaluates changes in venous capacity and outflow of the lower extremities. The test involves the placement of pressure cuffs at the level of the thigh and the calf. Each cuff is inflated to temporarily stop venous flow. Each one is then deflated to allow venous flow to resume. Venous waveforms are recorded throughout the procedure. Normal waveforms are characterized by a steady upslope after the cuff is inflated as the vein fills to capacity. After the cuff is deflated, there is a sharp downslope documenting rapid venous outflow. When there is an obstruction in the vein, as in deep vein thrombosis, the downslope of the line after cuff deflation is less steep, indicating minimal venous blood flow due to the obstruction. With the availability of ultrasound and computed tomographic scanning, the use of plethysmography is becoming much less frequent.

P

Normal Values

Normal venous waveforms

Possible Meanings of Abnormal Values

Deep vein thrombosis
Partial venous obstruction
Total venous obstruction

Contributing Factors to Abnormal Values

- Since nicotine constricts the blood vessels, smoking within 2 hours prior to the exam will affect the test results.
- The temperature of the testing area may alter the peripheral circulation, thus affecting the test results.

Interventions/Implications

Pretest
- Explain to the patient the purpose of the test and the procedure to be done.
- Inform the patient that the procedure is painless, but that no movement of the extremities can occur during the test.
- No fasting is required prior to the test.
- All clothing must be removed from the extremities.
- Obtain signed informed consent if required by the institution.

Procedure
- The patient is assisted into a supine position.
- Pressure cuffs are applied to the thigh and the calf of the affected leg.
- The calf cuff is inflated to 15 mm Hg and the thigh cuff is inflated to 55 mm Hg. The minimal pressure at the calf level allows monitoring of venous inflow. The thigh pressure obstructs the venous outflow and causes engorgement of the veins.
- The waveform is recorded as the veins fill to capacity.
- Once the waveform indicates full venous capacity has been reached, the pressure cuff on the thigh is deflated.
- The procedure is repeated for 3 to 5 waveforms.
- The procedure is repeated on the unaffected leg, which is used for comparison.

Posttest
- The cuffs are removed and the patient is allowed to dress.
- Ensure that each set of waveforms are labeled with the correct cuff site.
- Report abnormal findings to the primary care provider.

Pleural Biopsy

Test Description
Pleural biopsy is generally performed after the pleural fluid removed during a thoracentesis suggests infection, neoplasia, or tuberculosis. Determination of the actual nature of the problem can only be made by obtaining a biopsy of the tissue. In a pleural biopsy, a sample of pleural tissue is removed for histologic study. The tissue sample may be obtained by needle biopsy through the chest wall, as part of a thoracentesis, or by open biopsy during a thoracotomy. This discussion will be limited to that of needle biopsy of the pleura.

Normal Values
No abnormal cells or tissue present

Possible Meanings of Abnormal Values
Collagen vascular disease
Fungal disease
Malignancy
Parasitic disease

Tuberculosis
Viral disease

Interventions/Implications

Pretest

- Explain to the patient the purpose of the test and the procedure to be done. Explain to the patient that a local anesthetic will be used.
- Obtain baseline chest x-ray and coagulation tests (partial thromboplastin time, platelet count, prothrombin time).
- No fasting is required prior to the test.
- Obtain a signed informed consent.
- Obtain baseline vital signs.

Procedure

- The patient is assisted to a sitting position with the arms supported on a pillow on an overbed table.
- The skin is cleansed with an antiseptic and draped.
- A local anesthetic is administered.
- The needle is inserted through the posterior chest wall at the selected intercostal space, and into the biopsy site.
- The specimen is obtained and the needle removed.
- The tissue is placed in a container with a formaldehyde solution.
- Pressure is exerted on the biopsy site, followed by application of a sterile dressing.
- Gloves are worn throughout the procedure.

Posttest

- Assist the patient into a semi-Fowler's position.
- Monitor the patient's vital signs, breath sounds, and comfort level, and check the dressing for drainage every 15 to 30 minutes until stable.
- Observe for indications of hemothorax or pneumothorax: rapid, shallow respirations, dyspnea, air hunger, chest pain, cough, hemoptysis, and absence of breath sounds over area.
- Observe for signs of infection: elevated temperature, chest pain, yellow sputum, and abnormal breath sounds.
- Administer analgesics as needed.
- Provide emotional support as the patient awaits test results.
- Report abnormal findings to the primary care provider.

P

→ Clinical Alerts

- Possible complications include: bleeding, hemothorax, infection, and pneumothorax.

CONTRAINDICATIONS!

- Patients with bleeding disorders
- Patients unable to cooperate with the examination

Polysomnography (PSG, Sleep Study)

Test Description

Polysomnography (PSG) involves testing of sleep cycles and stages. Normally there are two states of sleep: nonrapid eye movement (NREM) sleep and rapid eye movement (REM) sleep. NREM sleep has 4 stages: drowsiness (Stage 1), light sleep (Stage 2), and deep sleep (Stages 3 and 4). A person with normal sleep usually has four or five 90-minute cycles in which NREM and REM alternate. PSG is performed to evaluate a variety of sleep problems including hypersomnia, excessive daytime sleepiness, narcolepsy, obstructive sleep apnea, and behavior disturbances or movements during sleep. Some medical conditions have been associated with increased risk for sleep-related breathing disorders, such as obesity, hypertension, stroke, and congestive heart failure.

There are two types of PSG. *Overnight polysomnography (oPSG)* is an overnight recording of the patient's sleep. *Multiple sleep latency testing (MSLT)* records multiple naps throughout a day. Numerous recordings are performed during PSG. These include:

- Audio monitoring to measure snoring sound levels
- Video monitoring to record nocturnal behavioral events (periodic limb movement, seizures, sleepwalking)
- Nasal/oral air flow measurement using thermistors to assist in diagnosis of obstructive sleep apnea and upper airway resistance syndrome
- Electrooculography to record the characteristic eye movements of REM sleep
- Electroencephalography to determine awake and sleep stages
- Electromyography to record muscle activity over the chin and anterior tibialis muscle
- Strain gauges placed over the thoracic and abdominal areas to measure respiratory movements
- Pulse oximetry to measure oxygen saturation/desaturation

THE EVIDENCE FOR PRACTICE

The American Sleep Disorders Association guidelines (2005) state:

- PSG is routinely indicated for the diagnosis of sleep related breathing disorders
- PSG is indicated for positive airway pressure (PAP) titration in patients with sleep related breathing disorders patients with neuromuscular disorders and sleep related symptoms
- PSG and a multiple sleep latency test performed on the day after the polysomnographic evaluation are routinely indicated in the evaluation of suspected narcolepsy
- PSG, with additional EEG derivations in an extended bilateral montage, and video recording, is recommended to assist with the diagnosis of paroxysmal arousals or other sleep disruptions that are thought to be seizure related
- PSG is indicated when a diagnosis of periodic limb movement disorder is considered because of complaints by the patient or an observer of repetitive limb movements during sleep and frequent awakenings, fragmented sleep, difficulty maintaining sleep, or excessive daytime sleepiness.

Normal Values

Usual or normal patterns of brain waves and muscle movements during sleep.
Pulse oximetry ≥90%
Oxygen desaturation episodes: <5/hour

Possible Meanings of Abnormal Values

Circadian rhythm disorders
Disorders of arousal
Disorders of sleep-wake transition
Idiopathic hypersomnia
Inadequate sleep hygiene
Narcolepsy
Nightmares
REM behavior disorder
Restless legs syndrome and periodic limb movement disorder
Sleep apnea
Sleep-related asthma
Sleep-related epilepsy
Upper airway resistance syndrome

Contributing Factors to Abnormal Values

- Use of alcohol, stimulants, and hypnotics may affect PSG results.
- Unfamiliar setting and numerous monitoring devices attached to the patient may interfere with sleep cycle.

Interventions/Implications

Pretest

- Explain to the patient the purpose of the test. Provide any written teaching materials available on the subject. Inform the patient that the test is usually done at night so as to reproduce normal sleep patterns.
- To prepare for the test, the patient should maintain a regular sleep-wake rhythm, avoid sleeping pills and alcohol, avoid stimulants (including medications for narcolepsy), and avoid strenuous exercise on the day of testing.
- No fasting is required before the test.

Procedure

- The patient rests comfortably on a bed in the test center.
- Electrodes are placed on the chin, the scalp, and the outer edge of the eyelids.
- Monitors to record heart rhythm and respirations are attached to the chest.
- Characteristic patterns from the electrodes are recorded while the patient is awake with eyes closed and during sleep.
- The time taken to fall asleep is measured as well as the time to enter REM sleep.
- Movements during sleep are recorded by video camera.

Posttest

- All monitoring devices are removed.
- Normal activities are resumed.
- Report abnormal findings to the primary care provider.

> **Clinical Alerts**

- Patient evaluation prior to PSG should include a thorough sleep history and physical examination, including the respiratory, cardiovascular, and neurologic systems.
  - Involve patient's sleep partner, if possible, when collecting sleep history.
  - Assess for occurrence of snoring, sleep apnea, nocturnal choking or gasping, restlessness, excessive daytime sleepiness, and leg movement.

Porphyrins (Coproporphyrin, Porphobilinogen [PBG], Uroporphyrin, Urinary Porphyrins)

Test Description

Several substances known as "porphyrins," including porphobilinogen (PBG), uroporphyrin, and coproporphyrin, are involved in the synthesis of heme of hemoglobin. Each of these steps requires the presence of a specific *enzyme*. If any of the enzymes are deficient (because of a genetic disease or interference by a toxic substance), the intermediate substances build up, and a type of porphyria results. With a disturbance of the heme synthesis pathway, as in the case of porphyria, large amounts of porphyrins are excreted. Since porphyrins are considered urine pigments, their presence causes the urine to be amber to burgundy in color.

Normal Values

Qualitative random sample
    coproporphyrins: 3–20 µg/dL
    porphobilinogen: Negative
    uroporphyrins: Negative
Quantitative 24 hour test
    coproporphyrins: 50–160 mg/24 hours or 0.075–0.24 µmol/24 hours (SI units)
    porphobilinogen: 0–1.5 mg/24 hours or 0–4.4 µmol/24 hours (SI units)
    uroporphyrins: Up to 50 mg/24 hours or up to 0.06 µmol/24 hours (SI units)

Possible Meanings of Abnormal Values

Increased

Cirrhosis of the liver
Infectious mononucleosis
Lead poisoning
Porphyrias
Viral hepatitis

Contributing Factors to Abnormal Values

- Pregnancy and menstruation may alter test results.
- Drugs which *increase* the porphyrin levels are: antibiotics (penicillin, tetracyclines), antiseptics (phenazopyridin), barbiturates, hypnotics, phenothiazines, procaine, sulfonamides.

Interventions/Implications

Pretest
- Explain 24-hour urine collection procedure to the patient.
- Stress the importance of saving *all* urine in the 24-hour period. Instruct the patient to avoid contaminating the urine with toilet paper or feces.
- Inform the patient of the presence of a preservative in the collection bottle.

Procedure

For qualitative (screening) tests
- Collect a random sample of at least 30 mL of urine during or immediately after an acute attack of porphyria, which is characterized by acute abdominal pain and neurologic changes.
- Protect the specimen from light and transport to the laboratory.

For quantitative (24 hour) tests
- Obtain the proper container containing the appropriate preservative from the laboratory.
- Begin the testing period in the morning after the patient's first voiding, which is discarded.
- Timing of the 24-hour period begins at the time the first voiding is discarded.
- *All* urine for the next 24 hours is collected in the container, which is to be kept refrigerated or on ice.
- If any urine is accidentally discarded during the 24-hour period, the test must be discontinued and a new test begun.
- The ending time of the 24-hour collection period should be posted in the patient's room.
- Gloves are worn whenever dealing with the specimen collection.

Posttest
- At the end of the 24-hour collection period, label and send the urine container on ice to the laboratory as soon as possible.
- Report abnormal findings to the primary care provider.

P

Positron Emission Tomography
(PET, Single Photon Emission Computed Tomography [SPECT])

Test Description

Positron emission tomography (PET) is a noninvasive radiographic method for studying blood flow and metabolic changes occurring in specific organs or regions of body tissues. Clinical applications of PET are in the areas of oncology (tumor staging, detection of recurrent tumors, or metastases), cardiology (determination of tissue viability after myocardial infarction, prediction of therapeutic success of bypass and angioplasty), and neurology (diagnosis of movement disorders, detection of seizure foci, investigation of dementia). Cancers for which PET is used for diagnosis and staging include: lung cancer, colorectal cancer, head and neck cancer, esophageal cancer, melanoma, and lymphoma. Brain tumors, musculoskeletal tumors, ovarian cancer, pancreatic cancer, and thyroid cancer can also be investigated with PET.

For PET studies, the patient receives an injection of a biochemical substance tagged with a radionuclide. This substance is a compound of complex sugars (called fluorodeoxyglucose or FDG) labeled with a short-lived isotope such as carbon-11, fluorine-18, gallium-68, nitrogen-13, or oxygen-15. As the radionuclide disintegrates, positively charged particles, called *positrons* are emitted. As the positrons are combined with the negatively charged electrons normally found in the tissue cells, they emit gamma rays which can be detected with a scanning device. The PET scanner then translates the emissions into color-coded images.

PET has several advantages. Although computed tomography (CT) and magnetic resonance imaging (MRI) are used to diagnose internal problems, their focus is on structural problems. PET and *SPECT (single photon emission computed tomography)* capture chemical and physiological changes related to metabolism, thus examining functional problems. There is minimal radiation dosage received by the patient from the radionuclide and the radiation of the PET scan itself is less than 25% of that required for a CT scan. A disadvantage of PET is that it is more costly than CT or MRI testing and the number of institutions with PET scanning capabilities is limited at this time. Typically, a diagnostic CT scan should precede PET to provide assistance in matching physiologic change noted with PET to the anatomic site noted with CT.

Normal Values

Normal patterns of tissue metabolism

Possible Meanings of Abnormal Values

Alzheimer's disease
Cerebrovascular accident
Coronary artery disease
Dementia
Epilepsy
Huntington's chorea
Malignant tumors
Metastatic tumors
Migraine headache
Myocardial infarction
Parkinson's disease
Pneumonia
Pulmonary edema
Schizophrenia

Contributing Factors to Abnormal Values

- Movement may blur the PET images.
- Drugs which may influence test results: sedatives, tranquilizers.

Interventions/Implications

Pretest

- Explain to the patient the purpose of the test and the procedure to be followed. Explain to the patient that movement is not allowed during the test. To assist with relaxation and to block any noises which occur during the testing, encourage the patient to listen to an audiotape during the procedure.

- Fasting for an average of 6 hours is required prior to the test. Gum, sugar, and caffeine must be avoided. Water is allowed.
- Instruct patients to refrain from vigorous exercise prior to the exam.
- CT films from previously completed exams need to be available for comparison with PET images.
- Obtain a signed informed consent.
- Preprocedure sedation may be ordered. If used, it cannot be given until 30 minutes post injection of the radioisotope, since it will affect glucose metabolism of the brain.
- The patient is instructed to void prior to the exam.

Procedure
- The patient is assisted to a supine position on the scanning table.
- An IV line is initiated.
- The patient is moved within the PET scanner.
- The radionuclide is administered either via the IV line or by inhalation of radioactive gas.
- Images are taken at various times, depending on the particular tissue being scanned.

Posttest
- Assist the patient to slowly rise from the lying position to avoid postural hypotension.
- Discontinue the IV site and check the site for bleeding.
- If a woman who is lactating *must* have this procedure, she should not breast feed the infant until the radionuclide has been eliminated, possibly for 3 days.
- Although the amount of diagnostic radionuclide excreted in the urine is low, the urine should not be used for any laboratory tests for the time period indicated by the nuclear medicine department.
- Gloves are worn whenever dealing with the urine.
- Encourage fluid intake to enhance elimination of the radionuclide from the body.
- Report abnormal findings to the primary care provider.

P

Clinical Alerts

- Patients who are diabetic should take their medications prior to the exam and eat a very small meal 4 hours prior to the exam.

CONTRAINDICATIONS!

- Patients who weigh >350 pounds
- Pregnant women
  - Caution: A woman in her childbearing years should undergo radiography only during her menses or 12 to 14 days after its onset to avoid any exposure to a fetus.
- Patients who are lactating
- Patients who are unable to cooperate due to age, mental status, pain, or other factors

Potassium, Blood

Test Description

Potassium (K^+) is the major cation in the intracellular fluid. It is also present in small amounts in the extracellular fluid. There is an inverse relationship between potassium and sodium. Potassium is responsible for maintenance of acid-base balance, regulation of cellular osmotic pressure, and electrical conduction in muscle cells, especially cardiac and skeletal muscles. Serum potassium levels are most often used in evaluating patients with cardiac dysrhythmias, renal dysfunction, mental confusion, and GI distress.

Patients with elevated serum potassium levels (*hyperkalemia*) have weakness, malaise, nausea, diarrhea, muscle irritability, oliguria, and bradycardia. *Hypokalemic* patients, those patients whose serum potassium level is below normal, experience mental confusion, anorexia, muscle weakness, paresthesias, hypotension, rapid weak pulse, and decreased reflexes.

It is important to note that hypokalemia enhances the effect of digitalis preparations, making the patient prone to digitalis toxicity. Many patients receive both digitalis and a diuretic which causes loss of potassium. The resultant hypokalemia can lead to potentially fatal cardiac dysrhythmias. Patients with hyperkalemia *or* hypokalemia may experience cardiac dysrhythmias.

Normal Values

3.5–5.0 mEq/L (3.5–5.0 mmol/L SI units)

P

Possible Meanings of Abnormal Values

Increased (Hyperkalemia)	Decreased (Hypokalemia)
Acidosis	Alkalosis
Acute renal failure	Chronic fever
Addison's disease	Chronic stress
Diabetes mellitus	Cushing's syndrome
Excessive potassium intake	Cystic fibrosis
Hypoaldosteronism	Diarrhea
Nephritis	Extensive burns
Sickle cell anemia	Hyperaldosteronism
Systemic lupus erythematosus	Hypothermia
Tissue necrosis	Liver disease
	Malabsorption
	Neoplasms
	Pyloric obstruction
	Renal tubular acidosis
	Salicylate intoxication
	Saline IV infusions
	Starvation
	Vomiting

Contributing Factors to Abnormal Values

- Use of a tourniquet during acquisition of the blood sample may alter test results. Use of a tourniquet and pumping of the patient's hand can increase the value by up to 20%.
- Hemolysis of the blood sample may alter test results.
- Drugs which may *increase* serum potassium levels: ACE-inhibitors, ARBs, azathioprine, beta blockers, cyclosporine, digoxin toxicity, epoetin, lithium, NSAIDs, potassium bicarbonate, potassium salts/supplements, spironolactone.
- Drugs which may *decrease* serum potassium levels: amphotericin, beta$_2$ agonists, beta blockers, cidofovir, cisplatin, corticosteroids, digoxin immune Fab, diuretics, fluconazole, foscarnet, insulin, itraconazole, licorice, lithium, theophylline, vitamin B$_{12}$.

Interventions/Implications

Pretest
- Explain to the patient the purpose of the test and the need for a blood sample to be drawn.
- No fasting is required before the test.

Procedure
- A 7-mL blood sample is drawn in a red-top collection tube, avoiding the use of a tourniquet, if possible.
- Gloves are worn throughout the procedure.

Posttest
- Apply pressure at venipuncture site. Apply dressing, periodically assessing for continued bleeding.
- Label the specimen and transport it to the laboratory.
- Report abnormal findings to the primary care provider.

P

→ Clinical Alerts

- Patients with low potassium levels should be informed of dietary sources of potassium: apricots, bananas, meats, potatoes, prunes, and tomatoes.
- Should IV replacement therapy of potassium be deemed necessary, the solution should be administered via an electronic infusion device.

Potassium, Urine

Test Description
Potassium is the major cation in the intracellular fluid. It is also present in small amounts in the extracellular fluid. There is an inverse relationship between potassium and sodium. Potassium is responsible for maintenance of acid-base balance, regulation of cellular osmotic pressure, and electrical conduction in muscle cells,

especially cardiac and skeletal muscles. Measurement of the amount of potassium excreted in the urine in a 24-hour period provides data regarding the electrolyte balance of the body. This knowledge aids in the diagnosis of adrenal and renal disorders.

Normal Values

25–123 mEq/24 hours (25–123 mmol/day SI units)

Possible Meanings of Abnormal Values

Increased	Decreased
Alkalosis	Acute renal failure
Chronic renal failure	Adrenal cortical insufficiency
Cushing's disease	Diarrhea
Dehydration	Excessive aldosterone activity
Diabetic ketoacidosis	Hyperkalemia
Excessive potassium intake	Malabsorption
Fever	Nephrotic syndrome
Hyperaldosteronism	Syndrome of inappropriate ADH
Hypokalemia	secretion (SIADH)
Renal tubular acidosis	
Salicylate intoxication	
Starvation	

Contributing Factors to Abnormal Values

- Drugs which may *increase* urinary potassium levels: acetazolamide, ammonium chloride, glucocorticoids, loop diuretics, mercurial diuretics, potassium, salicylates, thiazide diuretics.
- Drugs which may *decrease* urinary potassium levels: laxatives, licorice (contains a mineralocorticoid compound).

Interventions/Implications

Pretest
- Explain 24-hour urine collection procedure to the patient.
- Stress the importance of saving *all* urine in the 24-hour period. Instruct the patient to avoid contaminating the urine with toilet paper or feces.
- Inform the patient of the presence of a preservative in the collection bottle.

Procedure
- Obtain the proper container containing no preservative from the laboratory.
- Begin the testing period in the morning after the patient's first voiding, which is discarded.
- Timing of the 24-hour period begins at the time the first voiding is discarded.
- *All* urine for the next 24 hours is collected in the container, which is to be kept refrigerated or on ice.
- If any urine is accidentally discarded during the 24-hour period, the test must be discontinued and a new test begun.
- The ending time of the 24-hour collection period should be posted in the patient's room.
- Gloves are worn whenever dealing with the specimen collection.

Posttest
- At the end of the 24-hour collection period, label and send the urine container on ice to the laboratory as soon as possible.
- Report abnormal findings to the primary care provider.

 Prealbumin (PAB)

Test Description

Prealbumin is a plasma protein synthesized by the liver. It is considered the best marker for malnutrition. It has a half-life of 2 days, so prealbumin levels change very quickly and reflect the person's current nutritional status.

The test is most often used to help in diagnosis of protein-calorie malnutrition. It is important to assess prealbumin levels in chronically ill patients, in high-risk hospitalized patients, and prior to many surgical procedures. Finding and correcting nutritional deficits can prevent complications and improve patient outcomes. The test is also used to monitor the progress of patients who are receiving nutritional support such as parenteral nutrition.

Normal Values

16–35 mg/dL (160–350 g/L SI units)

Possible Meanings of Abnormal Values

Increased	Decreased
Corticosteroid use	Cancer
Hodgkin's disease	Chronic illness
Hypercortisolism	Hyperthyroidism
NSAID use (high-dose)	Infection
	Inflammation
	Liver disease
	Malnutrition

Contributing Factors to Abnormal Values

- Drugs that may *decrease* prealbumin levels: amiodarone, estrogens, oral contraceptives.
- Drugs that may *increase* prealbumin levels: anabolic steroids, androgens, carbamazepine, danazol, phenobarbital, prednisolone, progestins.
- Inflammation may cause prealbumin to be decreased.
- Renal failure may cause prealbumin to be *falsely increased.*

Interventions/Implications

Pretest
- Explain to the patient the purpose of the test and the need for a blood sample to be drawn.
- No fasting is required before the test.

Procedure
- A 7-mL blood sample is drawn in a red-top collection tube.
- Gloves are worn throughout the procedure.

Posttest
- Apply pressure at venipuncture site. Apply dressing, periodically assessing for continued bleeding.
- Label the specimen and transport it to the laboratory.
- Report abnormal findings to the primary care provider.

Clinical Alerts

- Patients with low prealbumin levels are likely to have decreased levels of other proteins in the body.
- Patients with low prealbumin levels need nutritional counseling and correction of the nutritional deficit.

Pregnancy Test, Serum
(Human Chorionic Gonadotropin [HCG])

Test Description

Human chorionic gonadotropin (HCG) is a hormone secreted exclusively by the placenta; thus, its measurement is useful in determining pregnancy. HCG is produced, and thus can be detected in the blood, 8 to 10 days after conception. This time period correlates with the implantation of the fertilized ovum into the uterine wall. The HCG level increases until it peaks at the twelfth week of gestation. It then decreases slowly during the remainder of the pregnancy. The hormone is no longer detectable approximately 2 weeks after delivery.

The test is performed by mixing the patient's serum with anti-HCG. If HCG is present in the patient's serum, it combines with and inactivates the anti-HCG antibodies. When indicator cells coated with HCG are then added, the cells do not clump since the anti-HCG antibodies have been inactivated. This indicates a positive pregnancy test. If clumping does occur, this means that anti-HCG antibodies have not been inactivated by HCG. Thus, the test is negative.

Elevated HCG levels can be found with various types of cancer, including lung, liver, ovarian, pancreatic, and testicular.

Normal Values

Qualitative (serum pregnancy): Negative
Quantitative:
  Males/Nonpregnant females: <5.0 IU/L (<5.0 mIU/mL SI units)
  Pregnancy (Weeks of gestation):
    Weeks 1–3   5–50 mIU/mL
    Week 4   5–425 mIU/mL

Week 5	20–7400 mIU/mL
Week 6	1000–56,000 mIU/mL
Weeks 7–8	7600–230,000 mIU/mL
Weeks 9–12	25,000–290,000 mIU/mL
Weeks 13–16	13,000–254,000 mIU/mL
Weeks 17–24	4000–166,000 mIU/mL
Weeks 24+	3400–117,000 mIU/mL

Possible Meanings of Abnormal Values

Increased	Decreased
Breast cancer	Abortion
Bronchogenic carcinoma	Ectopic pregnancy
Choriocarcinoma	Threatened abortion
Embryonal carcinoma	
Hydatidiform mole	
Liver cancer	
Malignant melanoma	
Multiple myeloma	
Ovarian tumors	
Pancreatic cancer	
Pregnancy	
Testicular cancer	

Contributing Factors to Abnormal Values

- Drugs which may cause *false-positive* results: anticonvulsants, antiparkinsonian agents, hypnotics, and tranquilizers (phenothiazines).
- *False-negative* results may occur if the test is performed too early in the pregnancy. It should be perform no earlier than 5 days after the first missed menstrual period.

P

Interventions/Implications

Pretest
- Explain to the patient the purpose of the test and the need for a blood sample to be drawn.
- No fasting is required before the test.

Procedure
- A 7-mL blood sample is drawn in a red-top collection tube.
- Gloves are worn throughout the procedure.

Posttest
- Apply pressure at venipuncture site. Apply dressing, periodically assessing for continued bleeding.
- Label the specimen and transport it to the laboratory.
- Report abnormal findings to the primary care provider.

Clinical Alerts

- A pregnancy test is considered to be about 98% accurate. When the test is negative but pregnancy is still suspected, the test should be repeated in 1 week.

Pregnancy Test, Urine
(Human Chorionic Gonadotropin [HCG])

Test Description
Human chorionic gonadotropin (HCG) is a hormone secreted exclusively by the placenta; thus its measurement is useful in determining pregnancy. HCG is produced, with levels in the blood rising as the pregnancy advances. A significant amount of HCG, in the form of alpha and beta subunits, is also excreted in the urine. The beta subunit is the most sensitive indicator of early pregnancy. A urine pregnancy test is usually positive within 5 to 7 days of conception.

Normal Values
Positive: Pregnancy
Negative: Nonpregnant

Possible Meanings of Abnormal Values

Increased	Decreased
Choriocarcinoma	Abortion
Ectopic pregnancy	Fetal demise
Embryonal carcinoma	Threatened abortion
Hydatidiform mole	
Pregnancy	
Testicular cancer	

Contributing Factors to Abnormal Values
- Drugs which may cause *false-positive* results: anticonvulsants, antiparkinsonian agents, hypnotics, and tranquilizers (phenothiazines).
- Presence of hematuria or proteinuria may cause *false-negative* results.
- *False-negative* results may occur if the test is performed too early in the pregnancy. It should be perform no earlier than 5 days after the first missed menstrual period.

Interventions/Implications
Pretest
- Explain to the patient the purpose of the test and the need for a urine sample to be collected.
- No fasting is required before the test.

Procedure
- An early-morning (first AM void) specimen is best, but a random urine can also be used.
- Gloves are worn when handling the specimen.

Posttest
- Label the specimen and transport it to the laboratory.
- Report abnormal findings to the primary care provider.

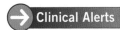

Clinical Alerts

- A pregnancy test is considered to be about 98% accurate. When the test is negative but pregnancy is still suspected, the test should be repeated in 1 week.

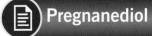

Pregnanediol

Test Description

Progesterone is a steroid sex hormone secreted by the corpus luteum, by the placenta during pregnancy, and by the adrenal cortex. The primary metabolite of progesterone is *pregnanediol*. This test is used to evaluate placental and ovarian function. Excretion of pregnanediol is typically high in pregnancy and low in luteal deficiency or placental insufficiency.

Normal Values

Male:	0–1.9 mg/24 hours (0–5.9 µmol/day SI units)
Female:	
Follicular phase:	0–2.6 mg/24 hours (0–8.1 µmol/day SI units)
Luteal phase:	2.6–10.6 mg/24 hours (8.1–33.1 µmol/day SI units)
Pregnancy:	
1st trimester:	10–35 mg/24 hours (31–109 µmol/day SI units)
2nd trimester:	35–70 mg/24 hours (109–218 µmol/day SI units)
3rd trimester:	70–100 mg/24 hours (218–312 µmol/day SI units)

P

Possible Meanings of Abnormal Values

Increased	Decreased
Adrenal hyperplasia	Amenorrhea
Biliary tract obstruction	Anovulation
Metastatic ovarian cancer	Breast neoplasms
Ovarian cyst	Fetal death
Ovulation	Hydatidiform mole
Pregnancy	Ovarian neoplasms
	Placental insufficiency
	Preeclampsia
	Threatened abortion
	Toxemia of pregnancy

Contributing Factors to Abnormal Values

- Drugs which may *increase* pregnanediol levels: corticotropin, methenamine mandelate.
- Drugs which may *decrease* pregnanediol levels: oral contraceptives, progesterones

Interventions/Implications

Pretest
- Explain 24-hour urine collection procedure to the patient.

- Stress the importance of saving *all* urine in the 24-hour period. Instruct the patient to avoid contaminating the urine with toilet paper or feces.
- Inform the patient of the presence of a preservative in the collection bottle.

Procedure
- Obtain the proper container containing 1 g of boric acid as preservative from the laboratory.
- Begin the testing period in the morning after the patient's first voiding, which is discarded.
- Timing of the 24-hour period begins at the time the first voiding is discarded.
- *All* urine for the next 24 hours is collected in the container, which is to be kept refrigerated or on ice.
- If any urine is accidentally discarded during the 24-hour period, the test must be discontinued and a new test begun.
- The ending time of the 24-hour collection period should be posted in the patient's room.
- Gloves are worn whenever dealing with the specimen collection.

Posttest
- At the end of the 24-hour collection period, label and send the urine container on ice to the laboratory as soon as possible.
- For female patients: On the laboratory slip, include the date on which the patient began her last menstrual period or, if pregnant, the approximate week of gestation
- Report abnormal findings to the primary care provider.

Pregnanetriol

P

Test Description

Pregnanetriol is involved in the synthesis of adrenal corticoids. It is a metabolite of 17-hydroxyprogesterone and is normally excreted in the urine in very small amounts. In adrenogenital syndrome, cortisol synthesis is blocked at the point at which 17-hydroxyprogesterone converts to cortisol. This results in a build up of 17-hydroxyprogesterone and increased amounts of its metabolite, pregnanetriol, are excreted in the urine.

The reduced plasma cortisol levels stimulate the secretion of ACTH, which normally leads to increased cortisol levels. However, since cortisol synthesis is impaired, pregnanetriol levels continue to rise instead. High levels of 17-hydroxyprogesterone and ACTH lead to virilization in females and sexual precocity in young males.

Normal Values

Adult:	0.1–1.6 mg/24 hours (0.3–4.8 µmol/day SI units)
Child:	0.3–1.1 mg/24 hours (0.9–3.3 µmol/day SI units)

Possible Meanings of Abnormal Values

Increased

Adrenocortical tumor
Adrenogenital syndrome

Congenital adrenocortical hyperplasia
Hirsutism
21-hydroxylase deficiency
Ovarian tumor
Stein-Leventhal syndrome
Virilization

Contributing Factors to Abnormal Values

- Exercise may alter test results

Interventions/Implications

Pretest

- Explain 24-hour urine collection procedure to the patient.
- Stress the importance of saving *all* urine in the 24-hour period. Instruct the patient to avoid contaminating the urine with toilet paper or feces.
- Inform the patient of the presence of a preservative in the collection bottle.
- Encourage the patient to avoid excessive physical activity during the testing period.

Procedure

- Obtain the proper container containing 1 g of boric acid as preservative from the laboratory.
- Begin the testing period in the morning after the patient's first voiding, which is discarded.
- Timing of the 24-hour period begins at the time the first voiding is discarded.
- *All* urine for the next 24 hours is collected in the container, which is to be kept refrigerated or on ice.
- If any urine is accidentally discarded during the 24-hour period, the test must be discontinued and a new test begun.
- The ending time of the 24-hour collection period should be posted in the patient's room.
- Gloves are worn whenever dealing with the specimen collection.

Posttest

- At the end of the 24-hour collection period, label and send the urine container on ice to the laboratory as soon as possible.
- Report abnormal findings to the primary care provider.

P

Proctosigmoidoscopy
(Anoscopy, Proctoscopy, Flexible Sigmoidoscopy)

Test Description

Proctosigmoidoscopy is the direct visualization of the distal sigmoid colon, the rectum, and the anus through the use of a flexible fiberoptic endoscope. This endoscope is a multilumen instrument which allows viewing of the organ linings, insufflation of air, aspiration of fluid, removal of foreign objects, obtaining of tissue biopsies, and passage of a laser beam for obliteration of abnormal tissue or control of bleeding. This procedure is performed when the patient has experienced lower abdominal pain, a change in bowel habits, or passage of blood, mucus, or pus in the stool.

THE EVIDENCE FOR PRACTICE

The U.S. Preventive Services Task Force (USPSTF) found good evidence that periodic fecal occult blood testing reduces mortality from colorectal cancer and fair evidence that sigmoidoscopy alone or in combination with fecal occult blood testing (FOBT) reduces mortality.

Normal Values

Normal sigmoid colon, rectum, and anus

Possible Meanings of Abnormal Values

Anal fissures
Anal fistula
Anorectal abscesses
Benign lesions
Crohn's disease
Hemorrhoids
Hypertrophic anal papilla
Irritable bowel syndrome
Polyps
Pseudomembranous colitis
Tumors
Ulcerative colitis

Contributing Factors to Abnormal Values

- Retention of barium following previous tests, active gastrointestinal bleeding, or inadequate colon preparation hinders successful completion of this test.

P

Interventions/Implications

Pretest

- Explain to the patient the purpose of the test. Provide any written teaching materials available on the subject. Inform the patient that pressure may be experienced during movement of the endoscope and during insufflation with air or carbon dioxide.
- Obtain a signed informed consent.
- The colon is prepared for the examination as follows:
  - clear liquid diet for 2 days prior to the test
  - an enema the morning of the test
- No fasting is required prior to the test.
- Resuscitation and suctioning equipment should be readily available.

Procedure

- The patient is assisted into the left lateral decubitus or knee-chest position on the endoscopy table.
- The physician inserts a well-lubricated index finger into the anus and rectum to palpate for tenderness. The finger is withdrawn and checked for the presence of blood, mucus, or stool.
- The sigmoidoscope is inserted into the anus and advanced into the distal sigmoid colon.
- During the procedure, insufflation of the bowel with air is used for better visualization.
- The sigmoid colon, rectum, and anus are visualized.

- Encourage the patient to take slow, deep breaths to induce relaxation and to minimize the urge to defecate.
- Biopsy forceps may be used to remove a tissue specimen, or a cytology brush may be used to obtain cells from the surface of a lesion. Removal of foreign bodies or polyps is accomplished, if needed.
- Videotaping of the procedure is often done via a camera attached to the endoscope.
- Gloves are worn throughout the procedure.

Posttest
- Monitor vital signs every 15 minutes until stable.
- Observe the patient for indications of bowel perforation: rectal bleeding, abdominal pain and distention, and fever.
- Inform the patient that passage of a large amount of flatus is normal after this procedure.
- Report abnormal findings to the primary care provider.

→ Clinical Alerts

- Possible complications include: Bleeding and perforation of the bowel.
- Diagnostic tests involving barium should be scheduled after the proctosigmoidoscopy is done.
- Double-contrast barium enema exam is often done in conjunction with proctosigmoidoscopy.

CONTRAINDICATIONS!

- Patients with acute diverticulitis
- Patients with suspected perforation of the colon
- Patients who are medically unstable
- Patients unable to cooperate with the exam

P

Progesterone

Test Description
Progesterone is a steroid sex hormone secreted via three sources:
- by the corpus luteum, which causes thickening of the endometrium in preparation for implantation of a fertilized egg
- by the placenta during pregnancy, which causes continued thickening of the endometrium for provision of nutrients for the developing fetus and decreased myometrial excitability and uterine contractions, and also prepares the breasts for lactation
- by the adrenal cortex in men

In females, progesterone converts proliferative endometrium to secretory endometrium and maintains pregnancy. In men, progesterone has no normal function except as an intermediate step in the synthesis of other steroid hormones. Measurement of progesterone levels is useful in studies of the corpus luteum and placental function, and for assessing ovulation.

Normal Values

Female:

Follicular phase:	0–1.5 ng/mL (0–4.7 nmol/L SI units)
Luteal phase:	2–30 ng/mL (6.3–94.5 nmol/L SI units)
Postmenopausal:	0–1.5 ng/mL (0–4.7 nmol/L SI units)
Pregnancy:	Peaks in third trimester as high as 200 ng/mL (630 nmol/L SI units)
Male:	0–1.0 ng/mL (0–3.2 nmol/L SI units)

Possible Meanings of Abnormal Values

Increased	Decreased
Adrenal hyperplasia	Adrenogenital syndrome
Adrenal neoplasms	Amenorrhea
Chorionepithelioma of ovary	Anovular menstruation
Corpus luteum cyst	Fetal death
Molar pregnancy	Menopause
Ovarian neoplasms	Menstrual disorders
Precocious puberty	Ovarian failure
Pregnancy	Placental insufficiency
Retained placental tissue	Preeclampsia
	Stein-Leventhal syndrome
	Threatened abortion
	Toxemia of pregnancy
	Turner's syndrome

Contributing Factors to Abnormal Values

- Hemolysis of the blood sample or having a radioactive scan within 1 week of the test may alter test results.
- Drugs which may *increase* progesterone levels: adrenocortical hormones, clomiphene, estrogens, ketoconazole, progesterones, tamoxifen.
- Drugs which may *decrease* progesterone levels: ampicillin, anticonvulsants, danazol, goserelin, leuprolide, oral contraceptives.

Interventions/Implications

Pretest
- Explain to the patient the purpose of the test and the need for a blood sample to be drawn.
- No fasting is required before the test.

Procedure
- A 7-mL blood sample is drawn in a red-top collection tube.
- Gloves are worn throughout the procedure.

Posttest
- Apply pressure at venipuncture site. Apply dressing, periodically assessing for continued bleeding.
- Label the specimen and transport it to the laboratory.
- On the laboratory slip, include the date on which the patient began her last menstrual period or, if pregnant, the trimester of the pregnancy.
- Report abnormal findings to the primary care provider.

Prolactin Level (PRL, Human Prolactin [HPRL], Lactogen, Lactogenic Hormone)

Test Description
Like growth hormone, prolactin (PRL) is secreted by the anterior pituitary gland. This hormone is responsible for growth of breast tissue and the promotion and maintenance of lactation. Determination of prolactin levels is used along with other tests, to:
- determine the cause of galactorrhea and amenorrhea
- determine the cause of headaches and visual disturbances
- diagnose infertility and erectile dysfunction in males
- diagnose infertility in females
- diagnose prolactinomas
- evaluate anterior pituitary function (along with other hormones)
- monitor treatment of prolactinomas and detect recurrences

Normal Values
Adult:	<20 ng/mL (<20 µg/L SI units)
Pregnancy:	10–300 ng/mL (10–300 µg/L SI units)

P

Possible Meanings of Abnormal Values

Increased	Decreased
Acromegaly	Gynecomastia
Addison's disease	Hirsutism
Amenorrhea	Hypogonadism
Anorexia nervosa	Osteoporosis
Breast stimulation	Pituitary infarction
Chronic renal failure	Pituitary necrosis
Cushing's syndrome	
Ectopic tumors	
Endometriosis	
Exercise	
Galactorrhea	
Hyperpituitarism	
Hypothalamic disorders	
Hypothyroidism	
Hysterectomy	
Lactation	
Pituitary tumors	

Polycystic ovary disease
Pregnancy
Sleep
Stress

Contributing Factors to Abnormal Values

- Prolactin levels are temporarily increased following exercise, stress, or a recent breast examination.
- Diagnostic tests using radioactive materials, recent surgery, or hemolysis of the blood sample may alter test results.
- Drugs which may *increase* prolactin levels: antipsychotics, cimetidine, clomipramine, cocaine, danazol, enalapril, furosemide, insulin, labetelol, megestrol, methyldopa, metoclopramide, morphine, oral contraceptives, phenytoin, risperidone, tricyclic antidepressants, verapamil.
- Drugs which may *decrease* prolactin levels: anticonvulsants, bromocriptine, calcitonin, cyclosporine, dexamethasone, estrogens, finasteride, levodopa, metoclopramide, morphine, nifedipine, octreotide, phenytoin, tamoxifen.

Interventions/Implications

Pretest

- Explain to the patient the purpose of the test and the need for a blood sample to be drawn.
- No fasting is required before the test.
- The patient should rest 30 minutes prior to the test.
- The sample should be drawn in the morning.

Procedure

- A 7-mL blood sample is drawn in a red-top collection tube.
- Gloves are worn throughout the procedure.

Posttest

- Apply pressure at venipuncture site. Apply dressing, periodically assessing for continued bleeding.
- Label the specimen and transport it to the laboratory.
- Report abnormal findings to the primary care provider.

Prostate Sonogram
(Prostate Ultrasound, Transrectal Sonogram)

Test Description

Ultrasonography is a noninvasive method of diagnostic testing in which ultrasound waves are sent into the body with a small transducer pressed against the skin. The transducer then receives any returning sound waves, which are deflected back as they bounce off various structures. The transducer converts the returning sound waves into electric signals that are then transformed by a computer into a visual display on a monitor.

The prostate sonogram is used in the early diagnosis of cancer of the prostate gland. It is used as an adjunct to digital examination of the prostate and to tests such as the prostate-specific antigen (PSA) test. The sonogram demonstrates the size and shape of the prostate gland and is thus helpful in monitoring patient response to therapy for prostate disease. It also provides guidance for prostate biopsy.

Normal Values

Normal size, shape, and consistency of the prostate gland

Possible Meanings of Abnormal Values

Benign prostatic hypertrophy
Perirectal abscess
Perirectal tumor
Prostate abscess
Prostate cancer
Prostatitis
Rectal tumor
Seminal vesicle tumor

Contributing Factors to Abnormal Values

- The transducer must be in good contact with the skin as it is being moved. A water-based gel is used to ensure good contact with the skin.
- Retained barium from previous tests or stool within the rectum will hinder accurate test results.

Interventions/Implications

Pretest
- Explain to the patient the purpose of the test. Provide any written teaching materials available on the subject. Note that rectal pressure will be felt during the test. Some discomfort may be experienced if a prostate biopsy is done.
- No fasting is required before the test.
- Some institutions may require a signed informed consent form to be completed, especially if prostate biopsy is to be done.
- For transrectal sonography, a small enema is administered 1 hour before the test.

Procedure
- The patient is assisted to a supine position on the ultrasonography table.
- A transabdominal sonogram and a suprapubic examination of the prostate are performed.
- The patient is then assisted to a knee-elbow or lateral decubitus position.
- The transducer is covered with a transparent cover, lubricated, and inserted into the rectum.
- The transducer is angled toward the prostate to provide good visualization of the gland.
- The sound waves are transformed into a visual display on the monitor. Printed copies of this display are made.
- Gloves are worn throughout the procedure.

Posttest
- Cleanse the patient's skin of any lubricant.
- Report abnormal findings to the primary care provider.

Clinical Alerts

- If a suspicious lesion is identified during the ultrasound or had previously been palpated during a digital rectal examination, or if the PSA (prostate specific antigen) testing was abnormal, a biopsy of the prostate may be done along with the prostate ultrasound. The ultrasound guides positioning of the needle for the biopsy to be done.

Prostate-Specific Antigen (PSA, Total PSA)

Test Description
Prostate-specific antigen (PSA) is a glycoprotein found only in the prostate epithelium. PSA is considered a reliable tumor marker for prostate cancer. Measurement of the PSA level is performed to screen patients for the presence of prostate cancer, to monitor the progression of the disease, and to monitor the response of the patient to treatment for prostate cancer.

Older men and African-American men typically have slightly higher normal PSA measurements. However, a PSA of 4 ng/mL and above is considered abnormally high and warrants further investigation. It is also important to note an upward trend in the PSA level. Even if the value is within the normal range, an increase of at least 0.75 ng/mL per year (high PSA velocity change) is considered abnormal and should be investigated. Additional diagnostic testing includes digital rectal examination, prostate sonogram, and possibly prostate biopsy.

Many national organizations do not recommend routine PSA testing. However, the American Urologic Association, the American Cancer Society, and the National Comprehensive Cancer Network suggest that all men have annual PSA tests beginning at age 50, and for high risk men, beginning at age 40 to 45. The test does have a high false positive rate, which may lead to unnecessary follow-up testing. Thus, patients must weigh the risk-benefit of the test in determining whether to have routine PSA testing.

THE EVIDENCE FOR PRACTICE
Recommendations from the American Cancer Society Workshop on Early Prostate Cancer Detection (2001) state:

The prostate-specific antigen (PSA) test and the digital rectal examination (DRE) should be offered annually beginning at age 50 to men who have a life expectancy of at least 10 years. Men at high risk (men of African descent [specifically, sub-Saharan African descent] and men with a first-degree relative diagnosed at a young age) should begin testing at age 45.

Information should be provided to patients about benefits and limitations of testing. Specifically, prior to testing, men should have an opportunity to learn about the benefits and limitations of testing for early prostate cancer detection and treatment.

Men who ask the clinician to make the testing decision on their behalf should be tested. A clinical policy of not offering testing, or discouraging testing in men who request early prostate cancer detection tests, is inappropriate.

Normal Values

Normal: <4 ng/mL (<4 µg/L SI units)

Possible Meanings of Abnormal Values

Increased

Benign prostatic hypertrophy
Cirrhosis
Impotence
Posturologic procedures
Prostate cancer
Prostate inflammation, trauma, or manipulation
Prostatitis
Recent sexual activity
Urinary retention
Urinary tract infection

Contributing Factors to Abnormal Values

- Falsely elevated PSA values occur following palpation of the prostate or any manipulation such as through cystoscopy, transrectal ultrasound, or prostatic biopsy.
- PSA values may be affected after recent urinary tract infection or bladder catheterization.
- Drug which may *increase* PSA level: allopurinol.
- Drug which may *decrease* PSA level: finasteride.

P

Interventions/Implications

Pretest
- Explain to the patient the purpose of the test and the need for a blood sample to be drawn.
- No fasting is required before the test.
- The blood sample is collected before palpation of the prostate during rectal examination.

Procedure
- A 7-mL blood sample is drawn in a red-top collection tube.
- Gloves are worn throughout the procedure.

Posttest
- Apply pressure at venipuncture site. Apply dressing, periodically assessing for continued bleeding.
- Label the specimen and transport it to the laboratory.
- Report abnormal findings to the primary care provider.

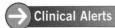

→ Clinical Alerts

- If the total PSA is elevated but the DRE is normal, the **_free PSA test_** may be ordered.
  - This test can help to distinguish between prostate cancer and non-cancer causes of elevated PSA.
  - PSA associated with cancer is more protein bound; free, or non-protein bound PSA increases in the case of benign prostatic hypertrophy.
  - Free PSA >27% has a lower likelihood of prostate cancer.

📄 Protein C (PC)

Test Description

After the process of hemostasis is completed, any excess amounts of clotting factors which remain are inactivated by fibrin inhibitors, such as antiplasmin, antithrombin III, and protein C (PC). This prevents clotting from occurring indiscriminately. PC is a protein produced in the liver and circulating in the plasma. Vitamin K is essential for its production. PC acts as an anticoagulant by inactivating coagulation factors V and VIII. Protein S serves as a cofactor to enhance this anticoagulant effect. Testing for PC is done when evaluating patients with recurrent thrombosis. When the level of protein C is found to be deficient, the patient is at increased risk of vascular thrombosis.

Normal Values

60–150%

Possible Meanings of Abnormal Values

Decreased

Acquired deficiency due to liver disease
Cirrhosis
Disseminated intravascular coagulation
Inherited deficiency
Pregnancy
Vitamin K deficiency

Contributing Factors to Abnormal Values

- Hemolysis of the blood sample and lipemia may alter test results.
- Drugs which may *decrease* protein C levels: antibiotics, asparaginase, estrogens, heparin, warfarin.

Interventions/Implications

Pretest

- Explain to the patient the purpose of the test and the need for a blood sample to be drawn.
- No fasting is required before the test.

Procedure
- A 7-mL blood sample is drawn in a light blue-top collection tube and placed immediately on ice.
- Gloves are worn throughout the procedure.

Posttest
- Apply pressure at venipuncture site. Apply dressing, periodically assessing for continued bleeding.
- Label the specimen and transport it on ice to the laboratory.
- Report abnormal findings to the primary care provider.

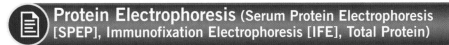

Protein Electrophoresis (Serum Protein Electrophoresis [SPEP], Immunofixation Electrophoresis [IFE], Total Protein)

Test Description

Total protein is composed of albumin and globulins. *Albumin*, which is synthesized in the liver, is essential in maintaining oncotic pressure. It transports various body substances, such as bilirubin, fatty acids, drugs, and hormones, which are bound to albumin while they are circulating in the bloodstream.

There are three primary types of *globulins:* alpha, beta, and gamma globulins. The *alpha globulins* are synthesized in the liver and include alpha$_1$ globulins, such as alpha$_1$ antitrypsin, alpha fetoprotein, and thyroxine-binding globulin, and alpha$_2$ globulins, including haptoglobin, ceruloplasmin, HDL, and alpha$_2$ macroglobulin. *Beta globulins* are also synthesized in the liver, and include transferrin, plasminogen, LDL, and the complement proteins. *Gamma globulins*, which are also called *immunoglobulins*, are produced by B-lymphocytes in response to stimulation by antigens, and include the IgA, IgD, IgE, IgG, and IgM antibodies. These are discussed in detail in the section "Immunoelectrophoresis."

Serum protein electrophoresis (SPEP) is a commonly used method of measuring albumin and each of the globulin types. It is used to identify patients with multiple myeloma and other serum protein disorders, inflammatory conditions, autoimmune disease, infection, or protein-losing conditions. SPEP is also used as a follow-up to other abnormal laboratory results, including total protein, albumin, and urine protein, low calcium levels, and low white and/or red blood cell counts. It can also be used to monitor disease progress and response to treatment.

Electrophoresis separates proteins based on their physical properties. The serum is placed on a special medium and a charge is applied, causing the various proteins to separate according to their electrical charge, molecular size, and shape. Albumin moves farthest away from the current, followed by the alpha globulins, beta globulins, and, finally, the gamma globulins. These groupings are then compared with patterns characteristic of specific disease entities.

A homogeneous spoke in a focal region of the gamma globulin grouping indicates a monoclonal gammopathy. Monoclonal gammopathies are associated with malignant or potentially malignant conditions, including multiple myeloma, Waldenström's macroglobulinemia, leukemia, heavy chain disease, and amyloidosis. Polyclonal gammopathies may be the result of any reactive or inflammatory

P

process. Once a monoclonal gammopathy is identified by SPEP, multiple myeloma must be differentiated from other causes. This can be done through a procedure called *immunofixation electrophoresis* (IFE). In IFE, specific proteins of interest can be identified by first fixing them into the gel with antibodies, then washing away all the other proteins prior to staining. Thus, it enhances the results of SPEP. IFE is usually ordered when SPEP shows the presence of an abnormal protein band that may be an immunoglobulin.

Normal Values

Total protein		6.0–8.0 g/dL (60–80 g/L SI units)
Albumin	58–74%	3.3–5.5 g/dL (33–55 g/L SI units)
Alpha$_1$ globulin	2–3.5%	0.1–0.4 g/dL (1–4 g/L SI units)
Alpha$_2$ globulin	5.4–10.6%	0.5–1.0 g/dL (5–10 g/L SI units)
Beta globulin	7–14%	0.7–1.2 g/dL (7–12 g/L SI units)
Gamma globulin	8–18%	0.8–1.6 g/dL (8–16 g/L SI units)

Possible Meanings of Abnormal Values

Total protein

Increased	Decreased
Macroglobulinemia	Acute cholecystitis
Multiple myeloma	Analbuminemia
Sarcoidosis	Glomerulonephritis
	Hodgkin's disease
	Hypertension
	Hypogammaglobulinemia
	Leukemia
	Nephrosis
	Peptic ulcer disease
	Ulcerative colitis

Albumin

Increased	Decreased
Acute pancreatitis	Acute cholecystitis
Dehydration	Analbuminemia
	Diabetes mellitus
	Gastrointestinal protein loss
	Glomerular protein loss
	Hepatic disease
	Hodgkin's disease
	Hyperthyroidism
	Inflammation
	Leukemia
	Malabsorption
	Malnutrition
	Peptic ulcer disease
	Pregnancy
	Protein-losing syndromes

P

Renal disease
Rheumatoid arthritis
Sarcoidosis
Stress
Systemic lupus erythematosus
Ulcerative colitis

Alpha globulin

Increased	Decreased
Acute infection	Alpha$_1$-antitrypsin deficiency
Acute inflammation	Cirrhosis
Carcinoma	Hemolytic anemia
Chronic glomerulonephritis	Hepatic disease
Cirrhosis	Hepatic metastases
Diabetes mellitus	Hyperthyroidism
Dysproteinemia	Malabsorption
Glomerular protein loss	Pulmonary emphysema
Hepatic damage	Scleroderma
Hodgkin's disease	Starvation
Hypoalbuminemia	Steatorrhea
Inflammatory disease	Viral hepatitis
Myocardial infarction	
Osteomyelitis	
Peptic ulcer disease	
Pregnancy	
Renal disease	
Rheumatoid arthritis	
Sarcoidosis	
Stress	
Systemic lupus erythematosus	
Ulcerative colitis	

Beta globulin

Increased	Decreased
Acute inflammation	Autoimmune disease
Analbuminemia	Hepatic disease
Diabetes mellitus	Leukemia
Dysproteinemia	Lymphoma
Glomerular protein loss	Malabsorption
Hypercholesterolemia	Malnutrition
Iron-deficiency anemia	Metastatic cancer
Multiple myeloma	Nephrosis
Nephrotic syndrome	Scleroderma
Obstructive jaundice	Starvation
Pregnancy	Systemic lupus erythematosus
Rheumatoid arthritis	Ulcerative colitis
Sarcoidosis	
Viral hepatitis	

Gamma globulin

Increased	Decreased
Advanced cancer	Agammaglobulinemia
Chronic hepatitis	Glomerular protein loss

P

Cystic fibrosis	Hypogammaglobulinemia
Hepatic disease	Leukemia
Hodgkin's disease	Lymphoma
Hypersensitivity reaction	Malabsorption
Leukemia	Nephrosis
Monoclonal gammopathy	Nephrotic syndrome
Multiple myeloma	Starvation
Rheumatoid arthritis	Ulcerative colitis
Sarcoidosis	
Severe infection	
Systemic lupus erythematosus	
Viral infections	
Waldenström's macroglobulinemia	

Contributing Factors to Abnormal Values

- Drugs which may alter test results include aspirin, corticosteroids, estrogens, penicillins, phenytoin, procainamide, oral contraceptives, progestins.
- Immunization within the previous 6 months can *increase* immunoglobulins.

Interventions/Implications

Pretest
- Explain to the patient the purpose of the test and the need for a blood sample to be drawn.
- No fasting is required before the test.

Procedure
- A 7-mL blood sample is drawn in a red-top collection tube.
- Gloves are worn throughout the procedure.

Posttest
- Apply pressure at venipuncture site. Apply dressing, periodically assessing for continued bleeding.
- Label the specimen and transport it to the laboratory.
- Report abnormal findings to the primary care provider.

Protein S

Test Description

After the process of hemostasis is completed, any excess amounts of clotting factors which remain are inactivated by fibrin inhibitors, such as antiplasmin, antithrombin III, and protein C. This prevents clotting from occurring indiscriminately. Protein S is a protein produced in the liver and circulating in the plasma. Vitamin K is essential for its production. Protein S serves as a cofactor to enhance the anticoagulant effect of protein C, which inactivates coagulation factors V and VIII. Testing for protein S is done when evaluating patients for hypercoagulability states such as recurrent thrombosis. When the level of protein S is found to be deficient, the patient is at increased risk of vascular thrombosis.

Normal Values

60–150%

Possible Meanings of Abnormal Values

Decreased

Acute consumption (as in disseminated intravascular coagulation)
Familial protein S deficiency
Pregnancy
Renal disease
Vitamin K deficiency

Contributing Factors to Abnormal Values

- Hemolysis of the blood sample may alter test results.
- Drugs that may *decrease* protein S levels: asparaginase, oral contraceptives, warfarin.

Interventions/Implications

Pretest
- Explain to the patient the purpose of the test and the need for a blood sample to be drawn.
- No fasting is required before the test.

Procedure
- A 7-mL blood sample is drawn in a light blue-top collection tube.
- Gloves are worn throughout the procedure.

Posttest
- Apply pressure at venipuncture site. Apply dressing, periodically assessing for continued bleeding.
- Label the specimen and transport it to the laboratory.
- Report abnormal findings to the primary care provider.

Prothrombin Fragment 1 + 2 (F1 + 2)

Test Description

During the process of hemostasis, intrinsic and extrinsic pathways lead to the activation of coagulation factor X. This leads to the conversion of prothrombin to thrombin. Thrombin then stimulates the formation of fibrin from fibrinogen. This fibrin, with the addition of fibrin stabilizing factor, forms a stable fibrin clot at the site of injury.

During the conversion of prothrombin to thrombin, prothrombin fragment 1 + 2 (F 1 + 2) is produced. Thus, F 1 + 2 is considered an indicator of prethrombosis or a hypercoagulable state. It is during this prethrombotic time that intervention with anticoagulants can best prevent thrombosis from occurring. Since thrombin itself is not measurable, F 1+ 2 provides a marker of thrombin generation. F 1+ 2 can also be used to monitor the effectiveness of anticoagulants.

Normal Values

7.4–103 µg/mL (0.2–2.8 nmol/L SI units)

Possible Meanings of Abnormal Values

Increased	Decreased
Disseminated intravascular coagulation	Anticoagulation therapy
Leukemia	
Post-myocardial infarction	
Severe liver disease	
Thrombosis	

Contributing Factors to Abnormal Values

- F 1 + 2 levels are increased in the very early postoperative period.
- Drugs that cause *decreased* F 1 + 2 levels: anticoagulants.

Interventions/Implications

Pretest
- Explain to the patient the purpose of the test and the need for a blood sample to be drawn.
- No fasting is required before the test.

Procedure
- A 7-mL blood sample is drawn in a light blue-top collection tube.
- Gloves are worn throughout the procedure.

Posttest
- Apply pressure at venipuncture site. Apply dressing, periodically assessing for continued bleeding.
- Label the specimen and transport it to the laboratory.
- Report abnormal findings to the primary care provider.

→ Clinical Alerts

- Possible complication: hematoma at site due to prolonged bleeding time.
- Teach patient to monitor the site. If the site begins to bleed, the patient should apply direct pressure and, if unable to control the bleeding, return to the laboratory or notify the primary care provider.

Prothrombin Time (PT, INR, Pro Time)

Test Description

The process of hemostasis involves numerous steps and the proper functioning of a variety of coagulating factors and other substances. The *prothrombin time (PT)* is used to evaluate how well the coagulation process is functioning. This test is useful for detecting bleeding disorders caused by either deficient or defective coagulation factors that compose the extrinsic system. These factors include fibrinogen (I), prothrombin (II), V, VII, and X. If the patient's blood is deficient in one of these factors, the patient's PT in seconds will be higher than the control PT in seconds (or less than the control if using percentages).

The PT is also used to monitor the effectiveness of anticoagulant therapy with warfarin sodium (Coumadin). This drug interferes with the production of vitamin K-dependent clotting factors, such as prothrombin.

The PT involves measuring the amount of time it takes for a clot to form in a plasma sample to which calcium and tissue thromboplastin have been added. A normal range for PT is 8.8 to 11.6 seconds, but varies according to the norms established by individual laboratories. Laboratories report the actual PT value along with the control value for reference. The goal of oral anticoagulant therapy is to maintain the PT at 1.5 to 2 times the control value (in seconds). Thus, a therapeutic goal, if receiving Coumadin, would be a PT of 24 seconds, or 25% of normal activity.

If the value falls below the therapeutic level for a patient on an oral anticoagulant, an increase in anticoagulation, and thus, dosage is needed. If the PT is greater than 30 seconds, the patient is at high risk for spontaneous bleeding. In the case of warfarin overdose with resultant hemorrhage, the antidote is vitamin K, which reverses the action of warfarin in 12 to 24 hours.

To provide standardization of PT reporting among different laboratories, the World Health Organization recommends the use of the *International Normalized Ratio (INR)* to express the intensity of therapy. Most laboratories now report both the PT and the INR.

Maintaining an INR of 2.0 to 3.0 is recommended for prophylaxis/treatment of venous thrombosis and thromboembolic complications associated with atrial fibrillation, for pulmonary embolism, for prophylaxis of systemic embolism after myocardial infarction, and for bioprosthetic cardiac valves. A higher INR of 2.5 to 3.5 is recommended for cardiac valve replacement which involves mechanical valves and antiphospholipid antibody syndrome. The frequency of testing to reach and maintain the recommended INR level is based upon the individual patient's clinical status.

P

Normal Values

8.8–11.6 seconds; 60–140% (varies according to laboratory)
Therapeutic level for anticoagulant therapy: 1.5–2 times the control value
INR for DVT prophylaxis and atrial fibrillation: 2.0–3.0
INR for mechanical valve: 2.5–3.5

Possible Meanings of Abnormal Values

Increased (in seconds)

Acute leukemia
Antiphospholipid antibody
Biliary obstruction
Congestive heart failure
Chronic pancreatitis
Disseminated intravascular coagulation

Factor deficiency (I/II/V/VII/X)
Hemorrhagic disease of the newborn
Hepatitis
Hypofibrinogenemia
Liver disease
Malabsorption
Obstructive jaundice
Oral anticoagulant therapy
Pancreatic cancer
Salicylate toxicity
Toxic shock syndrome
Vitamin K deficiency

Contributing Factors to Abnormal Values

- Hemolysis of the blood sample may alter test results.
- Diarrhea, vomiting, and alcohol ingestion may *increase* PT results.
- Intake of a high-fat diet may *decrease* PT results.
- Drugs which may *increase* PT results: antibiotics, acetaminophen, aspirin, chloral hydrate, chloramphenicol, cholestyramine, cimetidine, clofibrate, corticotropin, diuretics, ethanol, glucagon, heparin, indomethacin, kanamycin, levothyroxine, mefenamic acid, mercaptopurine, methyldopa, mithramycin, MAO inhibitors, nalidixic acid, neomycin, nortriptyline, phenylbutazone, phenytoin, propylthiouracil, quinidine, quinine, reserpine, streptomycin, sulfinpyrazone, sulfonamides, tetracyclines, tolbutamide, vitamin A, warfarin.
- Drugs which may *decrease* PT results: anabolic steroids, antacids, antihistamines, ascorbic acid, barbiturates, caffeine, chloral hydrate, colchicine, corticosteroids, digitalis, diuretics, griseofulvin, meprobamate, oral contraceptives, phenobarbital, rifampin, theophylline, xanthines.

Interventions/Implications

Pretest

- Explain to the patient the purpose of the test and the need for a blood sample to be drawn.
- Inform the patient that the PT test will probably be done on a daily basis until it is stabilized, followed by once every 4 to 6 weeks for long-term control.
- Obtain the blood sample prior to administration of any oral anticoagulant.
- No fasting is required before the test.

Procedure

- A 7-mL blood sample is drawn in a light blue-top collection tube.
- Gloves are worn throughout the procedure.

Posttest

- Apply pressure 3 to 5 minutes at venipuncture site. Apply dressing, periodically assessing for continued bleeding.
- Teach the patient to monitor the site. If the site begins to bleed, the patient should apply direct pressure and, if unable to control the bleeding, return to the laboratory or notify the primary care provider.
- Label the specimen and transport it to the laboratory immediately.
- Report abnormal findings to the primary care provider.

Clinical Alerts

- Possible complication: hematoma at site due to prolonged bleeding time.
- Spontaneous bleeding can occur with PT >30 seconds.
    - Assess patient for spontaneous bleeding: epistaxis, bleeding gums, low back pain from possible retroperitoneal bleeding, joint pain, bruising, petechiae, hematuria, or melena.
- Notify the patient of INR level and inform the patient of any dosage changes and date of next PT evaluation. Ensure that the patient understands any instructions.
- Inform patient that increased intake of green, leafy vegetables increases Vitamin K levels and will lower the INR.
- Discuss safety issues with the patient: prevention of falls, use of electric razors.

Pulmonary Function Tests (PFT, Spirometry)

Test Description

Pulmonary function testing (PFT) includes a series of measurements of pulmonary volume and capacity. These measurements are made by a spirometer, which is a breathing system that allows gas to be breathed in and out. An electrical recording is made of the gas amounts. Spirometry is used to determine the effectiveness of the movement of the lungs and chest wall. Test results provide information regarding the degree of obstruction to air flow and/or the restriction of the amount of air which can be inhaled. PFTs are typically ordered to evaluate signs and symptoms of lung disease such as cough, dyspnea, and hypoxemia; to assess progression of lung disease and response to treatment; to assess high-risk preoperative patients; and to screen people at high risk of pulmonary disease due to smoking or occupational exposure to substances toxic to the pulmonary system.

Some of the test findings are obtained through actual testing, while others are determined through calculation. The information obtained through PFT includes information regarding airway flow rates and regarding lung volumes and capacities.

Airway flow rate information is obtained primarily through two measurements. *Forced vital capacity (FVC)* is the amount of air which can be forcefully exhaled from a maximally inflated lung. *Forced expiratory volume in 1 second (FEV$_1$)* is the volume of air expelled during the first second of the FVC.

Lung volumes and capacities are also measured and/or calculated during pulmonary function testing. The relationships among the various volumes and capacities are shown in Table P-1

Four volume measurements are essential parts of the PFT.
- The *tidal volume (VT)* is the normal volume of air inspired and expired with each regular respiration.
- The *expiratory reserve volume (ERV)* is the maximal volume of air that can be exhaled after a normal expiration.
- *Residual volume (RV)* is the volume of air remaining in the lungs following forced expiration.

P

Table P-1	Pulmonary Function Testing

Lung Volumes			Lung Capacities	
Vital Capacity (VC) (IRV+VT+ERV)	Inspiratory Reserve Volume (IRV)	Inspiratory Capacity (IC) (IRV + VT)	Total Lung Capacity (TLC) (IRV+VT+ERV+RV) OR (VC + RV)
	Tidal Volume (VT)		
	Expiratory Reserve Volume (ERV)	Functional Residual Capacity (FRC) (ERV + RV)	
Residual Volume (RV)			

P

- The *inspiratory reserve volume (IRV)* is the maximal volume of air that can be inspired from the end of a normal inspiration.

  By combining two or more of these lung *volume* values, four lung *capacity* values can be calculated.
- The *inspiratory capacity (IC)*, which is the maximal amount of air that can be inspired after a normal expiration, is calculated by adding IRV and VT.
- *Functional residual capacity (FRC)*, the amount of air left in the lungs after a normal expiration, is calculated by adding ERV and RV.
- The *vital capacity (VC)*, which is the maximum amount of air which can be expired after a normal inspiration, is determined by adding the IRV, VT, and ERV.
- The *total lung capacity (TLC)*, the volume to which the lungs can be expanded with the greatest inspiratory effort, is calculated by adding the IRV, VT, ERV, and RV. Another way to determine TLC is to add the VC and RV values.

  When interpreting PFT results, three of these measures are of primary consideration: FVC, FEV_1, and the FEV_1/FVC ratio.
- A low FEV_1/FVC ratio indicates an *obstructive* pattern, whereas a normal value indicates either a restrictive or a normal pattern.
  - Examples of obstructive pattern causes include asthma, bronchitis, and emphysema

- If the FEV$_1$/FVC ratio is normal, a low FVC value indicates a *restrictive* pattern, whereas a normal value indicates a normal pattern.
  - Examples of restrictive pattern causes include pulmonary fibrosis, obesity, neuromuscular diseases, chest-wall deformities, and large pleural effusions.

Normal Values

A value is usually considered abnormal if it is less than 80% of the predicted value for that person. Values vary with age, height, sex.

Possible Meanings of Abnormal Values

Allergy
Asbestosis
Asthma
Bronchiectasis
Chest trauma
Chronic bronchitis
Chronic obstructive pulmonary disease
Emphysema
External compression (esophageal tumor, thyroid goiter)
Foreign body
Endobronchial tumor
Interstitial lung disease
Laryngeal obstruction
Myasthenia gravis
Pulmonary fibrosis
Pulmonary tumors
Respiratory infections
Sarcoidosis
Tracheomalacia

Contributing Factors to Abnormal Values

- Test results may be altered in the following situations or conditions: lack of patient cooperation during the testing, hypoxia, metabolic disturbances, pregnancy, gastric distention.

Interventions/Implications

Pretest

- Explain to the patient the purpose of the test and the procedure to be done.
- No fasting is required prior to the test, but the patient should not eat a heavy meal before the test.
- Instruct the patient to use no bronchodilators for 6 hours prior to the test, if ordered by the primary care provider.
- Instruct the patient not to smoke for 6 hours prior to the test.
- Measure the patient's height and weight.

Procedure
- The patient is in a sitting or standing position.
- The patient is fitted with a mouthpiece that is connected to the spirometer.
- A noseclip is used so that only mouth breathing is possible.
- The patient is instructed:
  - to breathe normally for 10 breaths. (VT)
  - to inhale deeply and then to exhale completely (VC).
    - This part of the test is usually repeated two additional times.
  - to breathe normally for several breaths and then to exhale completely (ERV).
  - to breathe normally for several breaths and then to inhale as deep as possible (IC).
  - to breathe normally into a spirometer containing a known concentration of an insoluble gas such as nitrogen. The point at which the concentration of gas in the spirometer is equal to that in the lungs is measured (FRC).
- Testing after administration of a bronchodilator may also be done to assess for improvement in function.

Posttest
- Assess patient for dizziness or weakness following the testing. Allow the patient to rest as needed.
- Report abnormal findings to the primary care provider.

→ **Clinical Alerts**

- Patients with asthma can use handheld peak flow meters to measure peak expiratory force (PEF) in order to assess the severity of asthma exacerbations and the response to treatment. Severity of asthma exacerbation is based on the following comparison of the PEF with the person's predicted or personal best value:
  - *Mild exacerbation*: PEF >80% of predicted or personal best
  - *Moderate exacerbation*: PEF 50–80% of predicted or personal best
  - *Severe exacerbation*: <50% of predicted or personal best
- The primary care provider and the patient (and, if applicable, parents) should work together to establish treatment and monitoring parameters based on the PEF results.
- Information on the National Asthma Education Program can be accessed at http://www.nhlbi.nih.gov/health/prof/lung/index.htm#asthma.

CONTRAINDICATIONS!

- Patients with acute coronary insufficiency, angina, or recent myocardial infarction
- Patients who are unable to cooperate due to pain, age, or mental status

Pyruvate Kinase (PK)

Test Description
Pyruvate kinase (PK) is a red blood cell glycolytic enzyme that helps convert glucose to energy when oxygen is low (anaerobic metabolism). Deficiency of this

enzyme is an inherited, autosomal recessive trait. PK deficiency is the second most frequent cause, after glucose-6-phosphate dehydrogenase (G-6-PD) deficiency, of congenital nonspherocytic hemolytic anemia. Thus, this test is performed to determine the cause of hemolytic anemia.

Normal Values

2.0–8.8 U/g of hemoglobin

Possible Meanings of Abnormal Values

Decreased

Congenital non-spherocytic chronic hemolytic anemia
Leukemia
Metabolic liver disease
Myelodysplastic syndromes
Pyruvate kinase deficiency
Sideroblastic anemia

Contributing Factors to Abnormal Values

- Hemolysis of the blood sample may alter test results.
- Recent blood transfusions may alter test results.

Interventions/Implications

Pretest
- Explain to the patient the purpose of the test and the need for a blood sample to be drawn.
- No fasting is required before the test.

Procedure
- A 7-mL blood sample is drawn in a green-top collection tube.
- Gloves are worn throughout the procedure.

Posttest
- Apply pressure at venipuncture site. Apply dressing, periodically assessing for continued bleeding.
- Label the specimen and transport it to the laboratory.
- Report abnormal findings to the primary care provider.

Rabies Antibody Test (Rabies Neutralizing Antibody Test)

Test Description

This test is used to determine whether a person has been infected with the rabies virus. Rabies is an acute viral infection of the central nervous system that affects animals such as bats, cats, dogs, skunks, and squirrels. The virus is present in the saliva of the infected animal, making transmission to humans possible through animal bites. The infection is fatal if symptoms appear before treatment is begun. Treatment involves the administration of rabies immunoglobulin (RIG) as soon as possible following exposure to neutralize the virus in the wound. RIG contains anti-rabies antibodies collected from donated human blood and confers passive immunity against rabies, an immediate though temporary protection against the progression of rabies infection.

Human diploid cell rabies vaccine is given intramuscularly at the same time as the RIG is given, and again at 3, 7, 14, and 28 days after the initial dose. This vaccine stimulates the body to produce its own antibodies against the rabies virus. This active immunity takes longer to develop but protects against development of rabies for a longer period of time.

This test is also used to measure the rabies neutralizing antibody titer to determine whether an individual who has received the human diploid cell rabies vaccine has developed adequate protection against the disease. This is especially important for individuals such as veterinarians, who work closely with animals. A rabies titer of at least 1:16 is considered protective.

Normal Values

Titer <1:16 is considered negative for rabies exposure
Titer ≥1:16 is considered as protective following vaccine administration

Possible Meanings of Abnormal Values

Increased
Immunity against rabies
Rabies

Interventions/Implications

R

Pretest
- Explain to the patient the purpose of the test and the need for a blood sample to be drawn.
- No fasting is required before the test.

Procedure
- A 7-mL blood sample is drawn in a red-top collection tube.
- Gloves are worn throughout the procedure.

Posttest
- Apply pressure at venipuncture site. Apply dressing, periodically assessing for continued bleeding.
- Label the specimen and transport it to the laboratory.
- Report abnormal findings to the primary care provider.

→ Clinical Alerts

- The animal's brain must be examined along with the patient's blood sample to determine presence of the rabies virus.

Radioactive Iodine Uptake (RAIU)

Test Description
The radioactive iodine uptake (RAIU) test evaluates thyroid function by measuring the amount of radioactive iodine (^{123}I or ^{131}I) that accumulates in the thyroid gland 6 and 24 hours after ingestion of the substance. A scanner measures the amount of radioactivity in the thyroid gland and, when compared with the original dose of radioactivity, provides a percentage of uptake. The RAIU is used in the diagnosis of hyperthyroidism and at times, hypothyroidism. It can also be used for evaluation of response to treatment/surgery for the conditions. The scan may also be useful in assessing the functional status of any palpable thyroid irregularities or nodules associated with a toxic goiter. Results of the RAIU are reviewed in conjunction with results of blood tests such as T_3, T_4, and TSH.

THE EVIDENCE FOR PRACTICE
The radioactive iodine uptake should be assessed prior to treatment for hyperthyroidism using radioactive iodine to ensure that the uptake is adequate at the time of therapy, to rule out the presence of a variant of thyroiditis or iodine contamination, and to help determine the dose of radioactive iodine.

Normal Values
After 6 hours:	3–16% absorbed by thyroid gland
After 24 hours:	8–29% absorbed by thyroid gland

Possible Meanings of Abnormal Values

Increased	Decreased
Early Hashimoto's thyroiditis	Hypothyroidism
Hyperthyroidism	Iodine overload
Hypoalbuminemia	Subacute thyroiditis
Iodine-deficient goiter	

Contributing Factors to Abnormal Values
- Any movement by the patient may alter quality of films taken.
- Test results may be affected by an iodine-deficient or iodine-excessive diet, other tests using iodine-based contrast within previous 2 weeks, and diarrhea.
- Drugs that *increase* uptake include barbiturates, estrogen, lithium, phenothiazines, and TSH.
- Drugs that *decrease* uptake include ACTH, antihistamines, corticosteroids, Lugol's solution, nitrates, potassium iodide, thyroid drugs, antithyroid drugs, tolbutamide.

Interventions/Implications

Pretest
- Explain to the patient the purpose of the test. Provide any written teaching materials available on the subject. Note that discomfort with this test is due to lying on a hard table

R

for an extended period of time. Reassure the patient that only trace amounts of the radionuclide are involved in the test.

- The patient must remain still while the scan is being performed.
- Fasting for 8 hours is required before the test.
- Obtain a signed informed consent.

Procedure

- Oral radioactive iodine is administered. The patient can resume eating 1 to 2 hours after ingesting the radionuclide.
- The patient is assisted to a supine position on the examination table.
- A scintillation camera is positioned over the patient's thyroid. This camera takes a radioactivity reading from the thyroid and transforms the information into a two-dimensional image.
- Scanning is done at 6 hours and again at 24 hours.
- Gloves are worn when handling the radionuclide.

Posttest

- If a woman who is lactating *must* have this scan, she should not breast feed the infant until the radionuclide has been eliminated, possibly for 3 days.
- Although the amount of diagnostic radionuclide excreted in the urine is low, the urine should not be used for any laboratory tests for the time period indicated by the nuclear medicine department.
- Gloves are worn when dealing with the urine.
- Encourage fluid intake by the patient to enhance excretion of the radionuclide.
- Report abnormal findings to the primary care provider.

Clinical Alerts

- No other radionuclide tests should be scheduled for 24 to 48 hours after the RAIU.

CONTRAINDICATIONS!

- Pregnant women
    - Caution: A woman in her childbearing years should undergo scanning only during her menses or 12 to 14 days after its onset to avoid any exposure to a fetus.
- Patients who are lactating
- Patients who are allergic to iodine, shellfish, or contrast medium
- Patients who are unable to cooperate because of age, mental status, pain, or other factors

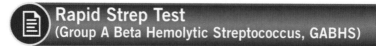

Rapid Strep Test
(Group A Beta Hemolytic Streptococcus, GABHS)

Test Description

The Rapid Strep Test is used to check for the presence of group A beta hemolytic streptococcal (GABHS) infection. This particular type of infection is usually easily treated with antibiotics. If untreated, the infection can lead to complications such as rheumatic fever and poststreptococcal glomerulonephritis. Conducting the test also allows the health-care provider the opportunity to avoid unnecessary use of antibiotics for viral infections, thus decreasing the incidence of antibiotic resistance.

The Rapid Strep Test has a sensitivity of approximately 95%. The test is conducted using commercial immunochemical antigen test kits which use antibody-antigen technology to identify the presence of group A streptococcus from a throat swab. The test only checks for the presence of GABHS; other causes of pharyngitis are not included in the test.

THE EVIDENCE FOR PRACTICE

Diagnosis of group A beta streptococcal (GABS) pharyngitis should be made by laboratory testing rather than clinically. The Rapid Strep Test is useful but does not have sufficient sensitivity to be used alone. The Rapid Strep Test followed by throat culture and sensitivity test has the highest positive predictive value that the patient actually has the illness.

Normal Values

Negative

Possible Meanings of Abnormal Values

Positive	Negative
Group A beta hemolytic streptococcal infection	No infection
	Viral infection
	False negative

Contributing Factors to Abnormal Values

- False negatives may occur if sample is taken from the uvula and soft palate due to dilution of the sample.
- Recent treatment with antibiotics.
- Gargling with some mouthwashes.

Interventions/Implications

Pretest
- Explain to the patient the purpose of the test.
- Note that the test is not painful, but may cause the patient to gag.

Procedure
- The patient may be seated, or if a child, held so as to immobilize the head.
- A tongue depressor is used to hold down the tongue. To minimize stimulating the gag reflex, the tongue depressor should be placed on the lateral portions of the tongue, rather than the center portion.
- Samples are taken from both tonsils and the posterior pharynx.

Posttest
- The patient may wish to drink water after the swab is taken.

- Explain to the patient when the test result will be available. If performed in the office setting, the result should be available in 10 to 20 minutes.
- If the test result is negative, explain the purpose of a follow-up culture and sensitivity test.

Clinical Alerts

- If the rapid strep test is positive, the patient needs to be treated with an antibiotic, such as penicillin or, if allergic to penicillin, erythromycin.
- If the rapid strep test is negative, a follow-up culture and sensitivity test is conducted to determine whether the rapid strep test result was a false negative result. It may take several days before the final culture report is available.
- A positive test result does not differentiate between individuals with an active strep infection and those who are carriers of strep bacteria who may currently have a viral infection.

CONTRAINDICATIONS!

Throat swabs are not to be done on any patient exhibiting signs of possible airway compromise due to such causes as epiglottis or peritonsillar abscess.

Red Blood Cell Count (RBC Count, Erythrocyte Count)

Test Description
The red blood cell (RBC) count is a measure of the number of red blood cells (erythrocytes) per cubic millimeter (mm^3) of blood. RBCs, which have a lifespan of 80 to 120 days, are produced by the bone marrow. These cells are important for the oxygen they carry on their hemoglobin molecules.

RBC production is stimulated by erythropoietin, a hormone secreted by the kidney. The amount of erythropoietin secreted increases whenever tissue hypoxia occurs. Such hypoxia occurs in individuals living at high altitudes or in people who smoke. The result is the production of an increased number of red blood cells, a condition known as *polycythemia*. If the number of RBCs is decreased below normal, the condition is known as *anemia*. There are several different types of anemia, with additional testing needed to differentiate among the various types.

Normal Values

Adult male:	$4.7–6.1 \times 10^6$/mm³ ($4.7–6.1 \times 10^{12}$/L SI units)
Female:	$4.2–5.4 \times 10^6$/mm³ ($4.2–5.4 \times 10^{12}$/L SI units)
Newborn:	$3.5–5.1 \times 10^6$/mm³ ($3.5–5.1 \times 10^{12}$/L SI units)
1–2 years:	$3.6–5.2 \times 10^6$/mm³ ($3.6–5.2 \times 10^{12}$/L SI units)
3–7 years:	$4.1–5.5 \times 10^6$/mm³ ($4.1–5.5 \times 10^{12}$/L SI units)
8–12 years:	$4.0–5.4 \times 10^6$/mm³ ($4.0–5.4 \times 10^{12}$/L SI units)

Possible Meanings of Abnormal Values

Increased	Decreased
Cardiovascular disease	Addison's disease
Chronic hypoxia	Alcohol abuse
Chronic lung disease	Anemias
Congenital heart defects	Bone marrow suppression
Cushing's disease	Chronic infection
Hemoconcentration	Chronic renal failure
Hepatic cancer	Hemodilution
High altitude	Hemolysis
Polycythemia vera	Hemorrhage
Smoking	Hodgkin's disease
	Hypothyroidism
	Leukemia
	Multiple myeloma
	Myelodysplasia
	Rheumatic fever
	Subacute bacterial endocarditis
	Systemic lupus erythematosus
	Vitamin deficiency
	(B$_6$, B$_{12}$, folic acid)

Contributing Factors to Abnormal Values

- Hemolysis of the sample may alter test results.
- Factors that may alter test results include: age, altitude, exercise, posture, and pregnancy.
- False low results have occurred in the presence of cold agglutinins.
- The extra fluid load experienced in pregnancy causes a falsely low RBC count.
- False high results occur with dehydration.
- Drugs that might *increase* RBC count: corticosteroids, cosyntropin, danazol, epoetin alfa, gentamicin, and thiazide diuretics.
- Drugs that might *decrease* RBC count: acetaminophen, acyclovir, allopurinol, amitriptyline, amphetamines, amphotericin B, antimalarials, antibiotics, barbiturates, captopril, chemotherapy, chloramphenicol, digoxin, donepezil, indomethacin, isoniazid, MAO inhibitors, phenobarbital, phenytoin, rifampin, tolbutamide, thrombolytics.

R

Interventions/Implications

Pretest
- Explain to the patient the purpose of the test and the need for a blood sample to be drawn.
- No fasting is required before the test.

Procedure
- A 7-mL blood sample is drawn in a lavender-top collection tube.
- Gloves are worn throughout the procedure.

Posttest
- Apply pressure at venipuncture site. Apply dressing, periodically assessing for continued bleeding.
- Invert and gently mix the sample with the anticoagulant in the collection tube.

- Label the specimen and transport it to the laboratory.
- Report abnormal findings to the primary care provider.

 Clinical Alerts

- Instruct patients diagnosed with polycythemia vera to maintain physical activity to prevent venous stasis with resultant venous thrombosis. This can occur because of the high viscosity of the blood in these patients.

Red Blood Cell Distribution Width (RDW)

Test Description
The red blood cell distribution width (RDW) is calculated by machine from the mean corpuscular volume (MCV) and the red blood cell count. It is a quantitative measure of anisocytosis, a condition in which the red blood cells are unequal in size. This assists in distinguishing iron deficiency anemia from thalassemia. Both conditions have a low MCV; however, iron deficiency anemia has a high RDW, whereas thalassemia has a normal RDW. The RDW may become abnormal before the MCV becomes abnormal and anemia is apparent.

Normal Values
11.5–14.5%

Possible Meanings of Abnormal Values

Increased
Alcohol abuse
Folic acid deficiency anemia
Hemolytic anemia
Iron deficiency anemia
Pernicious anemia
Sickle cell anemia

Contributing Factors to Abnormal Values
- Hemolysis of the sample may alter test results.
- Recent blood transfusion may alter test results.
- Drug which may *increase* RDW: epoetin.

Interventions/Implications
Pretest
- Explain to the patient the purpose of the test and the need for a blood sample to be drawn.
- No fasting is required before the test.

Procedure
- A 7-mL blood sample is drawn in a lavender-top collection tube.
- Gloves are worn throughout the procedure.

Posttest
- Apply pressure at venipuncture site. Apply dressing, periodically assessing for continued bleeding.
- Invert and gently mix the sample and the anticoagulant in the collection tube.
- Label the specimen and transport it to the laboratory.
- Report abnormal findings to the primary care provider.

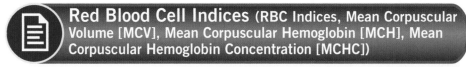

Red Blood Cell Indices (RBC Indices, Mean Corpuscular Volume [MCV], Mean Corpuscular Hemoglobin [MCH], Mean Corpuscular Hemoglobin Concentration [MCHC])

Test Description

Red blood cells (RBCs) transport oxygen via hemoglobin molecules. The amount of oxygen received by tissue depends on the number and function of RBCs and their hemoglobin concentration. The RBC indices are the mean corpuscular volume (MCV), the mean corpuscular hemoglobin (MCH), and the mean corpuscular hemoglobin concentration (MCHC). The indices are used to determine whether the RBCs are normal in size and whether they contain an appropriate amount of hemoglobin.

Mean Corpuscular Volume (MCV) is a measurement of the average RBC size. If the MCV is elevated, the RBCs are larger than normal, or *macrocytic* This occurs with macrocytic anemias such as those due to Vitamin B_{12} deficiency or folic acid deficiency. If the MCV is decreased, the RBCs are smaller than normal, or *microcytic*. Microcytic conditions include iron deficiency anemia and thalassemia. If the MCV is within normal range, the RBCs are considered *normocytic*. MCV is calculated thus:

$$MCV = \frac{\text{Hematocrit (in \%)} \times 10}{\text{RBC (in millions/mm}^3)}$$

Mean Corpuscular Hemoglobin (MCH) is a calculation of the amount of hemoglobin contained within the RBCs. MCH correlates with the MCV results. This is calculated thus:

$$MCH = \frac{\text{Hemoglobin (in g/dL)} \times 10}{\text{RBC (in millions/mm}^3)}$$

Mean Corpuscular Hemoglobin Concentration (MCHC) is the hemoglobin content relative to the size of the cell (hemoglobin concentration) per RBC. This is calculated thus:

$$MCHC = \frac{\text{Hemoglobin (in g/dL)} \times 100}{\text{Hematocrit}}$$

R

Decreased MCHC values are described as *hypochromic* and is found in iron deficiency anemia and thalassemia. Increased MCHC values, known as *hyperchromic,* are associated with hereditary spherocytosis. RBCs cannot hold more than 37 g/dL of hemoglobin, so even with macrocytic anemias, the cells will be *normochromic,* meaning they have a normal MCHC.

Examples of the various types of anemias include:

- *Normocytic/normochromic anemia,* in which the RBC indices are normal, but the RBC count is decreased. This can occur with hemorrhage and destruction by prosthetic heart valves.
- *Microcytic/hypochromic anemia,* in which the MCV and MCHC are both decreased. This occurs with iron deficiency anemia, lead poisoning, and thalassemia.
- *Macrocytic/normochromic anemia,* in which the MCV is elevated and the MCHC is normal. This occurs in Vitamin B_{12} and folate deficiencies.

Normal Values

MCV:	86–98 mm3	(86–98 fL SI units)
MCH:	28–33 pg/cell	(28–33 pg/cell SI units)
MCHC:	32–36 g/dL	(320–360 g/L SI units)

Possible Meanings of Abnormal Values

Mean corpuscular volume (MCV)

Mean corpuscular hemoglobin (MCH)

Increased	Decreased
Alcohol abuse	Anemia of chronic disease
Chronic liver disease	Iron deficiency anemia
Folic acid deficiency	Lead poisoning
Hypothyroidism	Malignancies
Myelodysplasia	Rheumatoid arthritis
Spherocytosis	Sickle cell anemia
Vitamin B_{12} deficiency	Sideroblastic anemia
	Thalassemia

Mean corpuscular hemoglobin concentration (MCHC)

Increased	Decreased
Infancy	Anemia of chronic disease
Spherocytosis	Iron deficiency anemia
	Lead poisoning
	Sideroblastic anemia
	Thalassemia

Contributing Factors to Abnormal Values

- False elevations of MCH and MCV may occur with hyperlipidemia.
- RBC indices may be falsely elevated in the presence of cold agglutinins.

- Drugs that may *increase* MCV: antimetabolites, colchicine, estrogens, heparin, nitrofurantoin, phenytoin, triamterene, trimethoprim.
- Drugs that may *increase* MCH: AZT, heparin, hydroxyurea, methotrexate, phenytoin.
- Drugs that may *increase* MCHC: heparin, oral contraceptives.

Interventions/Implications

Pretest
- Explain to the patient the purpose of the test and the need for a blood sample to be drawn.
- No fasting is required before the test.

Procedure
- A 7-mL blood sample is drawn in a lavender-top collection tube.
- Gloves are worn throughout the procedure.

Posttest
- Apply pressure at venipuncture site. Apply dressing, periodically assessing for continued bleeding.
- Label the specimen and transport it to the laboratory.
- Report abnormal findings to the primary care provider.

 Clinical Alerts

- Following analysis of the RBC indices, additional testing such as iron, ferritin, vitamin B_{12}, folate, transferrin or TIBC, will be needed.

R

 Red Blood Cell Survival Study (RBC Survival Study)

Test Description
Red blood cells (RBCs) normally remain in circulation until their national death at the end of their expected lifespan (80 to 120 days). However, in hemolytic diseases, RBC death occurs earlier than normal. The RBC survival study involves labeling a sample of the patient's RBCs with radioactive chromium. The labeled cells are reinjected into the patient and then monitored at regular intervals for several weeks through blood sampling. Scanning of the precordium, liver, and spleen is performed at the same intervals to look for possible sequestration of RBCs in the spleen. If this is occurring, splenectomy may be the treatment option.

Normal Values
Tagged ^{51}CR red cell half-life: 25–35 days

Possible Meanings of Abnormal Values

Decreased

Chronic lymphocytic leukemia
Congenital nonspherocytic hemolytic anemia
Elliptocytosis
Hemoglobin C disease
Hereditary spherocytosis
Idiopathic acquired hemolytic anemia
Paroxysmal nocturnal hemoglobinuria
Pernicious anemia
Sickle cell anemia
Sickle cell hemoglobin C disease
Uremia

Contributing Factors to Abnormal Values

- Any movement by the patient may alter quality of films taken.
- RBC survival may be *decreased* by recent blood transfusion, increased RBC production, active bleeding, leukocytosis, and thrombocytosis.

Interventions/Implications

Pretest

- Explain to the patient the purpose of the test. Provide any written teaching materials available on the subject. Note that the only discomfort involved with this test is due to the venipunctures. Reassure the patient that only trace amounts of the radionuclide are involved in the test.
- The patient must remain still while the scan is being performed.
- No fasting is required before the test.

Procedure

- A 20-mL blood sample is drawn and mixed with ^{51}Cr.
- The mixture is allowed to incubate at room temperature and is then reinjected into the patient.
- A 10-mL blood sample is drawn on the first day and then at regular intervals for the next 2 to 3 weeks.
- At the time each blood sample is drawn, a scan of the precordium, liver, and spleen is done to assess for RBC sequestration in the spleen.
- Gloves are worn during the radionuclide injection and blood sampling.

Posttest

- Report abnormal findings to the primary care provider.

CONTRAINDICATIONS!

- Pregnant women
  - Caution: A woman in her childbearing years should undergo scanning only during her menses or 12 to 14 days after its onset to avoid any exposure to a fetus.
- Patients who are unable to cooperate because of age, mental status, pain, or other factors.

Renal Biopsy (Kidney Biopsy)

Test Description

Renal biopsy, in which a sample of renal tissue is obtained for histologic study, is used to aid in the diagnosis of renal parenchymal disease. The tissue sample may be obtained by percutaneous needle biopsy through the skin, or by open biopsy through a surgical incision. This discussion will be limited to that of needle biopsy of the kidney.

Renal biopsy can be used in the diagnosis of such conditions as glomerulonephritis, pyelonephritis, and systemic lupus erythematosus. Considering the risk of damage to the kidney tissue during biopsy and the availability of alternative diagnostic tests such as ultrasonography and computer tomography (CT), the risk-benefit of performing this test must be carefully weighed.

Normal Values

No abnormal cells or tissue present

Possible Meanings of Abnormal Values

Acute glomerulonephritis
Amyloid infiltration
Chronic glomerulonephritis
Disseminated lupus erythematosus
Pyelonephritis
Rejection of kidney transplant
Renal cell carcinoma
Renal vein thrombosis
Wilms' tumor

Interventions/Implications

Pretest

- Explain to the patient the purpose of the test and the procedure to be done. Explain to the patient that a local anesthetic will be used. Transient pain may occur as the needle enters the kidney.
- Obtain baseline chest x-ray and coagulation tests (particle thromboplastin time, platelet count, prothrombin time).
- Fasting for 8 hours is required before the test.
- Obtain a signed informed consent.
- Obtain baseline vital signs.

Procedure

- The patient is assisted to a prone position with a sandbag beneath the abdomen to shift the kidneys to a posterior position.
- The skin is cleaned with an antiseptic and draped.
- A local anesthetic is administered.
- The patient is instructed to hold his breath as the biopsy needle is inserted through the back muscles and into the kidney capsule. The patient may then exhale.

R

- The specimen is obtained and the needle removed.
- Pressure is exerted on the biopsy site for 5 to 20 minutes, followed by application of a sterile pressure dressing.
- Gloves are worn throughout the procedure.

Posttest
- Send the specimen to the laboratory immediately.
- Assist the patient into a supine position. Bedrest is to be maintained for 24 hours to prevent bleeding.
- Monitor the patient's vital signs and comfort level, and check the dressing for drainage every 15 minutes for 4 hours, then every 30 minutes for 4 hours, then every hour for 4 hours, and finally, every 4 hours.
- Administer analgesics as needed.
- Encourage fluid intake. Monitor output, observing all urine for frank bleeding.
- Observe for indications of hemorrhage: decreased blood pressure, increased pulse, pallor, backache, flank pain, shoulder pain (from diaphragmatic irritation), and lightheadedness.
- Observe for signs of punctured bowel or liver: abdominal pain or tenderness, muscle guarding and rigidity, and decreased bowel sounds.
- Report abnormal findings to the primary care provider.

→ **Clinical Alerts**

- Possible complications include: hemorrhage, infection, and punctured liver, lung, bowel, aorta, or inferior vena cava.
- Strenuous activity should be avoided for at least 2 weeks after the procedure.

CONTRAINDICATIONS!

- Patients with bleeding disorders
- Patients with renal tumors, hydronephrosis, abscess, or advanced renal failure with uremia
- Patients with urinary tract infections
- Patients with only one kidney
- Patients who are unable to cooperate because of age, mental status, pain, or other factors

R

📄 **Renal Scan** (Kidney Scan)

Test Description
The renal scan is used to study the kidneys and ureters through the scanning and recording of the dispersion, clearance, and excretion of a radionuclide. This test is used to detect renal infarction, renal arterial atherosclerosis, renal trauma, renal tumors and cysts, and primary renal disease, such as glomerulonephritis. It is also used to monitor renal transplant rejection and to detect urologic problems in patients who are unable to have intravenous pyelography due to allergies to contrast dye.

Normal Values

Normal size, shape, and function of kidneys

Possible Meanings of Abnormal Values

Acute tubular necrosis
Congenital abnormalities
Excretory defects
Glomerulonephritis
Nephroureteral dilation
Pyelonephritis
Renal abscess
Renal cyst
Renal infarction
Renal ischemia
Renal obstruction
Renal transplant rejection
Renal tumor
Renovascular hypertension

Contributing Factors to Abnormal Values

- Any movement by the patient may alter quality of films taken.
- Presence of contrast material from previous exams may interfere with the test. Do not perform a renal scan within 24 hours after intravenous pyelography.

Interventions/Implications

Pretest
- Explain to the patient the purpose of the test. Provide any written teaching materials available on the subject. Note that discomfort involved with this test is primarily due to lying on a hard table for an extended period of time and the needle puncture. Reassure the patient that only trace amounts of the radionuclide are involved in the test.
- The patient must remain still while the scan is being performed.
- No fasting is required before the test. The patient needs to be well hydrated.
- Obtain a signed informed consent.

Procedure
- The radionuclide is administered by intravenous injection in a peripheral vein.
- The patient is assisted to a supine position on the examination table.
- A scintillation camera is positioned over the kidney area. This camera takes a radioactivity reading from the area and transforms the information into a two-dimensional image.
- Scans are obtained to record the passing of the radionuclide through the cortex and pelvis of each kidney.
- Gloves are worn during the radionuclide injection.

Posttest
- Check the injection site for redness or swelling.
- If a woman who is lactating *must* have this scan, she should not breast-feed the infant until the radionuclide has been eliminated, possibly for 3 days.

R

- Although the amount of diagnostic radionuclide excreted in the urine is low, the urine should not be used for any laboratory tests for the time period indicated by the nuclear medicine department.
- Gloves are worn when dealing with the urine.
- Encourage fluid intake by the patient to enhance excretion of the radionuclide.
- Report abnormal findings to the primary care provider.

CONTRAINDICATIONS!

- Pregnant women
    - Caution: A woman in her childbearing years should undergo scanning only during her menses or 12 to 14 days after its onset to avoid any exposure to a fetus.
- Patients who are lactating
- Patients who are unable to cooperate because of age, mental status, pain, or other factors

 ## Renin Activity, Plasma (Plasma Renin Assay [PRA])

Test Description
Renin is an enzyme that is produced, stored, and released by the juxtaglomerular cells of the kidneys. It is released in response to a decrease in blood flow through the kidneys. Renin plays a vital role in the regulation of blood pressure and fluid and electrolyte balance via the renin-angiotensin-aldosterone system.

Changes in position from recumbent to upright have been found to increase the renin level. Sodium intake also influences renin levels: high sodium intake decreases renin levels, while sodium depletion causes increased levels of renin to be released.

The measurement of plasma renin activity (PRA) is used in the differential diagnosis of hypertension. Hypertensive patients who have low renin activity probably have a fluid volume imbalance, whereas those with high renin activity probably are hypertensive because of the vasoconstrictive effects of angiotensin, a condition known as *renovascular hypertension*.

Patients with essential hypertension may have renin and aldosterone levels checked to evaluate if they are salt-sensitive, which causes a low renin with normal aldosterone levels. This helps to guide the primary care provider in choosing the correct medication for these patients. Salt-sensitive patients with low renin hypertension respond well to diuretic medications.

Normal Values

Normal sodium diet
Adult supine: 0.2–1.6 ng/mL/h (0.2–1.6 µg/L/h SI units)
Adult standing: 0.7–3.3 ng/mL/h (0.7–3.3 µg/L/h SI units)

Low sodium diet
Supine: Levels increase 2 times normal
Standing   Levels increase 6 times normal

R

Possible Meanings of Abnormal Values

Increased	Decreased
Addison's disease	Congenital adrenal hyperplasia
Bartter's syndrome	Cushing's syndrome
Chronic renal failure	Elderly
Cirrhosis	Essential hypertension
Erect posture for 4 hours	Fasting
Hemorrhage	High-sodium diet
Hypokalemia	Licorice ingestion
Hypovolemia	Primary hyperaldosteronism
Low-sodium diet	Volume overload
Malignant hypertension	Weight loss
Menstruation	
Nephropathy	
Pheochromocytoma	
Pregnancy	
Renovascular hypertension	
Secondary hyperaldosteronism	
Transplant rejection	

Contributing Factors to Abnormal Values

- The patient's position and diet may alter test results.
- Drugs that may *increase* plasma renin activity: ACE-inhibitors, albuterol, estrogens, furosemide, hydralazine, nifedipine, spironolactone, thiazides.
- Drugs that may *decrease* plasma renin activity: Beta blockers, clonidine, digoxin, indomethacin, licorice, methyldopa, prazosin, sodium-retaining steroids, salicylate.

Interventions/Implications

Pretest

- Explain to the patient the purpose of the test and the need for a blood sample to be drawn.
- Unless otherwise ordered, instruct the patient to follow a 3-g sodium diet for at least 2 weeks before the test. Explain to the patient that this is considered "normal" sodium intake.
- Fasting for 8 hours is required before the test.
- If possible, drugs that may affect test results should be withheld for at least 2 weeks before the test.

Procedure

- A 7-mL blood sample is drawn in a lavender-top collection tube.
- Gloves are worn throughout the procedure.

Posttest

- Apply pressure at venipuncture site. Apply dressing, periodically assessing for continued bleeding.
- Gently invert the specimen to mix the blood sample with the anticoagulant in the collection tube.
- Label the specimen and immediately transport it on ice to the laboratory.
- Report abnormal findings to the primary care provider.

Clinical Alerts

- Stimulation testing can also be done. For this, the patient significantly reduces sodium intake for 3 days prior to testing, and the blood is then drawn in both the recumbent and upright positions.
  - Supplemental potassium may be needed.
  - Patients with primary hyperaldosteronism will have increased aldosterone production associated with a decreased PRA. Patients with secondary hyperaldosteronism (that is, caused by kidney disease or renal vascular disease) will have increased plasma levels of renin and aldosterone.

Reticulocyte Count (Retic Count)

Test Description
A reticulocyte is an immature type of red blood cell (RBC). Its name comes from the fine network, or reticulum, which becomes visible on its surface when stained. After 1to 4 days in the bloodstream, the reticulocyte becomes a mature RBC. The reticulocyte count provides information regarding the rate of RBC production, and thus, bone marrow function.

If the bone marrow is responding as it should to a demand for more RBCs, it will allow for early release of reticulocytes, so the reticulocyte count will increase. Thus, when a patient hemorrhages, the reticulocyte count will increase in an attempt by the body to compensate for the blood loss. This is true in the case of a chronic blood loss as well. If, however, the bone marrow is unable to keep up with the increased demand for RBCs, or is not functioning properly, the reticulocyte count may be slightly elevated at first, but will then decrease as the bone marrow has inadequate production of RBCs.

The test is used in the differential diagnosis of anemia. If the reticulocyte count is within normal limits in a patient with anemia, the problem is most likely due to bone marrow dysfunction or a deficiency of erythropoietin.

Normal Values

Adult:	0.5–2 % red cells
Newborn:	3–7%
1 week:	1.8–4.6%
1 month:	0.1–1.7%
6 months:	0.7–2.3%
>6 months:	0.5–1.0%

Possible Meanings of Abnormal Values

Increased	Decreased
Effective treatment of anemia	Alcoholism
Erythroblastosis fetalis	Aplastic anemia
Hemolytic anemia	Bone marrow depression

R

Pregnancy
Sickle cell anemia
Thalassemia major

Cancer
Chronic infection
Cirrhosis of the liver
Folate deficiency
Iron deficiency anemia
Myelodysplasia
Myxedema
Pernicious anemia
Radiation therapy

Contributing Factors to Abnormal Values

- Hemolysis of the sample may alter test results.
- Falsely decreased values may occur after blood transfusion.
- Hemodilution of the test sample, owing to drawing the blood from the arm in which an IV is infusing, may alter test results.
- Drug which may *increase* test result: epoetin alfa.
- Drugs which may *decrease* test result: AZT, chemotherapy, chloramphenicol.

Interventions/Implications

Pretest
- Explain to the patient the purpose of the test and the need for a blood sample to be drawn.
- No fasting is required before the test.

Procedure
- A 7-mL blood sample is drawn in a lavender-top collection tube.
- Gloves are worn throughout the procedure.

Posttest
- Apply pressure at venipuncture site. Apply dressing, periodically assessing for continued bleeding.
- Invert and gently mix the sample with the anticoagulant in the collection tube.
- Label the specimen and transport it to the laboratory.
- Report abnormal findings to the primary care provider.

R

→ Clinical Alerts

- For patients with iron-deficiency iron, the reticulocyte count should be rechecked at least 7 days after starting iron therapy. The count should increase if there is appropriate response to the iron.

Retrograde Pyelography

Test Description
Retrograde pyelography is used to confirm findings found via excretory urography. The test involves examination of the kidneys using a contrast dye that is injected in a retrograde fashion. During a cystoscopic examination, a catheter is advanced

through each ureter and into the pelvis of the kidney. The renal pelvis is drained, and then a radiopaque iodine-based contrast medium is injected through the catheter into the kidney. The incidence of allergic reaction to the dye is reduced, since the dye is usually not absorbed when administered in this way. Radiographic films are taken throughout the procedure.

Normal Values

Normal size, shape, position of kidneys, ureters, and bladder

Possible Meanings of Abnormal Values

Bladder tumor
Congenital abnormalities
Hydronephrosis
Polycystic kidney disease
Prostatic enlargement
Renal calculi
Renal cysts
Renal tumor
Trauma
Ureteral calculi

Contributing Factors to Abnormal Values

- Retained barium, gas, or stool in the intestines may result in poor quality films.
- Any movement by the patient may alter quality of films taken.

Interventions/Implications

Pretest
- Explain to the patient the purpose of the test. Provide any written teaching materials available on the subject. Note that the test is uncomfortable due to the pressure experienced during injection of the dye.
- Check for allergies to iodine, shellfish, or contrast medium dye. Inform the radiologist of such possible allergy and obtain preprocedure medication as needed.
- Obtain a signed informed consent.
- Fasting for 8 hours is required before the test. The patient should be well hydrated before the beginning of the fasting period.
- A laxative the night before the test, or an enema or suppository the morning of the test may be ordered.
- Preprocedure sedation may be ordered.
- The procedure will usually be performed under local anesthesia.
- Resuscitation and suctioning equipment should be readily available.

Procedure
- The patient is placed in a dorsal lithotomy position. The test is usually performed during a cystoscopic examination in the surgical department.

- A catheter is advanced through the ureters and into the pelvis of each kidney.
- After draining the pelvis of each kidney, a radiopaque iodine-based contrast medium is injected through the catheter into each kidney.
- Radiographic films are taken throughout the procedure.
- Additional contrast dye may be instilled as the catheters are being removed from the ureters to allow for films of the ureters to be taken.
- Gloves are worn throughout the procedure.

Posttest
- Most allergic reactions to radiopaque dye occur within 30 minutes of administration of the contrast medium. Observe the patient closely for respiratory distress, hypotension, edema, hives, rash, tachycardia, and/or laryngeal stridor. Emergency resuscitation equipment must be readily accessible.
- Resume the patient's diet. Encourage fluid intake to decrease any dysuria that might be present.
- Observe for allergic reaction to the dye for 24 hours.
- Monitor vital signs at least every 4 hours for 24 hours.
- Observe for indication of infection, including elevated temperature, chills, flushing, tachycardia, and flank pain.
- Monitor urinary output for at least 24 hours. Assess for bladder distention. Observe the urine for clots or gross hematuria. Pink-tinged urine is expected immediately after the procedure.
- Assess the patient for discomfort, since bladder spasms may occur. If present, they are often treated with belladonna and opium (B&O) suppositories.
- Renal function should be assessed.
- Report abnormal findings to the primary care provider.

Clinical Alerts

- Possible complications include: Allergic reaction to dye, hematuria, perforation of ureter or bladder, sepsis, ureteral edema, and urinary tract infection.
- If barium studies are also ordered, they are to be performed *after* the retrograde pyelography has been successfully completed.

R

CONTRAINDICATIONS!

- Patients who are allergic to iodine, shellfish, or contrast medium dye.
- Pregnant women.
    - Caution: A woman in her childbearing years should undergo scanning only during her menses or 12 to 14 days after its onset to avoid any exposure to a fetus.
- Patients who are unable to cooperate because of age, mental status, pain, or other factors.
- Patients with renal failure or those susceptible to dye-induced renal failure (dehydrated patients).

Rheumatoid Factor (RF, Rheumatoid Arthritis Factor)

Test Description

Rheumatoid arthritis (RA) is a chronic progressive inflammatory condition of the connective tissue which mainly affects the small peripheral joints such as the fingers and wrists. Although the joint destruction is most often thought of when mentioning RA, it is a systemic disease that can affect other systems of the body as well. An autoimmune reaction occurs in the synovial tissue, leading to pain swelling, warmth, erythema, and lack of function in the affected joint. During the inflammatory process, antibodies team up with corresponding antigens to form immune complexes. These complexes are deposited in the synovial tissue, triggering the inflammatory reaction that leads to the damage seen in the joints of patients with RA.

One of the diagnostic tests for rheumatoid arthritis is the rheumatoid factor (RF) test. RF, an immunoglobulin, is present in more than 80% of patients with rheumatoid arthritis; however, a positive RF test can also occur in many other diseases. The antibody, which is produced by the synovium, appears in autoimmune and connective tissue diseases, and in chronic infections. Low titers suggest non-RA diagnoses and are seen in 4% of normal individuals and up to 20% of healthy elderly.

THE EVIDENCE FOR PRACTICE

According to the American Rheumatism Association criteria (Arnett, 1988), the criteria[*] for classification of RA include:

1. *Morning stiffness* (lasting at least 1 hour before maximal improvement)
2. *Arthritis of 3 or more joint areas* (simultaneously having soft tissue swelling or fluid)
3. *Arthritis of hand joints* (wrist, MCP, or PIP joints)
4. *Symmetric arthritis* (simultaneous involvement of same joint on both sides of body)
5. *Rheumatoid nodules* (subcutaneous nodules over bony prominences or extensor surfaces)
6. *Serum rheumatoid factor* (demonstration of abnormal amounts of serum RF)
7. *Radiographic changes* (those typical of RA on hand and wrist radiographs)

Normal Values

Qualitative: Negative
Quantitative: <60 U/mL (<60 kU/L SI units) (Nephelometry technique)
Titer <1:80

Possible Meanings of Abnormal Values

Increased

Allografts
Ankylosing spondylitis
Cancer
Cirrhosis
Cryoglobulinemia

---

[*]To be classified as having RA, the patient must meet at least 4 of the 7 criteria. Criteria 1 to 4 must have been present for at least 6 weeks.

Cytomegalovirus
Dermatomyositis
Hepatitis
Infectious mononucleosis
Influenza
Kidney disease
Liver disease
Lung disease
Malaria
Osteoarthritis
Periodontal disease
Rheumatoid arthritis
Rubella
Sarcoidosis
Scleroderma
Sjögren's syndrome
Subacute bacterial endocarditis
Syphilis
Systemic lupus erythematosus
Tuberculosis
Viral infections

Contributing Factors to Abnormal Values

- *False-positive* RF results may occur in the elderly and in individuals who have received numerous vaccinations and/or blood transfusions.
- Aspirin and NSAIDs do *not* interfere with testing for rheumatoid factor.

Interventions/Implications

Pretest
- Explain to the patient the purpose of the test and the need for a blood sample to be drawn.
- No fasting is required before the test.

Procedure
- A 7-mL blood sample is drawn in a red-top collection tube.
- Gloves are worn throughout the procedure.

Posttest
- Apply pressure at venipuncture site. Apply dressing, periodically assessing for continued bleeding.
- Label the specimen and transport it to the laboratory.
- Report abnormal findings to the primary care provider.

> ## Clinical Alerts
>
> - Typically the RF test is done along with testing for antinuclear antibody (ANA), C-reactive protein (CRP), erythrocyte sedimentation rate (ESR), and a complete blood count (CBC).
>   - Patients with RA frequently have anemia of chronic disease and an elevated ESR.

- RF may be used along with testing for Anti-SS-A (Ro) and Anti-SS-B (La) antibody to help with diagnosis of Sjögren's syndrome.

 ## Rubella Antibody Test (German Measles Test)

Test Description
Rubella, also known as the German measles or 3-day measles, is a virus that is not usually considered a serious condition. It usually causes fever and transient rash in children and adults who contract it. Rubella is serious, however, if a woman contracts the disease during the first trimester of pregnancy. It can cause miscarriage, stillbirth, and congenital defects such as deafness, microcephaly, and heart defects. Thus, it is extremely important for women considering pregnancy to be testing for susceptibility or immunity to rubella.

The rubella antibody test measures IgG and IgM antibody formation against the rubella virus. It can be used to diagnose rubella and to determine whether the person is immune to the virus. A diagnosis of rubella is made when a fourfold increase between the acute titer and the convalescent titer occurs. Demonstration of specific IgG on a serum sample is evidence of immunity to rubella.

Normal Values

Negative for IgM and IgG:	Susceptive to rubella
Positive for IgM:	Current or recent rubella infection
Positive for IgG:	Immunity to rubella

Possible Meanings of Abnormal Values

Positive	Negative
Immunity to rubella (IgG)	Susceptible to rubella
Rubella infection (IgM)	

Contributing Factors to Abnormal Values

- Hemolysis due to excessive agitation of the blood sample may alter test results.

Interventions/Implications
Pretest
- Explain to the patient the purpose of the test and the need for a blood sample to be drawn.
- No fasting is required before the test.

Procedure
- A 7-mL blood sample is drawn in a red-top collection tube.
- Gloves are worn throughout the procedure.

Posttest
- Apply pressure at venipuncture site. Apply dressing, periodically assessing for continued bleeding.
- Label the specimen and transport it to the laboratory.
- Report abnormal findings to the primary care provider.

Clinical Alerts

- Women considering pregnancy should be testing for immunity prior to pregnancy and be vaccinated against rubella if they are not immune.

Schilling Test (Vitamin B$_{12}$ Absorption Test)

Test Description
The Schilling test is used to evaluate the ability of the small intestine to absorb vitamin B$_{12}$. When vitamin B$_{12}$ is ingested, it combines with intrinsic factor from the gastric mucosa. It is then able to be absorbed in the ileum.

This test involves the oral administration of radioactive vitamin B$_{12}$. Nonradioactive vitamin B$_{12}$ is then administered intramuscularly (IM) to saturate the vitamin B$_{12}$ binding sites. A 24-hour urine specimen is collected. Normal patients will absorb and then excrete as much as 25% of the radioactive B$_{12}$, since they have intrinsic factor and can thus absorb the vitamin from the gastrointestinal tract. Patients who have pernicious anemia, in which intrinsic factor is lacking, absorb little if any of the oral dose of B$_{12}$, resulting in little or no radioactive material being excreted in the urine.

If the results of the Schilling test show low absorption of the radioactive vitamin B$_{12}$, the test is repeated along with intrinsic factor being given to rule out intestinal malabsorption. If the urinary excretion rises to normal levels, there is a lack of intrinsic factor. If urinary excretion remains low, malabsorption is probably the cause of the patient's anemia.

S

Normal Values
Excretion of 8% or more of test dose of radioactive B$_{12}$

Possible Meanings of Abnormal Values

Decreased
Hypothyroidism
Intestinal malabsorption
Liver disease
Pernicious anemia

Contributing Factors to Abnormal Values
- Receipt of radioactive nuclear material within 10 days of this test may alter test results.

- Conditions that may cause *decreased* excretion: diabetes, elderly, hypothyroidism, renal insufficiency.
- Drugs that may affect test results: laxatives.

Interventions/Implications

Pretest
- Explain to the patient the purpose of the test. Provide any written teaching materials available on the subject.
- Explain the 24-hour urine collection procedure to the patient. Stress the importance of saving *all* urine in the 24-hour period. Instruct the patient to avoid contaminating the urine with toilet paper or feces.
- Fasting for 12 hours is required before the test.
- No supplements containing vitamin B_{12} should be taken for at least 3 days prior the test.
- No laxatives should be used for 24 hours before the test.

Procedure

Stage I
- A capsule of radioactive vitamin B_{12} is administered orally.
- Next, nonradioactive B_{12} is administered IM to the patient.
- Obtain the proper container containing no preservative from the laboratory.
- Urine is to be collected for 24 hours.
- Gloves are worn whenever dealing with the specimen collection.

If test result from Stage I is below normal, Stage II is then conducted within 3 to 7 days.
- A capsule of radioactive vitamin B_{12} is administered orally, along with oral intrinsic factor.
- Next, nonradioactive B_{12} is administered IM to the patient.
- Obtain the proper container containing no preservative from the laboratory.
- Urine is to be collected for 24 hours.
- Gloves are worn whenever dealing with the specimen collection.

Posttest
- Label the container and transport it to the laboratory as soon as possible following the end of the 24-hour collection period.
- Report abnormal findings to the primary care provider.

S

→ Clinical Alerts

- If the patient is found to have pernicious anemia, treatment of monthly vitamin B_{12} injections will be needed.

CONTRAINDICATIONS!

- Pregnant women
    - Caution: A woman in her childbearing years should be exposed to radioactive substances only during her menses or 12 to 14 days after its onset to avoid any exposure to a fetus.
- Patients who are lactating
- Patients who are unable to cooperate because of age, mental status, pain, or other factors

Scrotal Ultrasound (Ultrasound of Testes)

Test Description

Ultrasonography is a noninvasive method of diagnostic testing in which ultrasound waves are sent into the body with a small transducer pressed against the skin. The transducer then receives any returning sound waves, which are deflected back as they bounce off various structures. The transducer converts the returning sound waves into electric signals that are then transformed by a computer into a visual display on a monitor.

With scrotal ultrasound, visualization of the scrotum and its contents is made possible. This test is used to assess for scrotal masses and infections, evaluation of scrotal pain and trauma, locate undescended testicles, and provide monitoring for patients with previously diagnosed testicular cancer.

THE EVIDENCE FOR PRACTICE

Gray-scale sonography is appropriate for evaluating whether a scrotal mass is cystic or solid. It can also document signs of epididymitis and a necrotic testicle, but it is much less sensitive to *early* changes in the testicle due to decreased or absent perfusion. Color Doppler ultrasound is a valuable test for evaluating perfusion to the testicle, with a sensitivity comparable to that of radionuclide scrotal imaging.

Normal Values

Normal size, shape, location, and perfusion of testicles.

Possible Meanings of Abnormal Values

Benign testicular tumors
Epididymitis
Hematocele
Hydrocele
Malignant testicular tumors
Orchitis
Pyocele
Scrotal hernia
Spermatocele
Testicular torsion
Undescended testicle (cryptorchidism)
Varicocele

Contributing Factors to Abnormal Values

- The transducer must be in good contract with the skin as it is being moved.

Interventions/Implications

Pretest
- Explain to the patient the purpose of the test. Provide any written teaching materials available on the subject. Note there is usually no discomfort involved with this test, unless there is tenderness due to infection or torsion.
- No fasting is required before the test.

S

Procedure
- The patient is assisted to a supine position on the ultrasonography table.
- The scrotum is supported by a towel or held in the examiner's hand.
- A coupling agent, such as a water-based gel, is applied to the area to be evaluated.
- A transducer is placed on the skin and moved as needed to provide good visualization of the scrotal contents.
- The sound waves are transformed into a visual display on the monitor. Printed copies of this display are made.
- Gloves are worn throughout the procedure.

Posttest
- Cleanse the patient's skin of remaining coupling agent.
- Report abnormal findings to the primary care provider.

 Clinical Alerts

- Testicular torsion is considered a surgical emergency. This finding must be reported immediately.

 ## Semen Analysis (Seminal Cytology, Sperm Count)

Test Description
Semen analysis is the most common diagnostic test used in an infertility workup. If testing indicates a low sperm count or other abnormalities, a second specimen is usually tested at least 7 days later. Abnormal semen analysis may require additional testing.

The analysis includes a semen volume, sperm count, determination of the percentage of normal sperm and sperm motility, and pH. The semen volume is usually 2 to 5 mL. Smaller volume indicates fewer sperm and larger volume may indicate diluted fluid, again with fewer sperm than normal. Either situation would affect fertility. The sperm count or density, is measured in millions of sperm per milliliter of semen. Below normal sperm counts are present in infertility.

Sperm motility is a measure of the percentage of moving sperm in a sample. Immobile or slowly moving sperm are problematic in terms of fertility. Analysis is done of 200 sperm to check for size, shape, and appearance. The more abnormal sperm present, the lower the likelihood of fertility.

THE EVIDENCE FOR PRACTICE
When the initial semen analysis is normal, a period of observation is warranted. The repeat semen analysis is delayed for 4 months in order to coincide with the spermatogenic cycle.

Normal Values
Volume:	2–5 mL
pH:	7.3–7.8
Color:	Grayish white
Sperm count:	20–250 million/mL

Motility: >60%
Normal sperm: >60%

Possible Meanings of Abnormal Values

Decreased
Cryptorchidism
Hyperpyrexia
Infertility
Klinefelter's syndrome
Orchitis

Contributing Factors to Abnormal Values

- Drugs that may *decrease* the sperm count: antineoplastic agents, azathioprine, cimetidine, estrogens, ketoconazole, methyltestosterone.

Interventions/Implications

Pretest
- Explain to the patient the purpose of the test and the need for a semen specimen.
- Instruct the patient to abstain from sexual intercourse and intake of alcohol for 2 to 3 days prior to the test.

Procedure
- Provide a specimen container.
- The best specimen is one collected in the primary care provider's office or laboratory by masturbation.
- If the patient prefers to collect the specimen at home a silastic condom with no lubricant may be used during coitus interruptus.

Posttest
- The specimen needs to remain at room temperature. Do not refrigerate.
- The specimen needs to be delivered to the laboratory within 1 hour of collection.
- Report abnormal findings to the primary care provider.

S

 Clinical Alerts

- A sperm analysis is recommended following a vasectomy. No sperm should be seen in such a sample.

 # Sentinel Lymph Node Biopsy

Test Description
Sentinel lymph node biopsy is used for staging of breast cancer or melanoma. In the past, if a patient was found to have breast cancer or melanoma, all of the lymph nodes serving the area were also excised, often causing residual pain, deformity, and

lymphedema. The concept of sentinel lymph node biopsy is that sentinel nodes are the first lymph nodes to receive lymph drainage from the cancer and thus are the most likely nodes to contain cancer if it has spread. If a sentinel node is removed and found to be free of cancer, the other nodes do not need to be removed. If the sentinel node contains cancer, a block dissection of all the lymph nodes in the area is performed.

To identify the sentinel lymph node(s), two types of materials are used. One is a radioactive substance injected into the breast or area surrounding a melanoma. The substance becomes trapped in the lymph node(s). A scanner is then used to find any radioactive lymph nodes. The other substance is a blue dye which is similarly injected. The surgeon follows the dye to identify the sentinel lymph node to be removed for study.

Normal Values

Normal lymphatic uptake

Possible Meanings of Abnormal Values

Lymphatic flow obstruction
Metastatic spread of cancer to lymph nodes

Interventions/Implications

Pretest
- Explain to the patient the purpose of the test and the procedure to be done. Provide any written teaching materials available on the subject. Note that discomfort involved with this test is primarily due to injection of the tracer substances. Reassure the patient that only trace amounts of the radionuclide are involved in the test.
- The patient must remain still while the scan is being performed.
- Fasting may be required before the procedure.
- Obtain a signed informed consent.

Procedure
- A radioactive tracer is injected into the breast or into the tissue surrounding the melanoma.
- The area is scanned, with repeat scanning done within 24 hours.
- In the operating room, the surgeon can use a handheld scanner to find the radioactive nodes. The one proximal to the area of cancer is considered the sentinel node.
- A blue dye is then injected into the breast or into the tissue surrounding the melanoma.
- The surgeon follows the dye to identify the first lymph node reached.
- The sentinel lymph node is removed and examined.
    - If negative, no further lymph node dissection is needed.
    - If positive, block dissection is usually done.
- Sterile surgical technique is followed throughout the procedure.

Posttest
- Monitor the patient for reaction to the blue dye.
- Explain to the patient that the dye may cause temporary coloring of the skin and may cause the urine to be blue for a short time.
- Provide emotional support before, during, and after the procedure.
- Report abnormal findings to the primary care provider.

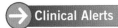

Clinical Alerts

- Possible complications include: bleeding, lymphedema, and wound infection

CONTRAINDICATIONS!

- Pregnant women
  - Caution: A woman in her childbearing years should undergo scanning only during her menses or 12 to 14 days after its onset to avoid any exposure to a fetus.
- Patients who are unable to cooperate because of age, mental status, pain, or other factors

 Sialography

Test Description

Sialography is the radiographic examination of the salivary ducts. The test is used to identify stones, tumors, strictures, infection, or inflammatory processes of the ducts. Any of the salivary ducts, including the sublingual, submaxillary, submandibular, and parotid ducts, may be studied. A baseline x-ray is taken, followed by insertion of a catheter in the duct to be studied. Contrast dye is injected through the catheter. Films are taken from several views. The patient is then given lemon juice to stimulate salivation and additional films are taken.

Normal Values

Normal salivary ducts

Possible Meanings of Abnormal Values

Calculi
Infection
Inflammation
Strictures
Tumors

Interventions/Implications

Pretest

- Explain to the patient the purpose of the test and the procedure to be followed. Inform the patient that some discomfort may be felt with insertion of the catheter into the duct and with injection of the contrast medium.
- Check for allergies to iodine, shellfish, or contrast medium dye. Inform the radiologist of any such allergy and obtain order for preprocedure medication.
- Obtain a signed informed consent.
- No fasting is required before the test.
- Instruct the patient to brush the teeth and rinse the mouth with mouthwash before the test to reduce bacterial flora.

S

Procedure
- The patient is assisted into a supine position on the radiology table.
- A baseline x-ray is taken to assess for presence of a ductal stone, which could prevent dye from entering the duct.
- A catheter is inserted through the mouth into the duct.
- Contrast dye is injected through the catheter, and x-rays are taken.
- The patient is then given lemon juice to drink to stimulate salivation.
- Additional x-rays are taken.
- Gloves are worn throughout the procedure.

Posttest
- Most allergic reactions to radiopaque dye occur within 30 minutes of administration of the contract medium. Observe the patient closely for respiratory distress, hypotension, edema, hives, rash, tachycardia, and/or laryngeal stridor. Emergency resuscitation equipment must be readily accessible.
- Encourage fluid intake to help eliminate the dye.
- A mild analgesic may be needed for pain and swelling at the site of the procedure.
- Report abnormal findings to the primary care provider.

CONTRAINDICATIONS!

- Patients with mouth infections
- Patients with allergies to iodine, shellfish, or contrast medium dye

Sims-Huhner Test (Cervical Mucus Sperm Penetration Test, Cervical Mucus Test, Fern Test, Postcoital Test)

Test Description
The Sims-Huhner test is a test for infertility in the male by determination of sperm quantity and motility in specimens obtained from the cervical canal after unprotected intercourse. The test is best performed 1 to 2 days before ovulation. At that time, two changes occur in the cervical mucus that enhance sperm survival. The elasticity of the cervical mucus, known as *spinnbarkheit (SBK)*, increases. Also, the cervical mucus contains more sodium at that time. This high sodium content can be determined by spreading the cervical mucus on a clean glass slide and allowing it to dry. A pattern of *arborization* or *ferning* occurs, which is the result of the salt and water interacting with mucus glycoproteins. Thus, the presence of excellent SBK and ferning are indications of ovulation.

The Sims-Huhner test involves the collection of an endocervical mucus sample. The total number of sperm and the number of motile sperm are reported. If the number of sperm present is adequate but they are not motile, the cervical environment is unsuitable for their survival. The test is done in conjunction with semen analysis with an infertility workup. The test is named after Harry M. Sims, a gynecologist who wrote about microscopic diagnosis of sterility in 1888, and

Max Huhner, a urologist who wrote of the value of sperm testing in sterility in 1913. The test is also done in suspected rape cases to document the presence of sperm.

Normal Values

Mucus tenacity: Adequate for sperm survival and penetration
Motile sperm: 6–20 per high-power field

Possible Meanings of Abnormal Values

Infertility
Suspected rape

Contributing Factors to Abnormal Values

- Cervical mucus specimen must be obtained within 2 to 4 hours after intercourse. Test results are unreliable when the specimen is collected more than 6 hours after coitus.

Interventions/Implications

Pretest

- Explain to the patient the purpose of the test and the need for a cervical mucus sample to be obtained.
- Obtain a signed informed consent if the procedure is being done for medicolegal purposes.
- For the test results to be most valid, lubricants are not to be used and the woman must not douche or take a tub bath after intercourse.
- In infertility workups, the male should abstain from ejaculation for 3 days before the test.
- The female should remain recumbent for 15 to 30 minutes following intercourse and then undergo testing within 1 to 5 hours.

Procedure

- The patient is assisted into the lithotomy position with the legs supported in stirrups, and draped for privacy.
- An unlubricated speculum is inserted into the vagina.
- The specimen is aspirated from the endocervix.
- Gloves are worn throughout the procedure.

Posttest

- Label the specimen and transport it to the laboratory immediately.
- Report abnormal findings to the primary care provider.

S

> ## Clinical Alerts
>
> - If the procedure is being conducted in the investigation of rape, the specimen collection must be witnessed, and the specimen placed in a sealed plastic bag. The bag is labeled as legal evidence and must be signed by every person handling the specimen.

Sinus Endoscopy

Test Description

Sinus endoscopy is performed to diagnose infection, structural defects, and other abnormalities of the sinuses. It can also involve therapeutic intervention, such as obtaining cultures, removal of polyps or draining of the sinuses. The procedure may be done under general anesthesia in an operating room or under local anesthesia in the ENT office. This discussion will be limited to that done under local anesthesia.

Normal Values

Normal sinuses

Possible Meanings of Abnormal Values

Sinus abnormalities
Cyst
Mucocele
Polyp
Sinusitis
Structural defects

Interventions/Implications

Pretest
- Explain to the patient the purpose of the test. Provide any written teaching materials available on the subject. Note that discomfort involved with this test is primarily due to the possibility of some discomfort and temporary gag reflex with insertion of the scope. Review possible complications of the procedure.
- Fasting may be required before the test.
- Obtain a signed informed consent.

Procedure
- The patient is usually awake and seated upright in a chair.
- A local anesthetic spray is applied to the nose.
- At times, viewing of the throat is also done. If so, local anesthetic spray is also applied to the posterior oropharnyx.
- The endoscope is inserted into a nostril and guided into the sinus cavities.
- Interventions such as obtaining cultures, biopsy, or polyp removal may be done.
- The scope is removed.
- Gloves are worn throughout the procedure.

Posttest
- A gauze pad is taped in place beneath the nose to collect any drainage.
- Monitor the patient for bleeding.
- Ensure there is no numbness of the throat and that swallowing is not impaired before allowing intake of liquids or solids.
- Report abnormal findings to the primary care provider.

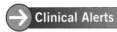

Clinical Alerts

- Possible complications include: Bleeding and cerebrospinal fluid (CSF) leakage.
  - Clear drainage may indicate a cerebrospinal fluid CSF leak and needs to be reported immediately.

CONTRAINDICATIONS!

- Patients who are unable to cooperate because of age, mental status, pain, or other factors.

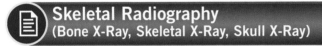

Skeletal Radiography
(Bone X-Ray, Skeletal X-Ray, Skull X-Ray)

Test Description

Radiography is the use of radiation (roentgen rays) to cause some substances to fluoresce and affect photographic plates. X-rays penetrate air easily; therefore areas filled with air, such as the lungs, appear very dark on the film. Conversely, bones appear almost white on the film because the x-rays cannot penetrate them to reach the x-ray film. Organs and tissues such as the heart appear as shades of gray because they have more mass than air but not as much as bone.

Skeletal radiography involves obtaining x-rays of any bone structure in the body. Examples include the spine or vertebral column, long bones, or the skull. The location of the x-ray may become even more precise, such as when an x-ray of the sella turcica, an area at the base of the skull, is ordered.

All x-rays of the skeletal system involve the same basic purposes, preparation, and patient education. They differ in the portion of the body to be studied and the positioning of the patient. The basic principle of position is that the part of the body that needs to be studied be next to the film.

The purpose of skeletal system radiography is to assess the bones for deformities, fractures, dislocations, tumors, and metabolic abnormalities, such as Paget's disease or osteoporosis. The bones are studied for their density, texture, and any erosion. Joint x-rays can reveal the presence of fluid, spur formation, narrowing, or changes in the joint structure. X-rays of the skull provide valuable information regarding the three groups of bones that comprise the skull (the vault, the mandible, and the facial bones) and possible abnormal contents of the skull, such as pituitary tumors.

S

THE EVIDENCE FOR PRACTICE

To determine whether an x-ray is needed for a suspected ankle fracture, the primary care provider can use the Ottawa Rules. An ankle x-ray, including AP, lateral, and mortise views, is recommended when the patient meets any of the following criteria:

1. Inability to bear weight immediately after the injury, *or*
2. Point tenderness over the medial malleolus, or the posterior edge or inferior tip of the lateral malleolus or talus or calcaneus, *or*
3. Inability to ambulate for four steps (Dalinka, Alazraki, Daffner, et al. 2005)

Normal Values

Normal bone structure, location, and density

Possible Meanings of Abnormal Values

Abnormal growth pattern
Arthritis
Bone metastases
Bone spurring
Cerebral hemorrhage
Degenerative arthritis changes
Fractures
Hematoma
Infection
Joint destruction
Joint effusion
Kyphosis
Osteomyelitis
Pituitary tumor
Primary bone tumor
Scoliosis
Sinusitis
Spondylosis

Contributing Factors to Abnormal Values

- Under- or overexposure of the film may alter film quality.
- When patients are unable to hold still, because of age, pain or mental status, the quality of the film may be affected.

Interventions/Implications

Pretest

- Explain to the patient the purpose of the test and the benefits and risks associated with the test. Provide any written teaching materials available on the subject. Note that no discomfort is associated with this procedure.
- No fasting is required before the test.
- Instruct the patient to remove all objects containing metal, such as jewelry or undergarments, as these will show on the film.

Procedure

- The patient's reproductive organs should be covered with a lead apron to prevent unnecessary exposure to radiation.
- Position the patient as ordered. The area to be evaluated must remain motionless during the procedure. Head bands, foam pads, or sandbags may be needed to immobilize the patient's head or extremity being evaluated.

Posttest

- No special physical posttest care is needed.
- Report abnormal findings to the primary care provider.

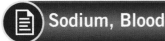

Sodium, Blood

Test Description

Of the electrolytes measured in the blood, sodium (Na^+) is the highest concentration. It is the major cation in the extracellular fluid (ECF). Sodium plays an important role in acid-base balance and promotes neuromuscular functioning. It maintains an inverse relationship with the potassium level of the blood.

Typically, the body uses what it needs from the person's sodium intake and any excess is excreted in the urine. This balance is regulated by several mechanisms. A problem with any of these can cause abnormal blood sodium levels. These mechanisms include production of hormones that increase (natriuretic peptides) or decrease (aldosterone) sodium losses in the urine, and production of antidiuretic hormone (ADH) to prevent water losses. Another mechanism is the use of thirst. When the blood sodium increases, the person will feel thirsty, with the resulting intake of water helping to return the blood sodium to a normal level.

Sodium concentration in the blood is closely related to the fluid balance of the body; in fact, its concentration stimulates the kidneys to compensate for changes in the body's fluid balance. For example, as water in the body increases, the concentration of sodium in the blood decreases. This stimulates the kidneys to compensate through conservation of sodium and excretion of water. This is accomplished through the work of aldosterone. If water in the body decreases, the concentration of sodium in the blood will increase. Antidiuretic hormone (ADH) is then activated, leading to conservation of water.

This test is performed when the patient has symptoms of sodium imbalance or disorders associated with abnormal sodium levels. A decreased level of sodium in the blood is known as hyponatremia. Signs of this imbalance include lethargy, confusion, abdominal cramping, apprehension, oliguria, rapid weak pulse, headache, decreased skin turgor, tremors, and possibly seizures and coma. *Hypernatremia* is the term given to blood sodium levels that are above normal. Signs of this imbalance include dry mucous membranes, fever, thirst, and restlessness.

S

Normal Values

135–145 mEq/L (135–145 mmol/L SI units)

Possible Meanings of Abnormal Values

Increased (Hypernatremia)	Decreased (Hyponatremia)
Cushing's disease	Acute renal failure
Dehydration	Addison's disease

Diabetes insipidus
Exchange transfusion with
   stored blood
Impaired renal function
Overuse of IV saline solutions
Primary aldosteronism
Too much oral salt intake
Tracheobronchitis

Burns (severe)
Chronic renal failure
Cirrhosis
Congestive heart failure
Diabetic acidosis
Diaphoresis
Diarrhea
Edema
Emphysema
Excessive non-electrolyte IV infusions
Gastrointestinal suctioning
Hyperglycemia
Hyperproteinemia
Hypothyroidism
Inadequate sodium intake
Ketonuria
Malabsorption
Nephrotic syndrome
Overdiuresis
Overhydration
Pyloric obstruction
Renal tubular acidosis
Syndrome of inappropriate ADH
Vomiting
Water intoxication

Contributing Factors to Abnormal Values

- Falsely low levels of sodium may be found in blood containing high levels of lipids (hyperlipidemia).
- Drugs that may *increase* the serum sodium level: ampicillin, anabolic steroids, antibiotics, cholestyramine, clonidine, corticosteroids, cough medications, diuretics (loop), doxorubicin, hypernatremic solutions, isosorbide, laxatives, methyldopa, oral contraceptives, progesterones, ramipril, sildenafil, tetracycline.
- Drugs that may *decrease* the serum sodium level: ACE-inhibitors, carbamazepine, carvediolol, chemotherapeutic agents, diuretics, lithium, nicardipine, NSAIDs, pimozide, SSRIs, sulfonylureas, triamterene, valproic acid, vasopressin.

Interventions/Implications

Pretest
- Explain to the patient the purpose of the test and the need for a blood sample to be drawn.
- No fasting is required before the test.

Procedure
- A 7-mL blood sample is drawn in a red-top collection tube.
- Gloves are worn throughout the procedure.

Posttest
- Apply pressure at venipuncture site. Apply dressing, periodically assessing for continued bleeding.
- Label the specimen and transport it to the laboratory.
- Report abnormal findings to the primary care provider.

→ **Clinical Alerts**

- Sodium levels <125 or >152 are considered critical values due to patients becoming symptomatic at these levels. The primary care provider needs to be notified immediately of such values.

Sodium, Urine

Test Description

Sodium (Na⁺) is the major cation in the extracellular fluid (ECF) of the body. It plays an important role in acid-base balance and promotes neuromuscular functioning. Although assessment of the serum sodium level is more common, the measurement of the urine sodium level via a 24-hour urine collection is also very important in determining the cause of abnormal blood sodium levels. It is also useful in assessing whether a patient is adhering to a sodium-restricted diet.

Determination of the sodium level in the urine assists the primary care provider with differential diagnosis when the sodium level in the blood is found to be low, an abnormality called *hyponatremia*. If the cause of this abnormality is due to inadequate sodium intake, the sodium level in the urine will also be low. However, if the cause is due to renal dysfunction, such as chronic renal failure, the sodium level in the urine will be high.

The maintenance of a normal urine sodium level is influenced by several factors, including the patient's dietary intake of sodium, the kidneys' ability to excrete sodium, and the effect of aldosterone (a mineralocorticoid hormone synthesized by the adrenal glands) and antidiuretic hormone (ADH, or vasopressin) which is released from the posterior pituitary. Aldosterone causes increased reabsorption of sodium in the distal tubules of the kidneys, leading to a lower level of sodium in the urine. ADH controls the reabsorption of water in the collecting ducts of the kidney, causing its return to the bloodstream. This results in decreased water in the urine and a corresponding increase in the urine sodium level. There is a diurnal variation of sodium excretion, with excretion being greater during daytime than during the night.

Normal Values

15–250 mEq/L/day (15–250 mmol/L/day SI units), depending on hydration status and daily intake of dietary sodium.

Possible Meanings of Abnormal Values

Increased	Decreased
Adrenal cortical insufficiency	Acute renal failure
Chronic renal failure	Congestive heart failure

S

Dehydration	Cushing's disease
Diabetic acidosis	Diabetes insipidus
Fever	Diaphoresis
Head trauma	Diarrhea
Hypothyroidism	Hypovolemia
Increased sodium intake	Inadequate sodium intake
Renal tubular acidosis	Liver disease
Salicylate intoxication	Malabsorption
Starvation	Nephrotic syndrome
Syndrome of inappropriate ADH	Prerenal azotemia
Toxemia of pregnancy	Primary aldosteronism
Use of diuretics	Pulmonary emphysema
	Pyloric obstruction

Contributing Factors to Abnormal Values

- Drugs that may *increase* urine sodium levels: loop diuretics.
- Drugs that may *decrease* urine sodium levels: corticosteroids.

Interventions/Implications

Pretest

- Explain 24-hour urine collection procedure to the patient.
- Stress the importance of saving *all* urine in the 24-hour period. Instruct the patient to avoid contaminating the urine with toilet paper or feces.
- No fasting is required before the test.

Procedure

- Obtain the proper container containing no preservative from the laboratory.
- Begin the testing period in the morning after the patient's first voiding, which is discarded.
- Timing of the 24-hour period begins at the time the first voiding is discarded.
- *All* urine for the next 24 hours is collected in the container, which is to be kept refrigerated or on ice.
- If any urine is accidentally discarded during the 24-hour period, the test must be discontinued and a new test begun.
- The ending time of the 24-hour collection period should be posted in the patient's room.
- Gloves are worn whenever dealing with the specimen collection.

Posttest

- At the end of the 24-hour collection period, label and send the urine container to the laboratory as soon as possible.
- Report abnormal findings to the primary care provider.

→ **Clinical Alerts**

- A 24-hour urine of <100 mEq/day reflects adherence to a sodium-restricted diet.

Somatomedin C (Insulin-Like Growth Factor-1 [IGF-1])

Test Description

Human growth hormone stimulates the secretion of peptide hormones produced in the liver known as somatomedins. These hormones are involved in cartilage and collagen formation, increased glucose metabolism, and amino acid transport in the diaphragm and heart. Somatomedin C, also known as insulin-like growth factor-1 (IGF-1) is affected by growth hormone activity. Thus, measurement of IGF-1 provides information regarding the amount of growth hormone present. This test is also useful in monitoring the patient's response to growth hormone treatment in pituitary dwarfism, and to evaluate the severity of acromegaly.

THE EVIDENCE FOR PRACTICE

Once acromegaly is suspected, measurement of serum insulin-like growth factor-1 (IGF-1) should be the next step. Acromegaly in the absence of high IGF-1 levels is extremely rare; therefore, this relationship makes IGF-1 an ideal screening test. IGF-1 is also useful for monitoring of treatment outcomes, such as after a surgical procedure or during treatment with octreotide or pegvisomant. (Cook, 2004)

Normal Values

16–24 years:	182–780 ng/mL (182–780 g/L SI units)
25–39 years:	114–492 ng/mL (114–492 g/L SI units)
40–54 years:	90–360 ng/mL (90–360 g/L SI units)
>54 years:	71–290 ng/mL (71–290 g/L SI units)

Possible Meanings of Abnormal Values

Increased	Decreased
Acromegaly	Anorexia nervosa
Gigantism	Chronic illness
Hyperpituitarism	Cirrhosis of the liver
Hypoglycemia	Delayed puberty
Liver cancer	Diabetes mellitus
Obesity	Dwarfism
Precocious puberty	Emotional deprivation syndrome
Pregnancy	Growth hormone deficiency
Wilms' tumor	Hypopituitarism
	Hypothyroidism
	Kwashiorkor
	Laron's dwarfism
	Malnutrition
	Physiologic stress
	Pituitary tumor

S

Contributing Factors to Abnormal Values

- Radioactive scans within 7 days before this test may falsely elevate test results.

- Drugs that may *increase* somatomedin C levels: corticosteroids.
- Drugs that may *decrease* somatomedin C levels: estrogens, octreotide, pegvisomant.

Interventions/Implications

Pretest

- Explain to the patient the purpose of the test and the need for a blood sample to be drawn.
- No fasting is required before the test.

Procedure

- A 7-mL blood sample is drawn in a red-top collection tube.
- Gloves are worn throughout the procedure.

Posttest

- Apply pressure at venipuncture site. Apply dressing, periodically assessing for continued bleeding.
- Label the specimen and transport it to the laboratory.
- Report abnormal findings to the primary care provider.

 Sputum Culture and Sensitivity (Sputum C & S)

Test Description

Sputum cultures are often used to aid in the differential diagnosis of bacterial, fungal, parasitic, and viral lower respiratory tract infections. However, the results obtained from such cultures can be misleading to the clinician if the sputum specimen is contaminated with the normal flora found in upper airway secretions. To assess acceptability of a sputum sample for culture, the laboratory first performs a Gram stain. Evidence of oropharyngeal contamination makes a specimen unsuitable for culture and a repeat sputum specimen collection is needed. Culture procedures differ depending on the organism suspected, thus the requisition slip should clearly indicate the suspected causative agent. Following culture, susceptibility or sensitivity testing is performed to guide the clinician in the selection of an appropriate antimicrobial agent.

Normal Values

The presence or absence of normal respiratory flora is reported.
No presence of disease-causing organisms in the sputum.

Possible Meanings of Abnormal Values

Bacterial infections (e.g., pneumonia, tuberculosis)
Fungal infections
Parasitic infections
Viral infections

Contributing Factors to Abnormal Values

- Contamination of the specimen, collection of saliva rather than sputum, and delay in specimen delivery to laboratory can alter test results.
- Initiating antimicrobial therapy prior to collection of the sputum can alter test results.

Interventions/Implications

Pretest
- The sputum should be collected before antimicrobial therapy is begun.
- Explain to the patient the purpose of the test and the procedure:
    - An early morning specimen is best, since sputum is most concentrated at that time.
    - The patient should brush the teeth and rinse the mouth with water before collecting the sputum to reduce contamination of the sample with normal upper respiratory tract flora.
    - The sputum must be from the bronchial tree. The patient must understand that this is different than saliva in the mouth.
    - Teach the patient how to expectorate sputum by taking three deep breaths and forcing a deep cough.
    - The sample is collected in a sterile sputum container.
- If tuberculosis is suspected, multiple morning specimens may be ordered.
- If the sputum is very thick, it can be thinned by inhaling nebulized saline or water, or by increasing fluid intake the evening before sample collection. Postural drainage and chest physiotherapy may also be helpful.

Procedure
- The patient should take several deep breaths and then cough deeply to obtain the specimen. At least one teaspoon of sputum is needed.
- Other ways to collect sputum include endotracheal suctioning, transtracheal aspiration, fiberoptic bronchoscopy, and gastric lavage.
- Following collection, the sample is sent to the laboratory. The laboratory determines the suitability of the specimen for culture by performing a Gram stain and microscopic evaluation. Sputum contaminated with upper respiratory secretions will contain an increased number of epithelial cells.
- Preliminary information about the primary microorganism present is also recorded during the initial microscopic examination.
- The sputum sample is then inoculated onto appropriate culture media and incubated.
- Final reports and susceptibility testing of most bacterial agents require 48 to 72 hours, whereas fungal cultures can take up to 4 weeks, and mycobacteria (i.e., tuberculous agents) cultures can take up to 6 weeks for a final report.

S

Posttest
- Label the specimen container and send to the laboratory as soon as possible. Note the suspected microorganism and any current antimicrobial therapy on the label. Do not refrigerate the specimen.
- Begin antimicrobial therapy as ordered *after* collection of the specimen.
- When available, report results of the cultural and sensitivity to the primary care provider so that modifications in drug therapy are made if needed.
- Report abnormal findings to the primary care provider.

→ Clinical Alerts

- The clinician must evaluate the significance of the types and numbers present of each microbe noted in the sputum C & S report.

Sputum Cytology

Test Description

Sputum cytology is used in the diagnosis of a variety of respiratory conditions. These include malignant conditions, as well as cellular changes of a premalignant nature, such as those seen with inflammation and inhaled toxins. Cytologic study of the sputum also assists in the diagnosis of tuberculosis, bacterial infection, parasitic infection, and viral infection.

Normal Values

Negative

Possible Meanings of Abnormal Values

Asbestosis
Asthma
Bacterial infections
Bronchiectasis
Cancer
Emphysema
Inflammatory disease
Lipid pneumonia
Parasitic infections
Pneumonitis
Tuberculosis
Viral infection

Contributing Factors to Abnormal Values

- Contamination of the specimen, collection of saliva rather than sputum, and delay in specimen delivery to laboratory can alter test results.

Interventions/Implications

Pretest
- Explain the procedure to the patient, stressing that:
    - An early morning specimen is best, since sputum is most concentrated at that time.
    - The patient should brush the teeth and rinse the mouth with water before collecting the sputum to reduce contamination of the sample with normal upper respiratory tract flora.
    - The sputum must be from the bronchial tree. The patient must understand that this is different from saliva in the mouth.
- Teach the patient how to expectorate sputum by taking three deep breaths and forcing a deep cough.
- If the sputum is very thick, it can be thinned by inhaling nebulized saline or water, or by increasing fluid intake the evening before sample collection. Postural drainage and chest physiotherapy may also be helpful.

Procedure
- The patient is instructed to take several deep breaths and then cough deeply to obtain the specimen. At least one teaspoon of sputum is needed.
- Other ways to collect sputum include endotracheal suctioning and fiberoptic bronchoscopy.
- Gloves are worn when handling the specimen.

Posttest
- Label the specimen container and send to the laboratory immediately.
- Report abnormal findings to the primary care provider.

 ## Stool Culture/Stool for Ova & Parasites

Test Description
The gastrointestinal (GI) tract contains many bacteria and fungi as its normal flora. When some of this normal flora is suppressed in some way, as with antibiotic use or immunosuppression, the remaining bacteria can become pathogenic. In addition, pathogens may enter the GI tract, causing symptoms such as persistent or bloody diarrhea, abdominal pain, and fever. Some pathogens cause symptoms directly and others, such as *Clostridium difficile*, cause symptoms through the toxins they produce.

People may be exposed to enteric pathogens in a variety of ways. For example, exposure may occur when traveling outside of the United States or through dietary intake of undercooked food or contaminated food and water. It is important to identify the pathogens to assist with treatment planning and prevention of complications.

A stool culture is done to isolate and identify organisms which might be causing GI symptoms. The culture is also warranted if there are leukocytes (WBCs) in the stool. In most laboratories, routine stool cultures are limited to screening for *Salmonella* and *Shigella* species, and *Campylobacter jejuni*. Testing for *E. coli* may require a special order.

Stool for ova and parasites tests for the presence of a parasite or worm-like infection of the intestine, or ova, the egg stage of a parasite's development. This test is indicated for patients who have recently traveled, those with persistent diarrhea, or when the diarrhea has been unresponsive to antimicrobial therapy. Testing typically enables identification of *Giardia lamblia* and *Entamoeba histolytica*.

THE EVIDENCE FOR PRACTICE
Any illness involving diarrhea that persists for greater than 7 days, especially in an immunocompromised patient, should prompt further testing of stool specimens.

Normal Values
Normal intestinal flora
Negative for pathogens

Possible Meanings of Abnormal Values

Positive
Bacterial enterocolitis
Parasitic enterocolitis
Protozoal enterocolitis

Contributing Factors to Abnormal Values

Drugs that may cause *false-negative* results: antibiotics, barium, bismuth, mineral oil.

Interventions/Implications

Pretest
- Explain to the patient the purpose of the test and the need for a stool sample to be collected.
- Instruct the patient to avoid contaminating the stool with toilet paper or urine. This can be done through use of a plastic collection receptacle in the toilet.
- No fasting is required before the test.

Procedure
- Obtain a 5-mL stool specimen in a plastic screw-cap container for the stool culture.
- Special vials for collection of stool to be tested for ova and parasites are commercially available. Such vials contain a fixative which allows the sample to remain at room temperature.
- An alternative method for obtaining stool is by inserting a cotton-tipped swab into the rectum approximately 1 in and rotating it to obtain a small specimen.
- Gloves are worn when dealing with the specimen collection.

Posttest
- The sample is labeled and transported to the laboratory as soon as possible after collection of the specimen.
- Report abnormal findings to the primary care provider.

→ **Clinical Alerts**

- Patients complaining of diarrhea for at least 2 weeks usually have stool analysis performed, often including stool for WBCs, stool culture, stool for ova and parasites, *Clostridium difficile*, and possibly Giardia.
- Follow-up stool analysis may be done if symptoms persist despite initial stool tests having negative results, or to demonstrate the pathogen is no longer present in the stool.

Stool for Occult Blood (Fecal Occult Blood Test [FOBT], Fecal Immunochemical Test [FIT])

Test Description
Bleeding in the gastrointestinal (GI) tract can occur as a result of some medications and many disease processes. Bleeding from the upper portion of the GI tract, such as from gastric ulcers, results in black, tarry stools. Bleeding from the lower GI tract, such as from hemorrhoids, usually causes bright red blood. Testing for occult blood

in the stool can detect blood loss of 5 mL/day or more. Most importantly is the need for detection of cancer of the GI tract, especially colorectal cancer. Early detection of this disease is essential to provide the best possible chance of survival.

Testing of stool for evaluation of possible cancer includes fecal occult blood testing (FOBT), fecal immunochemical testing (FIT), testing for immunochemical markers that may indicate cancerous growths, and testing for DNA markers that signal precancerous and cancerous growths.

There are now two methods for occult blood stool testing. One method is guaiac-based testing and the other is human hemoglobin-based testing. Guaiac-based FOBT detects heme perioxidase activity and is not specific for human hemoglobin. This can lead to false-positive results due to intake of some foods and medications prior to the test. Fecal immunochemical testing (FIT) is sensitive only to human hemoglobin, so that foods and medications are not likely to interfere with the test results. Currently, guaiac-based FOBT remains the most commonly used screening test, primarily due to cost and the fact that some insurers consider FIT to still be investigational. However, the American Cancer Society notes that "in comparison with guaiac-based tests for the detection of occult blood, immunochemical tests are more patient-friendly and are likely to be equal or better in sensitivity and specificity." (Smith, Cokkinides, and Eyre, 2003)

THE EVIDENCE FOR PRACTICE

The U.S. Preventive Services Task Force (USPSTF) strongly recommends that clinicians screen men and women 50 years of age or older for colorectal cancer. The USPSTF found good evidence that periodic FOBT reduces mortality from colorectal cancer.

Normal Values

Negative

Possible Meanings of Abnormal Values

Positive

Anal fissure
Colon polyp
Diaphragmatic hernia
Diverticulitis
Esophageal varices
Esophagitis
Gastritis
GI cancer (gastric, colon)
GI trauma, including surgery
Hemorrhoids
Inflammatory bowel disease (Crohn's disease, ulcerative colitis)
Peptic ulcer

Contributing Factors to Abnormal Values

- Red meats and foods with high perioxidase activity (beets, broccoli, cantaloupe, cauliflower, horseradish, parsnips, and turnips) cause *false-positive* test results with guaiac-based FOBT.

- Drugs that may cause *false-positive* results with guaiac-based FOBT: aspirin, boric acid, bromides, colchicine, iodine, iron preparations, nonsteroidal anti-inflammatory drugs (NSAIDs), potassium, reserpine, salicylates, steroids, thiazide diuretics.
- Drugs that may cause *false-negative* results with guaiac-based FOBT: ascorbic acid.

Interventions/Implications

Pretest
- Explain to the patient the purpose of the test and the need for a small sample of stool.
- No fasting is required before the test. For guaiac-based FOBT, the patient should follow a diet of no red meats or foods with high perioxidase activity (beets, broccoli, cantaloupe, cauliflower, horseradish, parsnips, and turnips) for 24 to 48 hours prior to the test.
- Aspirin and NSAIDs should be avoided for 2 days before the test.

Procedure

For guaiac smear
- A small amount of stool is smeared on the indicated area of commercially available FOBT cards. The sample can be obtained through digital rectal exam in the office or by the patient collecting a small amount of stool and smearing it with a wooden stick onto the card.
- The card cover is then closed.
- In the office, two drops of developing solution is then applied to the indicated areas.
- Patients completing the testing at home return the cards to the office for processing. Home testing includes sampling three consecutive stools.
- Gloves are worn when dealing with the specimen collection.

Posttest
- Once the developing solution is applied, the results are read in 30 to 120 seconds. The appearance of a blue color on the card indicates the presence of blood.
- Cards completed at home need to be tested within 14 days of collection.
- Report abnormal findings to the primary care provider.

 Clinical Alerts

S

- Stool testing for blood, via FOBT or FIT, is recommended to be done on an annual basis.
- Positive occult blood testing requires follow-up testing to determine the source of the bleeding.

 Sweat Test (Sweat Electrolytes)

Test Description
Cystic fibrosis is a hereditary disease that affects the exocrine glands of the body. The mucous glands produce very thick mucus, which is especially problematic in the lungs. There is also malfunctioning of the pancreatic exocrine gland. Sweat levels

of sodium, potassium, and chloride are abnormally elevated in children with cystic fibrosis and in genetic carriers of the disease.

This test involves the stimulation of sweat production by iontophoresis, the painless delivery of a small electrical current to the skin that causes the transportation of positive pilocarpine ions into the skin from gel pads applied to the skin. Once sweating has been stimulated, preweighed sodium chloride free filter paper is attached to the area and allowed to remain for 30 minutes to collect the sweat. Sweat sodium values of >90 mEq/L and chloride values of >60 mEq/L are indicative of cystic fibrosis.

Normal Values

Sodium
Normal:	<70 mEq/L
Abnormal:	>90 mEq/L
Equivocal:	70–90 mEq/L

Chloride
Normal:	<50 mEq/L
Abnormal:	>60 mEq/L
Equivocal:	50–60 mEq/L

Possible Meanings of Abnormal Values

Increased	Decreased
Addison's disease	Hypoaldosteronism
Adrenal insufficiency	Sodium depletion
Cystic fibrosis	
Diabetes insipidus	
Ectodermal dysplasia	
Glucose-6-phosphate-dehydrogenase deficiency	
Hypothyroidism	
Malnutrition	
Mucopolysaccharidosis	
Renal failure	

Contributing Factors to Abnormal Values

- Drugs that may *decrease* sweat chloride levels: mineralocorticoids.

Interventions/Implications

Pretest
- Explain to the patient/parent the purpose of the test and how it will be conducted.
- No fasting is required before the test.
- Obtain a signed informed consent.

Procedure
- Wash with distilled water and dry the site to be stimulated. The flexor surface of either forearm is the preferred site.

- A small amount of pilocarpine-soaked gauze is applied to the skin and attached to the positive electrode.
- A small amount of saline-soaked gauze is also applied to the skin and attached to the negative electrode.
- A 4 mA current is delivered in 15 to 20 second intervals for 5 minutes.
- Remove and discard the electrodes.
- Place a preweighed, dry gauze pad or filter paper on the site previously covered by the pilocarpine pad, cover it with plastic and seal the edges with water proof tape or cover the pad with paraffin.
- After 30 minutes, remove and discard the tape and plastic.
- Remove the gauze or filter paper with forceps and place it in a weighing bottle.
- Gloves are worn throughout the procedure.

Posttest
- Seal and label the bottle, and transport it to the laboratory immediately.
- Wash the iontophoresed area with soap and water, and dry thoroughly. Redness of the area will disappear within a few hours.
- Report abnormal findings to the primary care provider.

Clinical Alerts

- Resources for patients with cystic fibrosis and their families are available from the Cystic Fibrosis Foundation (www.cff.org).

Syphilis Serology (VDRL, RPR, FTA-ABS)

Test Description

Syphilis is a systemic, infectious disease caused by the spirochete *Treponema pallidum*. The organism is transmitted primarily through direct sexual contact. It can also be transmitted via the placenta from mother to fetus. If untreated, infected individuals can develop irreversible complications such as chronic inflammation of the joints, cardiovascular problems such as valvular involvement, and central nervous system problems such as mental illness and paralysis.

Laboratory diagnosis of syphilis can be made through direct and indirect tests. Direct tests, such as scraping of syphilis lesions, identify the causative organism. Indirect tests, such as the syphilis serologic tests, identify antibodies of the causative agent. These antibodies do not appear in the serum until 3 to 4 weeks after the appearance of the syphilis chancre, an ulcer located at the site where the organism initially enters the body.

The syphilis serology includes the VDRL, RPR, and FTA-ABS tests. The Venereal Disease Research Laboratory (VDRL) test and the rapid plasma regain (RPR) test are screening tests. In both of these tests, agglutination occurs in the presence of the syphilis antigen. Both of these tests have a high false-positive rate. Conditions such as infectious mononucleosis, rheumatoid arthritis, and malaria can cause false-positive reactions. Because of the high possibility of a false-positive result, any positive, or reactive VDRL or RPR test must be followed with a confirmatory test, such as the FTA-ABS. This test identifies the antibodies that are specific against *T. pallidum*. The FTA-ABS (fluorescent treponemal antibody absorption) test is the most sensitive test used to diagnose syphilis following a positive VDRL or RPR. This test will remain positive for life even if an individual has received appropriate treatment.

THE EVIDENCE FOR PRACTICE

The U.S. Preventive Services Task Force (USPSTF):

- Strongly recommends that clinicians screen persons at increased risk for syphilis infection.
  - Populations at increased risk for syphilis infection include men who have sex with men and engage in high-risk sexual behavior, commercial sex workers, persons who exchange sex for drugs, and those in adult correctional facilities.
  - Clinicians should use clinical judgment to individualize screening for syphilis infection based on local prevalence and other risk factors for those persons diagnosed with other sexually transmitted diseases.
- Strongly recommends that clinicians screen all pregnant women for syphilis infection.
- Recommends against routine screening of asymptomatic persons who are not at increased risk for syphilis infection.

Normal Values

Negative (Nonreactive)

Possible Meanings of Abnormal Values

Positive
Syphilis

Contributing Factors to Abnormal Values

- Hemolysis of the blood sample, presence of lipemia, and the intake of alcohol may alter test results.
- Conditions that can cause *false-positive VDRL or RPR* results: atypical pneumonia, brucellosis, HIV, infectious hepatitis, leprosy, Lyme disease, malaria, mononucleosis, pinta, pregnancy, systemic lupus erythematosus, typhus, yaws.
- The presence of antinuclear antibodies can cause *false-positive* RPR results.
- Conditions that can cause *false-positive FTA-ABS* results: diseases with increased or abnormal globins, patients with systemic lupus erythematosus, positive antinuclear antibodies (ANA), yaws, pinta, and pregnancy.

Interventions/Implications

Pretest

- Explain to the patient the purpose of the test and the need for a blood sample to be drawn.

- No fasting is required before the test.
- No alcohol is allowed for 24 hours before the test.

Procedure
- A 7-mL blood sample is drawn in a red-top collection tube.
- Gloves are worn throughout the procedure.

Posttest
- Apply pressure at venipuncture site. Apply dressing, periodically assessing for continued bleeding.
- Label the specimen and transport it to the laboratory.
- Report abnormal findings to the primary care provider.

→ **Clinical Alerts**

- Positive screening test results require follow-up confirmatory testing.
- Positive confirmatory test results should be followed with appropriate antibiotic therapy and education of the patient.
- Monitoring of RPR is helpful in assessing effectiveness of therapy.
- The VDRL test is most sensitive to detect syphilis during the middle stages; it is less sensitive during the earlier and later stages.
- A positive FTA-ABS will remain positive for life even if an individual has received appropriate treatment.

Testosterone

Test Description

Measurement of testosterone levels in the blood, when analyzed in conjunction with follicle-stimulating hormone (FSH) and luteinizing hormone (LH) levels, assists in the evaluation of gonadal dysfunction in both sexes.

In males, testosterone is the primary androgen secreted by the interstitial cells of the testes, known as Leydig cells. Testosterone promotes the growth and development of the male sex organs, contributes to the enlargement of voluntary muscle, stimulates the growth of axillary, facial, and pubic hair, and promotes spermatogenesis. Testosterone is evaluated in workups for impotency and infertility

In females, testosterone is secreted in small amounts by the ovaries and adrenal glands. Peak levels are noted at midcycle. The test is used for evaluation of ovarian tumors, hirsutism, and infertility.

Free or unbound testosterone is the active form; however, only in certain conditions such as hyperthyroidism is free measurement helpful. Typically, total testosterone is measured with highest levels found in the morning.

THE EVIDENCE FOR PRACTICE

The Endocrine Society Task Force:

- Recommends making a diagnosis of androgen deficiency only in men with consistent symptoms and signs and unequivocally low serum testosterone levels.
- Suggests the measurement of morning total testosterone level by a reliable assay as the initial test for the diagnosis of androgen deficiency in men.
- Recommends confirmation of the diagnosis by repeating the measurement of morning total testosterone and in some patients by measurement of free or bioavailable testosterone level, using an appropriate assay system.

Normal Values

Female
- Prepubertal child: 3–10 ng/dL (0.1–0.35 nmol/L SI units)
- Premenopause: 24–47 ng/dL (0.83–1.63 nmol/L SI units)
- Postmenopause: 7–40 ng/dL (0.24–1.4 nmol/L SI units)

Male
- Prepubertal child: 10–20 ng/dL (0.35–0.7 nmol/L SI units)
- Adult: 437–707 ng/dL (15.2–24.2 nmol/L SI units)

Possible Meanings of Abnormal Values

Increased (Male)	Decreased (Female)
Adrenal tumor	AIDS
Androgen secreting tumor	Bilateral cryptorchidism
Celiac sprue	Chronic renal failure
Cushing's syndrome	Cirrhosis
Hyperthyroidism	Congenital adrenal hyperplasia
Precocious puberty	Delayed puberty
Reifenstein's syndrome	Down syndrome
	Klinefelter's syndrome
	Myotonic dystrophy
	Primary hypogonadism
	Secondary hypogonadism

Increased (Females)

Adrenal tumor
Cushing's syndrome
Molar pregnancy
Obesity
Polycystic ovarian disease
Supplements (containing androgens)
Virilizing ovarian tumors

Contributing Factors to Abnormal Values

- Drugs that may *increase* testosterone levels in females: anticonvulsants, bromocriptine, clomiphene, danazol, estrogens, minoxidil, pravastatin, rifampin, tamoxifen.
- Drugs that may *increase* testosterone levels in males: bicalutamide, cimetidine, finasteride, lupron, nilutamide, phenytoin, pravastatin, rifampin, tamoxifen, valproic acid.

- Drugs that may *decrease* testosterone levels in males: carbamazepine, cimetidine, corticosteroids, cyclophosphamide, digoxin, estrogens, finasteride, gemfibrozil, goserelin, ketoconazole, leuprolide, narcotics, pravastatin, spironolactone, tetracycline, verapamil.

Interventions/Implications

Pretest
- Explain to the patient the purpose of the test and the need for a blood sample to be drawn.
- No fasting is required before the test.
- Sample should be drawn at 7 AM, when levels are highest.

Procedure
- A 7-mL blood sample is drawn in a collection tube.
- Gloves are worn throughout the procedure.

Posttest
- Apply pressure at venipuncture site. Apply dressing, periodically assessing for continued bleeding.
- Label the specimen and transport it to the laboratory.
- Report abnormal findings to the primary care provider.

→ **Clinical Alerts**

- Low testosterone levels, along with low LH and FSH levels, are diagnostic of secondary hypogonadism.

Therapeutic Drug Monitoring

Test Description

Therapeutic drug monitoring is used to manage individual patient drug therapy. Such testing is essential when there is a narrow margin of safety between therapeutic drug effect and drug toxicity. Examples of drugs requiring monitoring are aminophylline, digoxin, lithium, and phenytoin.

Oftentimes drugs being monitored are those that will need to be taken for the person's lifetime. Monitoring drug levels periodically assists the primary care provider in adjusting drug dosages to allow for changes in the person's condition and age. Drug monitoring can also identify patients who may not be taking their medication as prescribed and identify possible drug interactions.

Timing of blood collection is very important when conducting therapeutic drug monitoring. When a drug is taken, the serum level of the drug rises, peaks, and then begins to fall. Its lowest level, known as its trough, occurs just before the next dose. For the drug to be most effective the peak levels should be below toxic concentrations and the trough levels should remain in the therapeutic range. An example of using peak and trough levels is the monitoring done of patients receiving aminoglycosides.

These antimicrobials, which are used for severe infections, are nephrotoxic and ototoxic. Thus, it is essential that the serum drug level is high enough to treat the infection, yet low enough to avoid toxic complications.

Normal Values

Depends on specific drug being monitored and reference laboratory used

Possible Meanings of Abnormal Values

Increased	Decreased
Toxic drug levels	Subtherapeutic drug levels

Interventions/Implications

Pretest
- Explain to the patient the purpose of the test and the need for a blood sample to be drawn.
- No fasting is required before the test.

Procedure
- A 7- to 10-mL blood sample is drawn in the type of tube designated by the reference laboratory.
- Gloves are worn during the procedure.

Posttest
- Apply pressure at venipuncture site. Apply dressing, periodically assessing for continued bleeding.
- Label the specimen and transport it to the laboratory.
- Report abnormal findings to the primary care provider.

→ Clinical Alerts

- Assess for patient understanding regarding the medication dosing and determine whether the patient is taking the medication, and if so, whether correct dosing is being maintained.
- Discuss with the patient any changes needed in drug dosage or frequency of dosing based on the test results.

T

Thoracentesis (Pleural Fluid Analysis, Pleural Fluid Aspiration, Pleural Tap)

Test Description

Thoracentesis refers to the removal of fluid from the pleural cavity. This cavity is the space between the visceral pleura, which covers the lungs, and the parietal pleural which lines the chest cavity. In some conditions, such as inflammatory diseases of the lungs and neoplasms, a large amount of pleural fluid may accumulate in the pleural cavity, an assessment finding known as *pleural effusion*. Other substances, such as air (pneumothorax) or blood (hemothorax), may also be present in the pleural cavity.

Thoracentesis may be done for diagnostic purposes to determine the cause of the fluid production, or for therapeutic purposes to remove up to 1000 mL of fluid at any one time. The fluid is then analyzed for red and white blood cell counts, cytologic studies, bacterial and fungal cultures, and determination of glucose, lactic dehydrogenase, and protein levels. For patients with pleural effusion due to malignancy, intrapleural chemotherapy has the potential advantage of treating the underlying malignancy, in addition to treating the effusion.

The fluid is categorized as either an *exudate*, which is high-protein fluid that has leaked from blood vessels with increased permeability, or a *transudate*, a low-protein fluid leaked from normal blood vessels. An exudate may be caused by blocked lymphatic drainage, infection, neoplasm, pancreatitis, pulmonary infarction, rheumatoid arthritis, systemic lupus erythematosus, trauma, and tuberculosis. Transudate is caused by ascites, cirrhosis, congestive heart failure, hypertension, nephritis, and nephrosis.

Normal Values

Gross appearance:	Clear, odorless
Amount:	<20 mL
Specific gravity:	<1.016
Bacteria:	None
Cell counts:	Red blood cells: Few
	White blood cells: Few lymphocytes
Cytology:	No malignant cells present
Fibrinogen (clot):	None
Fungi:	None
Glucose:	Equal to serum level
Lactic dehydrogenase:	Equal to serum level
Protein:	<3 g/dL

Possible Meanings of Abnormal Values

Color
Milk colored: Chyle present
Cloudy fluid: Inflammation
Bloody fluid: Caused by hemothorax, traumatic tap

Bacteria (present)
Ruptured pulmonary abscess
Infection
Tuberculosis

Fungi (present)
Candidiasis

Coccidioidomycosis
Histoplasmosis

Glucose (decreased)
Bacterial infection
Malignancy
Metastasis
Nonseptic inflammation

Lactic dehydrogenase (increased)
Malignancy

Protein (increased)
Collagen vascular disease
Infection
Neoplasm
Pulmonary infarction
Trauma
Tuberculosis

Red blood cells (increased)
Chest trauma
Hemothorax
Neoplasm
Traumatic tap

White blood cells (increased)
Fungal effusion
Inflammation
Tuberculosis
Viral effusion

Contributing Factors to Abnormal Values

- Antimicrobial therapy, if started prior to the test, may decrease the bacterial count.
- Contamination of the specimen will alter white blood cell count.

Interventions/Implications

Pretest

- Explain to the patient the purpose of the test and the procedure to be done. Explain that a local anesthetic will be used, but that a pressure-like pain will occur as the needle pierces the pleura and as the fluid is being withdrawn. Explain that no movement, including deep breathing or coughing, can occur during the test.
- No fasting is required prior to the test.
- Complete blood count (CBC), platelet count, and coagulation studies are obtained.
- Obtain a signed informed consent.
- A chest x-ray or ultrasound is usually done before the test to locate the fluid and to avoid accidental puncture of the lung.
- Obtain baseline assessment information, including vital signs and weight.
- Pulse oximetry may be ordered for use throughout the procedure.

Procedure
- Assist the patient to a sitting position leaning forward with the arms supported on an overbed table. Provide support for the arms and head with pillows. If the patient cannot tolerate this position, an alternative position is lying on the unaffected side with the head of the bed elevated 30 to 45 degrees.
- Monitor vital signs every 15 minutes during the procedure.
- Sterile technique is used throughout the procedure.
- The area is cleansed and draped.
- A local anesthetic is administered.
- A 20-gauge or large needle attached to a 50-mL syringe and a three-way stopcock is inserted through the parietal pleura.
- When the pocket of fluid is reached, a 50-mL sample of the fluid is obtained.
- If additional fluid is to be drained, connect tubing between the cannula and the collection receptacle.
- A maximum of 1000 mL is allowed to drain slowly from the site. Rapid drainage, and thus hypovolemia, can be avoided by either raising the collection receptacle to slow the draining or by clamping the tubing.
- Throughout drainage of the pleural effusion, assess for respiratory distress: weakness, dyspnea, pallor, cyanosis, tachypnea, diaphoresis, hypotension, and blood-tinged frothy mucus. Treatment may be needed for bradycardia owing to vasovagal effect.
- Patients with pleural effusions caused by malignancies may have antineoplastic drugs injected into the pleural cavity through the stopcock prior to needle removal.
- When the procedure is complete, the needle is removed. A pressure dressing is applied.
- Gloves are worn throughout the procedure.

Posttest
- Turn the patient on the *unaffected* side for 1 hour to allow for lung expansion.
- Monitor vital signs until stable.
- Check the dressing frequently for drainage. Assess the puncture site for bleeding and the presence of crepitus. Assess breath sounds.
- Continue to observe the patient for any respiratory distress. A postprocedure chest x-ray may be ordered to assess for the presence of hemothorax, pneumothorax, tension pneumothorax, or accumulation of additional fluid.
- Label the specimen and transport it to the laboratory immediately.
- Report abnormal findings to the primary care provider.

T

→ **Clinical Alerts**

- Possible complications include: air embolism, hemothorax, pneumothorax, pulmonary edema, reaction to antineoplastic drugs, shock and hypovolemia

CONTRAINDICATIONS!

- Patients with bleeding disorders
- Patients who are unable to cooperate during the procedure

Thoracoscopy

Test Description

Thoracoscopy is a procedure in which small incisions are made in the chest wall and a thoracoscope is inserted. This procedure allows the physician to examine the parietal and visceral pleura, mediastinum, and pericardium. The procedure is done to obtain tissue and fluid samples, diagnose and stage cancer, remove fluid, and introduce medications into the pleural cavity. Although it is considered a surgical procedure, thoracoscopy results in a shorter hospital and recovery time than would occur with thoracotomy.

Normal Values

Normal appearance of structures; no infection or malignancy

Possible Meanings of Abnormal Values

Coccidioidomycosis
Empyema
Histoplasmosis
Inflammation
Metastatic cancer
Pleural effusion
Primary lung cancer
Tuberculosis

Interventions/Implications

Pretest

- Explain to the patient the purpose of the procedure. Provide any written teaching materials available on the subject. Note that discomfort involved with this procedure is primarily postprocedural incisional discomfort and presence of chest tube. Review possible complications of procedure.
- Fasting for 8 hours is required before the procedure.
- Preoperative blood tests, chest x-ray, and electrocardiogram are done.
- Skin preparation may be needed.
- Obtain a signed informed consent.

Procedure

- An intravenous line is initiated.
- The patient is given general anesthesia and placed in a lateral decubitus position.
- Several small incisions are made in the chest wall.
- The lung to be examined is deflated to allow space for examination of the pleura and the lung.
- An endoscope is inserted to carefully examine the lung and pleural cavity and to obtain tissue/fluid samples.
- After removal of the endoscope, all of the incisions but one are sutured closed.

T

- A chest tube is inserted into the remaining incision for drainage and to allow re-expansion of the lung.
- Sterile surgical technique is followed throughout the procedure.

Posttest

- Typical postoperative recovery is done in terms of vital sign assessment, monitoring of respiratory, cardiovascular, and neurological status, checking dressings and chest tube drainage, and monitoring for complications.
- Typical hospital stay postprocedure is 2 to 5 days.
- Strenuous activity, heavy lifting, and driving must be avoided for several weeks.
- Report abnormal findings to the primary care provider.

→ Clinical Alerts

- Possible complications include: air leak, bleeding, infection, pain or numbness at the incision sites, and pneumonia.
- Instruct patient to notify physician for presence of: dyspnea, chest pain, fever, hemoptysis, redness/drainage from incision.

CONTRAINDICATIONS!

- Patients with previous chest surgery.
- Patients with blood clotting problems.
- Patients with poor lung function.
- Patients who are unable to cooperate because of age, mental status, pain, or other factors.

Throat Culture

Test Description

A throat culture is used primarily to isolate and identify pathogens, especially group A beta-hemolytic streptococci (GABHS). This identification is important, since complications of such infections include rheumatic fever and glomerulonephritis. Although most sore throats are viral in nature, approximately 15% are caused by this particular type of streptococci. Symptoms exhibited by the patient with GABHS occur abruptly and may include fever, chills, headache, cervical lymphadenopathy, pharyngitis, and distinctive patches (exudate) on the throat. This test can be used in diagnosing glomerulonephritis, pharyngitis, scarlet fever, strep throat, and tonsillitis.

When a patient is suspected of having strep throat, a throat culture is ordered, or is performed following a negative Rapid Strep test. The test involves swabbing each tonsillar area and the posterior pharynx. The throat swab should be performed prior to the beginning of antibiotic therapy. A Gram stain of the specimen can be done and quickly reported. This provides basic information as to whether the organism is gram-positive or gram-negative. The throat swab is then cultured, that is, the organisms are allowed to grow in special culture media. In 48 to 72 hours, the organism is usually identified.

Once the specimen is obtained, the patient is often given a broad-spectrum antibiotic that is likely to be effective against strep throat. A repeat throat culture is sometimes done following completion of treatment.

Normal Values

Negative

Possible Meanings of Abnormal Values

Positive

Bacterial pathogens, such as GABHS, diphtheria, gonorrhea

Contributing Factors to Abnormal Values

- Drugs that may cause *false-negative* results: antibiotics.

Interventions/Implications

Pretest
- Explain to the patient the purpose of the test and the need for a swabbing of the throat to be done. Warn the patient of the possibility of gagging during the procedure.
- No fasting is required before the test.

Procedure
- The patient may be seated, or if a child, held so as to immobilize the head.
- A tongue depressor is used to hold down the tongue. To minimize stimulating the gag reflex, the tongue depressor should be placed on the lateral portions of the tongue, rather than the center portion.
- Swabbing is done of both tonsils and the posterior pharynx.

Posttest
- The patient may wish to drink water after the swab is taken.
- Explain to the patient when the test result will be available.
- Report abnormal findings to the primary care provider.

T

CONTRAINDICATIONS!

- Throat swabs are not to be done on any patient exhibiting signs of possible airway compromise due to such causes as epiglottis or peritonsillar abscess.

Thrombin Clotting Time (TCT, Thrombin Time [TT])

Test Description
During the process of hemostasis, intrinsic and extrinsic pathways lead to the activation of coagulation factor X. This leads to the conversion of prothrombin to thrombin.

Thrombin then stimulates the formation of fibrin from fibrinogen. This fibrin, with the addition of fibrin stabilizing factor, forms a stable fibrin clot at the site of injury.

Thrombin clotting time (TCT) measures the time it takes for a blood sample to clot when thrombin is added to the sample. TCT is longer than normal when there is an abnormality in the conversion of fibrinogen to fibrin. The test is used to assess for bleeding disorders, such as disseminated intravascular coagulation (DIC), and liver disease, and to monitor patients receiving fibrinolytic therapy.

Normal Values

15–20 seconds (varies with laboratory)

Possible Meanings of Abnormal Values

Increased	Decreased
Acute leukemia	Thrombocytosis
Afibrinogenemia	
DIC	
Dysfibrinogenemia	
Dysproteinemias (multiple myeloma)	
Liver disease	
Polycythemia vera	
Shock	
Stress	
Uremia	

Contributing Factors to Abnormal Values

- Hemolysis of the blood sample may alter test results.
- Drugs that may *increase* thrombin clotting time: asparaginase, heparin, streptokinase, urokinase.

Interventions/Implications

Pretest
- Explain to the patient the purpose of the test and the need for a blood sample to be drawn.
- No fasting is required before the test.
- Draw blood sample 1 hour before anticoagulant administration.

Procedure
- A 7-mL blood sample is drawn in a blue-top collection tube (containing sodium citrate)
- Gloves are worn throughout the procedure.

Posttest
- Apply pressure at venipuncture site. Apply dressing, periodically assessing for continued bleeding.
- Gently invert the top to mix sample with anticoagulant in tube.
- Label the specimen and transport it to the laboratory.
- Report abnormal findings to the primary care provider.

→ **Clinical Alerts**

- Possible complication: Hematoma at site due to prolonged bleeding time.
- Teach patient to monitor the site. If the site begins to bleed, the patient should apply direct pressure and, if unable to control the bleeding, return to the lab or notify the primary care provider.

 Thyroglobulin (Tg)

Test Description

Thyroglobulin is a thyroid glycoprotein that has a role in the synthesis of triiodothyronine (T_3) and thyroxine (T_4). Thyroglobulin is made by normal thyroid cells and/or by papillary and follicular thyroid cancer cells. The test, considered a tumor marker, is used to evaluate the effectiveness of treatment for thyroid cancer and to monitor tumor recurrence when the entire thyroid gland has been removed. It can also be ordered when a patient has symptoms of hyperthyroidism or has an enlarged thyroid gland.

THE EVIDENCE FOR PRACTICE

Measurement of serum thyroglobulin (Tg) in differentiated thyroid cancer (DTC) patients during pregnancy should be avoided. Serum Tg rises during normal pregnancy and returns to baseline levels postpartum. This rise is also seen in pregnant DTC patients with remnant normal thyroid or tumor tissue present and is not necessarily a cause for alarm. (NACB, 2002)

Normal Values

0–50 ng/mL (0–50 µg/L SI units)

Possible Meanings of Abnormal Values

Increased	Decreased
Goiter	Thyroid agenesis
Graves' disease	Thyroidectomy
Liver failure	
Metastatic thyroid carcinoma	

T

Contributing Factors to Abnormal Values

- Thyroglobulin levels increase in pregnancy.
- Drugs that may *increase* thyroglobulin level: levothyroxine.

Interventions/Implications

Pretest

- Explain to the patient the purpose of the test and the need for a blood sample to be drawn.
- No fasting is required before the test.

Procedure
- A 7-mL blood sample is drawn in a red-top collection tube.
- Gloves are worn throughout the procedure.

Posttest
- Apply pressure at venipuncture site. Apply dressing, periodically assessing for continued bleeding.
- Label the specimen and transport it to the laboratory.
- Report abnormal findings to the primary care provider.

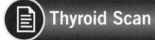

Thyroid Scan

Test Description
The thyroid scan involves administration of a radioactive isotope. Scanning of the thyroid gland is then conducted to assess the size, shape, position, and function of the thyroid. Areas in which there is increased uptake of the isotope are called *hot spots*. These areas are caused by hyperfunctioning thyroid nodules which are usually benign. *Cold spots* are nodules that do not take up the isotope. These areas have hypofunctioning tissue and are more likely to be malignant.

For patients who have had cancer of the thyroid, a *whole-body thyroid scan* may be performed periodically. Radioactive iodine (^{123}I) is administered to the patient and whole-body scanning is conducted. This not only provides evidence of how much thyroid tissue is left after surgery, but it also notes areas of possible metastasis of the thyroid cancer in other parts of the body.

Normal Values
Normal size, shape, position, and function of the thyroid gland
Equal uptake of isotope throughout the thyroid gland

Possible Meanings of Abnormal Values
Adenoma
Cyst
Goiter
Graves' disease
Hashimoto's thyroiditis
Hyperthyroidism
Hypothyroidism
Medullary carcinoma of thyroid
Multiple endocrine neoplasia
Papillary carcinoma of the thyroid
Plummer's disease
Thyroiditis

Contributing Factors to Abnormal Values
- Any movement by the patient may alter quality of films taken.

T

- Recent receipt of x-ray contrast agents or ingestion of iodine-containing foods will alter test results.
- Drugs that may alter test results: anticoagulants, antihistamines, corticosteroids, cough medicines, iodides, multiple vitamins, oral contraceptives, phenothiazines, salicylates, thyroid drugs.

Interventions/Implications

Pretest

- Explain to the patient the purpose of the test. Provide any written teaching materials available on the subject. Note that discomfort involved with this test is primarily due to lying on a hard table for an extended period of time and the needle puncture. Reassure the patient that only trace amounts of the radionuclide are involved in the test.
- Check for allergies to iodine.
- Medication that may alter test results should be withheld for 21 days before the test, if possible.
- The patient must remain still while the scan is being performed.
- Fasting for 8 hours is required before the test.
- Obtain a signed informed consent.

Procedure

- Oral radioactive iodine (preferably ^{123}I) is administered.
    - The IV route can also be used for isotope administration. If used, scanning can begin $^{1}/_{2}$ to 2 hours later.
- Scanning is done at 4 to 6 hours and again at 24 hours.
- The patient is assisted to a supine position on the examination table.
- A scintillation camera is positioned over the patient's thyroid. This camera takes a radioactivity reading from the body. This information is transformed into a two-dimensional picture of the thyroid.
- Gloves are worn during the radionuclide injection, if used.

Posttest

- Check the injection site for redness or swelling.
- If a woman who is lactating *must* have this scan, she should not breast-feed the infant until the radionuclide has been eliminated, possibly for 3 days.
- Although the amount of diagnostic radionuclide excreted in the urine is low, the urine should not be used for any laboratory tests for the time period indicated by the nuclear medicine department.
- Gloves are worn when dealing with the urine.
- Encourage fluid intake by the patient to enhance excretion of the radionuclide.
- Resume medications as taken before the test.
- Report abnormal findings to the primary care provider.

T

Clinical Alerts

- No other radionuclide tests should be scheduled for 24 to 48 hours.
- Monitor patients closely who have had thyroid surgery. Their ability to tolerate holding their medication prior to the test may depend on the extent of their surgery. For some patients, the medication will have to be continued throughout the testing period.

CONTRAINDICATIONS!

- Pregnant women
    - Caution: A woman in her childbearing years should undergo scanning only during her menses or 12 to 14 days after its onset to avoid any exposure to a fetus.
- Patients who are lactating.
- Patients who are allergic to iodine, shellfish, or contrast medium.
- Patients who are unable to cooperate because of age, mental status, pain, or other factors.

 Thyroid Sonogram (Ultrasonography of the Thyroid)

Test Description

Ultrasonography is a noninvasive method of diagnostic testing in which ultrasound waves are sent into the body with a small transducer pressed against the skin. The transducer then receives any returning sound waves, which are deflected back as they bounce off various structures. The transducer converts the returning sound waves into electric signals that are then transformed by a computer into a visual display on a monitor.

In thyroid ultrasonography, the size, shape, and position of the thyroid gland can be evaluated. This test is useful in distinguishing between a cyst and solid tumor of the thyroid gland, and can be used to provide guidance of needle positioning during fine needle aspiration of a suspicious nodule. It is also used to monitor the response of the thyroid gland to suppressive therapy treatment of hyperthyroidism.

THE EVIDENCE FOR PRACTICE

Use of the thyroid sonogram for routine screening of the general population is not recommended. Its use is recommended for high-risk patients (those with a history of familial thyroid cancer, multiple endocrine neoplasias, or external irradiation); for all patients with palpable thyroid nodules or multinodular goiter, and for those with adenopathy suggestive of a malignant lesion. (AACE/AME, 2006)

Normal Values

Normal size, shape, and position of the thyroid gland

Possible Meanings of Abnormal Values

Goiter
Thyroid cyst
Thyroid tumor

Contributing Factors to Abnormal Values

- The transducer must be in good contact with the skin as it is being moved. A water-based gel is used to ensure good contact with the skin.

Interventions/Implications

Pretest
- Explain to the patient the purpose of the test. Provide any written teaching materials available on the subject. Note that there is no discomfort involved with thyroid ultrasound. Some discomfort may be experienced if a biopsy is also performed.
- No fasting is required before the test.
- Signed informed consent is needed prior to biopsy being performed.

Procedure
- The patient is assisted to a supine position on the ultrasonography table. A pillow is placed beneath the shoulders and the neck is hyperextended.
- A coupling agent, such as a water-based gel, is applied to the area to be evaluated.
- A transducer is placed on the skin and moved as needed to provide good visualization of the thyroid gland.
- The sound waves are transformed into a visual display on the monitor. Printed copies of the display are made.

Posttest
- Cleanse the patient's skin of remaining gel.
- Report abnormal findings to the primary care provider.

 Thyroid-Stimulating Hormone (TSH, Thyrotropin)

Test Description

When thyroid hormone levels decrease in the bloodstream or the body is exposed to physiological or psychological stress, the hypothalamus is stimulated to release thyrotropin-releasing hormone (TRH). TRH in turn stimulates the production of thyroid-stimulating hormone (TSH) by the anterior lobe of the pituitary gland. TSH then stimulates production and release of triiodothyronine (T_3) and thyroxine (T_4). As levels of T_3 and free T_4 in the blood rise, the pituitary gland is stimulated to decrease TSH production via a negative feedback mechanism.

TSH release occurs in a diurnal pattern, with peaks occurring in the late evening and troughs occurring at midmorning. Measurement of the TSH level along with free T_4 is used for differential diagnosis of primary and secondary hypothyroidism. *Primary* type problems deal with the target organ (thyroid gland) itself, whereas *secondary* problems deal with abnormalities of the pituitary gland. For example, in primary hypothyroidism, the thyroid gland is hypoactive and producing abnormally low levels of free T_4 in the blood. The anterior pituitary gland senses the low serum T_4 levels and as a result, increases its release of TSH. This is an attempt to stimulate the thyroid gland to increase its production of T_3 and T_4. Since the thyroid gland is not responding to the stimulation, the TSH level keeps increasing. Measurement of TSH is also used to monitor patient response to treatment for thyroid disorders.

T

THE EVIDENCE FOR PRACTICE

The sensitive TSH assay is the single best screening test for hyperthyroidism, and in most outpatient clinical situations, the serum TSH is the most sensitive test for detecting mild (subclinical) thyroid hormone excess or deficiency.

Normal Values

0.4–4.0 µU/mL (0.4–4.0 mIU/L SI units)

Possible Meanings of Abnormal Values

Increased	Decreased
Anti-TSH antibodies	Graves' disease (treated)
Ectopic production (lung, breast cancer)	Hyperthyroidism
Hashimoto's thyroiditis	Multinodular thyroid gland
Hyperpituitarism	Organic brain syndrome
Hypothermia	Pituitary hypofunction
Pituitary adenoma	Secondary hypothyroidism
Primary hypothyroidism	
Subtotal thyroidectomy	
Thyroid hormone resistance	
Thyroiditis	

Contributing Factors to Abnormal Values

- Hemolysis of the blood sample may alter test results.
- Recent testing with radioactive isotope may affect test results.
- TSH levels are subject to a diurnal variation. Basal levels occur around 10 a.m. and highest levels occur around 10 p.m.
- Drugs that may *increase* TSH: amiodarone, amphetamines, clomiphene, inorganic iodides, lithium, methimazole, metoclopramide, morphine, nitroprusside, phenylbutazone, potassium iodide, propylthiouracil, radiographic dye, sulfonamides, sulfonylureas, thyroid-releasing hormone injection.
- Drugs that may *decrease* TSH: aspirin, dopamine, glucocorticoids, levodopa, phenytoin, thyroid hormones.

Interventions/Implications

Pretest
- Explain to the patient the purpose of the test and the need for a blood sample to be drawn.
- No fasting is required before the test.
- If possible, withhold medications that may affect test results.

Procedure
- A 7-mL blood sample is drawn in a red-top collection tube.
- Gloves are worn throughout the procedure.

Posttest
- Apply pressure at venipuncture site. Apply dressing, periodically assessing for continued bleeding.
- Label the specimen and transport it to the laboratory.
- Report abnormal findings to the primary care provider.

→ Clinical Alerts

- When a thyroid disorder is suspected clinically, a TSH level is obtained as an initial test.

- Amiodarone therapy causes thyroid dysfunction in 14% to 18% of the involved patients. Therefore, before initiation of such therapy, patients should have a baseline TSH measurement, and then they should be monitored at 6-month intervals during treatment.

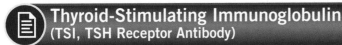

Thyroid-Stimulating Immunoglobulin
(TSI, TSH Receptor Antibody)

Test Description

Thyroid-stimulating immunoglobulin (TSI), formerly called long-acting thyroid stimulator, is an autoimmune antibody which binds to or near the thyroid-stimulating hormone (TSH) receptor site on thyroid cells. TSI mimics the action of TSH, stimulating the thyroid gland to release above normal levels of thyroid hormones. This test is used to assist in the diagnosis of Graves' disease, since the majority of patients with the disease have positive TSI.

Normal Values

Normal values are less than 130% of basal activity

Possible Meanings of Abnormal Values

Increased

Autoimmune thyroiditis
Graves' disease
Hyperthyroidism
Malignant exophthalmos

Contributing Factors to Abnormal Values

- Radioactive iodine preparations received within 24 hours of the test may alter test results.
- Hemolysis of the sample may alter test results.

Interventions/Implications

Pretest
- Explain to the patient the purpose of the test and the need for a blood sample to be drawn.
- No fasting is required before the test.

Procedure
- A 7-mL blood sample is drawn in a red-top collection tube.
- Gloves are worn throughout the procedure.

Posttest
- Apply pressure at venipuncture site. Apply dressing, periodically assessing for continued bleeding.

T

- Label the specimen and transport it to the laboratory.
- Report abnormal findings to the primary care provider.

 ## Thyroxine, Total (T$_4$, Total T$_4$)

Test Description
When thyroid hormone levels decrease in the bloodstream or the body is exposed to physiologic or psychologic stress, the hypothalamus is stimulated to release thyrotropin-releasing hormone (TRH). TRH in turn stimulates the production of thyroid-stimulating hormone (TSH) by the anterior lobe of the pituitary gland. TSH then stimulates production and release of triiodothyronine (T$_3$) and thyroxine (T$_4$) by the thyroid gland.

Thyroxine (T$_4$) is the most abundant of the thyroid hormones. There are two types of thyroxine: free thyroxine and the portion bound to plasma proteins (thyroxine-binding globulin). The total T$_4$ test measures both types of thyroxine. It is usually analyzed in conjunction with free thyroxine index and TSH levels to aid in the diagnosis of hyperthyroidism and hypothyroidism. It can also be used to monitor the effectiveness of drug therapy in these conditions.

Normal Values
4.5–11.2 µg/dL (58–144 nmol/L SI units)

Possible Meanings of Abnormal Values

Increased	Decreased
Early Hashimoto's disease	Hypoalbuminemia
Graves' disease	Hypothalamic failure
Hyperthyroidism	Hypothyroidism
Infancy (first 2 months)	Pituitary insufficiency
Pregnancy	
Toxic multinodular goiter	

Contributing Factors to Abnormal Values

- Hemolysis of the blood sample or having had a radionuclide scan within 1 week before the test may alter the test results.
- Drugs that may *increase* total T$_4$: amiodarone, amphetamines, clofibrate, estrogens, heparin, levodopa, methadone, oral contraceptives, progesterone, propranolol, thyroxine.
- Drugs that may *decrease* total T$_4$: anabolic steroids, asparaginase, aspirin, barbiturates, carbamazepine, chlorpromazine, corticosteroids, danazol, dopamine, furosemide, gold salts, iodides, isoniazid, lithium, methimazole, penicillin, phenylbutazone, phenytoin, potassium iodide, prednisone, propylthiouracil, reserpine, salicylates, sulfonamides, testosterone.

Interventions/Implications

Pretest
- Explain to the patient the purpose of the test and the need for a blood sample to be drawn.
- No fasting is required before the test.
- If possible, thyroid medications should be withheld for 1 month prior to this test. If this not possible, use of the medication should be noted on the laboratory slip.

Procedure
- A 7-mL blood sample is drawn in a red-top collection tube.
- Testing of newborns is done with a heel stick at least 3 days following birth.
- Gloves are worn throughout the procedure.

Posttest
- Apply pressure at venipuncture site. Apply dressing, periodically assessing for continued bleeding.
- Label the specimen and transport it to the laboratory.
- Resume medications as taken before the test.
- Report abnormal findings to the primary care provider.

 ## Thyroxine-Binding Globulin (TBG)

Test Description
Both of the thyroid hormones, triiodothyronine (T_3) and thyroxine (T_4) are present in the blood in two forms. These two forms are a "free" state that allows the hormone to be biologically active, and the portion bound to plasma proteins. This test measures the level of thyroxine-binding globulin (TBG), the primary protein carrier for both T_3 and T_4. It provides information to aid in the differential diagnosis of true thyroid disorders and those related to altered TBG levels.

Normal Values
1.3–2.0 mg/dL (radioimmunoassay technique)

Possible Meanings of Abnormal Values

Increased	Decreased
Acute intermittent porphyria	Acromegaly
Active hepatitis	Acute illness
Congenital TBG excess	Congenital TBG deficiency
Estrogen-secreting tumors	Hyperthyroidism
HIV	Low albumin levels (liver disease)
Hypothyroidism	Malnutrition
Liver disease	Nephrosis
Neonates	Nephrotic syndrome
Pregnancy	Stress
Subacute thyroiditis	Testosterone-producing tumors

Contributing Factors to Abnormal Values

- Hemolysis of the blood sample may alter test results.
- Drugs that may *increase* TBG results: clofibrate, estrogens, heroin, methadone, oral contraceptives, phenothiazines.
- Drugs that may *decrease* TBG results: androgens, phenytoin, prednisone, salicylates, testosterone, valproic acid.

Interventions/Implications

Pretest
- Explain to the patient the purpose of the test and the need for a blood sample to be drawn.
- No fasting is required before the test.
- If possible, withhold drugs affecting the test for 12 to 24 hours before the test.

Procedure
- A 7-mL blood sample is drawn in a red-top collection tube.
- Gloves are worn throughout the procedure.

Posttest
- Apply pressure at venipuncture site. Apply dressing, periodically assessing for continued bleeding.
- Label the specimen and transport it to the laboratory.
- Resume medications as taken before the test.
- Report abnormal findings to the primary care provider.

Thyroxine, Free (Free T$_4$, FT$_4$)

Test Description

When thyroid hormone levels decrease in the bloodstream or the body is exposed to physiologic or psychologic stress, the hypothalamus is stimulated to release thyrotropin- releasing hormone (TRH). TRH in turn stimulates the production of thyroid-stimulating hormone (TSH) by the anterior lobe of the pituitary gland. TSH then stimulates production and release of triiodothyronine (T$_3$) and thyroxine (T$_4$) by the thyroid gland.

Thyroxine (T$_4$) is the most abundant of the thyroid hormones. There are two types of thyroxine: free thyroxine and the portion bound to plasma proteins. Less than 0.05% of the total thyroxine is not bound to plasma proteins. This is known as "free thyroxine (FT$_4$)" and is the only type of thyroxine that is biologically active. This test is used to assist in diagnosing hyperthyroidism and hypothyroidism when thyroxine-binding globulin (TBG) levels are abnormal.

THE EVIDENCE FOR PRACTICE

According to the National Academy of Clinical Biochemistry (2002):

> *Patients with stable thyroid status:* When thyroid status is stable and hypothalamic-pituitary function is intact, serum TSH measurement is more sensitive than FT$_4$ for detecting mild (subclinical) thyroid hormone excess or deficiency.

Patients with unstable thyroid status: Serum FT$_4$ measurement is a more reliable indicator of thyroid status than TSH when thyroid status is unstable, such as during the first 2 to 3 months of treatment for hypo- or hyperthyroidism.

Normal Values

0.8–2.7 ng/dL (10–35 pmol/L SI units)

Possible Meanings of Abnormal Values

Increased	Decreased
Early Hashimoto's disease	Amyloidosis
Ectopic production	Goiter
Graves' disease	Hashimoto's thyroiditis
Hyperthyroidism	Hemochromatosis
Iodine-induced hyperthyroidism	Hypothyroidism
Thyroiditis	Scleroderma
Toxic multinodular goiter	

Contributing Factors to Abnormal Values

- A radionuclide scan within 1 week before the test may alter test results.
- Drugs that may *increase* FT$_4$ levels: amiodarone, androgens, carbamazepine, corticosteroids, danazol, estrogens, furosemide, heparin, oral contraceptives, phenytoin, propranolol, radiographic dyes, tamoxifen, thyroxine, valproic acid.
- Drugs that may *decrease* FT$_4$ levels: amiodarone, anabolic steroids, carbamazepine, corticosteroids, cytomel, estrogen, lithium, phenobarbital, phenytoin, ranitidine.

Interventions/Implications

Pretest
- Explain to the patient the purpose of the test and the need for a blood sample to be drawn.
- No fasting is required before the test.

Procedure
- A 7-mL blood sample is drawn in a red-top collection tube.
- Gloves are worn throughout the procedure.

Posttest
- Apply pressure at venipuncture site. Apply dressing, periodically assessing for continued bleeding.
- Label the specimen and transport it to the laboratory.
- Report abnormal findings to the primary care provider.

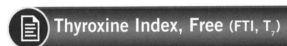

Thyroxine Index, Free (FTI, T$_7$)

Test Description

Free Thyroxine Index (FTI) is a mathematical computation used to estimate the free thyroxine index from the T$_4$ and T$_3$ uptake tests. The result indicates how much thyroid hormone is free and active in the blood. Unlike the T$_4$ alone, it is not affected by estrogen levels. Using the FTI is not as reliable as directly measuring the free T_4 in the blood. The calculation, also known as T_7, is:

$$FTI = (\text{Total } T_4 \times T_3 \text{ uptake } \%)/100$$

Normal Values

1.5–5.5

Possible Meanings of Abnormal Values

Increased	Decreased
Hyperthyroidism	Hypothyroidism

Contributing Factors to Abnormal Values

- Drugs that can *increase* FTI: amiodarone, carbamazepine, furosemide, oral contraceptives, phenobarbital, propranolol.
- Drugs that can *decrease* FTI: amiodarone, clomiphene, corticosteroids, iodide, lovastatin, methimazole, phenobarbital, phenytoin, primidone, salicylates.

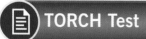

TORCH Test

Test Description

The TORCH test is a screening test conducted on newborn infants to evaluate possible congenital infection from one of the following: *T*oxoplasmosis, *O*ther, *R*ubella, *C*ytomegalovirus, *H*erpes virus. The "other" tests often included are those for syphilis or hepatitis. The test may also be done on women during pregnancy to screen for these diseases since they are likely to cause birth defects such as malformations, growth delay, and neurological problems.

T

Normal Values

Negative

Possible Meanings of Abnormal Values

Increased	
Presence of IgM antibodies	Congenital infection with the indicated virus
Presence of IgG antibodies	Transfer of antibodies from mother to newborn (mother has had past infection)

Contributing Factors to Abnormal Values

- Hemolysis of the blood cells caused by excessive agitation of the sample may alter test results.

Interventions/Implications

Pretest
- Explain to the patient the purpose of the test and the need for a blood sample to be drawn.
- No fasting is required before the test.

Procedure
- A 3-mL blood sample using blood from the infant's heel or umbilical cord or the mother's venous blood is drawn in a red-top collection tube.
- Gloves are worn throughout the procedure.

Posttest
- Apply pressure at venipuncture site. Apply dressing, periodically assessing for continued bleeding.
- Label the specimen and transport it to the laboratory.
- Report abnormal findings to the primary care provider.

 Clinical Alerts

- If a newborn's test result is positive, a definitive diagnosis will require additional testing. The mother will also need to be evaluated in order to interpret the newborn's blood tests.

 ## Total Carbon Dioxide Content
(Carbon Dioxide [CO_2] Content)

Test Description

Total carbon dioxide content of the blood consists of two sources. The first, accounting for more than 95% of the carbon dioxide, comes from bicarbonate (HCO_3), which is regulated by the kidneys. The other source (less than 5% of the total) is dissolved carbon dioxide and carbonic acid (H_2CO_3) which is regulated by the lungs. It is these substances that assist in maintaining the body's acid-base balance through its buffering system. Thus, measurement of the total carbon dioxide content of the blood provides a general indication of the body's buffering capacity.

T

Normal Values

20–29 mEq/L (20–29 mmol/L SI units)

Possible Meanings of Abnormal Values

Increased	Decreased
Alcoholism	Acute renal failure
Compensated respiratory acidosis	Compensated respiratory alkalosis
Emphysema	Dehydration
Fat embolism	Diabetic ketoacidosis
Hypoventilation	Diarrhea (severe)

Metabolic alkalosis	Head trauma
Nasogastric suctioning	High fever
Pneumonia	Hyperventilation
Primary aldosteronism	Malabsorption
Pyloric obstruction	Metabolic acidosis
Vomiting	Salicylate toxicity
	Starvation
	Uremia

Contributing Factors to Abnormal Values

- Use of a tourniquet or pumping of the patient's hand during acquisition of the blood sample may alter test results.
- Drugs that may *increase* total carbon dioxide content: aldosterone, antacids, barbiturates, corticotropin, cortisone, hydrocortisone, licorice, loop diuretics, mercurial diuretics, sodium bicarbonate.
- Drugs that may *decrease* total carbon dioxide content: acetazolamide, amiloride, ammonium chloride, aspirin, chlorothiazide diuretics, dimercaprol, metformin, methicillin, nitrofurantoin, pentamidine, salicylates, streptomycin, tetracycline, triamterene.

Interventions/Implications

Pretest
- Explain to the patient the purpose of the test and the need for a blood sample to be drawn.
- No fasting is required before the test.

Procedure
- A 7-mL blood sample is drawn. If the blood sample is drawn with electrolytes, a red-top collection tube is used. If the test is performed alone, a green-top collection tube is used.
- Gloves are worn throughout the procedure.

Posttest
- Apply pressure at venipuncture site. Apply dressing, periodically assessing for continued bleeding.
- Label the specimen and transport it to the laboratory immediately. If this is not possible, it should be placed on ice.
- Report abnormal findings to the primary care provider.

Total Iron-Binding Capacity (TIBC)

Test Description
Iron in the body is found in several locations. A large portion (approximately 65%) is carried in the red blood cells by hemoglobin. Another 4% is found in myoglobin in the skeletal muscle. Ferritin stores in the liver, bone marrow, and spleen account for almost 30% of the total iron. The remaining iron is in transit throughout the body, bound to transferrin and other iron binding serum proteins.

Total iron-binding capacity (TIBC) measures the total amount of iron that transferrin can bind. It is usually measured along with serum iron when investigating a possible iron deficiency anemia. When iron stores are low, the TIBC is usually higher than normal. The test can also be performed when iron overload is suspected. A calculation of serum iron divided by TIBC provides a percentage known as *transferrin saturation*, a useful indicator of iron status.

Normal Values

TIBC: 240–450 mcg/dl (43–81 μmol/L SI units)

Possible Meanings of Abnormal Values

Increased	Decreased
Iron deficiency anemia	Anemia of chronic disease
Pregnancy (late)	Cirrhosis
	Hemochromatosis
	Hemolytic anemia
	Hyperthyroidism
	Hypoproteinemia
	Inflammation
	Liver disease
	Malnutrition
	Nephrotic syndrome
	Pernicious anemia
	Sickle cell anemia

Contributing Factors to Abnormal Values

- Hemolysis of the sample may alter test results.
- Drugs that can *increase* TIBC: fluorides, oral contraceptives.
- Drugs that can *decrease* TIBC: ACTH, chloramphenicol, corticotropin, cortisone, dextran, steroids, testosterone.

Interventions/Implications

Pretest
- Explain to the patient the purpose of the test and the need for a blood sample to be drawn.
- Fasting is required for 12 hours before the test. Water intake is allowed.
- No iron supplements are to be taken with 24 to 48 hours of the testing.

Procedure
- Obtain the blood sample in the morning, usually after 10 AM, since iron levels vary throughout the day.
- A 7-mL blood sample is drawn in a red-top collection tube.
- Gloves are worn throughout the procedure.

Posttest
- Apply pressure at venipuncture site. Apply dressing, periodically assessing for continued bleeding.
- Label the specimen and transport it to the laboratory.

- Resume medications as taken before the test.
- Report abnormal findings to the primary care provider.

→ **Clinical Alerts**

- In iron deficiency anemia, iron is low and TIBC is increased, resulting in very low transferrin saturation.
- In iron overload, as seen with hemochromatosis, iron is high and TIBC is low or normal, resulting in high transferrin saturation.

Toxicology Screen (Drug Screen)

Test Description
Toxicology screening for drugs is used for determining the cause of acute drug toxicity in an unconscious person, to monitor compliance with treatment regimens for drug dependency, and to detect the presence of drugs in the body for employment or legal purposes. Blood or urine may be tested. Examples of drugs included in drug screens include amphetamines, barbiturates, benzodiazepines, cannabinoids, cocaine, ethanol, hypnotics, and narcotics.

Normal Values
Negative

Possible Meanings of Abnormal Values

Increased
Intake of tested substance
Toxicity

Contributing Factors to Abnormal Values

- *False-positive* results can occur with: cold remedies, cough medicines, ibuprofen, antibiotics.

Interventions/Implications
Pretest
- Explain to the patient the purpose of the test and the need for a blood sample or a urine sample to be collected.
- No fasting is required before the test.

Procedure
- If the test is to be used as legal evidence, have specimen collection witnessed.
- Follow institutional policy regarding handling of legal evidence.
- Gloves are worn throughout the procedure.

Blood testing
- Cleanse the venipuncture site and, if needed, the top of the collection tube, with povidone-iodine solution instead of alcohol.
- A 10-mL blood sample is drawn in a red-top collection tube.

Urine testing
- Obtain a 50-mL random urine specimen in a clean container. Cap tightly.

Posttest
- Apply pressure at venipuncture site. Apply dressing, periodically assessing for continued bleeding.
- Label the specimen and transport it to the laboratory.
- If being used as legal evidence, transport the specimen in a sealed plastic bag to the laboratory. The bag must be signed by each person handling the specimen.
- Report abnormal findings to the primary care provider.

 Clinical Alerts

- Any positive drug screen must be confirmed with more testing specific for the identified substance.

 Toxoplasmosis Antibody Test

Test Description
Toxoplasmosis is a disease caused by the protozoan organism *Toxoplasma gondii*. The organism can be acquired through ingestion of raw or poorly cooked meat. It is also found in the feces of cats. It is estimated that up to half of the adult population is infected with toxoplasmosis, but is asymptomatic. If symptoms do occur, they include fatigue, muscle pain, lymphadenopathy, and little or no fever.

The disease is not transmitted between humans, except through maternal-fetal transfer. If a woman is infected prior to conception, the fetus will not be affected by the organism. However, if the woman becomes infected during pregnancy, the unborn child is at risk for birth defects including mental retardation, hydrocephalus, microcephalus, and chronic retinitis. Fetal death may occur. The Centers for Disease Control recommends testing all pregnant women for toxoplasmosis prior to the twentieth week of pregnancy.

T

Normal Values
Titer <1:16   No previous infection

Possible Meanings of Abnormal Values
Titer 1:16–1:64   Past exposure
Titer >1:256   Recent infection
Titer >1:1024   Acute infection

Interventions/Implications

Pretest
- Explain to the patient the purpose of the test and the need for a blood sample to be drawn.
- Obtain a history regarding intake of raw or poorly cooked meat or contact with cats.
- No fasting is required before the test.

Procedure
- A 7-mL blood sample is drawn in a red-top collection tube.
- Gloves are worn throughout the procedure.

Posttest
- Apply pressure at venipuncture site. Apply dressing, periodically assessing for continued bleeding.
- Label the specimen and transport it to the laboratory.
- Report abnormal findings to the primary care provider.

→ **Clinical Alerts**

- Teach pregnant women to avoid contact with cat litter boxes. If that is not possible, the woman needs to wear gloves and clean the litter box every day, since the parasite found in cat feces needs one or more days after being passed to become infectious. Thorough handwashing afterward is essential.

Transesophageal Echocardiography (TEE)

Test Description

Ultrasonography is a noninvasive method of diagnostic testing in which ultrasound waves are sent into the body with a small transducer pressed against the skin. The transducer then receives any returning sound waves, which are deflected back as they bounce off various structures. The transducer converts the returning sound waves into electric signals that are then transformed by a computer into a visual display on a monitor.

In transesophageal echocardiography (TEE), a small transducer is attached to the end of a gastroscope. It is inserted into the esophagus, allowing high quality images to be taken from the posterior aspect of the heart. This allows for evaluation of thoracic, aortic, and cardiac disorders with less interference from chest wall structures.

THE EVIDENCE FOR PRACTICE

When TEE and MRI have been evaluated prospectively in adults with coronary heart disease, TEE is shown to be superior in evaluating intracardiac anatomy; MRI is superior for extracardiac anatomy and is slightly better than TEE for hemodynamic and functional evaluation. Taken individually, the two modalities provided similar overall diagnostic information, but when used in combination, they provide important complementary information in all diagnostic categories.

Normal Values

No cardiac abnormalities

Possible Meanings of Abnormal Values

Aortic aneurysm
Aortic dissection
Cardiac tumors
Cardiomyopathy
Congenital heart disease
Endocarditis
Intracardiac thrombi
Myocardial ischemia
Patent ductus arteriosus
Septal defects
Valvular disease

Interventions/Implications

Pretest
- Explain to the patient the purpose of the test. Provide any written teaching materials available on the subject. Note that there is minimal discomfort involved with this test.
- Fasting for 6 hours is required before the test.
- Obtain a signed informed consent.
- Have the patient remove any dentures or oral prostheses. Note any loose or capped teeth.
- Resuscitation and suctioning equipment should be available.

Procedure
- The patient is assisted to a left-lying position on the examination table.
- Cardiac monitoring, pulse oximetry, and vital sign monitoring are initiated. An IV infusion is begun, and a sedative such as midazolam is administered.
- The back of the patient's throat is sprayed with a topical anesthetic agent to suppress the gag reflex.
- The gastroscope is introduced into the mouth and with the patient swallowing, is advanced to the level of the right atrium of the heart.
- The sound waves are transformed into a visual display on the monitor. Printed copies of this display are made.

Posttest
- Monitor the vital signs and pulse oximetry until stable.
- Keep the patient supine until the sedation is ended. A narcotic antagonist such as naloxone may be administered to reverse the sedation.
- Do not allow food or fluid intake until the gag reflex has returned.
- Report abnormal findings to the primary care provider.

T

→ Clinical Alerts

- Possible complications include: cardiac arrhythmias, esophageal bleeding, esophageal perforation, and sore throat.

CONTRAINDICATIONS!

- Patients with esophageal pathology, including esophageal varices or strictures, or previous esophageal surgery.
- Patients with bleeding disorders.
- Patients who are unable to cooperate because of age, mental status, pain, or other factors.

 # Transferrin/Transferrin Saturation (Siderophilin)

Test Description

Transferrin is a plasma protein that is formed in the liver and has a half-life of 7 to 10 days. Its primary function is to transport iron from the mucosa of the intestines to iron storage sites in the body. Transferrin is capable of binding with more than its own weight in iron. One gram of transferrin can bind with 1.43 g of iron. TIBC (total iron-binding capacity) measures the total amount of iron that transferrin can bind. TIBC correlates with serum transferrin. Transferrin is responsible for 50% to 70% of the iron- binding capacity of serum.

Since transferrin is a protein and has a relatively short half-life, its level decreases very quickly in protein malnutrition. Because of this, measurement of transferrin is sometimes done as a way of assessing the patient's nutritional status. Because it is made in the liver, transferrin will be low with liver disease.

Transferrin saturation is a calculation that uses both the serum iron level and the total iron-binding capacity (TIBC). The test is used to aid in determining the cause of abnormal iron levels and abnormal TIBC levels. The percentage of saturation is calculated as follows:

$$(\text{Serum iron/TIBC}) \times 100 = \% \text{ of transferrin saturation}$$

Normal Values

Transferrin

Male:	215–365 mg/dL (2.15–3.65 g/L SI units)
Female:	250–380 mg/dL (2.5–3.8 g/L SI units)

Transferrin saturation
    20–50%

Possible Meanings of Abnormal Values

Transferrin

Increased	Decreased
Estrogen therapy	Acute inflammation
Iron deficiency anemia	Anemia of chronic disease
Pregnancy	Genetic defect
	Hemochromatosis
	Iron overload

Protein deficiency due to chronic
infection, chronic kidney disease,
chronic liver disease, malnutrition,
neoplasms, nephrosis, thermal burns

Transferrin saturation

Increased	**Decreased**
Hemochromatosis	Iron deficiency anemia
Hemosiderosis	Neoplasms
Thalassemia	Rheumatoid arthritis
	Uremia

Contributing Factors to Abnormal Values

- Elevations of transferrin levels may occur in the third trimester of pregnancy and in children aged 2 ½ to 10 years.
- Hemolysis of the sample, dietary intake of iron, and receipt of blood transfusions may alter test results.
- Drugs that may *increase* transferrin levels: carbamazepine, estrogens, oral contraceptives.
- Drugs that may *decrease* transferrin levels: cortisone.

Interventions/Implications

Pretest
- Explain to the patient the purpose of the test and the need for a blood sample to be drawn.
- Fasting is required for 12 hours before the test. Water intake is allowed.
- No iron supplements are to be taken within 24 to 48 hours of the testing.

Procedure
- Obtain the blood sample in the morning, usually after 10 AM, when serum iron levels peak.
- A 7-mL blood sample is drawn in a red-top collection tube.
- Gloves are worn throughout the procedure.

Posttest
- Apply pressure at venipuncture site. Apply dressing, periodically assessing for continued bleeding.
- Label the specimen and transport it to the laboratory.
- Report abnormal findings to the primary care provider.

T

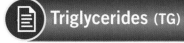

Triglycerides (TG)

Test Description
Triglycerides (TG) are synthesized in the liver from fatty acids, proteins, and glucose. They are stored in adipose tissue and muscle and can be retrieved when needed as an energy source. The triglyceride level is typically evaluated as part of a lipid panel. This panel includes total cholesterol, low-density lipoprotein (LDL), high-density lipoprotein (HDL), and triglycerides. Triglycerides are also used to calculate the LDL level:

$$LDL = Total\ Cholesterol - HDL - (Triglycerides/5)$$

Triglycerides are often measured to assess the balance between fat ingestion and fat metabolism. This is one aspect of evaluating coronary risk factors. High triglyceride levels are associated with a higher risk of heart disease and stroke. Often hypertriglyceridemia is seen concomitantly with diabetes and obesity, also cardiovascular disease risk factors.

THE EVIDENCE FOR PRACTICE

According to the third report of the National Cholesterol Education Program (NCEP) expert panel on detection, evaluation, and treatment of high blood cholesterol in adults (http://www.nhlbi.nih.gov/guidelines/cholesterol/atp3_rpt.htm):

- In all adults aged 20 years or older, a fasting lipoprotein profile (total cholesterol, LDL cholesterol, HDL cholesterol, and triglycerides) should be obtained once every 5 years.
- The treatment strategy for elevated triglycerides depends on the causes of the elevation and its severity.
    - For all persons with elevated triglycerides, the primary aim of therapy is to achieve the target goal for LDL cholesterol.
    - When triglycerides are *borderline high* (150 to 199 mg/dL), emphasis should also be placed on weight reduction and increased physical activity.
    - For *high triglycerides* (200 to 499 mg/dL), non-HDL cholesterol becomes a secondary target of therapy. Aside from weight reduction and increased physical activity, drug therapy can be considered in high-risk persons to achieve the non-HDL cholesterol goal.
    - If a high-risk person has high triglycerides or low HDL cholesterol, consideration can be given to combining a fibrate or nicotinic acid with an LDL-lowering drug.
    - In rare cases in which triglycerides are *very high* ($\geq$500 mg/dL), the initial aim of therapy is to prevent acute pancreatitis through triglyceride lowering. This approach requires very low fat diets ($\leq$15% of calorie intake), weight reduction, increased physical activity, and usually a triglyceride-lowering drug (fibrate or nicotinic acid). Only after triglyceride levels have been lowered to <500 mg/dL should attention turn to LDL lowering to reduce risk for coronary heart disease.

Normal Values

Normal:	<150 mg/dL (<1.70 mmol/L SI units)
Borderline high:	150–199 mg/dL (1.70–2.25 mmol/L SI units)
High:	200–499 mg/dL (2.26–5.64 mmol/L SI units)
Very high:	$\geq$500 mg/dL ($\geq$5.65 mmol/L SI units)

Possible Meanings of Abnormal Values

Increased	Decreased
Alcohol abuse	Abetalipoproteinemia
Cirrhosis	Brain infarction
Diabetes mellitus	Chronic obstructive pulmonary disease
Diet: low protein, high carbohydrate	Diet: low fat
Familial hyperlipoproteinemia	Hyperthyroidism
Glycogen storage disease	Malabsorption
Gout	Malnutrition
Hypertension	

Hypothyroidism
Myocardial infarction
Nephrotic syndrome
Pancreatitis
Renal disease

Contributing Factors to Abnormal Values

- Pregnancy and nonfasting blood samples will increase TG levels.
- Drugs that can *increase* TG levels: alcohol, beta-blockers, cholestyramine, corticosteroids, estrogens, oral contraceptives, thiazide diuretics.
- Drugs that can *decrease* TG levels: ascorbic acid, asparaginase, colestipol, clofibrate, dextrothyroxine, metformin, niacin.

Interventions/Implications

Pretest
- Explain to the patient the purpose of the test and the need for a blood sample to be drawn.
- Fasting for 12 hours is required before the test. Water is permitted.
- No alcohol is allowed for 24 hours before the test.

Procedure
- A 7-mL blood sample is drawn in a red-top collection tube.
- Gloves are worn throughout the procedure.

Posttest
- Apply pressure at venipuncture site. Apply dressing, periodically assessing for continued bleeding.
- Label the specimen and transport it to the laboratory.
- Report abnormal findings to the primary care provider.

 Clinical Alerts

- A triglyceride level of ≥150 mg/dL is one of the risk factors for metabolic syndrome. A higher intake of total fat, mostly in the form of unsaturated fat, can help to reduce triglycerides and raise HDL cholesterol in persons with the metabolic syndrome.
- Patients with diabetes whose blood glucose levels are uncontrolled will usually have very high triglyceride levels. Bringing the glucose levels under control will have an associated lowering effect on the triglycerides. Once the glucose levels are within normal limits, triglycerides should be reassessed to determine need for treatment.

T

 # Triiodothyronine, Free (Free T₃, FT₃)

Test Description
When thyroid hormone levels decrease in the bloodstream or the body is exposed to physiological or psychological stress, the hypothalamus is stimulated to release thyrotropin-releasing hormone (TRH). TRH in turn stimulates the production of

thyroid-stimulating hormone (TSH) by the anterior lobe of the pituitary gland. TSH then stimulates production and release of triiodothyronine (T_3) and thyroxine (T_4). Most of the thyroid hormone made in the thyroid is in the form of T_4. The body's cells convert the T_4 to T_3, which is the more active hormone.

There are two types of T_3: the free, or active, portion, and the portion bound to plasma proteins. Only a very small amount (<1%) of T_3 is free. Unlike the total T_3 level, the free T_3 level will not be affected by conditions that increase the levels of the plasma proteins. The free T_3 test may be ordered following an abnormal TSH and T_4 test, when a patient exhibits symptoms of hyperthyroidism, and to monitor effectiveness of treatment for hyperthyroidism.

Normal Values

260–480 pg/dL (4.0–7.4 pmol/L SI units)

Possible Meanings of Abnormal Values

Increased	Decreased
Hyperthyroidism	Acute illness
T_3 thyrotoxicosis	Chronic illness
Thyroid cancer	Congenital TBG deficiency
Thyroiditis	Hypothyroidism
	Thyroidectomy

Contributing Factors to Abnormal Values

- Drugs that can *increase* free T_3: amiodarone, clofibrate, cytomel, estrogens, methadone, oral contraceptives, phenothiazines, tamoxifen, terbutaline, thyroxine, valproic acid.
- Drugs that can *decrease* free T_3: amiodarone, anabolic steroids, androgens, antithyroid drugs, aspirin, atenolol, carbamazepine, cimetidine, corticosteroids, furosemide, lithium, phenytoin, propranolol, theophylline.

Interventions/Implications

Pretest
- Explain to the patient the purpose of the test and the need for a blood sample to be drawn.
- No fasting is required before the test.
- If possible, withhold any medications that may alter test results.

Procedure
- A 7-mL blood sample is drawn in a red-top collection tube.
- Gloves are worn throughout the procedure.

Posttest
- Apply pressure at venipuncture site. Apply dressing, periodically assessing for continued bleeding.
- Label the specimen and transport it to the laboratory.
- Resume medications as taken before the test.
- Report abnormal findings to the primary care provider.

Triiodothyronine, Total (T_3, Total T_3)

Test Description

When thyroid hormone levels decrease in the bloodstream or the body is exposed to physiological or psychological stress, the hypothalamus is stimulated to release thyrotropin-releasing hormone (TRH). TRH in turn stimulates the production of thyroid-stimulating hormone (TSH) by the anterior lobe of the pituitary gland. TSH then stimulates production and release of triiodothyronine (T_3) and thyroxine (T_4). Most of the thyroid hormone made in the thyroid is in the form of T_4. The body's cells convert the T_4 to T_3, which is the more active hormone.

There are two types of T_3: the free, or active, portion, and the portion bound to plasma proteins. About 99.7% of the T_3 is bound to plasma proteins, such as thyroxine-binding globulin (TBG). The T_3 test is usually ordered following an abnormal TSH and T_4 test. Conditions that increase the levels of the plasma proteins (TBG), such as pregnancy and liver disease, will falsely raise the total T_3 level. The free T_3 level will not be affected. Other testing may include thyroid antibodies and the T_3 uptake test.

This test may be ordered when a patient exhibits symptoms of hyperthyroidism. It is especially useful in the diagnosis of hyperthyroidism when the free T_4 is normal or borderline. It may also be used to monitor effectiveness of treatment for hyperthyroidism. If the T_3 is normal, the medication is controlling the condition.

Normal Values

100–200 ng/dL (1.54–3.08 nmol/L SI units)

Possible Meanings of Abnormal Values

Increased	Decreased
Hyperthyroidism	Acute illness
Pregnancy	Anorexia nervosa
T_3 thyrotoxicosis	Chronic illness
Thyroid cancer	Congenital TBG deficiency
Thyroiditis	Hypothyroidism
	Liver disease
	Renal failure
	Starvation
	Thyroidectomy

Contributing Factors to Abnormal Values

- Drugs that can *increase* T_3: amiodarone, clofibrate, cytomel, estrogens, methadone, oral contraceptives, phenothiazines, tamoxifen, terbutaline, thyroxine, valproic acid.
- Drugs that can *decrease* T_3: amiodarone, anabolic steroids, androgens, antithyroid drugs, aspirin, atenolol, carbamazepine, cimetidine, corticosteroids, furosemide, lithium, phenytoin, propranolol, theophylline.

Interventions/Implications

Pretest
- Explain to the patient the purpose of the test and the need for a blood sample to be drawn.
- No fasting is required before the test.
- If possible, withhold any medications that may alter test results.

Procedure
- A 7-mL blood sample is drawn in a red-top collection tube.
- Gloves are worn throughout the procedure.

Posttest
- Apply pressure at venipuncture site. Apply dressing, periodically assessing for continued bleeding.
- Label the specimen and transport it to the laboratory.
- Resume medications as taken before the test.
- Report abnormal findings to the primary care provider.

Clinical Alerts

- With elevated TSH levels:
  - If the T_3 and T_4 are normal: Mild (subclinical) hypothyroidism
  - If the T_3 and/or T_4 are low: Hypothyroidism
- With low TSH levels:
  - If the T_3 and T_4 are normal: Mild (subclinical) hyperthyroidism
  - If either the T_3 or T_4 is high: Hyperthyroidism
  - If the T_3 and T_4 are low or normal: Secondary hyperthyroidism due to pituitary dysfunction

Triiodothyronine Uptake Test
(T_3 Uptake, Resin T_3 Uptake)

Test Description
This test is an indirect measurement of the amount of unsaturated thyroxine-binding globulin (TBG) based on the total quantity of TBG present and the quantity of thyroxine (T_4) bound to it. During this test, a known quantity of radioactive T_3 and a resin are added to a sample of the patient's blood. The radioactive T_3 will bind with any available TBG sites. The percentage of radioactive T_3 that remains available to become attached to the resin after all available TBG sites have been filled is determined. This percentage is inversely proportional to the percentage of TBG saturation. A higher T_3 uptake means less TBG is available, possibly due to hyperthyroidism.

Normal Values
24–37%

Possible Meanings of Abnormal Values

Increased	Decreased
Congenital TBG deficiency	Acute hepatitis
Hyperthyroidism	Congenital TBG excess
Hypoproteinemia	Estrogen-secreting tumors
Malnutrition	Hypothyroidism
Nephrosis	Pregnancy
Nephrotic syndrome	
Renal failure	

Contributing Factors to Abnormal Values

- Drugs that can *increase* T_3 uptake (T_3U) values: anabolic steroids, barbiturates, corticosteroids, furosemide, heparin, phenylbutazone, phenytoin, salicylates, thyroxine, warfarin.
- Drugs that can *decrease* T_3U values: antithyroid agents, clofibrate, estrogens, oral contraceptives, thiazide diuretics.

Interventions/Implications

Pretest
- Explain to the patient the purpose of the test and the need for a blood sample to be drawn.
- No fasting is required before the test.

Procedure
- A 7-mL blood sample is drawn in a red-top collection tube.
- Gloves are worn throughout the procedure.

Posttest
- Apply pressure at venipuncture site. Apply dressing, periodically assessing for continued bleeding.
- Label the specimen and transport it to the laboratory.
- Report abnormal findings to the primary care provider.

T

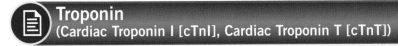

Troponin
(Cardiac Troponin I [cTnI], Cardiac Troponin T [cTnT])

Test Description
The troponins are proteins found in skeletal muscle and heart muscle. There are actually three types of troponin: C, I, and T. Subgroups of these, known as cardiac troponin I and cardiac troponin T, are specific to the heart muscle fibers. When there is damage to the heart muscle, the cardiac troponins are released into the blood. Thus, the two cardiac troponins are used to determine whether a person has had a myocardial infarction or some other injury to the heart muscle, such as when a cardiac contusion has occurred during chest trauma. Cardiac troponin is typically measured along with other cardiac biomarkers, such as CK, CK-MB, and myoglobin.

Following heart muscle damage, Tropinin I will increase in 3 to 6 hours, peak in 14 to 20 hours, and return to normal in 5 to 7 days. Tropinin T will increase in 3 to 12 hours, peak in 12 to 24 hours, and return to normal in 10 to 15 days. When a patient with chest pain presents to the emergency department, the cardiac troponin is immediately evaluated. It is then repeated 2 to 3 times in the first 12 to 16 hours, usually at 6 and 12 hours. Both of the cardiac troponins do not need to be checked. Typically an institution will perform one or the other.

It is important for health-care providers to use the troponin level as only one part of the clinical picture. The patient's history, physical assessment, and other test results, including electrocardiogram (ECG), must all be taken into consideration.

THE EVIDENCE FOR PRACTICE

Biomarkers of cardiac injury should be measured in all patients who present with chest discomfort consistent with acute coronary syndrome (ACS). A cardiac-specific troponin is the preferred marker, and if available, it should be measured in all patients.

Normal Values

Cardiac troponin I: <0.4 ng/mL (<0.4 μg/L SI units)
Cardiac troponin T: <0.2 ng/mL (<0.2 μg/L SI units)

Possible Meanings of Abnormal Values

Increased

Cardiotoxic drugs (chemotherapy, alcohol)
Congestive heart failure
Dermatomyositis
Kidney disease
Myocardial infarction
Myocarditis
Pericarditis
Polymyositis
Pulmonary embolism

Contributing Factors to Abnormal Values

- Unlike other cardiac markers which might also rise with damage to skeletal muscle, troponin levels are not generally affected by intramuscular injections, trauma, strenuous exercise, or medications.

Interventions/Implications

Pretest
- Explain to the patient the purpose of the test and the need for a blood sample to be drawn.
- No fasting is required before the test.

Procedure
- A 7-mL blood sample is drawn in a serum-separator collection tube.
- Gloves are worn throughout the procedure.

Posttest
- Apply pressure at venipuncture site. Apply dressing, periodically assessing for continued bleeding.
- Label the specimen and transport it to the laboratory.
- Report abnormal findings to the primary care provider.

Clinical Alerts

- Clinical interpretation of the troponin level is considered along with other laboratory information:
  - With an elevated troponin level in conjunction with an abnormal ECG, myocardial infarction is likely.
  - With an elevated troponin level and normal CK, CK-MB, and myoglobin, the cardiac muscle injury may have occurred more than 24 hours prior.
  - With a normal troponin and CK-MB and an elevated CK, the problem is most likely skeletal muscle related, rather than cardiac.

Tuberculin Skin Test (Mantoux Test, PPD Skin Test)

Test Description
The tuberculin skin test is used to screen for previous infection by the tubercle bacillus. The test is unable to differentiate between active tuberculosis (TB) and dormant TB. Tuberculin skin testing is a routine screening procedure for children, health-care workers, individuals at high risk of being infected, and individuals who are suspected of being infected with TB. Purified protein derivative (PPD) is administered intradermally. With the Mantoux test, the PPD is administered using a tuberculin syringe and a 25- or 26-gauge needle. The result is read in 48 to 72 hours. An area of *induration* (hardening) is measured. Redness (erythema) is not significant, and is thus not measured.

THE EVIDENCE FOR PRACTICE
According to the Centers for Disease Control, whether a reaction to the Mantoux tuberculin skin test is classified as positive depends on the size of the induration and the person's risk factors for TB (See http://www.cdc.gov/nchstp/tb/pubs/tbfactsheets/250005.pdf).

An induration of **5 mm or more** is considered a positive reaction for the following people:
- People with HIV infection
- Close contacts of people with infectious TB
- People with chest x-ray findings suggestive of previous TB disease
- People who inject illicit drugs and whose HIV status is unknown

An induration of **10 mm or more** is considered a positive reaction for the following people:
- People born in areas of the world where TB is common (foreign-born persons)
- People who inject illicit drugs but who are known to be HIV negative

- Low-income groups with poor access to health care
- People who live in residential facilities (e.g., nursing homes or correctional facilities)
- People with medical conditions that appear to increase the risk for TB (not including HIV infection), such as diabetes
- Children younger than 4 years old
- People in other groups likely to be exposed to TB, as identified by local public health officials

An induration of **15 mm or more** is considered a positive reaction for people with no risk factors for TB. In most cases, people who have a very small reaction or no reaction probably do not have TB infection.

Normal Values

Negative: Induration <5 mm

Possible Meanings of Abnormal Values

Positive

Active tuberculosis
Previous infection by tubercle bacilli

Contributing Factors to Abnormal Values

- Subcutaneous, rather than intradermal, injection of the PPD invalidates the test.
- Individuals with conditions which affect the immune system (cancer, recent chemotherapy, late-stage AIDS) may have a *false-negative* test result.
- Drugs that may *suppress* skin reactions when given within the past 4 to 6 weeks: corticosteroids, immunosuppressants, live vaccine virus such as measles, mumps, rubella, or polio.

Interventions/Implications

Pretest
- Explain to the patient the purpose of the test and the procedure to be performed.
- Obtain the patient's history regarding previous history of TB, previous PPD results, and previous BCG immunizations (see Contraindications).

Procedure
- The patient is placed in a sitting position, with the arm extended and supported on a flat surface.
- Cleanse the volar surface of the upper forearm with alcohol and allow to dry. Avoid nevi and other areas of pigmentation for injection of the PPD.
- Inject the PPD intradermally. A wheal should appear under the skin.
- Document the site of the injection.
- Gloves are worn throughout the procedure.

Posttest
- Measure any area of induration in 48 to 72 hours.
- Report abnormal findings to the primary care provider.

Clinical Alerts

- For a "2-step" TB test:
    - If the first Mantoux is negative, a second test is done is 1 to 2 weeks.
    - If the first Mantoux shows <5 mm induration, a second test is done on the other forearm at the time of the first reading.
    - If the first Mantoux is positive, a second Mantoux is not needed.
- Positive TB skin tests should be confirmed through further testing (sputum testing for acid-fast bacilli, chest x-ray).

CONTRAINDICATIONS!

- Patients with known active tuberculosis
- Patients who have received *bacilli Calmette-Guérin (BCG)*, an immunization against PPD. These patients will have a positive reaction to PPD, even though they have never had the TB infection.

 Upper Gastrointestinal and Small-Bowel Series (Gastric Radiography, Small-Bowel Study, Stomach X-ray, Upper GI Series)

Test Description

The upper gastrointestinal and small-bowel series is the fluoroscopic examination of the esophagus, stomach, and small intestine after ingestion of barium sulfate. During this procedure, a fluoroscopic screen is positioned over the structures being studied. These structures are then projected onto the fluoroscopic screen. The image remains on the monitor for continuous observation as the patient swallows barium and it passes into the stomach. The patient's position is changed throughout the exam to allow visualization of the structures and their function, including peristalsis. This test is especially useful in the evaluation of patients experiencing dysphagia, regurgitation, burning or gnawing epigastric pain, hematemesis, melena, and weight loss. Videotapes of the fluoroscopic procedure enable the movements to be studied at a later time.

U

Normal Values

Normal size, shape, position, and functioning of the esophagus, stomach, and small bowel

Possible Meanings of Abnormal Values

Achalasia/chalasia
Cancer: esophageal, gastric, duodenal
Congenital abnormalities
Diverticula: esophageal, duodenal
Esophageal motility disorders, such as spasms
Esophageal varices

Esophagitis

External compression by pancreatic and hepatic cysts and tumors

Gastric inflammatory disease

Gastric tumors

Gastritis

Hiatal hernia

Perforation of the esophagus, stomach, or small bowel

Polyps

Small-bowel tumors

Strictures

Ulcers: esophageal, gastric, duodenal

Contributing Factors to Abnormal Values

- Under- or overexposure of the film may alter film quality.
- When patients are unable to hold still, due to pain or mental status, the quality of the film may be affected.

Interventions/Implications

Pretest

- Explain to the patient the purpose of the test and the benefits and risks associated with the test. Provide any written teaching materials available on the subject. Note that no discomfort is associated with this procedure. The barium, although in a milkshake-type solution, may taste chalky.
- Fasting for 8 hours is required prior to the test.
- Instruct the patient to remove all objects containing metal, such as jewelry or undergarments, as these will show on the film.

Procedure

- The patient is first assisted to a supine position on the exam table.
- The table is tilted so that the patient is placed in an upright position for the first part of the procedure.
- The fluoroscopic screen is placed in front of the patient and the heart, lungs, and abdomen are viewed.
- The patient is instructed to take several swallows of a thick barium mixture while the videotape is made of the pharyngeal action.
- As the patient then continues to drink the barium mixture, in addition to the fluoroscopic viewing, spot films are made of the esophageal area from a variety of angles.
- The patient is then instructed to finish drinking the barium mixture, while films are made of the filling of the stomach and the emptying of the stomach into the duodenum.
- The small intestine is observed for passage of barium, with films made at 30 to 60 minute intervals until the barium reaches the ileocecal valve.

Posttest

- Resume the patient's diet and medications as taken prior to the test.
- Encourage fluid intake to promote excretion of the barium.
- Instruct the patient on the need to evacuate all of the barium. Administer a cathartic as ordered. Check all stools for presence of barium, explaining to the patient that the stools will be white initially and return to normal color following passage of all of the barium.
- Notify the primary care provider if the barium is not expelled within 2 to 3 days.

- Provide emotional support as the patient awaits the test results.
- Report abnormal findings to the primary care provider.

Clinical Alerts

- If cholangiography and/or a barium enema test are ordered, these should be completed *before* the barium swallow is performed. Otherwise the barium sulfate ingested during the barium swallow may obscure the films made during the other exams.
- Possible complication: fecal impaction due to retention of barium.

CONTRAINDICATIONS!

- Pregnant women
  - Caution: A woman in her childbearing years should undergo radiography only during her menses or 12 to 14 days after its onset to avoid any exposure to a fetus.
- Patients with intestinal obstruction
- Patients with a perforated viscus (gastrografin, a water-soluble contrast medium, would be used in place of barium)
- Patients who are unable to cooperate due to age, mental status, pain, or other factors
- Patients with unstable vital signs

Urea Nitrogen, Blood (Blood Urea Nitrogen, BUN)

Test Description
Urea is produced in the liver as a result of protein metabolism. Urea nitrogen is the nitrogen portion of urea. Urea is transported in the blood to the kidneys, where it is excreted. Since urea is cleared from the bloodstream by the kidneys, measurement of the level of urea nitrogen in the blood is an appropriate test of renal function, specifically that of glomerular function. The blood urea nitrogen (BUN) is usually determined in conjunction with the creatinine level in assessing renal function. Both of these parameters should be assessed prior to administration of any nephrotoxic medication. The normal ratio of BUN to creatinine ranges from 6:1 to 20:1.

Normal Values
Adult:	7–20 mg/dL (2.5–7.1 mmol/L SI units)
Elderly:	Slightly increased
Child:	5–18 mg/dL (1.8–6.4 mmol/L SI units)

U

Possible Meanings of Abnormal Values

Increased	Decreased
Acute glomerulonephritis	Alcohol abuse
Acute myocardial infarction	Celiac disease
Congestive heart failure	Diet inadequate in protein
Diabetes mellitus	Hemodialysis
Diarrhea	Hepatitis
Gastrointestinal bleeding	Increased antidiuretic
High-protein diet	hormone (ADH)
Mercury poisoning	Late pregnancy
Nephrotic syndrome	Liver failure
Obstructive uropathy	Malnutrition
Renal disease	Nephrosis
Severe dehydration	Overhydration
Severe infection	Pregnancy
Shock	

Contributing Factors to Abnormal Values

- False elevation of BUN with hemolysis of blood sample.
- Drugs which may *increase* the BUN: ACE-inhibitors, acetaminophen, acyclovir, allopurinol, amantadine, aminoglycosides, amiodarone, amphotericin B, antidepressants, antibiotics, ARBs, beta-blockers, diuretics, hydroxyurea, methysergide, NSAIDs, radiopaque contrast dye, streptokinase.
- Drugs which may *decrease* the BUN: chloramphenicol, streptomycin.

Interventions/Implications

Pretest
- Explain to the patient the purpose of the test and the need for a blood sample to be drawn.
- No fasting is required before the test.
- Instruct the patient to avoid a diet high in red meat prior to the test.

Procedure
- A 7-mL blood sample is drawn in a red-top collection tube.
- Gloves are worn throughout the procedure.

Posttest
- Apply pressure at venipuncture site. Apply dressing, periodically assessing for continued bleeding.
- Label the specimen and transport it to the laboratory.
- Report abnormal findings to the primary care provider.

Clinical Alerts

- If the BUN is elevated, check with the primary care provider prior to administering any nephrotoxic medication.
- Before receiving intravascular iodinated contrast material, patients meeting one or more of the following criteria should have BUN and creatinine testing completed:
  - Known creatinine level ≥1.5

- Age 60 and over
- Personal or family history of renal disease
- Personal history of diabetes mellitus
- History of collagen vascular disease, such as lupus
- Currently taking certain medications: metformin, nephrotoxic antibiotics

 ## Uric Acid, Blood

Test Description
Uric acid is produced by the breakdown of purines, chemicals that are the building blocks for DNA and RNA. They enter the circulation from digestion of foods or from normal breakdown and turnover of cells in the body. Part of the uric acid is excreted in the feces, but most uric acid is excreted in the urine. Excess serum uric acid can become deposited in joints and soft tissues, causing gout, an inflammatory response to the deposition of the urate crystals. Conditions in which there is rapid turnover of cells and/or slowing of uric acid excretion by the kidneys may cause elevated serum uric acid levels (*hyperuricemia*). The most common causes of accumulation of uric acid are an inherited tendency to overproduce uric acid and impaired kidney function that results in decreased ability to excrete uric acid.

Normal Values
Female: 2.3–6.6 mg/dL (137–393 µmol/L SI units)
Male: 3.6–8.5 mg/dL (214–506 µmol/L SI units)

Possible Meanings of Abnormal Values

Increased (hyperuricemia)	Decreased (hypouricemia)
Acute leukemia	Acromegaly
Acute infectious mononucleosis	Celiac disease
Alcoholism	Fanconi's syndrome
Anemia	Hodgkin's disease
Congestive heart failure	Liver disease
Dehydration	Neoplasms
Down's syndrome	Renal tubular defects
Eclampsia	Syndrome of inappropriate
Fasting	ADH secretion (SIADH)
G6PD deficiency	Wilson's disease
Glomerulonephritis	Xanthinuria
Gout	
Hypoparathyroidism	
Hypothyroidism	
Lead poisoning	
Lymphomas	

U

Malnutrition
Neoplasms
Nephritis
Preeclampsia
Polycythemia vera
Purine ingestion (excessive)
Renal failure
Trauma
Underexcretion of uric acid
Uremia

Contributing Factors to Abnormal Values

- Drugs which may *increase* uric acid levels: acetaminophen, ampicillin, ascorbic acid, beta-blockers, caffeine, chemotherapeutic agents, cyclosporine, diltiazem, diuretics, epinephrine, G-CSF, isoniazid, levodopa, lisinopril, methyldopa, niacin, NSAIDs, phenothiazines, rifampin, salicylates, sildenafil, theophylline, warfarin.
- Drugs which may *decrease* uric acid levels: acetazolamide, allopurinol, aspirin (high dose), chlorpromazine, corticosteroids, enalapril, estrogens, griseofulvin, lisinopril, lithium, mannitol, marijuana, probenecid, salicylates, verapamil, vinblastine.

Interventions/Implications

Pretest
- Explain to the patient the purpose of the test and the need for a blood sample to be drawn.
- Fasting is usually required for 4 to 8 hours prior to the test, depending on reference laboratory used.
- Assess the patient's dietary history for intake of purine-rich foods.

Procedure
- A 7-mL blood sample is drawn in a red-top collection tube.
- Gloves are worn throughout the procedure.

Posttest
- Apply pressure at venipuncture site. Apply dressing, periodically assessing for continued bleeding.
- Label the specimen and transport it to the laboratory.
- Report abnormal findings to the primary care provider.

U

Clinical Alerts

- If the uric acid in the blood is found to be high, instruct the patient to increase the fluid intake to prevent renal stones from forming. Alcohol should be avoided, in that it inhibits the excretion of urate crystals.
- Dietary sources high in purines include: anchovies, asparagus, caffeine-containing beverages, legumes, mushrooms, spinach, yeast, and organ meats such as liver and kidneys.

Uric Acid, Urine

Test Description

Uric acid is produced by the breakdown of purines, chemicals that are the building blocks for DNA and RNA. They enter the circulation from digestion of foods or from normal breakdown and turnover of cells in the body. Part of the uric acid is excreted in the feces, but most uric acid is excreted in the urine. Excess urinary uric acid can precipitate into urate stones in the kidneys. Thus, this test is used to evaluate gout, to determine whether there is an overexcretion of uric acid, and to determine whether renal calculi may be due to hyperuricosuria.

Normal Values

250–650 mg/24 hours (1.48–4.43 mmol/24 hours SI units)

Possible Meanings of Abnormal Values

Increased	Decreased
Chronic myelogenous leukemia	Acidosis
Gout	Alcoholism
High-purine diet	Folic acid deficiency
Infection	Glomerulonephritis
Liver disease	Lead poisoning
Nephrolithiasis	Renal disease
Polycythemia vera	Urinary obstruction
Sickle cell anemia	
Wilson's disease	
Trauma	

Contributing Factors to Abnormal Values

- Drugs which may *increase* uric acid excretion: ascorbic acid, aspirin (high doses), cytotoxic drugs, phenylbutazone (high doses), probenecid (high doses), radiographic dyes, sulfinpyrazone.
- Drugs which may *decrease* uric acid excretion: aspirin (low doses), diuretics, phenylbutazone (low doses), probenecid (low doses).

Interventions/Implications

Pretest

- Explain 24-hour urine collection procedure to the patient.
- Stress the importance of saving *all* urine in the 24-hour period. Instruct the patient to avoid contaminating the urine with toilet paper or feces.
- Inform the patient of the presence of a preservative in the collection bottle.

Procedure

- Obtain the proper container containing appropriate preservative from the laboratory.
- Begin the testing period in the morning after the patient's first voiding, which is discarded.

U

- Timing of the 24-hour period begins at the time the first voiding is discarded.
- *All* urine for the next 24 hours is collected in the container, which is to be kept refrigerated or on ice.
- If any urine is accidentally discarded during the 24-hour period, the test must be discontinued and a new test begun.
- The ending time of the 24-hour collection period should be posted in the patient's room.
- Gloves are worn whenever dealing with the specimen collection.

Posttest

- At the end of the 24-hour collection period, label and send the urine container on ice to the laboratory as soon as possible.
- Report abnormal findings to the primary care provider.

 Clinical Alerts

- If the uric acid level in the urine is found to be high, instruct the patient on a low purine diet. Dietary sources high in purines include: anchovies, asparagus, caffeine-containing beverages, legumes, mushrooms, spinach, yeast, and organ meats such as liver and kidneys.

Urinalysis (Routine Urinalysis, U/A)

Test Description
The urinalysis is a routine screening test which is usually done as a part of a physical examination, during preoperative testing, and upon hospital admission. It is used in the diagnosis of infections of the kidneys and urinary tract and also in the diagnosis of diseases unrelated to the urinary system.

The urinalysis consists of several components including: appearance, bilirubin, blood, color, glucose, ketones, leukocyte esterase, nitrites, odor, pH, protein, specific gravity, urobilinogen, and microscopic examination of sediment (bacteria, crystals, epithelial casts, fatty casts, granular casts, hyaline casts, red blood cells and casts, white blood cells and casts). Many of the component tests within the urinalysis are performed via dipstick method, with abnormalities further investigated by viewing microscopically.

In general, if the urine sample is left standing too long, bacteria begin to split urea into ammonia, resulting in alkaline urine. Should this occur, test results regarding protein and the microscopic examination of casts will be inaccurate. A delay in testing may also result in falsely low glucose, ketone, bilirubin, and urobilinogen values and falsely elevated bacteria levels.

APPEARANCE

The appearance of the urine refers to the clarity of the fluid. Deviations from the normal appearance of urine may indicate the presence of infection or hematuria.

Normal Values

Clear to slightly hazy

Possible Meanings of Abnormal Values

- *Cloudy* urine may be due to the presence of bacteria, fat, red blood cells, or white blood cells, or change in pH.
- *Smokey* urine may be due to the presence of blood.

Contributing Factors to Abnormal Values

- If the urine sample is left standing too long, bacteria begin to split urea into ammonia, resulting in alkaline urine. Alkaline urine (pH above 7.0) results in turbid urine.
- Contamination of the sample with vaginal secretions may affect its appearance.

COLOR

In general, the color of the urine should correspond to the specific gravity of the urine. For example, dilute urine with its low specific gravity is almost colorless, whereas concentrated urine, with a high specific gravity, is dark yellow to amber in color. There are many factors which can affect the color of the urine, including food, drugs, and various conditions.

Normal Values

Light yellow to amber

Possible Meanings of Abnormal Values

Color of urine	Condition/Substance/Drugs
Blue/Green	Bacterial infections, pseudomonal UTI Drugs: amitriptyline, IV cimetidine, indomethacin, methocarbamol, methylene blue, IV promethazine, triamterene
Brown/Black	Alkaptonuria, melanotic tumor, bile pigments, methemoglobin Drugs: anticoagulants, cascara (with acidic urine), chloroquine, ferrous sulfate, levodopa, methyldopa, methocarbamol, metronidazole, nitrofurantoin, quinine, salicylates, senna, sulfonamides
Dark yellow to amber	Concentrated urine, presence of bilirubin Foods such as carrots Drugs: cascara
Light straw/Very pale yellow	Alcohol, large fluid intake, dilute urine
Orange	Presence of bile, fever Drugs: anticoagulants, fluorescein sodium, phenazopyridine, phenothiazines
Orange-yellow	Drugs: sulfasalazine (in alkaline urine)

U

Pink	Drugs: anticoagulants, doxorubicin, ibuprofen, phenytoin, salicylates
Purple	Drugs: phenothiazines
Red	Excessive exercise, porphyria Foods such as beets, rhubarb, blackberries Drugs: anticoagulants, cascara (with alkaline urine), deferoxamine mesylate, doxorubicin, ibuprofen, methyldopa, phenazopyridine, phenolphthalein (in some laxatives), phenothiazines, phenytoin, rifampin, salicylates, senna (with alkaline urine)
Red-Brown	Drugs: levodopa, phenytoin
Red-Orange	Drugs: rifabutin, rifampin
Rust	Drugs: phenothiazines, sulfonamides
Yellow	Drugs: nitrofurantoin, riboflavin, sulfonamides

Contributing Factors to Abnormal Values

- Urine tends to darken in color upon standing, thus urine specimens should be transported to the laboratory immediately after collection.

ODOR

Another portion of the routine urinalysis, is the assessment of the urine's odor. The normal odor of urine is due to its acidic content. Various conditions, medications, and foods may cause changes in odor of the urine.

Normal Values

Aromatic

Possible Meanings of Abnormal Values

Condition/Substance	Odor
Food (asparagus, garlic)	Musty
Ketonuria	Sweet/fruity
Maple syrup urine disease	Burnt sugar
Oathouse urine disease (methionine malabsorption)	Brewery odor Musty, mousey
Phenylketonuria	Stale fish
Trimethylaminuria	Fishy
Tyrosinemia	Fish/foul-smelling
Urinary tract infection	

Contributing Factors to Abnormal Values

- If the urine sample is left standing too long, bacteria begin to split urea into ammonia, resulting in alkaline urine and an ammonia odor.
- Drugs which may alter urine odor: antibiotics, estrogens, paraldehyde, vitamins.

Use of a reagent dipstick provides rapid screening of the urine for: specific gravity, pH, leukocyte esterase, nitrites, protein, glucose, ketones, urobilinogen, and bilirubin.

SPECIFIC GRAVITY

The routine urinalysis also includes the determination of the specific gravity of the urine. The *specific gravity* is a measure of the concentration of the urine compared to the concentration of water, which is 1.000. The higher the specific gravity, the more concentrated the urine. This test value is an indication of the kidneys' ability to concentrate and excrete urine. The specific gravity is normally lower in the elderly due to a decreased ability to concentrate urine. There is a condition, known as **fixed specific gravity,** in which the specific gravity remains at 1.010, without variance from specimen to specimen. This is usually indicative of severe renal damage.

Normal Values

Adult:	1.005–1.030 (random sample usually 1.015–1.025)
Elderly:	Decreased
Infant:	1.001–1.018 (through age 2)

Possible Meanings of Abnormal Values

Increased	Decreased
Acute glomerulonephritis	ADH deficiency (diabetes insipidus)
Congestive heart failure	Chronic pyelonephritis
Dehydration	Cystic fibrosis
Diabetes mellitus	Diuretics
Diarrhea	High fluid intake
Excessive fluid loss	
Fever	
Increased secretion of ADH	
(due to trauma, stress, drugs)	
Liver failure	
Low fluid intake	
Nephrosis	
Toxemia of pregnancy	
Vomiting	

Contributing Factors to Abnormal Values

- The specific gravity may be increased when the urine sample has been contaminated with stool or toilet paper.
- Drugs which may *increase* specific gravity: albumin, dextran, glucose, isotretinoin, penicillin, radiopaque contrast media, sucrose.
- Drugs which may *decrease* specific gravity: aminoglycosides, lithium.

pH

The determination of the pH of the urine provides information regarding the acid-base status of the patient. Urine is considered alkaline when the pH is greater than 7.0, and is found in such conditions as urinary tract infection. When the urine pH is less than 7.0, or acidic in nature, the cause may be such problems as diarrhea or starvation. There is an inverse relationship between the pH of the urine and the ketone (acetone) level in the urine.

Normal Values

4.6–8.0 with a mean of 5.0–6.0 (diet dependent)

Possible Meanings of Abnormal Values

Increased (alkaline)	Decreased (acidic)
Bacteriuria	Alkaptonuria
Chronic renal failure	Dehydration
Fanconi's syndrome	Diabetes mellitus
Metabolic alkalosis	Diarrhea
Pyloric obstruction	Fever
Respiratory alkalosis	Metabolic acidosis
Renal tubular acidosis	Phenylketonuria
Respiratory acidosis	Renal tuberculosis
Urinary tract infection	Urinary tract infection
Starvation	

Contributing Factors to Abnormal Values

- Foods which may *increase* the pH, making the urine more alkaline: most fruits and vegetables.
- Foods which may *decrease* the pH, making the urine more acidic: cranberry juice, eggs, meats, pineapple juice, high protein diets.
- Drugs which may *increase* the pH, making the urine more alkaline: acetazolamide, amiloride, antibiotics, potassium citrate, sodium bicarbonate.
- Drugs which may *decrease* the pH, making the urine more acidic: ammonium chloride, ascorbic acid, diazoxide, methenamine mandelate, metolazone.

LEUKOCYTE ESTERASE

Leukocyte esterase is an enzyme released from white blood cells when bacteria are present in the urine. Testing the urine for leukocyte esterase is considered a screening test for the presence of white blood cells in the urine. A positive reaction warrants further investigation to determine whether a urinary tract infection truly exists.

This test has been found to be very sensitive, meaning false-negative findings are extremely rare. Thus, a negative dipstick finding requires no further evaluation, unless the patient demonstrates signs and symptoms of a urinary tract infection. Any positive findings with this test should be verified by a urine culture.

Normal Values

Negative

Possible Meanings of Abnormal Values

Positive
Bacteriuria

Contributing Factors to Abnormal Values

- *False-negative* results may occur when there is ascorbic acid or protein in the urine.
- *False-positive* results may occur when there is contamination of urine sample with vaginal secretions.

NITRITES

The substance nitrate, which is derived from dietary metabolites, is normally found in the urine. When gram-negative bacteria are present in the urine, nitrate is converted to nitrite. The presence of nitrite in the urine, then, is an indication that bacteria are also present. This test is used in conjunction with a dipstick test for leukocyte esterase to screen for the presence of bacteria during a routine urinalysis. It is important to note that the presence of some types of bacteria do not lead to a positive nitrite. Thus, a negative nitrite does not rule out the presence of a urinary tract infection, especially if the patient is symptomatic.

The conversion of nitrate to nitrite by bacteria requires the microorganism to be in contact with the nitrate for some time. Thus, the test is best conducted on the first urine specimen of the morning. Any positive findings with this test should be verified by a urine culture.

Normal Values

Negative

Possible Meanings of Abnormal Values

Positive
Bacteriuria

Contributing Factors to Abnormal Values

- *False-negative* results may occur due to:
  - presence of yeasts or gram-positive bacteria, since these microorganisms do not convert nitrate to nitrite
  - inadequate nitrate levels in the urine due to diet lacking in green vegetables
  - extremely large numbers of bacteria in urine
  - high specific gravity of urine
  - fresh voided specimen or urine withdrawn from a urinary catheter
- *False-positive* results may occur due to contamination of sample by gram-negative bacteria.
- Drugs which may cause *false-negative* results: ascorbic acid (high level in the urine), antibiotics.

PROTEIN

In the individual with normal renal function, there is no protein in the urine. This is due to the glomerular filtrate membrane of the kidney being impervious to the large protein molecules. In the case of renal dysfunction, as in glomerulonephritis, the membrane is damaged, allowing the protein to pass through and be excreted in the urine. Thus, this test is one way to assess the patient for renal disease. It should be noted, however, that a small percentage of the population may have what is known as *orthostatic or postural proteinuria*, which is a benign condition. However, if random urine samples are consistently positive for protein, it is suggested that further testing, including the collection of a 24-hour urine sample, be conducted.

Normal Values

Negative

Possible Meanings of Abnormal Values

Increased
Diabetes mellitus
Emotional stress
Exercise
Glomerulonephritis
Malignant hypertension
Multiple myeloma
Orthostatic proteinuria
Preeclampsia
Premenstrual state
Pyelonephritis
Systemic lupus erythematosus

Contributing Factors to Abnormal Values

- False-positive results may occur if the urine is highly alkaline or highly concentrated. If the urine sample is left standing too long, bacteria begin to split urea into ammonia, resulting in alkaline urine.
- *False-positive* after receiving radiopaque contrast dye.
- *False-positive* results may occur after eating large amounts of protein.
- *False-negative* results may occur if the urine is highly dilute.
- Drugs which may *increase* the protein level in the urine: acetazolamide, amikacin, aminoglycosides, amphotericin B, aspirin, auranofin, basiliximab, carbamazepine, carvedilil, cephalosporins, cisplatin, diazoxide, doxorubicin, gold preparations, indinavir, lithium, nephrotoxic medications, probenicid, radiopaque contrast media, sulfonamides, venlafaxine.

U

GLUCOSE

Glucose filtered by the kidneys is normally reabsorbed by the proximal convoluted tubule. The kidney has a "renal threshold" for glucose. As long as the blood glucose level is less than the renal threshold, no glucose will be present in the urine. However, if the blood glucose level is greater than the renal threshold, all of the glucose will not be able to be reabsorbed and will instead be excreted into the urine.

As a part of the routine urinalysis, the urine is screened for the presence of glucose. This screening is typically accomplished through use of a reagent strip is dipped into the urine sample. The chemical reaction results in color changes which correspond to the level of glucose in the urine. Normally, there should be no glucose present in the urine, although occasionally a trace amount will occur during pregnancy. Should glucose be found in the urine (usually when serum glucose is >180 mg/dL), a condition known as *glycosuria*, diabetes mellitus is suspected. However, further testing must be done to positively diagnose this condition.

Normal Values

Negative

Possible Meanings of Abnormal Values

Increased

Acromegaly
Cushing's syndrome
Diabetes mellitus
Fanconi's syndrome
Galactose intolerance
Gestational diabetes
Hyperalimentation
Infection
Lowered renal threshold for glucose (pregnancy)
Multiple myeloma
Pheochromocytoma
Proximal tubular dysfunction
Stress

Contributing Factors to Abnormal Values

- Drugs which may cause *increased* levels of glucose in the urine: ammonium chloride, asparaginase, carbamazepine, corticosteroids, lithium, nicotinic acid, phenothiazines, thiazide diuretics.
- Drugs which may cause *false-positive* results: cephalosporins, chloral hydrate, chloramphenicol, corticosteroids, indomethacin, isoniazid, nalidixic acid, nitrofurantoin, penicillin, probenecid, streptomycin, sulfonamides, tetracyclines, sugars other than glucose (lactose, fructose, galactose, pentose)
- Drugs which may cause *false-negative* results: cancer metabolites.
- Drugs which may cause *either* false-positive or false-negative results: ascorbic acid, levodopa, methyldopa, phenazopyridine hydrochloride, salicylates.

KETONES

U

Normally, glucose is used by the cells of the body for energy. This use of glucose as an energy source can only occur if the glucose is able to enter the cell with the assistance of insulin. When insulin is lacking, as in the patient with uncontrolled diabetes mellitus, glucose is unable to enter the cell, resulting in the need for an alternate energy source. The body then turns to the metabolism of fatty acids for energy. As fatty acids are metabolized, three ketone bodies are formed and later excreted in the urine: acetoacetic acid, acetone, and beta hydroxybutyric acid. Thus, testing for the presence of ketones in the urine (ketonuria) is assistive in the diagnosis of diabetes mellitus, as well as in evaluating conditions associated with ketoacidotic states, such as starvation.

Normal Values

Negative

Possible Meanings of Abnormal Values

Increased

Alcoholism
Anorexia
Diabetes mellitus
Diarrhea
Fasting
Fever
High protein diet
Hyperthyroidism
Postanesthesia
Pregnancy
Starvation
Vomiting

Contributing Factors to Abnormal Values

- Diets high in fat and protein and low in carbohydrates may alter test results.
- Drugs which may cause *false-positive* results: bromosulfophthalein, isoniazid, levodopa, phenazopyridine, phenothiazines, phenolsulfonphthalein.

UROBILINOGEN

Bilirubin, which is one of the components of bile, is formed in the liver, spleen, and bone marrow. It is also formed as a result of hemoglobin breakdown. One type of bilirubin, conjugated (direct) bilirubin, is changed into urobilinogen by intestinal bacteria in the duodenum. The majority of urobilinogen is excreted in the stool. The liver reprocesses the remaining urobilinogen into bile. A very small amount is excreted in the urine. An increase in urobilinogen is indicative of hepatic dysfunction or a hemolytic process. Urobilinogen levels are typically highest during the early to mid-afternoon. Thus, should dipstick testing for urobilinogen be positive, the collection of a 2-hour urine would be most appropriate between 1 and 3 P.M.

Normal Values

Negative or 0.1–1.0 Ehrlich units/dL

Possible Meanings of Abnormal Values

Increased	**Decreased**
Acute hepatitis	Biliary obstruction
Cirrhosis	Inflammatory disease
Cholangitis	Renal insufficiency
Hemolytic anemia	Severe diarrhea
Severe ecchymosis	
Severe infection	

Contributing Factors to Abnormal Values

- *False-positive* test results may occur in porphyria.

- Drugs which may *increase* urobilinogen levels: acetazolamide, bromosulfoph-thalein, cascara, chlorpromazine, phenazopyridine, phenothiazines, sulfonamides.
- Drugs which may *decrease* urobilinogen levels: antibiotics.

BILIRUBIN

Bilirubin, which is one of the components of bile, is formed in the liver, spleen, and bone marrow. It is also formed as a result of hemoglobin breakdown. There are three types of bilirubin: total, direct (conjugated), and indirect (unconjugated). Normally, direct, or conjugated, bilirubin is excreted by the gastrointestinal (GI) tract, with only minimal amounts entering the bloodstream.

Direct bilirubin is water soluble and is the only type of bilirubin able to cross the glomerular filter. Although it is the only type of bilirubin which could be found in the urine, it is usually not detectable in the urine, since it is converted to urobilinogen in the intestine. However, should jaundice occur due to obstruction or liver disease, the direct bilirubin is unable to reach the GI tract. It instead enters the bloodstream, where it is eventually filtered out by the kidneys and excreted in the urine. Thus, an increased level of direct bilirubin in the urine is indicative of some type of hepatic or obstructive problem.

Normal Values

Negative (routine screening procedure)
No more than 0.2 mg/dL (<0.34 μmol/L SI units)

Possible Meanings of Abnormal Values

Increased
Cirrhosis of the liver
Hepatitis
Obstructive jaundice

Contributing Factors to Abnormal Values

- Drugs which may cause *false-positive* results: phenazopyridine, phenothiazines, salicylates.
- Drug which may cause *false-negative* results: ascorbic acid.
- Exposure of the specimen to light may affect test results.

Microscopic examination of sediment in the urine includes observation of bacteria, casts, crystals, red blood cells, and white blood cells.

BACTERIA

Tests for the presence of leukocyte esterase and nitrites in the urine are conducted to determine whether bacteria are present in the urine. Bacteria may also be noted via the microscopic examination of the urine. Should bacteria be found during a routine urinalysis, culture, and sensitivity testing of the urine should be done to determine the organism and to provide assistance in determining appropriate antimicrobial therapy.

Normal Values

Negative

Possible Meanings of Abnormal Values

Increased
Urinary tract infection

Contributing Factors to Abnormal Values

- Contamination of specimen by inadequate cleansing of the external genitalia may cause *false-positive* results.

CASTS

Casts are collections of gel-like protein material which result from the agglutination of cells and cellular debris. They form in, and take the shape of, the renal tubules. Epithelial cells in the renal tubules are the components of *epithelial casts*. *Fatty casts* are formed from fat droplets. When the cellular material in epithelial cells and white blood cells breaks down, the resulting granular particles form *granular casts*. *Hyaline casts* are formed from protein, and thus indicate the presence of proteinuria.

Normal Values

Epithelial:	No casts, occasional epithelial cells
Fatty:	No casts
Granular:	No casts
Hyaline:	1–2 casts per low-power field

Possible Meanings of Abnormal Values

Type of cast	Condition
Epithelial casts	Acute tubular necrosis
	Eclampsia
	Glomerulonephritis
	Heavy metal poisoning
	Interstitial nephritis
	Nephrosis
	Tubular damage
Fatty casts	Chronic renal disease
	Diabetes mellitus
	Glomerulonephritis
	Hypothyroidism
	Nephrotic syndrome
Granular casts	Acute renal failure
	Chronic lead poisoning
	Chronic renal failure
	Glomerulonephritis
	Malignant hypertension
	Pyelonephritis
	Renal tuberculosis
	Strenuous exercise
	Toxemia of pregnancy

U

Hyaline casts	Acid urine
	Chronic renal failure
	Congestive heart failure
	Glomerulonephritis
	Proteinuria
	Pyelonephritis
	Strenuous exercise
	Trauma to glomerular capillary membrane

Contributing Factors to Abnormal Values

- Urine allowed to stand too long without refrigeration will become alkaline due to bacterial conversion of urea into ammonia. Should this occur, casts may disintegrate, resulting in inaccurate test results.

CRYSTALS

The accumulation of certain substances in the urine leads to the formation of crystals. They may also form when urine is allowed to stand at room temperature before testing or be caused by several drugs. A few crystals present in the urine have little clinical significance. However, it is problematic when numerous crystals form, resulting in the formation of renal stones. For example, numerous calcium oxalate crystals, resulting from hypercalcemia, may form calcium oxalate stones. Knowing the composition of the renal stone aids the health-care provider in determining appropriate treatment modalities.

Normal Values

A few may be normally present

Possible Meanings of Abnormal Values

Increased
Renal stone formation
Urinary tract infection

Contributing Factors to Abnormal Values

- Allowing urine sample to stand at room temperature prior to testing may alter test results.
- Drugs that cause crystal formation in the presence of acidic urine: acetazolamide, aminosalicylic acid, ascorbic acid, nitrofurantoin, theophylline, thiazide diuretics.

RED BLOOD CELLS AND CASTS

The microscopic examination of sediment also serves to determine whether any blood is present in the urine, a condition known as *hematuria*. The urine is observed for both red blood cells and red blood cell casts. When red blood cells are present in the urine, it usually indicates damage to the renal glomeruli, which allows red blood cells to enter the urine. Since there are several interfering factors, such as trauma incurred during catheterization, which might also cause blood to be present in the urine, it is suggested that a fresh urine specimen be collected and the presence of blood be verified.

Red blood cell casts, aggregates of cells formed in the renal tubules, may also be found in the urine. Their presence usually indicates the blood is of glomerular origin, something which may occur in patients with a variety of conditions.

Normal Values

Cells: 0–2 per high-power field
Casts: None

Possible Meanings of Abnormal Values

Increased: Red blood cells	Increased: Red blood cell casts
Acute tubular necrosis	Acute inflammation
Benign familial hematuria	Blood dyscrasias
Benign prostatic hypertrophy	Collagen disease
Benign recurrent hematuria	Glomerulonephritis
Calculi	Goodpasture's syndrome
Foreign body	Malignant hypertension
Glomerulonephritis	Renal infarction
Hemophilia	Scurvy
Hemorrhagic cystitis	Sickle cell anemia
Interstitial nephritis	Subacute bacterial endocarditis
Polycystic kidneys	Vasculitis
Pyelonephritis	
Renal trauma	
Renal tuberculosis	
Renal tumor	
Subacute bacterial endocarditis	
Systemic lupus erythematosus	
Urinary tract infection	

Contributing Factors to Abnormal Values

- Hematuria may occur due to: tissue trauma from urinary catheterization, strenuous exercise, smoking, and contamination with menstrual flow.
- Drugs which may *cause hematuria*: acetylsalicylic acid, amphotericin B, bacitracin, indomethacin, methenamine, methicillin, phenylbutazone, salicylates, sulfonamides, warfarin.
- *False-positive* results may occur after intake of certain foods, such as beets, blackberries, and rhubarb.
- *False-negative* results may occur in the presence of ascorbic acid.

WHITE BLOOD CELLS AND CASTS

A few white blood cells are normally found in the urine. If more than five white blood cells per high-power field are present, a urinary tract infection should be suspected and further testing conducted. White blood cell casts are aggregates of white blood cells which collect in the renal tubules. These casts are seen most often in patients with acute pyelonephritis.

Normal Values

Cells: 4–5 per high-power field
Casts: None

Possible Meanings of Abnormal Values

Increased: White blood cells	Increased: White blood cell casts
Cystitis	Acute pyelonephritis
Pyogenic infection	Glomerulonephritis
	Lupus nephritis
	Nephrotic syndrome
	Renal inflammatory processes

Contributing Factors to Abnormal Values

- If the urine is contaminated with vaginal discharge, test results may be inaccurate.

Pretest Nursing Care

- Explain to the patient the purpose of the routine urinalysis and the need for a urine sample to be obtained.
- No fasting is required prior to the test.

Procedure

- Testing the first morning urine specimen, when the urine is concentrated, is preferred.
- A minimum sample of 15 mL of urine is required.
- A clean-catch midstream technique to obtain the urine sample is recommended to prevent contamination of the specimen.
- A clean-catch kit containing cleansing materials and a sterile specimen container is given to the patient.
    - Male patients should cleanse the urinary meatus with the materials provided or with soap and water, void a small amount of urine into the toilet, and then void directly into the specimen container.
    - Female patients should cleanse the labia minora and urinary meatus, cleansing from front to back. While keeping the labia separated, the female should void a small amount into the toilet and then void directly into the specimen container.
- Instruct patients to avoid touching the inside of the specimen container and lid.
- For the portions of the urinalysis which involve use of dipstick testing, a reagent strip is dipped into the urine specimen. After a period of time specified by the manufacturer of the dipstick, the color of the reagent pad is compared with a color chart provided by the manufacturer.
- Gloves are worn throughout the procedure.

Posttest Nursing Care

- Label the urine specimen and transport it to the laboratory immediately. The urine needs to be examined within 2 hours.
- If urine is collected via an indwelling urinary catheter, a syringe and needle is used. Remove the needle prior to transferring the urine to the specimen cup to avoid damage to any microscopic sediment which may be present.
- Report abnormal findings to the primary care provider.

→ Clinical Alerts

- Additional testing which may be indicated based on abnormal urinalysis results.

Urine Culture and Sensitivity (Urine for C & S)

Test Description
The urine is normally a sterile body fluid. Although a few bacteria reside in the urethra, in the absence of infection, bacteria should not normally be present in the urine.

When a patient is suspected of having a urinary tract infection (UTI), a urine sample for culture and sensitivity is ordered. The urine specimen should be obtained prior to the beginning of antibiotic therapy. This test involves several components. First, a Gram stain of the specimen can be done and quickly reported. This provides basic information as to whether the organism is gram-positive or gram-negative. Next, the urine is cultured, that is, the organisms are allowed to grow in special culture media. In 48 to 72 hours, the organism is usually identified. The sensitivity portion of the test involves the testing of the organism to identify drugs to which the organism is sensitive or resistant.

Once the specimen is obtained, the patient is usually given a broad-spectrum antibiotic which is likely to be effective against most UTIs. After the urine culture and sensitivity results are available, the antibiotic in use should be verified as to its appropriateness according to the sensitivity report.

THE EVIDENCE FOR PRACTICE
The screening tests used commonly in the primary care setting (dipstick analysis and direct microscopy) have poor positive and negative predictive value for detecting bacteriuria in asymptomatic persons. Urine culture is the gold standard for detecting asymptomatic bacteriuria.

Normal Values
No growth

Possible Meanings of Abnormal Values
Probable sample contamination with bacterial counts <10,000/mL
Urinary tract infection with bacterial counts >100,000/mL

Contributing Factors to Abnormal Values
- Improper collection technique may alter test results.
- Drugs which may *decrease* bacterial counts: antibiotics.

Interventions/Implications
Pretest
- Explain to the patient the purpose of the test and the need for a urine sample.
- No fasting is required prior to the test.

Procedure
- At least 5 mL of urine is needed for this test.
- Use of clean-catch midstream technique is recommended to prevent contamination of the specimen.

- A clean-catch kit containing cleansing materials and a sterile specimen container is given to the patient.
- Male patients should cleanse the urinary meatus with the materials provided or with soap and water, void a small amount of urine into the toilet, and then void directly into the specimen container.
- Female patients should cleanse the labia minora and urinary meatus, cleansing from front to back. While keeping the labia separated, the female should void a small amount into the toilet and then void directly into the specimen container.
- Instruct patients to avoid touching the inside of the specimen container and lid.
- Other methods for obtaining the urine specimen include catheterization of the patient solely to obtain the specimen, obtaining the sample from an indwelling urinary catheterization, or, in the case of patients with urinary diversions, obtaining the sample through the stoma. In neonates and infants, suprapubic aspiration may be necessary. A disposable pouch (U bag) is also used with infants and young children.
- Gloves are to be worn by the health care worker whenever dealing with the specimen.

Posttest
- Label the specimen. It must be transported to the laboratory immediately or placed on ice.
- Report results of the culture and sensitivity to the primary care provider so that modifications in drug therapy are made if needed.

→ **Clinical Alerts**

- Some facilities automatically conduct a C & S on any urine specimen with positive leukocytes and/or nitrites on urinalysis; others require a separate order from the primary care provider after review of the urinalysis results.

 Urobilinogen, Fecal

Test Description

Bilirubin, which is one of the components of bile, is formed in the liver, spleen, and bone marrow. It is also formed as a result of hemoglobin breakdown. There are three types of bilirubin: total, direct (conjugated), and indirect (unconjugated).

Direct, or conjugated, bilirubin is converted to *urobilinogen* by intestinal bacteria in the duodenum. The majority of urobilinogen is excreted in the stool. The liver reprocesses the remaining urobilinogen into bile. A very small amount is excreted in the urine.

The fecal urobilinogen level is dependent upon the amount of conjugated bilirubin excreted in the bile salts into the intestine. Fecal urobilinogen levels decrease when obstructive jaundice (as from gallstones) or hepatic jaundice occurs, since the bilirubin is unable to reach the intestines for excretion and instead enters the bloodstream for excretion by the kidneys.

There must also be adequate numbers of bacteria present in the intestine to breakdown the bilirubin into urobilinogen. With inadequate bacterial presence, as

U

occurs following oral antibiotic therapy, the decreased urobilinogen in the feces results in a light-colored stool.

Normal Values

30–200 mg/100 g of feces (50–300 mg/24 hours)

Possible Meanings of Abnormal Values

Increased	Decreased
Hemolytic anemias	Aplastic anemia
Hemolytic jaundice	Complete biliary obstruction
	Hepatic jaundice
	Obstructive jaundice
	Oral antibiotic therapy
	Severe liver disease

Contributing Factors to Abnormal Values

- Drugs which may *increase* fecal urobilinogen levels: salicylates, sulfonamides.
- Drugs which may *decrease* fecal urobilinogen levels: broad-spectrum antibiotics.

Interventions/Implications

Pretest
- Explain to the patient the purpose of the test and the need for collection of stool for 48 hours.
- The patient should take no antibiotics for 1 week prior to the test.
- No fasting is required prior to the test.
- Instruct the patient to avoid contaminating the stool with toilet paper or urine.

Procedure
- Collect the stool specimen and place it in a dry, clean, urine-free container provided by the laboratory.
- Gloves are worn throughout the procedure.

Posttest
- Cover the specimen, label the container, and transport it to the laboratory immediately.
- Report abnormal findings to the primary care provider.

📄 Uroflowmetry (Urine Flow Studies, Urodynamic Studies)

Test Description

Uroflowmetry is a noninvasive procedure which is used to detect dysfunctional voiding patterns. The test includes the measurement of the voiding duration, amount, and rate using a urine flowmeter, an instrument into which the patient voids. For the most accurate evaluation of urine flow patterns, recording of each voiding for 2 to 3 days should be performed. Uroflowmetry is usually performed in conjunction with other urinary tract testing, such as cystometry. Although the urethral pressure profile test is more often used, uroflowmetry is useful for testing patients in whom urinary catheterization is contraindicated.

Normal Values

The following values are usually based on a minimum urine volume of 200 mL for adults and 100 mL for children under age 14:

	Female	Male
>age 64	10 mL/sec	9 mL/sec
age 46–64	15 mL/sec	12 mL/sec
age 14–45	18 mL/sec	21 mL/sec
age 8–13	15 mL/sec	12 mL/sec
<age 8	10 mL/sec	10 mL/sec

Possible Meanings of Abnormal Values

External sphincter dysfunction
Hypotonia of detrusor muscle
Outflow obstruction (urethral stricture, prostatic cancer, benign prostatic hypertrophy)
Stress incontinence

Contributing Factors to Abnormal Values

- Drugs such as urinary spasmolytics and anticholinergics may alter test results.
- Contamination of the flowmeter by toilet paper or stool will alter test results.

Interventions/Implications

Pretest
- Explain to the patient the purpose of the test.
- Instruct the patient to void into the urine flowmeter. No toilet paper or stool can be allowed to enter the flowmeter funnel, or the test results will be altered.
- No fasting is required prior to the test.

Procedure
- When the patient feels the urge to void, a normal voiding position should be assumed. Voiding should occur directly into the urine flowmeter; the bladder is to be completely empty.
- Serial recordings of each voiding over 2 to 3 days are usually performed.

Posttest
- Uroflowmeter recordings are analyzed and displayed graphically by the instrument.
- Report abnormal findings to the primary care provider.

U

Uroporphyrinogen-I-Synthase

Test Description

Uroporphyrinogen-I-synthase is an enzyme found in red blood cells which is necessary for the conversion of porphobilinogen to uroporphyrinogen during the production of heme. This test is used to diagnose acute intermittent porphyria (AIP), during both latent and active phases. Acute intermittent porphyria (AIP) is one of the porphyrias, a group of diseases involving defects in heme metabolism that results in excessive secretion of porphyrins and porphyrin precursors. AIP manifests itself by abdominal pain, neuropathies, and constipation. Most importantly, it can be used to detect individuals affected with AIP prior to the occurrence of any acute episodes, episodes which can be fatal.

Normal Values

2.10–4.30 mU/g of hemoglobin

Possible Meanings of Abnormal Values

Decreased

Acute intermittent porphyria

Contributing Factors to Abnormal Values

- Hemolysis due to rough handling of the sample.
- False positive due to failure to freeze sample.
- Failure to fast prior to the test.
- Hemolytic and hepatic diseases may *increase* uroporphyrinogen-I-synthase levels.
- Low-carbohydrate diets, alcohol intake, infection, and certain drugs may *decrease* uroporphyrinogen-I-synthase levels.

Interventions/Implications

Pretest

- Explain to the patient the purpose of the test and the need for a blood sample to be drawn.
- The patient needs to fast for 12 to 14 hours before the test.
- Explain to the patient that abstinence from alcohol is needed for 24 hours prior to the test. Intake of water is allowed.

Procedure

- A 10-mL blood sample is drawn in a green-top collection tube.
- Gloves are worn throughout the procedure.

Posttest

- Apply pressure at venipuncture site. Apply dressing, periodically assessing for continued bleeding.
- Handle blood sample gently.
- Label the specimen and transport it on ice to the laboratory immediately.
- Include the patient's hemoglobin on the laboratory slip.
- Report abnormal findings to the primary care provider.

> ### → Clinical Alerts
>
> - When suspecting AIP, urine porphyrin studies should also be done.
> - If the patient is found to have acute intermittent porphyria, provide teaching regarding factors which have been found to precipitate acute episodes, including: drugs and hormones (barbiturates, chlordiazepoxide, ergot, estrogens, glutethimide, griseofulvin, meprobamate, methyprylon, phenytoin, steroid hormones, and sulfonamides), low-carbohydrate diets, alcohol consumption, and infections.

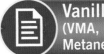

Vanillylmandelic Acid and Catecholamines
(VMA, Dopamine, Epinephrine, Norepinephrine, Metanephrine, Normetanephrine)

Test Description

The major catecholamines are *dopamine*, secreted from nerve endings, and *epinephrine* and *norepinephrine*, secreted from the adrenal medulla and from nerve endings. These hormones play a vital role in the "fight or flight" response of the body which occurs with stimulation of the sympathetic nervous system. The metabolite of epinephrine, *metanephrine*, and the metabolite of norepinephrine, *normetanephrine*, may also be measured. The end-product of epinephrine and norepinephrine metabolism is *vanillylmandelic acid (VMA)*.

In patients with unexplained hypertension, a catecholamine-secreting tumor of the adrenal medulla, known as *pheochromocytoma*, is suspected. By measuring 24-hour urinary levels of catecholamines, metanephrines, and VMA, the increased levels of catecholamines released by such a tumor can be found much more readily than through periodic plasma levels. Elevated VMA levels also occur with other catechlolamine-secreting tumors, such as neuroblastoma and ganglioneuroma.

Normal Values

Vanillylmandelic acid (VMA):	1.4–6.5 mg/24 hours (7.1–32.7 µmol/day SI units)
Catecholamines:	Total: 14–110 µg/24 hours
Dopamine:	65–400 µg/24 hours (424–2612 nmol/day SI units)
Epinephrine:	1.7–20 µg/24 hours (9.3–109 nmol/day SI units)
Norepinephrine:	12.1–85.5 µg/24 hours (72–505 nmol/day SI units)
Metanephrines, total:	0.0–0.9 mg/24 hours (0.0–4.9 µmol/day SI units)
Normetanephrine:	105–354 µg/24 hours (573–1933 nmol/day SI units)

V

Possible Meanings of Abnormal Values

Increased	Decreased
Acute anxiety	Anorexia nervosa
Exercise	Familial dystonia
Ganglioblastoma	Idiopathic orthostatic hypertension
Ganglioneuroma	

Neuroblastoma
Pheochromocytoma
Stress

Contributing Factors to Abnormal Values

- Drugs which may *increase* urinary VMA/catecholamine levels: acetaminophen, aminophylline, caffeine, chloral hydrate, disulfiram, epinephrine, erythromycin, ethanol, insulin, levodopa, lithium, methenamine mandelate, methyldopa, nicotinic acid, nitroglycerin, quinidine, tetracyclines.
- Drugs which may *decrease* urinary VMA/catecholamine levels: clonidine, disulfiram, guanethidine sulfate, imipramine, MAO inhibitors, phenothiazines, reserpine, salicylates.
- Foods/products which may interfere with test results: alcohol, coffee, tea, tobacco (including use of nicotine patch), bananas, citrus fruits, and vanilla.

Interventions/Implications

Pretest
- Explain 24-hour urine collection procedure to the patient.
- Stress the importance of saving *all* urine in the 24-hour period. Instruct the patient to avoid contaminating the urine with toilet paper or feces.
- Inform the patient of the presence of a preservative in the collection bottle.
- Instruct the patient to avoid excessive physical activity and stress during the testing period.
- The patient should avoid alcohol, coffee, tea, tobacco (including use of nicotine patch), bananas, citrus fruits, and vanilla for 3 days prior to the test.
- If possible, withhold medications which may alter test results for at least 3 days. These include: clonidine, L-dopa, methocarbamol, monoamine oxidase inhibitors, reserpine, salicylates.
    - Diuretics, ACE-inhibitors, calcium channel blockers, alpha blockers, and beta blockers cause minimal or no interference.

Procedure
- Obtain the proper container containing hydrochloric acid as preservative from the laboratory.
- Begin the testing period in the morning after the patient's first voiding, which is discarded.
- Timing of the 24-hour period begins at the time the first voiding is discarded.
- *All* urine for the next 24 hours is collected in the container, which is to be kept refrigerated or on ice.
- If any urine is accidentally discarded during the 24-hour period, the test must be discontinued and a new test begun.
- The ending time of the 24-hour collection period should be posted in the patient's room.
- Gloves are worn whenever dealing with the specimen collection.

Posttest
- At the end of the 24-hour collection period, label and send the urine container on ice to the laboratory as soon as possible.
- Resume diet and medications as taken prior to the testing period.
- Report abnormal findings to the primary care provider.

Varicella-Zoster (Chickenpox) Antibody Test

Test Description

Chickenpox is caused by the varicella-zoster virus (VZV), a member of the herpesvirus family. It is highly contagious and can be spread by direct contact, droplet transmission, and airborne transmission. The incubation period is 10 to 21 days from exposure to the virus until the appearance of pox—fluid-filled blisters that burst and form crusts. The blisters often appear first on the face, trunk, or scalp and spread to the rest of the body. People are contagious beginning 1 to 2 days before pox appear and remain contagious until all blisters are crusted. Children commonly complain of fever, headache, abdominal ache, and loss of appetite 1 to 2 days before the pox appear.

Most cases of chickenpox occur in children younger than 10 and are usually mild. However, serious complications such as encephalitis, pneumonia, and other invasive bacterial infections, and even death sometimes occur, especially in those who are immunocompromised or are taking chemotherapy or steroids. Adults and older children usually get sicker than younger children do. Women who acquire chickenpox during pregnancy are at risk for congenital infection of the fetus. Newborns are at risk for severe infection if they are exposed and their mothers are not immune.

The American Academy of Pediatrics (AAP) recommends the traditional chickenpox vaccine for children over 12 months. Those age 13 years and older who have not received the vaccine and have not had chickenpox should get 2 doses 4 to 8 weeks apart. Children who receive the vaccine before age 13 only need to receive 1 dose.

Providing immunity to VZV through vaccination is important for future health. When a person has the VZV infection, the virus remains latent in sensory nerve roots. Later, usually when the person is immunocompromised or is elderly, the virus can reactivate in the form of herpes zoster, also known as shingles. This is a painful vesicular rash which follows a dermatomal pattern, with the pain often continuing for months or years after the rash resolves.

The varicella-zoster antibody test measures IgG and IgM antibody formation against VZV. It can be used to diagnose chickenpox and to determine whether the person is immune to the virus either from having had the chickenpox infection or from having been vaccinated. A diagnosis of chickenpox is made when a fourfold increase between the acute titer and the convalescent titer occurs (a period of 10 to 14 days). Demonstration of specific IgG on a serum sample is evidence of immunity to chickenpox.

V

Normal Values

Negative for IgM and IgG:	Susceptible to varicella-zoster
Positive for IgM:	Current or recent varicella-zoster infection
Positive for IgG:	Immunity to varicella-zoster

Possible Meanings of Abnormal Values

Positive	Negative
Immunity to varicella-zoster (IgG)	Susceptible to varicella-zoster
Varicella-zoster infection (IgM)	

Contributing Factors to Abnormal Values

- Hemolysis due to excessive agitation of the blood sample may alter test results.

Interventions/Implications

Pretest
- Explain to the patient the purpose of the test and the need for a blood sample to be drawn.
- No fasting is required before the test.

Procedure
- A 7-mL blood sample is drawn in a red-top collection tube.
- Gloves are worn throughout the procedure.

Posttest
- Apply pressure at venipuncture site. Apply dressing, periodically assessing for continued bleeding.
- Label the specimen and transport it to the laboratory.
- Report abnormal findings to the primary care provider.

Video Capsule Endoscopy (VCE)

Test Description

Video capsule endoscopy (VCE) was approved for use in 2001. It involves the patient swallowing a miniature high-resolution camera that is propelled through the gastrointestinal (GI) tract by peristalsis. Data is picked up through sensors attached to the skin and recorded in a portable data recorder.

The major clinical application of VCE is in the evaluation of obscure GI bleeding. Typically, patients with obscure GI bleeding (noted through recurrent iron deficiency anemia or positive fecal occult blood testing) undergo esophagogastroduodenoscopy (EGD) and colonoscopy. However, these procedures are unable to visualize the majority of the small intestine. Currently, intraoperative endoscopy is used to visualize the small intestine, but it involves exploratory laparotomy and general anesthesia. Use of VCE provides a noninvasive way to view the entire small intestine. Limitations of VCE are that biopsy and therapeutic interventions are not able to be performed.

Normal Values

Normal anatomy of GI tract

Possible Meanings of Abnormal Values

Abnormalities of the small intestine
Angiodysplasia
Angioectasia
Carcinoma
Crohn's disease

Erosion
Obscure GI bleeding
Polyp
Stricture
Ulcer

Contributing Factors to Abnormal Values

- Too rapid movement of capsule through the GI tract may provide inadequate visualization of the entire small intestine.
- Very slow movement of the capsule through the small intestine may prevent the entire small intestine from being visualized before the battery pack shuts down.

Interventions/Implications

Pretest

- Explain to the patient the purpose of the test. Provide any written teaching materials available on the subject. Note that there is no discomfort with the test.
- Fasting for 12 hours is required before the test.
- The patient must refrain from taking any medications that could delay gastric emptying.
- No bowel preparation is necessary.
- Obtain a signed informed consent.

Procedure

- Eight sensors are attached to the patient's abdomen.
- A belt holding a data recorder and battery pack is applied to the patient's waist.
- The patient swallows the video capsule with a small amount of water.
- The patient is allowed to participate in usual daily activities.
- Clear liquids are allowed beginning 2 hours after capsule ingestion, and a light meal is allowed 4 hours later.

Posttest

- The patient returns after 8 hours for removal of the data recorder. Images are downloaded and processed.
- Report abnormal findings to the primary care provider.

→ Clinical Alerts

- Potential complications include: capsule retention if there is an obstruction or stricture and capsule failure.
- Patients should avoid magnetic resonance imaging (MRI) and radio transmitters until the video capsule is passed in the stool (in 10 to 48 hours).
- Instruct patients to notify the primary care provider if nausea, vomiting, or abdominal pain occurs, or if they do not pass the capsule within 1 week.

CONTRAINDICATIONS!

- Patients with known or suspected GI obstruction, strictures, or fistulae
- Patients with Zenker diverticulum or swallowing disorders

- Patients who are pregnant
- Patients with multiple previous abdominal surgeries
- Patients who cannot or refuse to undergo surgery
- Patients who are unable to cooperate because of age, mental status, pain, or other factors
- Patients with implanted pacemakers or defibrillators (relative contraindication)

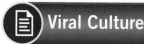

Viral Culture

Test Description

A viral culture involves collecting a small sample of body tissue or fluid and placing it in a cell culture. The virus is allowed to replicate to help with identification of the specific virus. It is best for samples to be collected during the acute phase of a condition.

Sources of specimens for culturing include blood, cerebrospinal fluid (CSF), respiratory secretions, stool, tissue, urine, eyes, and lesions of the oral mucosa, rectal mucosa, skin, and genitals. The types of viruses able to be detected include adenovirus, cytomegalovirus, herpes simplex virus, influenza, mumps, respiratory syncytial virus (RSV), varicella-zoster virus, and enteroviruses such as coxsackie virus and poliovirus. The length of time from specimen collection until diagnosis varies from hours to days, depending on the virus and the culture method used.

Normal Values

No virus isolated

Possible Meanings of Abnormal Values

Viral infection (identified virus)

Contributing Factors to Abnormal Values

- Use of wooden shaft and calcium alginate swabs will interfere with the culture.
- *False-negative* results may occur if specimen collection is done at times other than the acute phase of the illness/condition.

Interventions/Implications

Pretest
- Explain to the patient the purpose of the test and how the specimen is to be collected.

Procedure
- Use proper specimen collection swab or container as indicated by reference laboratory.
- General technique guidelines include:
  - Blood: Collect 5 mL of blood in a green-top heparinized collection tube.
  - CSF: Collect 1 mL of CSF in a sterile tube with a leak-proof cap.
  - Stool: Collect a sample of stool $\frac{1}{2}$ to 1 in. in diameter in a clean, dry container, or use viral swab.

- Urine: Collect clean midstream catch urine in sterile container.
- Oral mucosa: Swab posterior oropharynx with dry, sterile swab for throat culture.
- Rectal mucosa: Swab is inserted 2 in into rectum and rubbed on the mucosa.
- Eye: A viral swab can be used to collect conjunctival material.
- Skin/genital lesions: Vesicular fluid can be aspirated or the vesicle can be open and the swab rubbed on the base of the open lesion.
- Gloves are worn during specimen collection.

Posttest
- Check with reference laboratory regarding need to refrigerate specimen.
- Label the specimen, noting the exact source. Also include patient age, relevant vaccinations, and relevant clinical history.
- Report abnormal findings to the primary care provider.

Clinical Alerts

- Whenever a viral etiology is suspected and whenever appropriate, acute and convalescent serum should be collected for viral serology tests.

Vitamin B$_{12}$ (Cyanocobalamin)

Test Description

Vitamin B$_{12}$ is a water-soluble vitamin obtained from dietary animal sources. It is necessary for DNA synthesis, red blood cell production, and neural function. In order for Vitamin B$_{12}$ to be absorbed from the gastrointestinal tract, the *intrinsic factor*, a glycoprotein secreted by the parietal cells in the stomach, must be present. If the intrinsic factor is lacking, vitamin B$_{12}$ will not be absorbed, and pernicious anemia, a type of macrocytic anemia, will occur. Testing for vitamin B$_{12}$, along with testing for folic acid, is used to diagnose macrocytic anemia.

Normal Values

Normal: 205–876 pg/mL (151–646 pmol/L SI units)

Possible Meanings of Abnormal Values

Increased	Decreased
Chronic renal failure	Alcoholic hepatitis
Congestive heart failure	Aplastic anemia
Diabetes	Cancer
Leukemia	Folate deficiency
Leukocytosis	Hemodialysis
Liver disease	Hypothyroidism
Liver metastasis	Inflammatory bowel disease
Obesity	Malabsorption
Uremia	Malnutrition

V

Pancreatitis
Parasites
Pernicious anemia
Pregnancy
Smoking
Vegetarianism

Contributing Factors to Abnormal Values

- Hemolysis of the sample may interfere with test results.
- Prolonged exposure of the sample to light may alter test results.
- Patients who have received radiographic dyes within 7 days prior to the test may have altered test results.
- Drugs which may *increase* vitamin B_{12} levels: ascorbic acid, chloral hydrate, estrogens, omeprazole, and ingestion of vitamin A.
- Drugs which may *decrease* vitamin B_{12} levels: alcohol, anticonvulsants, antimalarials, ascorbic acid, antineoplastic agents, cholestyramine, colchicine, diuretics, metformin, neomycin, oral contraceptives, ranitidine, rifampin.

Interventions/Implications

Pretest

- Explain to the patient the purpose of the test and the need for a blood sample to be drawn.
- Fasting overnight is required prior to the test. Water intake is allowed.
- Testing for vitamin B_{12} should be performed prior to the Schilling test.
- A baseline hematocrit should be obtained.

Procedure

- A 7-mL blood sample is drawn in a red-top collection tube.
- Gloves are worn throughout the procedure.

Posttest

- Apply pressure at venipuncture site. Apply dressing, periodically assessing for continued bleeding.
- Protect the sample from light by immediately placing the tube in a paper bag.
- Label the specimen and transport it to the laboratory.
- Report abnormal findings to the primary care provider.

V → Clinical Alerts

- Testing for Vitamin B_{12} is usually done in conjunction with other tests for anemia, including, folic acid, iron, ferritin, TIBC.
  - Other types of anemia, such as macrocytic anemia due to folic acid deficiency, can occur concomitantly with Vitamin B_{12} deficiency.
- If the Vitamin B_{12} deficiency is due to lack of intrinsic factor, treatment consists of intramuscular injections of Vitamin B_{12}. Typical treatment schedule is daily injections for 1 week, then weekly for 1 month, then monthly for life.
- Patients may need folic acid and iron supplementation to replenish stores.
- Vitamin B_{12} comes primarily from animal products, including eggs and dairy products. B_{12} supplements may be needed for people who follow a strict vegetarian diet.

West Nile Virus Testing

Test Description

The West Nile virus is an organism from the flavivirus family. Although originally identified in eastern Africa in 1937, West Nile virus has been present in the United States only since 1999. The most common hosts are birds, with mosquitoes being the carriers from the birds to humans. Thus, highest incidence of the virus occurs during warm weather when mosquito population is greatest. The virus may also be spread through blood transfusions and organ transplants, and possibly through breast milk.

For most people infected with West Nile virus, no symptoms are noted. Some people will have relatively mild flu-like symptoms. These symptoms, lasting up to 6 days, include fever, headache, decreased appetite, sore throat, nausea and vomiting, diarrhea, and muscle aching. In a very small number of people, especially those who are immunocompromised, are pregnant, or are elderly, the illness can be life-threatening. Symptoms progress to muscle weakness or paralysis, stiff neck, confusion, and possible loss of consciousness. At this point, patients are diagnosed with West Nile encephalitis or West Nile meningitis.

Because symptoms involving the central nervous system are present, diagnostic testing often includes CT scan or MRI scan of the head, along with a lumbar puncture for testing of the cerebrospinal fluid (CSF). The most accurate method to diagnose West Nile virus is testing of the patient's blood or CSF for antibodies against the virus. Nonspecific IgM antibodies are first assessed to check on current or recent infection. If this test is positive, IgM antibodies specific to West Nile virus are assessed. IgG antibodies are also assessed. Positive IgG antibodies with a low IgM level indicate previous and not likely current infection with West Nile virus. Although antibody testing is helpful for diagnosis, it does not predict disease severity. Newer testing which is highly specific for West Nile virus is PCR (polymerase chain reaction) testing.

Normal Values

Negative for West Nile virus antibody

Possible Meanings of Abnormal Values

Positive

West Nile virus

Contributing Factors to Abnormal Values

- *False-positive* results may occur in patients exposed to St. Louis encephalitis.

Interventions/Implications

Pretest

- Explain to the patient the purpose of the test and the procedure.
- Assess patient risk factors for infection with West Nile virus, including travel to areas with mosquito infestation.

Procedure

- A 7-mL blood sample is drawn in a red-top collection tube, or a 2-mL sample of CSF is obtained via lumbar puncture.
- Gloves are worn throughout the procedure.

Posttest

- Apply pressure at specimen collection site. Apply dressing, periodically assessing for continued bleeding or CSF leakage.
- Label the specimen and transport it to the laboratory.
- Report abnormal findings to the primary care provider.

→ **Clinical Alerts**

- If initial IgM testing is negative but symptoms persist, repeat testing may be done.
- Treatment for West Nile virus is primarily supportive and symptomatic.
- Prevention of the illness is recommended through use of mosquito repellent, eliminating areas where mosquitoes breed, preventing mosquitoes from entering the home, and avoiding outdoor activities at times when mosquitoes are most prevalent (evening).

Wet Mount for Vaginal Secretions (KOH/Wet Mount)

Test Description
This test involves the microscopic examination of vaginal discharge. It is the most important test for the diagnosis of vaginal infections, which may cause vaginal itching, pain, odor, and discharge. Wet mount analysis should be performed with all symptomatic patients and with asymptomatic patients when an abnormal discharge is detected. The discharge is mixed with saline and with potassium hydroxide (KOH) and then viewed under the microscope. The test provides immediate results so that treatment can be initiated as soon as possible.

Normal Values
Negative

Possible Meanings of Abnormal Values
Bacterial vaginosis
Candida vaginitis
Trichomonas vaginitis

Contributing Factors to Abnormal Values

- Douching within 24 hours of the test may affect test results.

Interventions/Implications

Pretest
- Explain to the patient the purpose of the test. Provide any written teaching materials available on the subject.
- Instruct the patient to not douche for 24 hours before the procedure.
- No fasting is required before the test.

Procedure
- Prepare a slide by using a grease pencil to draw a line down the middle of a glass slide. An alternative method is to have two separate slides.
- Prepare the slide with saline and KOH
  - Two drops of 0.9% saline are placed on the left side of the slide.
  - Two drops of 10% KOH on the right side of the slide.
- The patient is assisted into lithotomy position with her feet in the stirrups.
- The vaginal speculum is inserted and opened.
- Two separate swabs of vaginal fluid are obtained from the posterior aspect of the lateral vaginal walls.
  - The first sample is applied to the saline side of the slide by making 2 to 3 rotations to dilute the sample.
  - The second sample is applied to the KOH side of the slide, making 10 to15 rotations to assure a concentrated sample.
- Immediately after mixing the sample with the KOH, take a "quick whiff" of the mixture. A fishy odor suggests bacterial vaginosis or *Trichomonas*.
- Apply cover slips to both portions of the slide.
- Gloves are worn during the pelvic examination.

Posttest
- The slide is first viewed under low power (4X–10X objective setting).
  - Scan the saline sample for presence of white blood cells (WBCs) and motile pear-shaped organisms representing *Trichomonas*; also scan for yeast buds and pseudohyphae.
  - Scan the KOH sample for mycelia or pseudomycelia (suggestive of fungal infection).
- The slide is then viewed under high power (≥ 40X objective setting).
  - Inspect the saline sample for clue cells (bacterial vaginosis), WBCs, *Lactobacillus*, spores, mycelia, and trichomonads.
  - Analyze the KOH sample for confirmation of the presence of fungal infection.
- Report abnormal findings to the primary care provider.

W

→ Clinical Alerts

- Patients who continue to be symptomatic despite treatment should be retested, along with obtaining a vaginal culture.

White Blood Cell Count and Differential (Basophil Count, Eosinophil Count, Leukocyte Count, Lymphocyte Count, Monocyte Count, Neutrophil Count, WBC Count and Differential)

Test Description

The purpose of white blood cells is to protect the body from the threat of foreign agents, such as bacteria. All blood cells, including white blood cells, red blood cells, and platelets, originate from a common stem cell. Blood cell differentiation takes place in the bone marrow. This differentiation results in the development of the phagocytic white blood cells and the immune white blood cells.

The phagocytic white blood cells, which include granulocytes and monocytes, play an important role in the process of *phagocytosis,* the digestion of cellular debris. The *granulocytes* are so named because of their granular appearance. They are also called *polymorphonuclear leukocytes* (polys) because of their multilobed nucleus. The three types of granulocytes are neutrophils, eosinophils, and basophils. Monocytes, along with lymphocytes, are considered *mononuclear leukocytes,* since their nuclei are not multilobed. They are also called *nongranulocytes.*

Neutrophils are the first white blood cells to arrive at an area of inflammation. They begin working to clear the area of cellular debris through the process of phagocytosis. Neutrophils have a lifespan of approximately 4 days. Mature neutrophils are distinguishable by their segmented appearance, thus they are often called "segs." Immature neutrophils, which are nonsegmented, are known as "bands" or "stabs." In the case of an acute infectious process, the body reacts quickly by releasing the neutrophils before they have reached maturity. When this increase in bands is found, it is known as a *shift to the left.* As the infection or inflammation resolves and the immature neutrophils are replaced with mature cells, the return to normal is called a *shift to the right.* This term is also used to mean that the cells have more than the usual number of nuclear segments. This may be seen in liver disease, pernicious anemia, megaloblastic anemia, and Down syndrome.

Eosinophils play an important role in the defense against parasitic infections. They also phagocytize cell debris, but to a lesser degree than neutrophils, and do so in the later stages of inflammation. They are also active in allergic reactions.

Basophils release histamine, bradykinin, and serotonin when activated by injury or infection. These substances are important to the inflammatory process since they increase capillary permeability and thus increase the blood flow to the affected area. Basophils are also involved in producing allergic responses. In addition, the granules on the surface of basophils secrete the natural anticoagulating substance, heparin. This provides some balance to the clotting and coagulation pathways.

Monocytes, which live months or even years, are not considered phagocytic cells when they are in the circulating blood. However, after they are present in the tissues for several hours, monocytes mature into macrophages, which are phagocytic cells.

The immune white blood cells, which include the *T lymphocytes,* or T cells, and the *B lymphocytes,* or B cells, mature in lymphoid tissue and migrate between the blood and lymph. They play an integral part in the antibody response to antigens. The lymphocytes have a lifespan of days or years, depending on their type. (See Lymphocyte Immunophenotyping)

The white blood cell count and differential test, which is included in a complete blood count, includes two components. The "white blood cell count" denotes the total number of white blood cells (leukocytes) in 1 mm³ of blood. The "differential" denotes the percentage of basophils, eosinophils, lymphocytes, monocytes, and neutrophils within a sample of 100 white blood cells. Since the differential percentages always equal 100%, an increase in the *percentage* of one type of white blood cell causes a mandatory decrease in the *percentage* of at least one other type of white blood cell. Also included are the absolute values for normal counts of each of the five types of white blood cells.

Normal Values

White blood cell count

Adult:	4500–10,500/mm³ or 4.5–10.5 × 10⁹/L (SI units)
Child 6–12 years:	4500–13,500/mm³ or 4.5–13.5 × 10⁹/L (SI units)
Child 2–6 years:	5000–15,500/mm³ or 5.0–15.5 × 10⁹/L (SI units)
Child < 2 weeks:	5000–21,000/mm³ or 5.0–21.0 × 10⁹/L (SI units)
Newborn:	9000–30,000/mm³ or 5.0–21.0 × 10⁹/L (SI units)

Differential	*Percentages*	*Absolute Counts*
Basophils	0.5–1%	15–100 cells/mm³
Eosinophils	1–4%	<450 cells/mm³
Lymphocytes	20–40%	1000–4000 cells/mm³
Monocytes	2–8%	<850 cells/mm³
Segmented Neutrophils	40–60%	3000–7000 cells/mm³
Band Neutrophils	0–3%	<350 cells/mm³

Possible Meanings of Abnormal Values

Basophils

Increased (Basophilia)	**Decreased (Basopenia)**
Certain skin diseases	Acute infection
Chicken pox	Adrenocortical stimulation
Chronic myelogenous leukemia	Graves' disease
Chronic sinusitis	Irradiation
Irradiation	Pregnancy
Measles	Shock
Myeloproliferative disorders	Stress
Myxedema	
Postsplenectomy	
Smallpox	
Ulcerative colitis	

Eosinophils

Increased (Eosinophilia)	**Decreased (Eosinopenia)**
Addison's disease	Adrenocortical stimulation
Allergic disease	Cushing's disease
Cancer of lung, stomach, ovary	Severe infection

W

Chronic myelogenous leukemia
Hodgkin's disease
Irradiation
Parasitic infections (trichinosis)
Pernicious anemia
Polycythemia
Rheumatoid arthritis
Scarlet fever
Scleroderma
Systemic lupus erythematosus
Ulcerative colitis

Shock
Stress
Trauma

Lymphocytes

Increased (Lymphocytosis)

Addison's disease
Chronic lymphocytic leukemia
Crohn's disease
Cytomegalovirus
Drug hypersensitivity
Infectious mononucleosis
Pertussis
Serum sickness
Thyrotoxicosis
Toxoplasmosis
Typhoid
Ulcerative colitis
Viral disorders (mumps, rubella,
  rubeola, hepatitis, varicella)

Decreased (Lymphocytopenia)

Acute tuberculosis
Adrenocortical stimulation
AIDS
Aplastic anemia
Congestive heart failure
Hodgkin's disease
Irradiation
Lymphosarcoma
Myasthenia gravis
Obstruction of lymphatic drainage
Renal failure
Stress
Systemic lupus erythematosus

Monocytes

Increased (Monocytosis)

Brucellosis
Chronic inflammatory disorders
Chronic ulcerative colitis
Hodgkin's disease
Myeloproliferative disorders
Subacute bacterial endocarditis
Syphilis
Tuberculosis
Viral infections

Decreased (Monocytopenia)

Acute stress reaction
Overwhelming infection

Neutrophils

Increased (Neutrophilia)

Acidosis
Acute hemolysis of red blood cells
Acute pyogenic infections
Cancer of liver, GI tract, bone marrow
Eclampsia
Emotional/physical stress
  (exercise, labor)
Gout
Hemorrhage

Decreased (Neutropenia)

Anaphylactic shock
Anorexia nervosa
Aplastic anemia
Hypersplenism
Irradiation
Leukemia
Pernicious anemia
Rheumatoid arthritis
Rickettsial infection

W

Myeloproliferative diseases
Poisoning by chemicals,
    drugs, venom
Rheumatic fever
Septicemia
Stress
Thyroid storm
Tissue necrosis (surgery, burns,
    myocardial infarction)
Uremia
Vasculitis

Septicemia
Systemic lupus erythematosus
Viral infection (measles, rubella,
    infectious mononucleosis, hepatitis)

Contributing Factors to Abnormal Values

- Stress, excitement, exercise, and labor may increase neutrophils.
- Stressful conditions can decrease the eosinophil count.
- Drugs which *increase* the number of basophils: antithyroid therapy.
- Drugs which *decrease* the number of basophils: antineoplastic agents, glucocorticoids.
- Drugs which *increase* the number of eosinophils: digitalis, heparin, penicillin, propranolol hydrochloride, streptomycin, tryptophan.
- Drugs which *decrease* the number of eosinophils: corticosteroids.
- Drugs which *decrease* the number of lymphocytes: antineoplastic agents, corticosteroids.
- Drugs which *decrease* the number of monocytes: glucocorticoids, immunosuppressive agents.
- Drugs which *increase* the number of neutrophils: endotoxin, epinephrine, heparin, histamine, steroids.
- Drugs which *decrease* the number of neutrophils: analgesics, antibiotics, antineoplastic agents, antithyroid drugs, phenothiazines, sulfonamides.

Interventions/Implications

Pretest
- Explain to the patient the purpose of the test and the need for a blood sample to be drawn.
- No fasting is required before the test.

Procedure
- A 7-mL blood sample is drawn in a lavender-top collection tube.
- The tourniquet must not be in place longer than 60 seconds.
- Gloves are worn throughout the procedure.

Posttest
- Apply pressure at venipuncture site. Apply dressing, periodically assessing for continued bleeding.
- Label the specimen and transport it to the laboratory.
- Report abnormal findings to the primary care provider.

W

→ **Clinical Alerts**

- White blood cell counts and eosinophil counts tend to be lower in the morning and higher in the evening. Thus, repeat tests should be done at the same time each day to provide accurate comparisons.

Wound Culture and Sensitivity (Wound C & S)

Test Description
When a patient is suspected of having a wound infection, a wound culture is ordered. The test involves swabbing the interior of the wound. The specimen collection should be performed prior to the beginning of antibiotic therapy. This test involves several components. First, a Gram stain of the specimen can be done and quickly reported. This provides basic information as to whether the organism is gram-positive or gram-negative. Next, the swab is cultured, that is, the organisms are allowed to grow in special culture media. In 48 to 72 hours, the organism is usually identified. The sensitivity portion of the test involves the testing of the organism to identify antibiotics to which the organism is sensitive or resistant.

Once the specimen is obtained, the patient is usually given a broad-spectrum antibiotic which is likely to be effective against typical wound infections. After the wound culture and sensitivity results are available, the antibiotic in use should be verified as to its appropriateness according to the sensitivity report.

Normal Values
Negative

Possible Meanings of Abnormal Values

Positive
Wound infection

Contributing Factors to Abnormal Values
- Drugs which may cause *false-negative* results: antibiotics.

Interventions/Implications
Pretest
- Explain to the patient the purpose of the test.

Procedure
- Swab the site with the cotton-tipped end of a culturette.
- The swab needs to be of the interior of the wound itself, not of the skin surrounding the wound.
- Gloves are worn throughout the procedure.

Posttest
- Place the swab in the culturette tube.
- Label the specimen, noting source of specimen, and transport it to the laboratory immediately.
- Report abnormal findings to the primary care provider.

W

→ **Clinical Alerts**

- Open wounds are cultured using aerobic culture tubes. Anaerobic culture tubes are used if drainage is aspirated from a closed wound.

Appendices

TYPICAL GROUPINGS OF BLOOD/URINE TESTS

The following lists are included to provide a quick reference of the blood and urine tests to consider for use in various clinical situations. The lists are meant to provide the health-care provider with possible testing options within a category. It is the health-care provider's responsibility to choose the test(s) most appropriate for the particular patient situation based upon thorough history-taking and physical examination and sound clinical judgment. The lists are general in nature; they may not be all-inclusive of all available testing.

ADRENAL FUNCTION TESTS

Adrenocorticotropic hormone
Adrenocorticotropic hormone stimulation test
Aldosterone
Cortisol, blood
Cortisol, urine
Dexamethasone suppression test
17-hydroxycorticosteroids
17-ketosteroids
Pregnanetriol
Renin activity, plasma
Vanillylmandelic acid and catecholamines

ANEMIA DIAGNOSIS

Blood smear
Complete blood cell count
Ferritin
Folic acid
Free erythrocyte protoporphyrin

Glucose-6-phosphate dehydrogenase
Iron
RBC indices
RBC distribution width
Reticulocyte count
Schilling test
Total iron-binding capacity
Transferrin
Transferrin saturation
Vitamin B$_{12}$

CARDIAC MARKERS

Asparate aminotransferase (AST)
Creatine kinase (CK) and isoenzymes
Lactic dehydrogenase (LDH, LD)
Myoglobin
Troponin

CHEMISTRY PROFILE

Alanine aminotransferase (ALT)
Albumin
Alkaline phosphatase (ALP)
Asparate aminotransferase (AST)
Bilirubin, total
Calcium, blood
Carbon dioxide content, total
Chloride, blood
Creatinine, blood
Glucose, blood
Potassium, blood
Protein, total
Sodium, blood
Urea nitrogen, blood

COAGULATION STUDIES

Anti-thrombin III
Bleeding time
Coagulation factor assay
D-dimer test
Euglobulin lysis time
Fibrin degradation products
Fibrinogen
Partial thromboplastin time
Plasminogen
Protein C

Protein S
Prothrombin time
Thrombin clotting time

DIABETES MELLITUS TESTING

Anti-insulin antibody test
Glucose, blood
Glucose tolerance test
Glycosylated hemoglobin
Insulin
Microalbumin

DISSEMINATED INTRAVASCULAR COAGULATION (DIC) SCREEN

Antithrombin III
Bleeding time
Coagulation factors
D-dimer
Fibrin degradation products
Fibrinogen
Fibrinopeptide A
Partial thromboplastin time
Platelet count
Prothrombin time
Thrombin time

ELECTROLYTES

Anion gap
Calcium, blood
Calcium, urine
Carbon dioxide content, total
Chloride, blood
Chloride, urine
Magnesium
Phosphorus
Potassium, blood
Potassium, urine
Sodium, blood
Sodium, urine

LIPID ANALYSIS

Apolipoprotein A & B
Cholesterol
High-density lipoprotein
Low-density lipoprotein
Triglycerides

LIVER FUNCTION TESTS

Alanine aminotransferase (ALT)
Albumin
Alkaline phosphatase (ALP)
Aspartate aminotransferase (AST)
Bilirubin
Gamma glutamyl transferase (GGT)
5′-Nucleotidase
Lactate dehydrogenase
Prothrombin time

PANCREATIC ENZYMES

Amylase, serum
Amylase, urine
Lipase

PLATELET ACTIVITY TESTS

Bleeding time
Platelet aggregation test
Platelet count
Platelet, mean volume

RENAL FUNCTION TESTS

Creatinine, blood
Creatinine clearance
Osmolality, blood
Osmolality, urine
Urea nitrogen, blood
Uric acid, blood
Uric acid, urine

RHEUMATOID ARTHRITIS TESTS

Antinuclear antibody (ANA)
C-reactive protein
Erythrocyte sedimentation rate
Rheumatoid factor

THYROID FUNCTION TESTS

Free thyroxine index (FTI)
Thyroglobulin
Thyroid-stimulating hormone (TSH)
Thyroid-stimulating immunoglobulin (TSI)
Thyroxine-binding globulin
Thyroxine, free (free T_4)

Thyroxine, total (T_4)
Triiodothyronine, free (free T_3)
Triiodothyronine, total (T_3)
Triiodothyronine uptake test

TORCH TEST

Cytomegalovirus (CMV)
Herpes simplex antibody
Rubella antibody titer
Toxoplasmosis antibody test

TUMOR MARKERS

Acid phosphatase
Alpha-fetoprotein (AFP)
BRCA 1/2
Carcinoembryonic antigen (CEA)
CA-15-3
CA 19-9
CA 125
Prostate specific antigen (PSA)
Thyroglobulin

THE ENDOCRINE SYSTEM: SIGNALS & FEEDBACK

The endocrine system can seem rather confusing if one simply tries to memorize individual tests and conditions. It can be simplified if one understands the typical process of endocrine functioning and the feedback mechanism needed to keep hormones at normal levels. Once this understanding is achieved, interpretation of test results and clinical decision-making are facilitated.

The endocrine system and the nervous system work together to regulate responses to stimuli from the internal and external environment. The process that occurs from stimuli to response is consistent for most of the hormones. A stimulus from inside or outside the body causes the hypothalamus to release a "releasing factor," which in turn causes the pituitary to release a trophic hormone. This hormone then acts on the target organ, causing it to release a hormone that provides the physiologic response. This process can be used to illustrate what happens in the case of stress causing the eventual release of the "stress hormone" cortisol.

Table App B-1

Process		Example	
Stimulus (internal or external)		Stress (emotional or physical)	
Affects	Hypothalamus	Affects	Hypothalamus
Releases	Releasing factor	Releases	Corticotropic releasing factor
Affects	Pituitary gland	Affects	Pituitary Gland
Releases	Trophic hormone	Releases	ACTH (Adrenocorticotropic Hormone)
Affects	Target organ	Affects	Adrenal Gland
Releases	Hormone	Releases	Cortisol
Achieves	Physiologic response	Achieves	Increased energy due to glucose production

There is also a *feedback mechanism* involved in this process. The hypothalamus monitors the level of the body's hormones, in the above case, cortisol. If the system is working as it should, if cortisol levels increase above normal, the hypothalamus recognizes this and signals the pituitary to decrease release of ACTH. This in turn, provides less stimulation to the adrenal gland, resulting in less cortisol production and the return to normal cortisol levels. If, on the other hand, cortisol levels fall below normal, the hypothalamus signals the pituitary gland to increase ACTH release to stimulate the adrenal gland to increase cortisol release.

Once the process of achieving a physiologic response through the secretion of hormones is clearly understood, the application of this knowledge to treatments for conditions can occur. This is best illustrated by looking at what happens with the thyroid normally, and in the patient with hypothyroidism who is receiving thyroid hormone supplementation. First the normal process of thyroid functioning:

Table App B-2	Normal Functioning		
Process		**Example**	
Stimulus (internal or external)		Low T_4 level	
Affects	Hypothalamus	Affects	Hypothalamus
Releases	Releasing factor	Releases	Thyrotropic releasing hormone (TRH)
Affects	Pituitary gland	Affects	Pituitary gland
Releases	Trophic hormone	Releases	Thyroid-simulating hormone (TSH)
Affects	Target organ	Affects	Thyroid gland
Releases	Hormone	Releases	T_4
Achieves	Physiologic response	Achieves	Increased T_4 levels with improved physiologic functioning

In the case of the person with hypothyroidism, the underlying problem can occur in any of the organs involved in the hormonal process. If the problem is with the target organ (the thyroid gland), it is called *primary* hypothyroidism. If the problem involves the pituitary gland, it is *secondary* hypothyroidism, and if the problem lies with the hypothalamus, it is *tertiary* hypothyroidism. In the following example, the patient has primary hypothyroidism, in other words, the problem is a hypofunctioning thyroid gland. When the thyroid gland is not functioning normally, it does not respond as well to TSH, and thus does not release normal amounts of T_4. Due to the feedback mechanism, the pituitary secretes increasing amounts of TSH to try to stimulate the thyroid gland to release the T_4. So, testing results indicative of a hypofunctioning thyroid gland would be an increased TSH level and a decreased T_4 level.

When the person is receiving the correct dosage of supplemental T_4, the feedback to the hypothalamus is that there is now a normal level of T_4. The pituitary responds by reducing the amount of TSH back to a normal level. If the dosage is inadequate, the TSH continues to be elevated and an increase in medication dosage is warranted. If the dosage is too high, the TSH will fall below normal and indicates the need to decrease the dosage. These scenarios are shown below.

Table App B-3	Treatment of Primary Hypothyroidism (Hypofunctioning Thyroid Gland)		
Problem	Medication Dosage Too Low	Medication Dosage Too High	Medication Dosage Correct
TRH level	Increased	Decreased	Normal
TSH level	Increased	Decreased	Normal
T_4 level	Decreased	Increased	Normal
Treatment needed	Increase dosage, continue monitoring	Decrease dosage, continue monitoring	Maintain current dose, continue monitoring

Monitoring of thyroid replacement can easily be accomplished through periodically checking TSH levels.

SAFETY OF

THE PATIENT

Patient safety is without question an essential component of health care. Considering the complexity of the health-care system and the patient conditions with which providers must deal, the risk of error can be high. Safety standards and guidelines are designed to minimize this risk.

JCAHO NATIONAL PATIENT SAFETY GOALS

The Joint Commission on Accreditation of Healthcare Organizations (JCAHO) has developed National Patient Safety Goals for 2007. The goals are available at http://www.jointcommission.org/PatientSafety/NationalPatientSafetyGoals/07_npsg_facts.htm. Those goals and requirements applicable to laboratory and diagnostic testing will be discussed. The provider is referred to the JCAHO website for more detailed information.

Goal 1: Improve the Accuracy of Patient Identification

Requirement 1A: Use at least two patient identifiers when providing care, treatment or services. Prior to collection of blood and other types of samples, the patient is to be identified by two methods other than by room number. For example, asking the patient to state his/her full name and also checking the patient's identification band would be appropriate. In addition, all specimen contains are to be labeled with the patient's name and other identifying information while in the presence of the patient.

Requirement 1B: Prior to the start of any invasive procedure, conduct a final verification process, (such as a "time out,") to confirm the correct patient, procedure and site using active-not passive-communication techniques. This verification process must be done in the location where the procedure will be done, just prior to starting the procedure. For example, if a patient is to have a biopsy of a right breast mass, just prior to the procedure in the procedure room, the provider should verify the patient's name, verify with the patient that a biopsy is to be taken of the right breast, and also verify this information by reviewing the written order for the procedure. There is to be written documentation that the verification has been done. This documentation can be through use of a simple checklist which becomes a part of the medical record. If there is a difference between what the provider states and what the patient states, there must be a system in place for reconciling the difference. Should the provider need to leave the area after verifying the above information, identity must be re-established prior to the procedure. Marking the site of the procedure (in this case, the right breast) is required if the provider is not in constant attendance with the patient.

Goal 2: Improve the Effectiveness of Communication Among Caregivers

Requirement 2A: For verbal or telephone orders or for telephonic reporting of critical test results, verify the complete order or test result by having the person receiving the information record and "read-back" the complete order or test result. For example, if a nurse reports a critically high INR result to a physician, the physician is to repeat back the INR value and the order for medication change and any other treatment. The nurse is to write down the order and read it back to the physician, after which the physician is to confirm the accuracy of the order.

Requirement 2B: Standardize a list of abbreviations, acronyms, symbols, and dose designations that are not to be used throughout the organization. JCAHO notes the following as the "Official Do Not Use List", but organizations can expand this list as they deem appropriate.

Table App C-1	
"Do Not Use"	**Instead, Write**
U, u	Unit
IU	International unit
Q.D., QD, q.d., qd	Daily
Q.O.D., QOD, q.o.d., qod	Every other day
Trailing zero (as in 5.0 mg)	5 mg
Lack of leading zero (.5 mg)	0.5 mg
MS	Morphine sulfate
MSO_4, $MgSO_4$	Magnesium sulfate

Requirement 2C: Measure, assess and, if appropriate, take action to improve the timeliness of reporting, and the timeliness of receipt by the responsible licensed caregiver, of critical test results and values. This item requires that an organization define the acceptable length of time between the ordering of critical tests and the reporting of the results; also the time between the availability of test results and receipt of the results by the caregiver. A back-up reporting system is required to avoid delays if the responsible caregiver is not available.

Requirement 2E: Implement a standardized approach to "hand-off" communications, including an opportunity to ask and respond to questions. "Hand-off" communication occurs when there is a change in responsibility for the patient's care. This includes shift change reports, reports between areas when a patient is transferring from one area to another (including from a procedure and returning back to a hospital unit), providers transferring on-call responsibility, and the reporting of critical test results to provider offices. JCAHO requires the following to be included in any "hand-off" communication:

- up-to-date information regarding the patient's care, treatment and services, condition and any recent or anticipated changes,
- a process for verification of the received information, including repeat-back or read-back, as appropriate, and

- an opportunity for the receiver of the hand-off information to review relevant patient historical data, which may include previous care, treatment and services.

Goal 7: Reduce the Risk of Health Care-Associated Infection

Requirement 7A: Comply with current Center for Disease Control and Prevention (CDC) hand hygiene guidelines. The most current CDC guidelines are available at: http://www.cdc.gov/handhygiene/.

Requirement 7B: Manage as sentinel events all identified cases of unanticipated death or major permanent loss of function associated with a health care-associated infection. A "root cause analysis" is conducted of such cases to include analysis of why the patient acquired an infection and based on that knowledge, why the patient died or suffered permanent loss of function. It is important with diagnostic testing to inform patients, especially those who are immunocompromised of the signs/symptoms of infection, so that if any begin to occur after a procedure, the patient will know to notify the provider, and hopefully prevent sentinel events from occurring.

Goal 13: Encourage Patients' Active Involvement in their Own Care as a Patient Safety Strategy

Requirement 13A: Define and communicate the means for patients and their families to report concerns about safety and encourage them to do so. Patients need be informed about the procedures they are to undergo and what to expect before, during, and after the procedure. They should be encouraged to report anything which might deviate from the expectations so that possible errors or advanced events can be avoided. For example, if a patient is to undergo a diagnostic test involving a radiopaque contrast, the patient should be informed about the symptoms of an allergic reaction. If any of the symptoms begin to occur, the patient will know to immediately notify the provider.

COMMUNICATION OF TEST RESULTS

In addition to JCAHO requirements for reporting of critical test values, there are other considerations in the communication of test results. This deals with the communication of test results between the health-care provider and the patient. The provider needs to be familiar with the regulations concerning the privacy of patients' health information. This is contained within the Health Insurance Portability and Accountability Act of 1996 (HIPAA), which is available at *http://www.hhs.gov/ocr/hipaa/*. Under this Act, patients can request that their health-care provider take steps to ensure that their communications with the patient are confidential. For example, if a patient does not wish for others in his/her household to know he/she has sought health care, the patient may request that all communication be made through a work or cellular phone number. In most instances, a patient's health information cannot be shared without the patient's written permission. For example, a patient may complete and sign a form at the provider's office listing only those individuals with whom information may be shared. Information cannot be released to a relative or friend not included on the list. The patient may also indicate whether messages may be left at home or work.

In addition to complying with HIPAA restrictions, the provider must also ensure that patients are informed of test results. If patients are unable to be reached by telephone, communication in writing may be required. Patients should not assume that "no news is good news." Patients should be encouraged to call the provider's office requesting test results if they have not been contacted in a reasonable amount of time. This time may vary depending on the test; for example, final reports for a culture to diagnose tuberculosis may take 1 to 6 weeks to receive final results. In this way, if the provider has not reviewed a test result by the time a patient calls for the results, the result can be obtained and communicated to the patient. Documentation of this reporting should be included in the medical record.

Another potential safety issue involves regular screening tests. A patient may be seen by the provider for a preventive health visit, or for a periodic follow-up on a condition such as diabetes or hyperlipidemia. The provider recommends a screening test to be done which may not be scheduled for several months. Patient follow-through on such appointments may be limited. To assist patients to remember to have the test done, some offices or testing facilities send reminder cards to the patient. Another option is registering through a reminder service such as that offered by the College of American Pathologists (http://www.MyHealthTestReminder.com)

SAFETY OF THE HEALTH-CARE PROVIDER

The safety of the health-care provider is of concern to not only local health-care facilities, but also governmental agencies such as the U.S. Department of Labor Occupational Safety and Health Administration (OSHA). The World Health Organization (WHO) notes the need for health-care workers to use universal precautions with all patients, at all times, regardless of diagnosis. OSHA describes universal precautions as a concept in which all human blood and certain human body fluids are treated as if known to be infectious for human immunodeficiency virus (HIV), hepatitis B virus (HBV), and other bloodborne pathogens.

The Centers for Disease Control and Prevention (CDC) have published recommendations for preventing the transmission of bloodborne pathogens in health-care settings. Their recommendations for universal precautions include:

- The routine use of appropriate barrier precautions to prevent skin and mucous membrane exposure when contact with blood or other body fluids is anticipated.
    - Universal precautions apply to blood, any fluids containing visible blood, semen, vaginal secretions, tissues, cerebrospinal fluid, synovial fluid, pleural fluid, peritoneal fluid, pericardial fluid, and amniotic fluid.
    - Barrier precautions include the use of gloves, masks, protective eyewear, face shields, gowns, and/or aprons.
- The thorough and immediate washing of hands and other skin surfaces contaminated with blood or other body fluids.
- The prevention of injuries from sharps such as needles

Special precautions for individuals dealing with laboratory and diagnostic testing include:

- Using leak-proof containers for specimen transport;
- Using appropriate barrier precautions, especially gloves and protective eyewear;
- Washing the hands after glove removal and after specimen processing;
- Using mechanical pipetting only; and
- Decontamination of surfaces and equipment contaminated with blood or body fluids.

RESOURCES

- Centers for Disease Control & Prevention (http://www.cdc.gov/ncidod/dhqp/bp_universal_precautions.html)
- Occupational Safety & Health Administration (http://www.osha.gov)
- World Health Organization (http://www.who.int)

EVIDENCE-BASED PRACTICE

Evidence-based practice (EBP) is the combining of research with one's clinical judgment and the patient's preferences and values to make decisions in clinical practice. EBP involves taking the current best evidence obtained through clinical research and applying it to specific clinical cases to improve patient care. Other terms are noted in the literature (evidence-based medicine, evidence-based health care, evidence-based nursing), but regardless of the term used, the focus is the same: basing clinical decision making on research, not habit.

HISTORICAL PERSPECTIVE

Beginning in 1992, a series of articles were published in the *Journal of the American Medical Association (JAMA)* called "Users' Guides to Evidence-based Medicine." The initial article noted a new paradigm for medical practice was emerging. It stated, "Evidence-based medicine de-emphasizes intuition, unsystematic clinical experience, and pathophysiologic rationale as sufficient grounds for clinical decision-making, and stresses the examination of evidence from clinical research." (AMA, 1992)

In 1997, the Agency for Health Care Policy and Research (AHCPR), now known as the Agency for Healthcare Research and Quality (AHRQ) established 12 Evidence-based Practice Centers (EPCs) in an effort to promote evidence-based practice in everyday health care. These centers are responsible for developing evidence reports based on rigorous, comprehensive synthesis and analysis of the scientific literature related to topics related to health care. (AHRQ, 2006)

In 2001, the Institute of Medicine (IOM) released its vision and recommendations for a new health-care system for the twenty-first century. According to the IOM, one of the ten rules for redesign of the system is that decision making be *evidence based*. The report states "Patients should receive care based on the best available scientific knowledge. Care should not vary illogically from clinician to clinician or from place to place." (IOM, 2001). The IOM called for AHRQ to identify 15 or more common priority conditions and then work with stakeholders to develop plans to improve care for each of these conditions.

The original articles in *JAMA* pointed out misapprehensions about evidence-based medicine, stating "Recognizing the limitations of intuition, experience, and understanding of pathophysiology in permitting strong inferences may be misinterpreted as rejecting these routes of knowledge." (AMA, 1992) On the contrary, these qualities continue to be important for clinical decision making. This view is supported by Sigma Theta Tau International's Position Statement on Evidence-Based Nursing, which emphasizes inclusion of the latest research and consensus of expert opinion, along with personal judgment, in the decision-making process involved in the planning and provision of nursing care. (Sigma Theta Tau, 2005). White (2004) emphasizes that in evidence-based practice, the health-care provider must integrate the evidence with one's clinical expertise and apply it to the patient, a person who has unique personal characteristics and a unique clinical situation which also must be taken into consideration.

THE EBP PROCESS

The EBP process consists of formulating the clinical question, searching for the evidence, critically appraising the evidence, and then putting it into practice. (DiCenso, Guyatt, and Ciliska, 2005; Melnyk and Fineout-Overholt, 2005) It is suggested that the clinical question be formulated in PICO format. This format includes the *P*atient population of interest, the *I*ntervention of interest, the *C*omparison of interest, and the *O*utcome of interest. Using this format helps to narrow the search for evidence to that which is most relevant to the particular situation. (Melnyk and Fineout-Overholt, 2005) For example, a 65-year-old patient seen in clinic states she has seen advertisements for a vaccine for shingles and asks whether she should receive it. The clinical question here would be "For patients 65 years and older, does the use of a vaccine reduce the future risk of herpes zoster compared with patients who have not received the vaccine?" The steps of the EBP process, including use of PICO format, are shown in Fig. E-1.

When critically appraising the evidence, the clinician needs to be aware of the hierarchy, or levels, of evidence being used. There are numerous such hierarchies in use, with the basic format of these being that the higher on the hierarchy evidence is placed, the more likely it is to provide information of a cause-and-effect relationship. The highest level of evidence is that of large, randomized clinical trials (RCTs), whereas the lowest level of evidence is that of expert opinion. The gradations of evidence between these two levels vary with the particular taxonomy, but often include small RCTs, nonrandomized studies, systematic reviews of qualitative studies, and single qualitative studies. (Melnyk and Fineout-Overholt, 2005)

It is not expected that the health-care provider will have the time and resources to obtain and analyze numerous research studies, meet with content experts, and develop clinical guidelines for each patient who is seen. Rather, the provider needs to know where to find the evidence, such as clinical practice guidelines or systematic reviews, and then be able to determine whether the evidence is valid for use with a particular patient situation. A systematic review of the literature in a particular area also highlights gaps in current knowledge, areas in which conclusive research is lacking. Such findings can help focus future research agendas and lead to further refinement of clinical practice guidelines.

There are numerous resources readily available, with periodic updates done to ensure the latest information is available to the provider. AHRQ provides several such resources for the health-care provider. Clinical Practice Guidelines are available online at *http://www.ahrq.gov/clinic/epcix.htm.* AHRQ also sponsors the National Guideline Clearinghouse *(http://www.guideline.gov)* which provides evidence-based clinical practice guidelines related to many clinical problems. The National Guideline Clearinghouse (NGC) is a central repository for clinical practice guidelines originating from any source. While the NGC provides a summary of each guideline's background and essential elements,

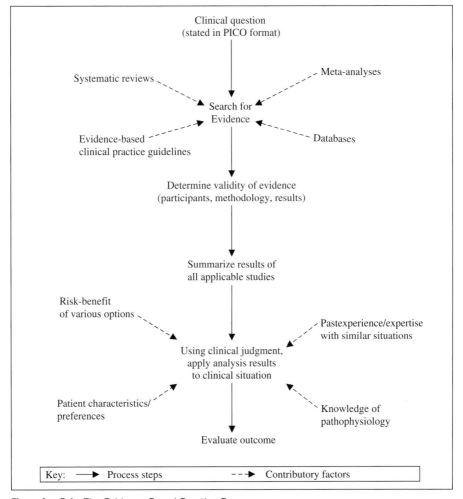

Figure App E-1. The Evidence-Based Practice Process

the actual guideline documents are available electronically from the source organization via links from the NGC website. Numerous other resources are available which provide guidelines and/or systematic reviews, including the Institute for Clinical Systems Improvement (*http://www.icsi.org/guidelines_and_more/*), the Cochrane Collaboration *(www.cochrane.org)*, and BMJ Clinical Evidence *(www.clinicalevidence.com)*. A useful internet search tool is SUMSearch, available through the University of Texas Health Science Center at San Antonio (*http://sumsearch.uthscsa.edu/*). Use of SUMSearch is advantageous in that the clinician need only to enter a query once and SUMSearch will then query a number of sources, primarily the National Library of Medicine (NLM), DARE (Database of Abstracts of Review of Effectiveness), and NGC.

With evidence-based practice, there is also an emphasis on *patient* outcomes, rather than on *disease-oriented* outcomes. For example, in recent years, testing for homocysteine was recommended in some patients, as it had been found that homocysteine levels were elevated in patients with cardiovascular disease. The suggestion was that finding elevated homocysteine levels was essential, so that treatment could then be initiated to lower the homocysteine levels. This was at first a worthy goal, but what current research has demonstrated is that even if the homocysteine level is lowered, the risk of a cardiac event is not lowered. Thus, the treatment of an elevated homocysteine level with folic acid is now in question. (American Dietetic Association, 2005) On the other hand, research *has* documented the importance of controlling lipid levels and glucose levels for a myriad of reasons, with national guidelines available for the health-care provider to use in making clinical decisions. These guidelines can be found through the National Guideline Clearinghouse or directly from the following sites:

- *Third Report of the National Cholesterol Education Program (NCEP) Expert Panel on Detection, Evaluation, and Treatment of High Blood Cholesterol in Adults from the National Heart, Lung and Blood Institute of the National Institutes of Health.* This report is available at: *http://www.nhlbi.nih.gov/guidelines/cholesterol/atp3_rpt.htm*
- *American Diabetes Association Standards of Medical Care in Diabetes.* Available at: *http://care.diabetesjournals.org/content/vol30/suppl_1/*

Screening for various conditions can be confusing and at times, controversial for the health-care provider. Some screenings are very beneficial, while others result in much higher cost (risk) than any perceived benefit due to needed follow-up of false-positive findings. AHRQ provides easy access to the work of the U.S. Preventive Services Task Force (USPSTF) at http://www.ahrq.gov/clinic/prevenix.htm. This group systematically reviews all available evidence regarding the effectiveness of clinical preventive services and provides its recommendation for provision of the particular service. The USPSTF grades its recommendations according to one of five classifications reflecting the strength of evidence and magnitude of net benefit (benefits minus harms). The classifications include A (strongly recommends), B (recommends), C (makes no recommendation), D (recommends against), and I (insufficient evidence to recommend for or against). The group grades the quality of evidence as good, fair, or poor. An example of this system is the recommendation by the USPSTF for a one-time screening for abdominal aortic aneurysm by ultrasound in men aged 65–75 who have ever smoked. The rationale for this recommendation is that "The USPSTF found good evidence that screening for AAA and surgical repair of large AAAs (5.5 cm or more) in men aged 65 to 75 who have ever smoked (current and former smokers) leads to decreased AAA-specific mortality." (USPSTF, 2005)

Consumers expect their health-care providers to use the most current recommendations for diagnostic and treatment options. The challenge for the provider is to bring evidence-based practice into the room with the patient, and to demonstrate the use of clinical practice guidelines or the consideration of systematic reviews in the planning of the patient's care. Evidence, not habit, is essential for provision of quality health care.

REFERENCES

Agency for Healthcare Research and Quality (AHRQ). (2006). Evidence-based practice centers: Synthesizing scientific evidence to improve quality and effectiveness in health care. Available at http://www.ahrq.gov/clinic/epc/. Accessed February 3, 2007.

American Dietetic Association. Disorders of lipid metabolism evidence-based nutrition practice guideline. Chicago (IL): American Dietetic Association; 2005 Aug. Available at: http://www. guideline.gov/summary/summary.aspx?doc_id=9533&nbr=005083&string=homocysteine. Accessed February 14, 2007.

American Medical Association (AMA). Users' guides to evidence-based medicine. *JAMA.* 1992 Nov 4;268(17):2420–5.

DiCenso, A, Guyatt, G, Cilka, D. *Evidence-Based Nursing: A Guide to Clinical Practice*. St. Louis: Elsevier Mosby; 2005.

Institute of Medicine (IOM) Committee on Quality of Health Care in America. *Crossing the Quality Chasm: A New Health System for the 21st Century*. Washington, DC: National Academy Press; 2001.

Melnyk, BM, Fineout-Overholt, E. *Evidence-Based Practice in Nursing & Healthcare: A Guide to Best Practice*. Philadelphia: Lippincott Williams & Wilkins; 2005.

Sigma Theta Tau International. Position Statement on Evidence-based Nursing (2005). Available at: http://www.nursingsociety.org/research/main.html. Accessed February 3, 2007.

U.S. Preventive Services Task Force (USPSTF). Screening for Abdominal Aortic Aneurysm. Release Date: February 2005. Available at: http://www.ahrq.gov/clinic/uspstf/uspsaneu.htm. Accessed February 17, 2007.

White, B. Making evidence-based medicine doable in everyday practice. *Fam Prac Manag*. 2004;11(2):51–58.

BIBLIOGRAPHY

AACE/AAES Thyroid Carcinoma Task Force. AACE/AAES medical/surgical guidelines for clinical practice: management of thyroid carcinoma. *Endocr Pract.* 2001;7(3):202–20.

AACE/AAES Task Force on Primary Hyperparathyroidism. The American Association of Clinical Endocrinologists and the American Association of Endocrine Surgeons position statement on the diagnosis and management of primary hyperparathyroidism. *Endocr Pract.* 2005;11(1):49–54.

AACE/AME Task Force on Thyroid Nodules. American Association of Clinical Endocrinologists and Associazione Medici Endocrinologi medical guidelines for clinical practice for the diagnosis and management of thyroid nodules. *Endocr Pract.* 2006;12(1):63–102.

AACE Hypertension Task Force. American Association of Clinical Endocrinologists medical guidelines for clinical practice for the diagnosis and treatment of hypertension. *Endocr Pract.* 2006;12(2): 193–222.

AACE Menopause Guidelines Revision Task Force. American Association of Clinical Endocrinologists medical guidelines for clinical practice for the diagnosis and treatment of menopause. *Endocr Pract.* 2006;12(3):315–37.

AACE National Guidelines Task Force. American Association of Clinical Endocrinologists medical guidelines for the clinical use of dietary supplements and nutraceuticals. *Endocr Pract.* 2003;9(5):417–70.

AACE Thyroid Task Force. American Association of Clinical Endocrinologists medical guidelines for clinical practice for the evaluation and treatment of hyperthyroidism and hypothyroidism. *Endocr Pract.* 2002;8(6):457–69.

Adler DG, Baron TH, Davila RE, et al. ASGE guideline: the role of ERCP in diseases of the biliary tract and the pancreas. *Gastrointest Endosc.* 2005;62(1):1–8.

Akinpelu D, Reddy S, Gonzalez JM. Treadmill and pharmacologic stress testing. Available at: http://www.emedicine.com/med/topic2961.htm. Accessed October 1, 2006.

Al-Ashkar F, Mehra R, Mazzone PJ. Interpreting pulmonary function tests: recognize the pattern, and the diagnosis will follow. *Clev Clin J Med.* 2003;70(10):866–81.

Albertsen PC. Prostate-specific antigen: how to advise patients as the screening debate continues. *Clev Clin J Med.* 2005;72(6):521–27.

Ali A, Santisi JM, Vargo J. Video capsule endoscopy: A voyage beyond the end of the scope. *Clev Clin J Med.* 2004;71(5):415–25.

American Academy of Family Physicians (AAFP). *Summary of Recommendations for Clinical Preventive Services. Revision 6.2.* Leawood, KS: American Academy of Family Physicians (AAFP); 2006.

American Academy of Pediatrics. Lead exposure in children: prevention, detection, and management. *Pediatrics.* 2005;116(4):1036–46.

American Academy of Pediatrics, Committee on Infectious Disease. Recommended childhood and adolescent immunization schedule—United States, 2007. *Pediatrics.* 2007;119(1):207–8.

American Cancer Society Guidelines for the Early Detection of Cancer. Available at: http://www.cancer.org/docroot/PED/content/PED_2_3X_ACS_Cancer_Detection_Guidelines_36.asp. Accessed September 15, 2006.

American College of Cardiology Foundation, American Heart Association. *ACC/AHA Guidelines for the Management of Patients with Unstable Angina and Non-ST-Segment elevation myocardial Infarction. A report of the American College of Cardiology/American Heart Association Task Force on Practice Guidelines.* Bethesda, MD: American College of Cardiology Foundation (ACCF); Mar 2002. Available at: http://www.acc.org/qualityandscience/clinical/guidelines/unstable/incorporated/index.htm.

American College of Emergency Physicians (ACEP). Clinical policy: critical issues in the evaluation and management of patients presenting to the emergency department with acute headache. *Ann Emerg Med.* 2002;39(1):108–22.

American College of Emergency Physicians. Clinical policy: critical issues in the evaluation and management of adult patients presenting with suspected lower-extremity deep venous thrombosis. *Ann Emerg Med.* 2003;42(1):124–35.

American College of Obstetricians and Gynecologists (ACOG). *Management of Herpes in Pregnancy.* Washington, DC: American College of Obstetricians and Gynecologists (ACOG); 1999.

American College of Obstetricians and Gynecologists (ACOG). *Neural tube defects.* Washington, DC: American College of Obstetricians and Gynecologists (ACOG); (ACOG practice bulletin; no. 44), 2003.

American College of Obstetricians and Gynecologists (ACOG). *Perinatal Viral and Parasitic Infections.* Washington, DC: American College of Obstetricians and Gynecologists (ACOG); (ACOG practice bulletin; no. 20), 2000.

American College of Obstetricians and Gynecologists (ACOG). *Prenatal diagnosis of fetal chromosomal abnormalities.* Washington, DC: American College of Obstetricians and Gynecologists (ACOG); 2001.

American College of Obstetricians and Gynecologists. Revised Cervical Cancer Screening Guidelines Require Reeducation of Women and Physicians. Available at: http://www.acog.org/from_home/publications/press_releases/nr05-04-04-1.cfm. Accessed September 11, 2006.

American College of Radiology (ACR), Expert Panel on Cardiovascular Imaging. *Suspected congenital heart disease in the adult.* Reston, VA: American College of Radiology (ACR); 2002.

American Diabetes Association (ADA). Diagnosis and classification of diabetes mellitus. *Diabetes Care.* 2004;27:S5–S10.

American Diabetes Association (ADA). Standards of medical care in diabetes. I. Classification and diagnosis. *Diabetes Care.* 2006;29(Suppl 1):S4–5.

American Diabetes Association (ADA). Standards of medical care in diabetes. II. Screening for diabetes. *Diabetes Care.* 2006;29(Suppl 1):S5–7.

American Diabetes Association (ADA). Standards of medical care in diabetes. V. Diabetes care. *Diabetes Care.* 2006;29(Suppl 1):S8–17.

American Diabetes Association (ADA). Standards of medical care in diabetes. VI. Prevention and management of diabetes complications. *Diabetes Care.* 2006;29(Suppl 1):S17–26.

American Gastroenterological Association. American Gastroenterological Association medical position statement: evaluation of liver chemistry tests. *Gastroenterology.* 2002;123(4):1364–6.

American Heart Association. Homocysteine, folic acid and cardiovascular disease. Available at: http://www.americanheart.org/presenter.jhtml?identifier=4677. Accessed October 15, 2006.

American Heart Association. Stent Procedure. Available at: http://www.americanheart.org/presenter.jhtml?identifier-4721. Accessed October 15, 2006.

Arnett FC, Edworthy SM, Bloch DA, et al. The American Rheumatism Association 1987 revised criteria for the classification of rheumatoid arthritis. *Arthritis Rheum.* 1988;31(3):315–324.

Bast RC, Ravdin P, Hayes DF, et al. 2000 update of recommendations for the use of tumor markers in breast and colorectal cancer: clinical practice guidelines of the American Society of Clinical Oncology. *J Clin Oncol.* 2001;19(6):1865–78.

Bhasin S, Cunningham GR, Hayes FJ, et al. Testosterone therapy in adult men with androgen deficiency syndromes: An Endocrine Society clinical practice guideline. *J Clin Endocrinol Metab.* 2006;91(6):1995–2010.

Bluemke DA, Gatsonis CA, Chen MH, et al. Magnetic resonance imaging of the breast prior to biopsy. *JAMA*. 2004;292(22):2735–2742.

Bonin E, Brammer S, Brehove T, et al. *Adapting your practice: Treatment and recommendations for homeless patients with asthma*. Nashville, TN: Health Care for the Homeless Clinicians' Network, National Health Care for the Homeless Council, Inc., 2003.

Borg B, Herts BR, Masaryk TJ. Imaging in practice: Imaging in acute brain infarction. *Clev Clin J Med*. 2005;72(7):579–584.

Branson BM, Handsfield HH, Lampe MA, et al. Centers for Disease Control and Prevention (CDC). Revised recommendations for HIV testing of adults, adolescents, and pregnant women in health-care settings. *MMWR Recomm Rep*. 2006;22;55(RR-14):1–17.

Brigham and Women's Hospital. *Common gynecologic problems: a guide to diagnosis and treatment*. Boston, MA: Brigham and Women's Hospital; 2002. Available at: http://www.guideline.gov/summary/summary.aspx?doc_id=3486&nbr=002712&string=pelvic+AND+ultrasound. Accessed October 29, 2006.

Brigham and Women's Hospital. *Menopause: a guide to management*. Boston, MA: Brigham and Women's Hospital; 2005. Available at: http://www.guideline.gov/summary/summary.aspx?doc_id=7010&nbr=004219&string=estrogen. Accessed October 29, 2006.

Carey, WD. *A guide to commonly used liver tests*. 2003, Cleveland Clinic website. Available at: http://www.clevelandclinicmeded.com/diseasemanagement/gastro/livertests/livertests.htm. Accessed October 15, 2006.

Carman TL, Fernandez BB Jr. A primary care approach to the patient with claudication. *Am Fam Physician*. 2000;15;61(4):1027–32, 1034.

Centers for Disease Control and Prevention. Diseases characterized by genital ulcers. Sexually transmitted diseases treatment guidelines 2006. *MMWR Morb Mortal Wkly Rep*. 2006;4;55(RR-11):14–30.

Chaturvedi S, Bruno A, Feasby T, et al. Carotid endarterectomy—an evidence-based review: Report of the Therapeutics and Technology Assessment Subcommittee of the American Academy of Neurology. *Neurology*. 2005. 65(6):794–801.

Chémali KR, Tsao B. Electrodiagnostic testing of nerves and muscles: when, why, and how to order. *Clev Clin J Med*. 2005;71(1):37–48.

Chemical inhalants/carbon monoxide inhalation. Philadelphia, PA: Intracorp; 2004. Available at: http://www.guideline.gov/summary/summary.aspx?doc_id=5942&nbr=003911&string=carboxy-hemogobin. Accessed September 15, 2006.

Clinical policy: Critical issues in the evaluation and management of adult patients presenting with suspected pulmonary embolism. *Ann Emerg Med*. 2003;41(2):257–70.

Cohen J, Safdi MA, Deal SE, et al. Quality indicators for esophagogastroduodenoscopy. *Gastrointest Endosc*. 2006;63(Suppl 4):S10–5.

Cook DM. AACE medical guidelines for clinical practice for the diagnosis and treatment of acromegaly. *Endocr Pract*. 2004;10(3):213–25.

Cook NR, Buring JE, Ridker PM. The effect of including C-reactive protein in cardiovascular risk prediction models for women. *Ann Intern Med*. 2006;145:21–29.

Dalinka MK, Alazraki NP, Daffner RH, et al. Expert Panel on Musculoskeletal Imaging. *Imaging evaluation of suspected ankle fractures*. [online publication]. Reston, VA: American College of Radiology (ACR); 2005. Available at: http://www.acr.org/s_acr/bin.asp?CID=1206&DID=11774&DOC=FILE.PDF. Accessed December 16, 2006.

Dellinger RP, Carlet JM, Masur H, et al. Surviving Sepsis Campaign guidelines for management of severe sepsis and septic shock. *Crit Care Med*. 2004;32(3):858–73.

Desch CE, Benson AB III, Somerfield MR, et al. Colorectal cancer surveillance: 2005 update of an American Society of Clinical Oncology practice guideline. *J Clin Oncol*. 2005;23(33):8512–9.

Detterbeck FC, DeCamp MM Jr, Kohman LJ, et al. Lung cancer. Invasive staging: the guidelines. *Chest.* 2003;123(Suppl 1):167S–75S.

Dienstag JL, McHutchison JG. American Gastroenterological Association medical position statement on the management of hepatitis C. *Gastroenterology.* 2006;130(1):225–30.

Dumot, JA. ERCP: Current uses and less-invasive options. *Clev Clin J Med.* 2006;73(5):418–442.

Eniu A, Carlson RW, Aziz Z, et al. Breast cancer in limited-resource countries: treatment and allocation of resources. *Breast J.* 2006;12(Suppl 1):S38–53.

Erlinger TP, Platz EA., Rifai N, et al. C-reactive protein and the risk of incident colorectal cancer. *JAMA.* 2006;291(5):585–590.

Cameron D, Gaito A, Harris N, et al. Evidence-based guidelines for the management of Lyme disease. *Expert Rev Antiinfect Ther.* 2004;2(Suppl 1):S1–13.

Fennerty, MB. *Helicobacter pylori:* Why it still matters in 2005. *Clev Clin J Med.* 2005;72(Suppl 2): S1–S7.

Fletcher B, Berra K, Ades P, et al. Managing abnormal blood lipids: a collaborative approach. *Circulation.* 2005;15;112(20):3184–209.

Frost SD, Brotman DJ, Michota FA. Rational use of D-dimer measurement to exclude acute venous thromboembolic disease. *Mayo Clin Proc.* 2003;78:1385–1391.

Fye KH. Rheumatic disease: How to use the lab in the workup. *Consultant.* Mar 2004;369–377.

Galgiani JN, Ampel NM, Blair JE, et al. Coccidioidomycosis. *Clin Infect Dis.* 2005;41(9):1217–23.

Green RM, Flamm S. AGA technical review on the evaluation of liver chemistry tests. *Gastroenterology.* 2002;123(4):1367–84.

Greer FR, Shannon M. Infant methemoglobinemia: the role of dietary nitrate in food and water. *Pediatrics.* 2005;116(3):784–6.

Grossfeld GD, Litwin MS, Wolf JS Jr, et al. Evaluation of asymptomatic microscopic hematuria in adults: The American Urological Association best practice policy—part II: patient evaluation, cytology, voided markers, imaging, cystoscopy, nephrology evaluation, and follow-up. *Urology.* 2001;57(4):604–10.

Grossman, ZD. The uses of PET and PET/CT in cancer staging. *Patient Care.* July, 2006; 30–37.

Guerrant RL, Van Gilder T, Steiner TS, et al. Practice guidelines for the management of infectious diarrhea. *Clin Infect Dis.* 2001;32(3):331–51.

GUIPCAR Group. Clinical practice guideline for the management of rheumatoid arthritis. Madrid: Spanish Society of Rheumatology; 2001. Available at: http://www.guideline.gov/guidelines/ ftngc-2909-GUIPCAR.pdf. Accessed September 15, 2006.

Harrison JK, Valente AM, Crowley AL, et al. Clinical use of cardiac magnetic resonance imaging. *Adv Stud Med.* 2005;5(7):351–9.

Heart Failure Society of America. Evaluation and management of patients with acute decompensated heart failure. *J Card Fail.* 2006;12(1):e86–103.

Henschke CI. Survival of patients with Stage I lung cancer detected on CT screening. *N Engl J Med.* 355: 2006;1763–71, 1822–24.

Hepatitis Foundation International. The ABCs of hepatitis. Available at: http://www.hepfi.org/education/ estore_info.html. Accessed September 12, 2006.

Heseltine P. Fecal immunochemical test: Improving detection of colorectal cancer with the new generation occult blood test. *Clinical Laboratory News.* January, 2007;8–10.

Hobbs, RE. Using BNP to diagnose, manage, and treat heart failure. *Clev Clin J Med.* 2003;70(4): 333–336.

Horner JB, Einstein DM, Herts BR. Imaging in practice: A patient with acute flank pain. *Clev Clin J Med* 2005;72(12):1102–1104.

Institute for Clinical Systems Improvement (ICSI). Acute pharyngitis. Bloomington, MN: Institute for Clinical Systems Improvement (ICSI); May 2005. Available at: http://www.icsi.org/knowledge/detail.asp?catID=29&itemID=147. Accessed October 21, 2006.

Institute for Clinical Systems Improvement (ICSI). *Chronic obstructive pulmonary disease.* Bloomington, MN: Institute for Clinical Systems Improvement (ICSI); Jan. 2007. Available at: http://www.icsi.org/chronic_pulmonary_disease/chronic_pulmonary_disease_2286.html. Accessed June 13, 2007.

Institute for Clinical Systems Improvement (ICSI). *Diagnosis and management of basic infertility.* Bloomington, MN: Institute for Clinical Systems Improvement (ICSI); Jul 2004. Available at: http://www.icsi.org/knowledge/browse_category.asp?catID=29&StartAlpha=I&EndAlpha=I&page=1. Accessed October 29, 2006.

Institute for Clinical Systems Improvement (ICSI). *Diagnosis of breast disease.* Bloomington, MN: Institute for Clinical Systems Improvement (ICSI); 2005 Nov. Available at: http://www.icsi.org/knowledge/browse_category.asp?catID=29&StartAlpha=B&EndAlpha=B&page=1. Accessed October 29, 2006.

Institute for Clinical Systems Improvement (ICSI). *Emergency and inpatient management of asthma.* Bloomington, MN: Institute for Clinical Systems Improvement (ICSI); Mar 2006. Available at: http://www.icsi.org/knowledge/detail.asp?catID=29&itemID=1988. Accessed December 20, 2006.

Jafri SZ, Choyke PL, Bluth EI, et al. Expert Panel on Urologic Imaging. Radiologic investigation of patients with renovascular hypertension. [online publication]. Reston (VA): American College of Radiology (ACR); 2005. Available at: http://www.acr.org/s_acr/bin.asp?CID=1202&DID=11823&DOC=FILE.PDF. Accessed September 14, 2006.

Januzzi JL Jr. Natriuretic peptide testing: a window into the diagnosis and prognosis of heart failure. *Clev Clin J Med.* 2006;73(2):149–157.

Januzzi, JL Jr. Utility of amino-terminal pro-brain natriuretic peptide testing for prediction of one-year mortality in patients with dyspnea treated in the emergency department. *Arch Intern Med.* 2006;166:315–20.

K/DOQI, National Kidney Foundation. K/DOQI clinical practice guidelines for bone metabolism and disease in children with chronic kidney disease. *Am J Kidney Dis.* 2005 Oct;46(4 Suppl 1):S1–121.

Kellogg N. The evaluation of sexual abuse in children. *Pediatrics.* 2005;116(2):506–12.

Kessenich CR. Osteoporosis in primary care: The role of biochemical markers and diagnostic imaging. *Amer J Nurse Pract.* 2000;4(2):24–29.

Kucik, CJ, Martin, GL, Sortor, BV: Common intestinal parasites. *Am Fam Physician.* 2004;69:1161–8.

Kushida CA, Littner MR, Morgenthaler T, et al.: Practice parameters for the indications for polysomnography and related procedures: an update for 2005. *Sleep.* 28(4):499–521, 2005.

Lab Tests Online. Available at: http://labtestsonline.org/index.html.

Laughlin S, Montanera W. Central nervous system imaging. *Postgraduate Medicine.* 1998;104(5):73–88.

Lentz SR, Haynes WG. Homocysteine: Is it a clinically important cardiovascular risk factor? *Clev Clin J Med.* 2004;71(9):729–34.

Levine MS, Bree RL, Foley WD, et al. *Expert Panel on Gastrointestinal Imaging. Imaging recommendations for patients with dysphagia.* [online publication]. Reston, VA: American College of Radiology (ACR); 2005. Available at: http://www.acr.org/s_acr/bin.asp?CID=1207&DID=11772&DOC=FILE.PDF. Accessed January 3, 2007.

Mansi IA, Reddy P, Carden D: Cardiac troponins: Caveats and controversies in analysis and interpretation. *Johns Hopkins Adv Studies Med.* 2005;5(8):428–435.

March of Dimes. Chorionic Villus Sampling. Available at: http://www.marchofdimes.com/professionals/681_1165.asp. Accessed November 3, 2006.

Mayo Clinic. Amniocentesis: Answers to common questions. Available at: http://www.mayoclinic.com/ health/amniocentesis/PR00144. Accessed November 3, 2006.

Medical Advisory Panel for the Pharmacy Benefits Management Strategic Healthcare Group. *The pharmacologic management of chronic obstructive pulmonary disease.* Washington, DC: Veterans Health Administration, Department of Veterans Affairs; 2002 Sep. Available at: http://www.guideline.gov/ summary/summary.aspx?doc_id=5186&nbr=003568&string=alpha1+AND+antitrypsin. Accessed October 28, 2006.

Medline Plus. Available at: http://www.nlm.nih.gov/medlineplus/.

Moeschler JB, Shevell M. American Academy of Pediatrics Committee on Genetics. Clinical genetic evaluation of the child with mental retardation or developmental delays. *Pediatrics.* 2006;117(6): 2304–16.

Nash DT. C-reactive protein: A promising new marker of cardiovascular risk? *Consultant.* Apr. 1, 2005;453–460.

National Academy of Clinical Biochemistry (NACB). NACB: *Laboratory support for the diagnosis and monitoring of thyroid disease.* Washington, DC: National Academy of Clinical Biochemistry (NACB); 2002. Available at: http://www.nacb.org/lmpg/thyroid_LMPG_PDF.stm. Accessed September 18, 2006.

National Heart, Lung, and Blood Institute, National Institutes of Health, US Department of Health and Human Services. *Third Report of the National Cholesterol Education Program (NCEP) Expert Panel on Detection, Evaluation, and Treatment of High Blood Cholesterol in Adults (Adult Treatment Panel III).* Bethesda, MD: U.S. Department of Health and Human Services, Public Health Service, National Institutes of Health, National Heart, Lung and Blood Institute; May 2001. Available at: http://www.nhlbi.nih.gov/guidelines/cholesterol/atp3_rpt.htm. Accessed June 3, 2006.

National Kidney Foundation. K/DOQI clinical practice guidelines for bone metabolism and disease in chronic kidney disease. *Am J Kidney Dis* 2003;42(4 Suppl 3):S1-201.

NCI Bethesda System 2001. Available at: http://www.bethesda2001.cancer.gov/terminology.html. Accessed September 15, 2006.

Nowack, WJ. Polysomnography: Overview and clinical application. Mar. 29, 2005. Available at: http://www.emedicine.com/neuro/topic566.htm. Accessed December 29, 2006.

O'Connell TX, Horita TJ, Kasravi B: Understanding and interpreting serum protein electrophoresis. *Amer Fam Physician.* 2005;71(1), 105–112.

Older RA, Choyke PL, Bluth EI, et al. Expert Panel on Urologic Imaging. *Acute onset of scrotal pain (without trauma, without antecedent mass).* [online publication]. Reston, VA: American College of Radiology (ACR); 2005. 4 p. Available at: http://www.acr.org/s_acr/bin.asp?CID=1202&DID= 11831&DOC=FILE.PDF. Accessed October 1, 2006.

Otchy D, Hyman NH, Simmang C, et al. Practice parameters for colon cancer. *Dis Colon Rectum.* 2004;47(8):1269–84.

Pandolfino JE, Kahrilas PJ. American Gastroenterological Association medical position statement: clinical use of esophageal manometry. *Gastroenterology.* 2005;128(1):207–8.

Parkin, CG, Brooks, N. Is postprandial glucose control important? Is it practical in primary care settings? *Clinical Diabetes.* 2002;20:71–76.

Plevritis SK, Kurian AW, Sigal BM, et al. Cost-effectiveness of screening BRCA 1/2 mutation carriers with breast magnetic resonance imaging. *JAMA.* 295(20):2374–2384, 2006.

Polson J, Lee WM. AASLD position paper: The management of acute liver failure. *Hepatology.* 2005;41(5):1179–97.

Practice guidelines for perioperative blood transfusion and adjuvant therapies: An updated report by the American Society of Anesthesiologists Task Force on Perioperative Blood Transfusion and Adjuvant Therapies. *Anesthesiology.* 2006;105(1):198–208.

Quest Diagnostics. Patient Health Library. Available at: http://www.questdiagnostics.com.

Rapp DE, Gerber GS. A "slightly high" PSA: When should you call the urologist? *Consultant.* Apr. 1, 2005;437–442.

Recommendations from the American Cancer Society Workshop on Early Prostate Cancer Detection, May 4–6, 2000 and ACS guideline on testing for early prostate cancer detection: update 2001. *CA Cancer J Clin.* 2001;51(1):39–44.

Richmond B. DXA scanning to diagnose osteoporosis: Do you know what the results mean? *Clev Clin J Med.* 2003;70(4):353–60.

Rivera MP, Detterbeck F, Mehta AC. Diagnosis of lung cancer: The guidelines. *Chest.*123(Suppl 1): 2003;129S–36S.

Roberts EA, Schilsky ML. A practice guideline on Wilson disease. H*epatology.* 2003;37(6):1475–92.

Ros PR, Bree RL, Foley WD, et al. *Expert Panel on Gastrointestinal Imaging. Acute pancreatitis.* [online publication]. Reston, VA: American College of Radiology (ACR); 2006. Available at: http://www.acr.org/ s_acr/bin.asp?CID=1207&DID=11769&DOC=FILE.PDF. Accessed November 29, 2006.

Rosenfield AT, Choyke PL, Bluth E, et al. Expert Panel on Urologic Imaging. *Acute onset flank pain, suspicion of stone disease.* [online publication]. Reston, VA: American College of Radiology (ACR); 2005. Available at: http://www.acr.org/s_acr/bin.asp?CID=1202&DID=11826&DOC= FILE.PDF. Accessed November 15, 2006.

Royal College of Obstetricians and Gynaecologists (RCOG). *Hormone replacement therapy and venous thromboembolism.* London, UK: Royal College of Obstetricians and Gynaecologists (RCOG); Jan 2004. Available at: http://www.rcog.org.uk/resources/Public/pdf/HRT_Venous_ Thromboembolism_no19.pdf. Accessed October 15, 2006.

Rumberger, JA, Brundage, BH, Rader, DJ, et al. Electron beam computed tomographic coronary calcium scanning: A review and guidelines for use in asymptomatic persons. *Mayo Clin Proc.* 1999;74:243–252.

Sacks D, Bakal CW, Beatty PT, et al. Position statement on the use of the ankle brachial index in the evaluation of patients with peripheral vascular disease. A consensus statement developed by the Standards Division of the Society of Interventional Radiology. *J Vasc Interv Radiol.* 2003;14(9 Pt 2):S389.

Sarodia BD, Mehra R, Golish JA: A 52-year-old man with excessive daytime sleepiness. *Clev Clin J Med.* 2002;69(3):193–208.

Screening for abdominal aortic aneurysm: Recommendation statement. *Ann Intern Med.* 2005;142(3): 198–202.

Screening for coronary heart disease: Recommendation statement. *Ann Intern Med.* 2004;140(7): 569–72.

Screening for hepatitis C virus infection in adults: Recommendation statement. *Ann Intern Med.* 2004;140(6):462–4.

Screening for osteoporosis in postmenopausal women: Recommendations and rationale. *Am Fam Physician.* 2002;66(8):1430–2.

Screening for ovarian cancer: Recommendation statement. U.S. Preventive Services Task Force. *Am Fam Physician.* Feb 15;2005;71(4):759–62.

Screening for type 2 diabetes mellitus in adults: Recommendations and rationale. *Ann Intern Med.* 2003;138(3):212–4.

Scudder L. Using evidence-based information. *The Journal for Nurse Practitioners.* 2006;2(3): 180–185.

Seehusen DA, Asplund CA, Johnson DR, et al. Primary evaluation and management of statin therapy complications. *South Med J.* 2006;99(3):250–254.

Selman JE. CT, MRI, Doppler, or EEG: When—and when not—to use a specific imaging test. *Cortlandt Forum.* Nov. 2003;23–29.

Semelka RC. When to refer for body MRI: a user's guide. Available at: http://www.medscape.com/ viewprogram/4731_pnt. Accessed November 15, 2006.

Sheeler RD, Houston MS, Radke S, et al. Accuracy of rapid strep testing in patients who have had recent streptococcal pharyngitis. *J Am Board Fam. Pract*. 2002;15(4):261–5.

Shoup AG: Electronystagmography. Oct. 19, 2005. Available at: http://www.emedicine.com/ent/ topic373.htm. Accessed November 1, 2006.

Shyyan R, Masood S, Badwe RA, et al. Breast cancer in limited-resource countries: diagnosis and pathology. *Breast J*. 2006;12(Suppl 1):S27–37.

Siegel CA, Surivawinata AA, Silas AM, et al. Liver Biopsy 2005: When and how? *Clev Clin J Med*. 2005;72(3):199–224.

Silverstein J, Klingensmith G, Copeland K, et al. Care of children and adolescents with type 1 diabetes: A statement of the American Diabetes Association. *Diabetes Care*. 2005;28(1):186–212.

Simerville JA, Maxted WC, Pahira JJ: Urinalysis: a comprehensive review. *Amer Fam Physician*. 2005;71(6):1153–1162.

Sin DD, Man, SFP, McWilliams A, et al. Progression of airway dysplasia and C-reactive protein in smokers at high risk of lung cancer. *Am J Respir Crit Care Med*. 2006;173:535–539.

Smith RA, Cokkinides V, Eyre HJ. American Cancer Society guidelines for the early detection of cancer, 2003. *CA Cancer J Clin*.53(1):27–43.

Smith RA, Saslow D, Sawyer KA, et al. American Cancer Society guidelines for breast cancer screening: update 2003. *CA Cancer J Clin*. 2003;53(3):141–69.

Society of American Gastrointestinal Endoscopic Surgeons (SAGES). *SAGES guidelines for diagnostic laparoscopy*. Los Angeles, CA: Society of American Gastrointestinal Endoscopic Surgeons (SAGES); Mar 2002. Available at: http://www.sages.org/sagespublication.php?doc=12. Accessed November 15, 2006.

Standards for breast conservation therapy in the management of invasive breast carcinoma. *CA Cancer J Clin*. 2002;52(5):277–300.

Stanford W, Yucel EK, Bettmann MA, et al. Expert Panel on Cardiovascular Imaging. *Acute chest pain: no ECG or enzyme evidence of myocardial ischemia/infarction*. [online publication]. Reston (VA): American College of Radiology (ACR); 2005. Available at: http://www.acr.org/s_acr/bin.asp?CID= 1208&DID=11751&DOC=FILE.PDF. Accessed September 1, 2006.

Szmitko PE, Verma S. C-reactive protein and the metabolic syndrome: useful addition to the cardiovascular risk profile? *JCMS*. 2006;1:66–69.

Taylor Z, Nolan CM, Blumberg HM. Controlling tuberculosis in the United States. Recommendations from the American Thoracic Society, CDC, and the Infectious Diseases Society of America. *MMWR Recomm Rep*. 2005;54(RR-12):1–81.

Terasawa T, Blackmore CC, Bent S, et al. Systematic review: Computer tomography and ultrasonography to detect acute appendicitis in adults and adolescents. *Ann Intern Med*. 2004;141:537–546.

The Reference Laboratory at the Cleveland Clinic. Available at: http://referencelab.clevelandclinic.org/

Tunkel AR, Hartman BJ, Kaplan SL, et al. Practice guidelines for the management of bacterial meningitis. *Clin Infect Dis*. 2004;39(9):1267–84.

U.S. Food and Drug Administration Center for Devices and Radiological Health. New device approval: StarClose vascular closure system—P050007. Available at: http://www.fda.gov/cdrh/mda/ docs/p050007.html. Accessed November 25, 2006.

U.S. Preventive Services Task Force. Genetic risk assessment and BRCA mutation testing for breast and ovarian cancer susceptibility: recommendation statement. *Ann Intern Med*. 2005;6;143(5): 355–61.

U.S. Preventive Services Task Force. Screening for breast cancer: recommendations and rationale. *Ann Intern Med*. 2002;3;137(5 Part 1):344–6.

U.S. Preventive Services Task Force. Screening for colorectal cancer: recommendations and rationale. *Ann Intern Med.* 2002;16;137(2):129–31.

U.S. Preventive Services Task Force (USPSTF). Screening for asymptomatic bacteriuria: recommendation statement. Rockville (MD): Agency for Healthcare Research and Quality (AHRQ); Feb. 2004. Available at: http://www.ahrq.gov/clinic/uspstf/uspsbact.htm. Accessed September 25, 2006.

U.S. Preventive Services Task Force (USPSTF). *Screening for gonorrhea: recommendation statement.* Rockville, MD: Agency for Healthcare Research and Quality (AHRQ); 2005. Available at: http://www.ahrq.gov/clinic/uspstf/uspsgono.htm. Accessed September 28, 2006.

U.S. Preventive Services Task Force (USPSTF). *Screening for iron deficiency anemia–including iron supplementation for children and pregnant women.* Rockville, MD: Agency for Healthcare Research and Quality (AHRQ); 2006. Available at: http://www.ahrq.gov/clinic/uspstf/uspsiron.htm. Accessed October 15, 2006.

U.S. Preventive Services Task Force (USPSTF). *Screening for pancreatic cancer: recommendation statement.* Rockville, MD: Agency for Healthcare Research and Quality (AHRQ); Feb 2004. Available at: http://www.ahrq.gov/clinic/uspstf/uspspanc.htm. Accessed September 29, 2006. Accessed December 1, 2006.

U.S. Preventive Services Task Force. *Screening for syphilis infection: recommendation statement.* Rockville, MD: Agency for Healthcare Research and Quality (AHRQ); Jul 2004. Available at: http://www.ahrq.gov/clinic/uspstf/uspssyph.htm. Accessed September 28, 2006.

U.S. Preventive Services Task Force (USPSTF). *Screening for Rh(D) incompatibility: recommendation statement.* Rockville, MD: Agency for Healthcare Research and Quality (AHRQ); Feb 2004. Available at: http://www.ahrq.gov/clinic/uspstf/uspsdrhi.htm. Accessed November 12, 2006.

Vakil N, Fendrick AM. How to test for *Helicobcter pylori* in 2005. *Clev Clin J Med.* 2005;72(Supp 2), S8–S13.

Veterans Health Administration, 2006 Department of Defense. *VHA/DoD clinical practice guideline for the management of chronic kidney disease and pre-ESRD in the primary care setting.* Washington, DC: Department of Veterans Affairs (U.S.), Veterans Health Administration; May 2001. Available at: http://www.oqp.med.va.gov/cpg/ESRD/ESRD_Base.htm. Accessed August 30, 2006.

White B. Making evidence-based medicine doable in everyday practice. *Fam Prac Manag.* 2004;11(2):51–58.

Who Named It? Available at http://www.whonamedit.com/index.cfm.

Winawer S, Fletcher R, Rex D, et al. Gastrointestinal Consortium Panel. Colorectal cancer screening and surveillance: clinical guidelines and rationale. Update based on new evidence. *Gastroenterology.* 2003;124(2):544–60.

Wolkov HB, Constine LS, Yahalom J, et al. *Staging evaluation for patients with Hodgkin's Disease.* [online publication]. Reston, VA: American College of Radiology (ACR); 2005. Available at: http://www.acr.org/s_acr/bin.asp?CID=1229&DID=11885&DOC=FILE.PDF. Accessed December 20, 2006.

Wright TC Jr, Cox JT, Massad LS, et al. 2001 Consensus guidelines for the management of women with cervical cytological abnormalities. *JAMA.* 2002;24;287(16):2120–9.

Zuber TJ. Endometrial biopsy. *Am Fam Physician.* 2001;1;63(6):1131–5.

Zubrod G, Holman JR. Novel biochemical markers of cardiovascular risk: a primary care primer. *Consultant.* October 2004;1509–13.

INDEX